COSMETICS:

Their Principles and Practices

COSMETICS:

Their Principles and Practices

BY

RALPH G. HARRY, F.R.I.C.

Certificate of the Royal Institute of Chemistry in the Chemistry and Microscopy of Foods, Drugs and Waters, Pharmacognosy, Pharmacology and Therapeutics; Associate of the Royal Photographic Society

1956

CHEMICAL PUBLISHING CO., INC.

212 Fifth Avenue New York 10, N.Y.

Cosmetics:
Their Principles and Practices

ISBN: 978-0-8206-0162-5

Chemical Publishing Company:
www.chemical-publishing.com
www.chemicalpublishing.net

First American Edition: Chemical Publishing New York 1956

Printed in the United States of America

THIS BOOK IS AFFECTIONATELY DEDICATED

TO

MY WIFE

MY PARENTS

AND TO

MY DAUGHTERS

PATRICIA AND SHEILA

Patents

In this book, certain formulations and processes have been included in the interests of science, notwithstanding the existence of actual or potential patent rights.

In so far as such substances are protected by Letters Patent, their inclusion in this book neither conveys nor implies licence to manufacture. Each manufacturer should ascertain for himself the patent position existing in that country and at that time.

"I look with pleasure on my book however defective, and deliver it to the world with the spirit of a man that has endeavoured well. That it will immediately become popular I have not promised to myself; a few wild blunders and risible absurdities, from which no work of multiplicity was ever free, may for a time furnish folly with laughter and harden ignorance in contempt; but useful diligence will at last prevail, and there never can be wanting some who distinguish desert ......
... that a writer will sometimes be hurried by eagerness to the end; that what is obvious is not always known and what is known is not always present, that sudden fits of inadvertency will surprise vigilance, slight avocations will seduce attention, and causal eclipses of the mind darken learning, and that the writer shall often in vain trace his memory at the moment of need, for that which yesterday he knew with intuitive readiness and which will come uncalled into his thoughts tomorrow ..."

Dr. Johnson (1755).

PREFACE

EXTENSIVE developments in the cosmetic and toilet industry in the past decade have rendered desirable the writing of a completely new work dealing with modern cosmetic discoveries.

In these developments the 1939–45 war played an important part. In the direct military sphere of influence, the operation of armies in the Far Eastern theatre of warfare necessitated an exhaustive study of the properties and efficacy of insect repellents and over 4000 compounds were studied in this connection. In the fields of military and naval aviation, and in naval warfare, it became necessary to study the efficacy and safety of sun-screening agents, since men marooned on life rafts or in the desert might be subject to very severe solar exposure without shelter. Flashburn creams designed to protect exposed skin surfaces against burns were adopted by the U.S. Army for issue to tank crews and flame throwers. On the battlefield also, camouflage creams (" Commando Make-Up ") and anti-sunburn lipsticks were employed.

Stringent precautionary measures were necessary to ensure the safety of Allied Secret Service Agents operating behind the enemy lines. The use by Allied agents of white or perfumed soap or of shaving creams or toothpastes of different colour, perfume or physical characteristics, or in tubes of different metal or different design would inevitably have led to enquires. Within a few days of the battle of El Alamein, toilet preparations captured from the enemy were under examination with a view to producing, as a matter of urgency, simulative preparations.

On the Home Front, special toilet soaps and barrier creams were developed for use in shell-filling factories and—in conjuntion with suitable protective clothing and hygienic measures—proved to be of value in reducing the incidence of tetryl dermatitis. At the same time the value of cosmetics as a morale builder became recognised. [It was claimed that cosmetics served to combat fatigue and that a dressing room in a factory might improve efficiency by as much as 10–15 per cent. (Report of the Office of Civilian Supply to the U.S. Director of Economic Stabilisation, 1943.)]

All these developments, necessarily have had repercussions in the cosmetic field. In the field of industrial organic chemicals an almost bewildering range of compounds has been synthesised for use by the cosmetic industry, some of these as insect repellents, others emulsifiers, detergents, antioxidants, preservatives, etc. Outstanding examples are the non-ionic emulsifiers; and antiseptics effective when incorporated into soaps such as "Hexachlorophene" (G–11) and "Actamer".

Considerable thought has been given to the general "lay-out" of this book with a view to making it as rational and helpful as possible. With this object in mind, cosmetic and toilet preparations have been classified into groups in so far as they are used on the face, hair, eyes, teeth, body, etc. In the text dermatological considerations are discussed first and in the light of such discussion, consideration is given to the *raison d'être* for the formulation of the preparation under discussion. That the cosmetician cannot be too well acquainted with the mode of action of the preparation formulated is well exemplified by the comparatively recent discovery of the potential hazard to the eye mucosa occasioned by the use of certain surface-active materials in shampoos (*see* Chapter 22), and the specific anti-thyroid action of Resorcinol (Chapter 21).

Whilst every attempt has been made to present formulae which typify the present trend in cosmetic formulation (and ones which will yield satisfactory products) it should not be assumed that formulae taken directly, without experiment, from any textbook—no matter how good—will yield the preparation most desirable for marketing.

Four factors have to be taken into account:

(1) variations in the quality of raw materials;
(2) equipment available and skill and experience of operator;
(3) cost of the product (including overheads, packaging, distribution and advertising, together with any government taxation) in relation to selling price;
(4) if the product is to be packaged in a metal tube (and this form of packaging has many advantages) the potential "corrosion" hazard involved.

In the last named instance, the potential corrosion hazard is of great importance. In terms of organic and physical chemistry, no cosmetic cream is "simple" in composition and the true complexity of such preparations is exemplified in Chapter 9.

When such products are packed into a metal tube, the metal wall of the tube may be attacked and the dissolved metal pass into solution in the cosmetic preparation, as a result either of direct chemical or electrochemical attack, and we have the phenomenon we term "corrosion", which may result in the occurrence of one or more of the following effects:

(1) discoloration of the product, (*a*) by formation of heavy metal compounds, (*b*) by oxidation, (*c*) by reduction of any incorporated colouring material;

(2) hardening of the product through formation of metallic salts or soaps ;

(3) destruction of the wall of the tube either in the form of localised pin-holing which allows seepage of the contents of the tube, or more generalised corrosion ;

(4) formation of toxic compounds in the product, for example, lead salts in dentifrices.

The problem of forecasting the degree of hazard and of taking steps to inhibit, or at least minimise it, in any particular formulation is difficult ; the problem is considerably influenced not only by the formula *per se*, but also by the presence of traces of impurities in the components of the formulation which may act as corrosion activators, the conditions of storage, and naturally, the composition of the tube itself (not only in respect of its major metallic elements, but also in respect of minor elements which may be present).

Only tests in the laboratory upon the finalised product in question (including its perfume and/or flavour) can assess the actual degree of hazard involved.

With the availability of water-soluble derivatives of lanolin and beeswax, differing in their hydrophilic balance and available under a range of numbers and of non-ionic emulsifiers whose very complexity defies giving them a correct and simple chemical designation, it is no longer possible to present a cosmetic textbook which is representative of the industry *without* the inclusion of proprietary materials. Proprietary materials are therefore included in this edition.

In preparing this work, I acknowledge with appreciation my indebtedness to :

Professor W. T. Astbury, M.A., Sc.D., F.R.S., of the Department of Biomolecular Structure, The University, Leeds, for permission to reproduce X-ray diffraction photographs of human hair and for the diagrams of primary and secondary folds in stretched and unstretched hair.

Professor J. H. Schulman, O.B.E., Sc.D., F.R.S., of the Department of Colloid Science, The University, Cambridge, for permission to utilise researches on emulsions and transparent dispersions.

Professor G. Weddell, M.D., D.Sc., of the Department of Anatomy, The University, Oxford, and to The British Council and British Medical Bulletin for permission to reproduce certain material on cutaneous sensibility published in the *British Medical Bulletin.*

To the British Medical Association and to the American Medical Association and to the editors and publishers of the following journals for permission to utilise material appearing in their respective journals :

American Perfumer; *Archives of Dermatology and Syphilology*; *British Journal of Dermatology*; *British Journal of Experimental Pathology*; *British Medical Journal*; *Drug & Cosmetic Industry*; *Journal American Dental Association*; *Journal American Pharmaceutical Association*; *Manufacturing Chemist*; *Soap and Sanitary Chemicals*; *Transactions of the Faraday Society*; *Journal of Colloid Science*; *Proceedings of the Royal Society of Medicine*.

The co-operation of *Mr. S. L. Mayham* and of the *U.S. Toilet Goods Association* and of *Mr. M. G. deNavarre* and *The U.S. Society of Cosmetic Chemists* in allowing reproduction of certain matter published in the *Proceedings of the Scientific Section of the T.G.A.* and in the *Journal of The Society of Cosmetic Chemists* is acknowledged with appreciation; appropriate recognition is given where such matter has been utilised, both to the authors concerned and to the Journal.

In particular my thanks are due to Griffin, Behrens and Cross and to the Society of Cosmetic Chemists for permission to quote extensively in Chapter 44 from hygrosopicity data on the use of hygroscopic agents in cosmetics.

In conclusion I would like to express my thanks to the following for their co-operation in allowing reproduction of material (formulae illustrations, etc.), Edward Arnold (Publishers) Ltd., Lea and Febiger, Philadelphia, William Heinemann Medical Books Ltd., and to:

Mr. J. E. Andre (American Alcolac Corporation); Dr. Louis C. Barail (United States Testing Co.); Mr. Wayne E. Dorland; Dr. John H. Draize (Division of Pharmacology, U.S. Food and Drug Administration, Washington); Drs. Joseph J. Eller and William Eller; Dr. Ralph Liggett Evans; Mr. L. D. Grady (The New Jersey Zinc Co.); Dr. W. C. Griffin (Atlas Powder Co.); Dr. Lloyd W. Hazelton (Hazelton Laboratories); Mr. I. R. Hollenberg (Van Dyke & Co. Inc.); Dr. Van Huysen; Dr. Emil G. Klarmann (Lehn & Finke); Dr. E. P. Laug (Division of Pharmacology, U.S. Food and Drug Administration, Washington); Dr. Matthew Luckiesh (Director, "Lighting Research Laboratory", General Electric Co., Ohio); Dr. Everett G. McDonough; Dr. R. W. Phillips (Assistant Professor in Dental Materials, Indiana School of Dentistry); Dr. R. S. Rose (Atlas Chemical Co.); Mr. H. L. Sanders (Ninol Laboratories); Dr. I. C. Schoonover (U.S. National Bureau of Standards); Dr. Marion B. Sulzberger; Dr. M. L. Tainter; Dr. H. W. Zussman.

Also: Atlas Chemical Company, Wilmington, Delaware; A. Boake Roberts & Co. Ltd., London; Croda Ltd., Goole, Yorks; Dow Chemical Company, Midland, Michigan; E. I. du Pont de Nemours; Firmenich & Cie., Geneva; Givaudan & Co., Geneva and New York;

Fries Bros. Inc., New York; Goldschmidt Chemical Corporation, New York; Imperial Chemical Industries Ltd., England; Monsanto Ltd., London and St. Louis; Proctor and Gamble Co. Ltd.; R. T. Vanderbilt, New York.

Finally, I should like to acknowledge my wife's help in typing and indexing the manuscript.

RALPH G. HARRY.

CONTENTS

IN FAVOUR OF COSMETICS

THE SKIN

THE CARE OF THE FACE

THE CARE OF THE MOUTH

THE CARE OF THE EYES

THE CARE OF THE HAIR

THE CARE OF THE BODY

THE CARE OF THE HANDS

COSMETIC FACTS AND FALLACIES

GENERAL ASPECTS OF COSMETIC FORMULATION

LIST OF ILLUSTRATIONS

IN FAVOUR OF COSMETICS

"... *Cosmetics at first glance might be considered to be non-essential; they are not.*

I think that if a woman looks good, she feels good, and if she feels good, she works better...."

By the Parliamentary Secretary to the Board of Trade (*Soap Perfum. Cosm.*, Nov. 1947, p. 1087).

THE moderate use of reputable cosmetic and toilet preparations has earned the approval of the majority of modern dermatologists. In the first place it is true to state that the use of modern cosmetics, together with the introduction of artificial silk, has done more to remove class distinction and give every girl a fair chance than centuries of social reform. With the availability of good cosmetics at reasonable prices, and the introduction of synthetic imitation jewellery, silk and other textile colours, it is possible for a girl of very little worldly wealth to compete with those more fortunate.

From earliest antiquity, woman has adorned her face and body by the application of coloured earths and perfumed ointments.

Excavation of the tombs of the Pharaohs has shown that the colouring of the skin around the eyes was practised in their days. The use of Malachite (a green copper ore) as an eye-shadow was practised as far back as 5000 B.C. whilst kohl (a fine powder used to darken the eyes) was used about 3400 B.C.

Apart from adornment of the eyes, hair dyeing must have been in vogue at an early date as evidenced by the red hair dye of the mummy of Hentawi (18th Dynasty, i.e. about 1580 B.C.).

It was the custom also for dancing girls to bear upon their heads perfumed ointments, the contents of which would flow down over their bodies whilst dancing and distribute their pleasant odour.

"Ointments and perfume rejoice the heart" (Proverbs xxvii. 9), but we have evidence also of other cosmetic arts, for it is stated (2 Kings ix. 30) that: "When Jehu was come to Jezreel, Jezebel heard of it; and she painted her face and tired her head, and looked out at a window". It does not concern us that the ancients of the day regarded her with prejudiced and jaundiced eye. The fact remains that Jezebel had sense enough to realise that colour is attractive whether purchased from a paint pot, or "natural".

In a broad translation we are told that the poet Ovid advised: "Rouge a pale cheek, a red one powder. Each maiden knows that art's allowed her."

So far as face creams are concerned, the best known of the cosmetic creams, "cold cream", is believed to have been invented by Galenus, a physician in Rome in the second century, although many people consider that he may have obtained it originally from Hippocrates who was the source of much of Galen's inspiration.

During the intervening centuries, the use of cosmetics steadily increased to such an extent that, in 1770, the following Act was introduced into the English Parliament:

"That all women of whatever age, rank, profession, or degree, whether virgins, maids or widows that shall from and after such Act, impose upon, seduce and betray into matrimony, any of His Majesty's subjects, *by the scents, paints, cosmetic washes,* artificial teeth, false hair, Spanish wool, iron stays, hoops, high-heeled shoes, bolstered hips, *shall incur the penalty of the law in force against witchcraft and* like misdemeanours and that *the marriage upon conviction shall stand null and void.*"

In spite of the terrible penalties in force at that time, against witchcraft and the fact that the Act, so far as can be ascertained, *has never been repealed but is still legally in force,* the use of cosmetics steadily expanded.

The use of cosmetics is, however, by no means confined to the female sex. Even in biblical days it was the custom to anoint the head of men of high office with perfumed "ointments", and the head of Jesus was so anointed as a tribute.

Today the use of male cosmetics embraces hair oils, creams and lotions, brushless and saponaceous shaving creams, pre-shave and after-shave lotions and powders, tooth powders, tooth pastes, denture cleansers, insect repellents, sunburn preparations and so on.

Psychologically, it must be realised that there is a marked difference in the mental make-up of men and women, and a dab of lipstick, a flick of the powder-puff or a new dress may prove of more value to a tired and depressed housewife or office worker than a cartload of medicine.

In the *Report of the Office of Civilian Supply to the U.S. Director of Economic Stabilisation* (1943), the following statement is made concerning cosmetics: "Psychiatrists maintain that cosmetics serve to counteract fatigue and that a dressing room in a factory may improve efficiency to the extent of 10 to 15 per cent. British experience substantiates this contention. At the beginning of the 1939-45 War, the manufacture of cosmetics was restricted to 25 per cent. of the peacetime production. It was discovered that the civilian population was growing depressed and war factory records were steadily declining. When cosmetic stations were established in the industries the production curve soared upwards immediately and increased numbers of women came flocking to the war factories for work. The effect was so striking that the restricting order for the nation as a whole was relaxed to 50 per cent. of the peacetime level."

The announcement that the British Prison Commissioners have decided to allow women prisoners the use of cosmetics (*Perfum. essent. Oil. Rec.*, Sept. 1946, p. 231) is a further proof, *if proof were needed*, that "Cosmetics" have become an *essential* part of our modern life.

The best definition of the term "Cosmetic" is that contained in the U.S. Federal Food, Drug and Cosmetic Act of 1938, which stipulates that the term cosmetic means (1) articles intended to be rubbed, poured, sprinkled or sprayed on, introduced into, or otherwise applied to the human body or any part thereof for cleansing, beautifying, promoting attractiveness or altering the appearance, and (2) articles intended for use as a component of any such articles; except that such term shall not include soap.

Cosmetic preparations may exert a four-fold action, namely, decorative, psychological, social and clinical.

Decorative. The aim of cosmetic preparations is to enhance the general appearance by minimising facial defects and unobtrusively directing attention towards individual qualities. That, in practice, this aim is not always achieved is due almost entirely to the lack of artistic skill on the part of the user. Properly applied, there is not the slightest shadow of doubt that cosmetics can achieve an astonishing transformation in an otherwise uninteresting face.

Psychological. The psychological value of cosmetic preparations should not be underestimated. The mental effects of hyperhidrosis may be out of all proportion to its severity and the use of deodorants has achieved general scientific approval. Many individuals suffer from distressing skin affections and in such cases the skilful use of cosmetics can often disguise, or at least minimise, the appearance of such a condition and can completely alter the sufferer's outlook on life. Grey hair is commonly associated, often erroneously, with old age. In these days of increasing business competition the appearance of grey hair may jeopardise an individual's future and, particularly in the case of a woman, may destroy her chance of marriage. By the skilful use of hair dyes this condition may be concealed.

Social. The availability of cosmetics, the increasing interest in one's appearance engendered by beauty salons and hairdressers, and the introduction of synthetic jewellery and textiles has probably done as much as anything else to break down artificial distinctions of class.

Clinical. Although there is no evidence that the skin can be really "fed" by cosmetic creams,[1] the application of emollient creams supplies a very valuable check to *premature ageing* of the skin in that such preparations assist in maintaining the suppleness of the outer skin layer and prevent, or at least minimise, "skin chapping" (with consequent risk of bacterial infection) and wind-burn, both of which lead to earlier ageing of the skin. In delaying this *they do therefore delay the onset of wrinkles although they do not prevent the ultimate wrinkling of the skin.*

Indeed, this was rapidly realised by the U.S. War Department who utilised cosmetics not only for camouflage but also for preventing skin chapping, sunburn, etc. Soldiers in desert areas and in climes of extreme cold were supplied with "chap sticks", since it was discovered that in dry desert climates the lips would crack badly even in temperatures of 110° F. (*Perfum. essent. Oil Rec.*, Dec. 1943, p. 328).

Powders possess soothing and cooling properties and are of value in preventing skin maceration and infection in regions of the body subject to heavy perspiration. The desirable improvement in hygiene produced by the introduction of dentifrices requires no elaboration. The value of sun screens in the case of persons exposed to excessive sunlight is becoming increasingly realised. Whilst the moderate exposure of the human organism to sunlight is beneficial, if carried to excess detrimental results accrue. Many irritable skin conditions are exacerbated and there is evidence that the development of malignant growths may be encouraged. The investigation of suitable sun-screening preparations is a specialised branch in which the cosmetician has blazed the trail. The dermatologist and pharmacist have been quick to adopt the pioneer work of the cosmetician in developing new emulsified ointment bases and lotions with the result that many of these preparations are not only more aesthetic in use but are more therapeutically effective.

The position of the dermatologist with regard to cosmetics was well summed up by Dr. W. J. O'Donovan in giving evidence in a Court case (*Perfum. essent. Oil Rec.*, April 1938, p. 140), who on being asked whether he regarded cosmetics as a curse replied: "Neither I, nor any of my colleagues, consider cosmetics as a curse. We always write or speak with approval of the opinion of Professor Sabouraud of Paris—the greatest dermatologist in Europe—that *women are indebted to cosmetics and that, on the whole, their introduction has been beneficial to their skins.*"

[1] See Chapter 10 for a more detailed discussion on this point.

CHAPTER I

THE SKIN

Calculation of Weight of the Skin—Histology of Skin—The Epidermis, Qualitative Analysis of Growth of Epidermis, Anatomy of Cutaneous Sensibility, the Vessels of the Skin, the Sebaceous Glands, the Freezing Point of Skin and the effect of washing thereon—Colour of Skin—Dermatoglyphics—The Skin Mosaic—The Molecular Structure of Skin—Skin Respiration—Biodynes—*p*H of Skin and its possible significance—Bioelectric Phenomena of Skin—"Nutritional Index"—Endocytines—Skin Blemishes: Freckles, Lentigines, Moles, Warts, Boils, Miliaria—Cosmetic Treatment of Skin Blemishes—Bleaching Creams—Chemical Components of the Skin—Functions of the Skin—Skin Enzymes—The Ageing of Skin—Cosmetics and the Ageing of Skin.

HISTOLOGY OF SKIN

THE skin is an important organ of the body and not merely a covering for the sub-adjacent structure. It is, in fact, one of the largest organs in the human body. Leider (*J. Invest. Derm.*, 1949, **12**, 187) gives the following formula and constants for calculating the weight of the skin:

Area of skin (in sq. cms) = (body weight in kgm) $^{0.425}$ × (height, in cms) $^{0.725}$ × 71·84. The thickness of the skin (including a little fat), has been taken to average 0·15 cm and its specific gravity as 1·25.

Thus for a man of 11 stone in weight and of height 5 ft. 6 in. (70 kg. and 170 cm.) the *area of the skin is* 16,000 sq. cm., *the volume* 2400 cc. *and weight* 3000 g., i.e. *about* 6·6 lb. It possesses a most complex structure and is conveniently classified into three layers:

(*a*) The EPIDERMIS, or cuticle.
(*b*) The CORIUM, often called the dermis.
(*c*) The SUBCUTANEOUS tissue, or hypoderm.

The EPIDERMIS may be further subdivided for convenience, but it should be remembered that in this case no definite separation of layers exists and that our subdivisions represent changes in cell structure as they move towards the surface, such layers often merging almost imperceptibly into the next. For descriptive and recognition purposes, it is convenient to classify the epidermis into five subdivisions: [1]

[1] Some authorities have divided the epidermis into four divisions, reckoning prickle and basal cell as one, which accounts for variations in the literature. (*See also* The Molecular Structure of Skin.)

(1) STRATUM CORNEUM.

(2) STRATUM LUCIDUM.

(3) STRATUM GRANULOSUM (GRANULAR LAYER).

(4) STRATUM MALPIGHII (MALPIGHIAN LAYER), prickle cell layer.

(5) STRATUM GERMINATIVUM (GERMINAL LAYER), basal layer.

The STRATUM CORNEUM or superficial portion of the horny layer consists of several layers of flattened cells lying in lamellae. These have no nuclei and are composed of keratin, their thickness differing in different parts of the body according to the degree of protection required. They are thickest on the palms of the hands and soles of the feet (some 0·4 to 0·6 mm. thick), but are exceptionally thin on the face, a point to be remembered in considering the possible penetration of cosmetic substances. (*See* Skin Penetration.)

These cells are constantly being shed, and contain an epidermic fatty material which renders them supple and waterproof.

A complete explanation of the problem of *keratinisation* as we proceed from the innermost to the outermost cells of the skin is still required, but it certainly becomes very marked as the cells migrate from the corium with its copious blood supply. The function of vitamin in the procedure is not quite explained, but it is instructive to note that Wolbach and Howe (1925) brought about keratinisation in rats by reducing their vitamin A intake, even in epithelia not normally subject to keratinisation. Cowgill, Stucky and Rose (*Arch. Path.* (*Lab. Med.*), 1929, **7**, 197) also recorded cutaneous changes produced by vitamin deficiency.

Since that time a number of investigators have shown the necessity of an adequate vitamin A supply if normal skin health, and even its histological appearance, is to be preserved. It is likely that the skin is one of the first organs to show evidence of vitamin deficiency, even before the other organs of the body [consider the fact that the skin responds immediately to traces of food to which it is allergic though other organs show no change]. There is reason to believe that vitamin A, B complex and possibly vitamin C may be of importance in this connection. (*See* Chapters 3 and 4.)

Priestley (*Bull. Post. Grad. Comm. Univ. Sydney*, Dec. 1947, **3**, 217) stresses the fact that the epidermis is a rapidly growing tissue throughout life and that, from our knowledge of the requirements of growing cells, one would expect such cells to exhibit the effects of vitamin and other deficiencies to a marked degree, which, he states, they do.

The usual method of administering vitamin concentrates is by the mouth and this is, so far as we know at present, the most effective method of administration. Vitamins can, however, be shown to exert effects when applied percutaneously and this question is discussed in detail in Chapter 4 which deals with skin penetration and skin nutrition.

The STRATUM LUCIDUM lies immediately below the stratum corneum, and may be regarded as intermediate in structure between the horny outer corneous layer and the granular layer. It is best seen in sections of the sole of the foot where this layer appears as an almost transparent line, or oil-like streak. Around the cells of this layer, and also in their contents, drops of an oily liquid, termed eleiden, are found.

The STRATUM GRANULOSUM, or granular layer, owes its name to the fact that in stained sections, granules of keratohylin may be seen. These refract incident light and help to give the white appearance to the skin. The thickness of this layer may vary from one to four cells deep, and like the stratum corneum is thickest on the palm of the hand and sole of the foot. With the exception of the red portion of the lip and the bed of the nail, this layer is found throughout the skin.

The STRATUM MALPIGHII, Malpighian layer so named after its discoverer, or as it is sometimes termed, prickle cell layer, varies in thickness, being thickest where the stratum corneum is well developed, and vice versa. The cells of this layer are polygonal and are peculiar in that they radiate a network of fine protoplasmic threads which pass across the intercellular spaces and join up with similar protoplasmic threads of contiguous cells. Thus the whole layer is in organic connection. From their appearance these cells have been likened to a prickly pear. Hence the origin of the term prickle cell layer.

The STRATUM GERMINATIVUM consists of a single row of columnar cells having oval nuclei. These are also joined together and to overlying cells by protoplasmic processes. This layer is constantly in a state of evolution, new cells being produced by the usual process of cell division or *mitosis*. The daughter cells do not divide in the normal state but are pushed away towards the surface. When formed, they are polygonal and nucleated, but in moving outwards they are flattened by pressure. They become horny partly by evaporation and by conversion of their protoplasm into keratinised tissue, and in their outward journey pass through the stages or *stratums* denoted above, until they finally take their place as non-nucleated stratified cells in the stratum corneum. This borderline between Malpighian layer and the corium contains the characteristic pigment of the skin which is associated with racial and individual differences. (*See* Melanin.)

QUALITATIVE ANALYSIS OF THE GROWTH OF EPIDERMIS. Hoffmann (*Arch. Path.* (*Lab. Med.*), 1949, **47**, 37) states that advanced mathematics show that if the duration of mitosis is taken as half an hour, then the time sequence of differentiation of epidermal cells in the scalp is: 3100 hours as a basal cell, 2900 hours as a prickle cell and 1900 hours as a granular cell.

The EPIDERMIS rests upon the DERMIS (sometimes called CORIUM), the dense fibrous layer beneath it, into which it fits by a series of inter-papillary processes or digitations. The papillae are finger-like projections which interlock with the irregularities of the epidermis.

The DERMIS (or Corium), consists of dense fibrous tissues containing strands of elastic tissue together with blood vessels, lymphatics, nerves, tactile corpuscles and hair follicles.

Priestley (*Bull Post. Grad. Comm. Univ. Sydney*, Dec. 1947, **3**, 217), has stressed that the epidermis and the dermis are totally different structures. The dermis, so far as we can see, being essentially a condensed connective tissue with no sharp demarcation from the underlying alveolar tissue. The epidermis consists of epidermal cells without connective tissue and without vessels. These cells differ visually, and doubtless chemically, from the stratum germinativum through to the completely keratinised stratum corneum, but, whilst the histological appearances have been well studied, little is known of the changing chemical structure or of the complete mechanism of the changes. A feature of the epidermis is its extraordinary speed of ageing, the cells changing in a relatively few layers from the protoplasmic cells of the germinal layers, through the granular layers of the Malpighian layers to the squames of the corneous layer.

Collagen is the principal protein of the dermis; other important proteins are *elastin*, of whose chemistry little is known, and *reticulin*, about which we appear to know even less. Priestley (*Bull. Post. Grad. Comm. Univ. Sydney*, Dec. 1947, **3**, 217) has drawn attention to the fact that for the formation of collagen in the skin (essential to the healing of wounds and ulcers), several factors are necessary, including an adequate supply of ascorbic acid (vitamin C), together with certain amino acids, notably methionine. How this latter protein acts we do not know, for skin proteins apparently contain but little methionine. This fact may account for satisfactory results obtained by the administration of adequate protein in wound treatment.

The dermis is conveniently classed into two further layers namely:

(*a*) The *Papillary Layer* containing conical processes, capillary loops, and nerve terminations, which provide us with our sense of touch and are thus most abundant where the sense of touch is most keen, finger-tips, toes, genital organs, nipples. This layer passes almost imperceptibly into (*b*) The *Reticular Layer* which is traversed by vessels, nerves, hair follicles, etc., and in which the fibrous bundles are more numerous. It was formerly believed that it was the elastic fibres which accounted for the amazing elasticity of the skin in such conditions as pregnancy. It is now known that actually these fibres stand little strain and rupture in pregnancy, the elasticity of the skin being chiefly due to its involuntary skin muscles.

Nerves of the Skin (The Anatomy of Cutaneous Sensibility)

Since the skin is in direct contact with the outside world, one would expect that Nature would provide a specialised system of warning signals to indicate when the body is in contact with heat, cold and other external influences which might otherwise do it injury. This is, in fact, the case, but the anatomy of cutaneous sensibility is too complex to discuss within the scope of this book. It has been generally conceded by competent observers that four primary sensations can be aroused through the skin, namely, *touch*, *cold*, *warmth* and *pain*. Other sensations—as for example the sense of smoothness, itching and tickling, etc.—are considered to be the result of a combination of two or more of the primary sensations impinging simultaneously on the central nervous system. Our knowledge of such systems and of their mechanism has been considerably advanced in recent years through the researches of Dr. Weddell (Reader in Human Anatomy at the University of Oxford).

In 1940, Wollard, Weddell and Harpman (*J. Anat., Lond.*, 1940, **74,** 413) in combined physiological and histological studies established the fact that pain is subserved in the skin by specific nerve terminals and further that, pressure, warmth, touch, cold and pain are represented in the skin by specific nerve terminals in punctate form as originally contended by Frey (*Ber. sachs. Ges.* (*Akad.*), Wiss Lpz, 1897, **49,** 462), but that the theory of punctate sensibility must be interpreted from a three-dimensional point of view, i.e. specific receptors lie at different depths beneath the skin.

Figure 1 summarises in diagrammatic form Weddell's conception of cutaneous innervation.

It now appears certain that the sensation of cold is subserved by Krause end-bulbs and touch by Meissner's corpuscles, as well as by Merkel's discs and by hairs. Pressure is subserved by Pacinian corpuscles. The position as regards warmth is not so definite but it is probable that the sensation of warmth is subserved by Ruffini's nerve endings.

The *Subcutaneous Layer*, or hypoderm, consists of loose fibrous tissue containing masses of fat cells. Histologists have now ceased to regard this as a separate and independent structure but rather as the lowest layer of the corium, in which masses of fat cells occur. This layer serves as a protective cushion for the vital underlying structures, as a support for the Pacinian bodies, nerve trunks, coil glands and blood vessels and, being a bad conductor of heat, prevents excessive loss of heat from the body.

The Vessels of The Skin

The Sweat Glands are tubular in character and of about 1/300th in. in diameter, being coiled back upon themselves to form a convoluted body. Commencing in the deeper layers of the dermis, they extend through the epidermis and culminate at the surface. (*See also* Chapter 30.)

According to the estimates of Krause (in Wagner's *Handwörterbuch der Physiologie*, 1844, **2**, 131) and more recently those of Taniguchi and Kamiyama (in Y. Kuno's *The Physiology of Human Perspiration*, 1934, p. 7), the human body contains about 2,380,000 sweat glands. The true sweat glands (known as the *eccrine* or *small coil* glands) secrete only water and water-soluble substances, no portion of the cell structure entering into their content. These glands are found distributed all over the body except on the margin of the lips and certain portions of the sex organs. These sweat glands are very largely concerned in the regulation of body temperature, evaporation of their contents leading to a loss of heat. In a normal healthy person such loss is automatic, unless the surrounding air is hot or very moist, in which case, if evaporation is insufficient to prevent a sharp rise in temperature, distress may occur. The function of these sweat glands is complementary to that of the kidneys and they probably assist in maintaining the elasticity of the skin (in conjunction with the secretion of the sebaceous glands—" sebum ". *See* Chapter 20).

The sweat glands are commonly divided into two types, the *eccrine* glands discussed above and the *apocrine* (or *large coil* glands) which are connected with a hair follicle and are, in general, limited to the underarm, breasts and genital regions of the body. These secrete nitrogenous and fatty substances in addition to water and salt and contain portions of the inner cell layer. As mentioned in Chapter 30, these glands are actually secondary sexual characteristics and in earlier days at least, played an important part in sexual attraction. Even today, it is not possible to state that they have ceased to have an influence, even though this may be subconscious.

The Sebaceous Glands are lobular structures situated in the dermis and are connected with hair follicles (except in the glans penis, prepuce,

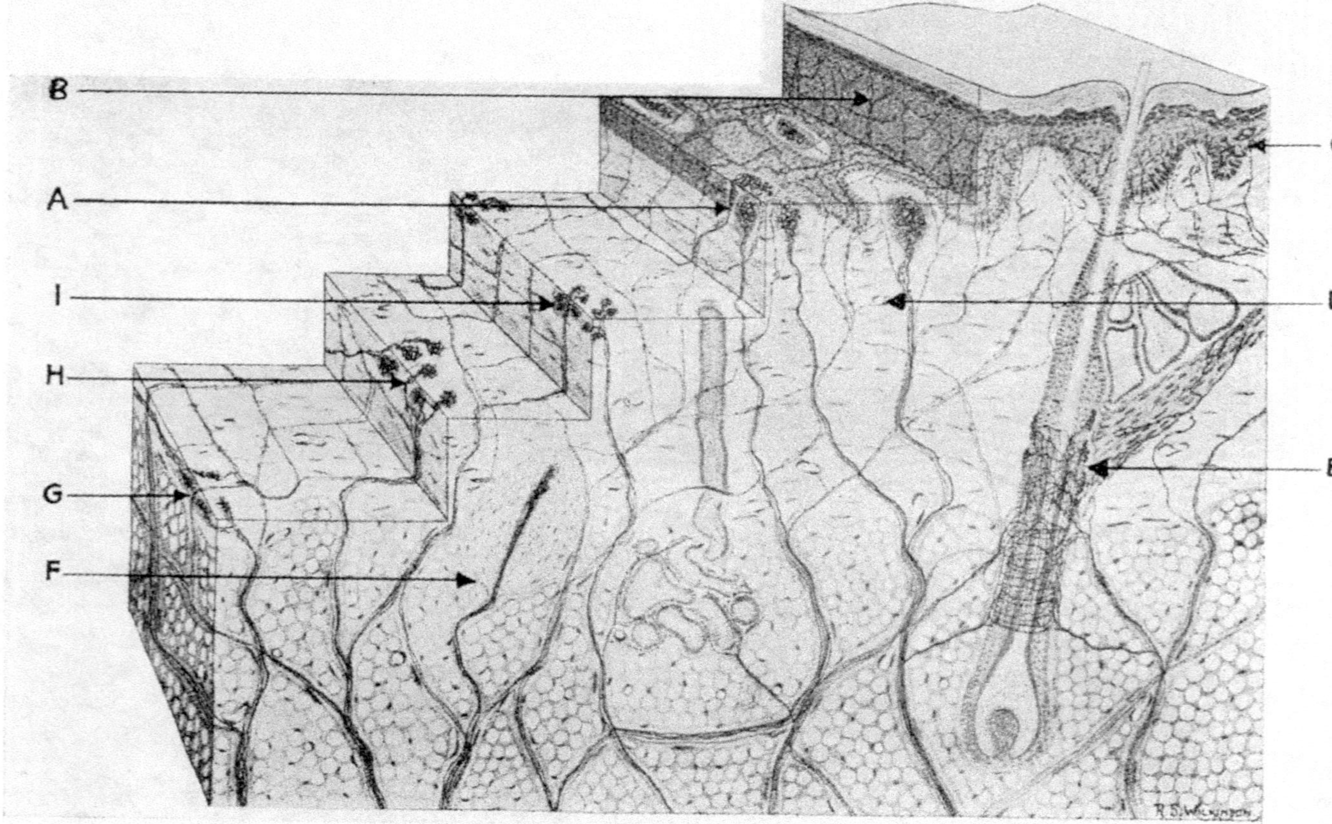

[*By courtesy of the British Medical Bulletin.*

FIG. 1.—Weddell's conception of cutaneous innervation.

See foot of opposite page for key.

labia minora and the red border of the lips). They secrete a fatty substance termed *sebum* which keeps the skin surface (and through capillary attraction the hair shaft) soft and supple. (*See* Chapter 20.) They are influenced by the secretion of the endocrine glands and, at puberty, become very active. After middle-age, however, their activity usually decreases.

Prolonged soaking of the skin in alkaline solutions, surface-active agents or solvents for sebum, may, by removing this sebaceous layer, render the skin more prone to dryness and " chapping ".

The Freezing Point of Skin and the Effect of Washing Thereon

Although very accurate determinations of the living skin's freezing-point have never been made, this point is not far from − 0·53° C. When skin is cooled, however, it rarely freezes at its true freezing point but exhibits to a remarkable degree the property of supercooling. Because of this property it is unusual for the skin to freeze unless its surface temperature is reduced below − 5° C., and it often happens that this temperature is lowered to as much as − 20° C. without the occurrence of freezing. Freezing begins with difficulty, but once started spreads rapidly throughout all the chilled tissue. Such supercooling is a very important form of protection against the injurious physical effects which would otherwise follow freezing. Sir Thomas Lewis (*Brit. med. J.*, 20 Dec. 1941) states that it has been found that supercooling displays itself in greater degree in skin that remains unwashed. Washing the skin encourages, whilst rubbing the skin with spirit and anointing it with oil, discourages freezing. The capacity to supercool appears, it is stated, to be connected with the relative dryness of the horny layer of the skin, and it is a well-known fact that Arctic explorers leave their skins unwashed.

The above points should be borne in mind in the formulation of protective creams for persons whose hands are exposed to extreme cold.

Fig. 1.—**A**, groups of Meissner's corpuscles subserving the sensation of touch; **B** shows beaded nerve-nets subserving pain (probably fast pain); **C** shows Merkel's discs subserving touch; **D** shows beaded nerve-fibres derived from nerve-nets subserving pain and associated with blood-vessels (probably slow pain); **E** shows nerve terminals around the sheath of a hair subserving touch; **F** shows a pacinian corpuscle subserving pressure; **G** shows a group of Ruffini endings subserving warmth; **H** and **I** show groups of Krause's end-bulbs subserving cold (these lie at somewhat variable depths beneath the skin-surface). *Note.*—The organised endings are accompanied in every instance by fine-beaded nerve-fibres subserving pain.

The Colour of the Skin

The colour of the skin is due to the presence of five pigments, three of which, melanin, melanoid and carotene are extravascular, whilst the other two are the oxyhaemoglobin and reduced haemoglobin of the blood. Edwards and Duntley (*Amer. J. Anat.*, 1939, **65**, 1), have pointed out that differences in the amounts and concentrations of these pigments account for the varying colour of the skin in different regions of the body.

Melanin is the most important of the skin pigments and is present in the form of dark brown granules in the lower strata of the Malpighian layer.

Melanin pigment formation is stimulated by exposure to ultraviolet light and is of definite physiological importance since it protects the lower layers of the skin against the injurious effects of excessive light. In mulattos and negroes the amount of melanin present is much higher than in the white races and it is probably this factor which contributes to the resistance of the black races to sunlight.

Increased formation of melanin also occurs in association with certain skin diseases, in certain types of poisoning, for example, arsenical, and in certain parts of the body in pregnancy.

A very comprehensive review of the pigment melanin has been presented by Peck (*J. Soc. cosmet. Chem.*, July 1947, pp. 33 ff.). Peck points out that modern investigators agree that the formation of pigment in the melanoblasts of ectodermal and mesodermal origin is due to the oxidation of a colourless propigment by an enzyme. Fuerth has shown that this melanogen is most probably a cyclic protein component and amongst others proposed tyrosine as the melanogen. Free tyrosine has been demonstrated in the circulation of the higher vertebrates, but tyrosinase has been found in insects and coldblooded animals only, and there is no positive evidence that tyrosine is the mother substance of melanin in man or animals.

Bloch ("Das Pigment", in *Jadassohn J.: Handbuch der Haut-und Geschlechtskrankheiten*, Berlin: Julius Springer, 1927, Vol. 1), showed that another aromatic amino acid, namely, B-3-4-dioxyphenylalanine, is the probable propigment in warmblooded animals. The main support for this assumption was his discovery of the reaction to dioxyphenylalanine in the melanoblasts. This reaction consists in the change of dioxyphenylalanine into a melanin which Bloch was able to study under the microscope and, moreover, to show that this reaction was specific only for B-3-4-dioxyphenylalanine and could not be elicited with tyrosine, or other related dioxyphenyl derivatives. Moreover, there is no reaction to dioxyphenylalanine in albinotic skin or in vitiligo.

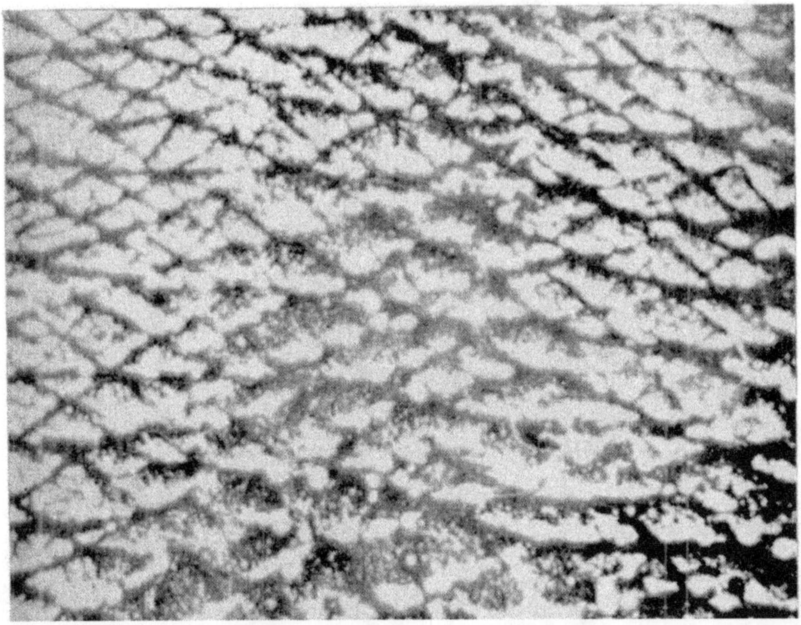

(*a*) Back of human hand (× 10).

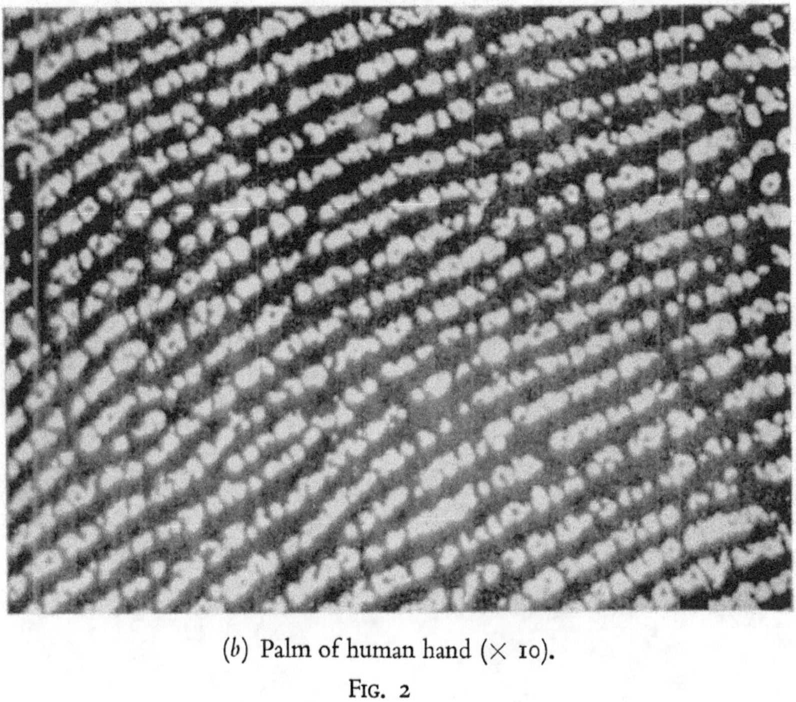

(*b*) Palm of human hand (× 10).

FIG. 2

(Illustrations by the Author.)

Peck draws attention to the fact that one cannot refute the assumption of the propigment function of dioxyphenylalanine on the ground that its presence has not been demonstrated in the animal body, since deeper understanding of biological processes has shown that an intermediary substance can easily escape analytic detection and yet form a pivotal phase in the course of the enzymatic process. Other criticisms raised against Bloch's assumption of a specific dioxyphenylalanine oxidase, have been based upon the fact that there are other catalytic systems of wider distribution that convert dioxyphenylalanine into melanin, for example, polyphenolase (an enzyme of almost ubiquitous occurrence in living matter), tyrosinase, etc. The mechanism of the formation of melanin from tyrosine was elucidated by Raper (*Biochem. J.*, 1927, **21**, 89). The enzymes responsible for the formation of melanin may be summarised diagrammatically :

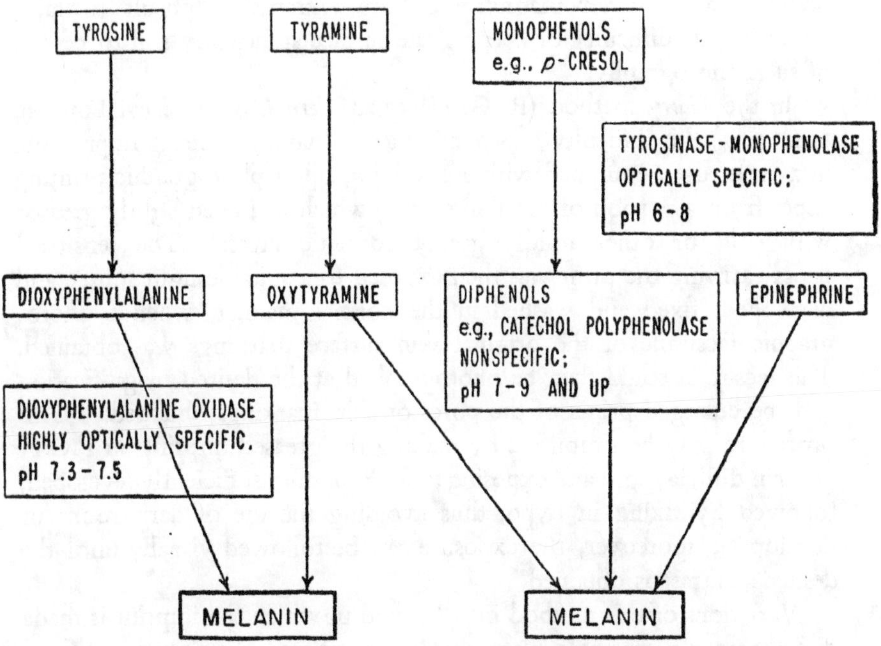

[*By courtesy of Dr. Samuel Peck.*

FIG. 3.—Enzymes responsible for the formation of melanin.

It is interesting to note that in an investigation into occupational leukoderma by Oliver, Schwartz and Warren (*J. Amer. med. Assoc.*, 1939, **113**, 927 ; Public Health Reports, 21 June, 1940, **55**, 1111-30, U.S.A.), it was found that the monobenzyl ether of hydroquinone contained as an antioxidant in the rubber gloves of the workers was responsible for the depigmentation of the skin. Experiments on both white and coloured human subjects carried out by Peck and Sobotka (*J. invest. Derm.*, 1941, 4, No. 4) showed that application of this monobenzyl compound in the form of an ointment or ether-suspension produced leukoderma and further that histological examination of the depigmented areas revealed a negative reaction for dioxyphenylalanine and an almost complete disappearance of the melanin.

[Modern methods of controlling skin pigmentation by the use of cosmetic preparations containing suitable sun screens will be found under Sunburn Preparations ; *see also* Freckles and the Use of Bleaching Creams, at the end of the chapter.]

Dermatoglyphics

Dermatoglyphics, i.e. the study of the surface markings (or ridges) of the skin, is complicated by the fact that direct photographs of any desired feature under magnification are extremely difficult to take, owing to the difficulty of keeping the surface sufficiently still to permit of such photography.

In the *Harry* method (R. G. Harry, *Modern Cosmeticology*, London, 1944, p. 4) this difficulty was overcome by making a direct impression, in a dark room equipped with a safe-light, upon photographic printing paper from a portion of the skin surface which had been lightly greased with cold or other mildly greasy cosmetic cream. The sensitised paper carrying the print was then exposed to a suitable light source and developed, fixed and washed in the normal manner, when a photographic facsimile of the original skin surface markings was obtained. This facsimile could then be photographed at the desired magnification and the enlarged prints of the pores or skin markings obtained. [This procedure may be simplified by making the greased imprint on P.O.P. paper in dull daylight and exposing to sunlight until sufficiently developed, followed by fixing in hypo, thus avoiding the use of dark room or developer ; moreover, the exposure can be followed visually until the desired contrast is obtained.

Variations of this method may be used in which the imprint is made directly upon a sensitised plate, this being exposed, developed and fixed and an enlargement made directly from the negative. Alternatively, solutions or creams containing substances which react with the sensitised paper or plate may be used to obtain the original skin print, the subsequent procedure being essentially the same as that described previously.]

The value of the use of cosmetic creams in such impressions is that there is no aesthetic or professional objection to their use ; they do not stain, and they may be used on sensitive regions of the body or where the keratin layer is very thin, such as the face.

The photographs of skin prints in Figure 2 demonstrate :

(*a*) The scaly, snake-skin like appearance of the corneous layer and also the apertures of the sebaceous glands.

(*b*) The patterning and frequency of the apertures of the sweat ducts.

The author has also studied various methods of making impressions by the use of cellulose nitrate and acetate, and of various plastics dissolved in volatile solvents in which a solution of the substance used is applied to the skin surface, allowed to evaporate and then peeled off. The objection to such methods is that, during evaporation of the solvent, air-bubbles may arise from the warm skin giving misleading pin-holed impressions. To obviate this, and still obtain rapid "impression-moulding", the author studied the use of hot waxes as impression materials. Hot dental wax was found the best of the waxes tried for this purpose. This was applied to the skin surface, allowed to set for a moment and then detached. To facilitate examination of this wax impression under a low-power microscope, it was dusted with fine carbon black.

Such methods may be used to calculate the number of sweat glands in a given area, etc. Skin markings ("finger-prints"), are of course of great value from the criminological aspect and Mitchell (*The Scientific Detective and the Expert Witness*, 1931) has pointed out that it has been proved that the pore openings upon the skin ridges are distinctive in size, shape and position, and that they vary widely as do the patterns themselves in different individuals. Removal of these patterns by pumice stone, burning, or peeling does not destroy them, for the new skin will continue to show the same pattern as the old. It is stated that the number of such pores, in the palmar surfaces, ranges from 9-28 per sq. cm. Gates (*Human Genetics*, New York : Macmillan, 1946) points out that the skin pattern of the finger pads and palm remains constant throughout the lifetime of the individual but varies from person to person *even in identical twins* and Gates concludes that every finger print *is unique and beyond the control of heredity*. [In order to obliterate the finger print pattern, the underlying dermis as well as the epidermis must be destroyed. If the epidermis only is burned with acid or scraped, the pattern is reproduced with identical details when the skin regenerates.]

The Skin Mosaic

So far the skin has been considered as a homogeneous entity, whereas genetically it is nothing of the kind, but rather a *mosaic*, a kind of patch-work quilt, as E. Meirowsky has shown (*Brit. J. Derm.*, 1942, **54**, 99-121 ; 129-153), containing qualities inherited from one parent in certain parts of the skin and of qualities from the other parent in other parts, each of these regions being dependent upon the person's genes.[1]

Meirowsky has drawn attention to the fact that cross-breeding experiments made by numerous research workers (Sunn, Schneider and Webb (1923), Kossigi (1926), Nachtsheim (1929), C. E. Blunu (1936)) have revealed that certain special genes are responsible for the location of markings, and that other heritable, and perhaps not heritable, factors *modify* and *regulate* their size and shape,[2] for example, Schindelka (*Handbuch tieraerztl. Chirurgie*, 6, Leipzig, 1903) experimented by crossing a long-haired and a hairless dog with striking proof of such an inherited mosaic. It resulted in sharply defined regions of the skin, some of which were naked and others hairy.

Numerous references in the literature confirm the presence of such a skin pattern governed in different localities by different genes, and it is obvious that these factors must be taken into account in studying hair poverty, varying areas of susceptibility on the skin surface (allergy, dermatitis, eczema), and in the measurement of surface biochemical phenomena.

The Molecular Structure of Skin and Related Tissues

So far we have discussed the diversity of the various cells and layers of the skin which are, at least superficially, evident. However, recent work by Astbury and other workers have shown that, in the last resort, all these types of structure are derived from a single master molecular group.

The application of X-ray diffraction patterns to the study of the keratin molecule will be found more fully discussed in Chapter 23 dealing with Permanent Waving.

Astbury ("The Molecular Structure of Skin, Hair and Related Tissues", *Brit. J. Derm.*, Jan. 1950, **62**, 1-15) has pointed out that the elastic properties of mammalian hairs applies also to horn nails, hedgehog spines, porcupine quills, whalebone (but not to avian and reptilian keratin[3]);

[1] See *Heredity and Hair Affections*, Chapter 20.

[2] *See* A. E. Cockayne, *Inherited Abnormalities of the Skin and its Appendages*, London: Humphrey Milford, 1933; E. Meirowsky, *Arch. Derm. Syph., Wien*, 1919, **127**, 1; Chas. Darwin, *Variations in Animals and Plants*, London: J. Murray, 1868.

[3] An X-ray diagram of feather keratin (diagrams of essentially the same type are given also by birds' beaks and claws, tortoise-shell, "snakes' scales", and lizards' claws, all of which may be described for convenience as "feather keratin") shows that this structure is not so divorced from mammalian keratin as a preliminary inspection of their diffraction patterns might suggest; on examining the matter more closely it is seen that the feather structure is after all of a disguised beta-type analogous not indeed to unstretched but to *stretched* human (i.e. mammalian) hair. The avian and reptilian family constitutes therefore a beta-subgroup of the k-m-e-f group mentioned on facing page.

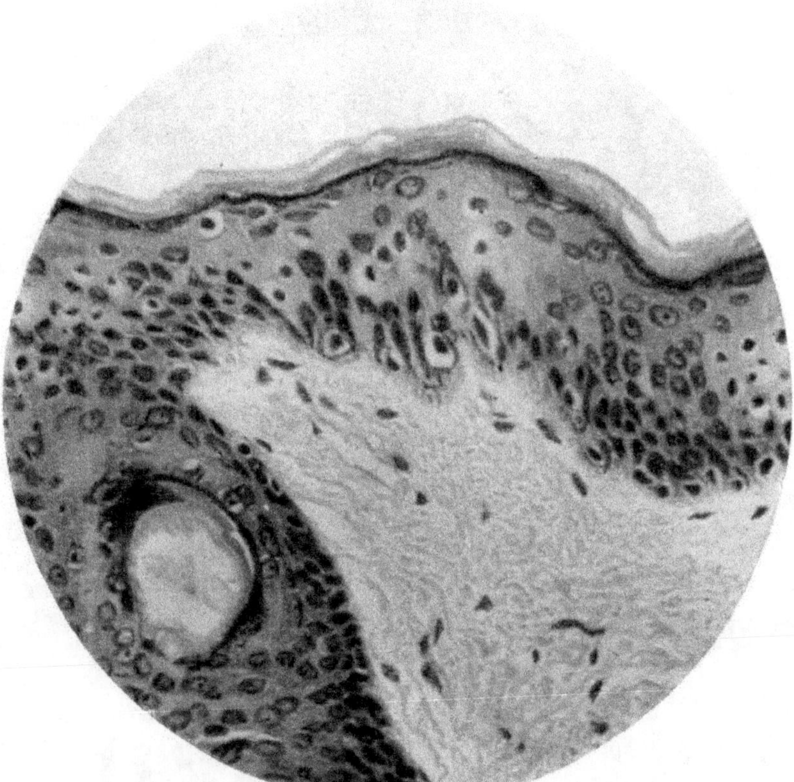

Fig. 4.—Vertical section of skin of cheek of adult female.
(From the Author's collection. × 400.)

i.e. they are "*all of a family*" (*molecularly speaking*), differing not in kind but only in degree. This remarkable relationship turns out to be only the foreshadowing of a much wider and deeper master plan. X-ray diagrams of essentially the keratin type are found also with the other fibrous proteins of the epidermis, the chief muscle protein, myosin and two other recently discovered muscle components, paramyosin, and tropomyosin, the blood-clotting proteins fibrinogen and fibrin and most recently—bacterial flagella. All these differ considerably in detail; nevertheless X-rays show that in the last resort they are all derived from a single master plan which Astbury and his co-workers have called the keratin-myosin-epidermis-fibrinogen (k-m-e-f) group. The molecular plan, common to all of them when they are in the unstretched state, is the folded alpha-structure and likewise, when they are stretched, they pass into a common beta-form. Astbury points out: "What we are saying in effect is that epidermal protein, hair protein and muscle protein are basically the same thing, or at least the same idea. Myo-epithelial tissue is equivalent to both skin and muscle, a hair is by way of being a 'vulcanised' muscle fibre, and it may be no exaggeration to describe bacterial flagella as 'monomolecular' hairs or muscles—and it matters little in the fundamental sense which name we use." [The X-ray structures of stretched and unstretched hair keratin is more fully discussed in Chapter 23.]

Skin Respiration

Continuous chemical changes are proceeding in living matter of all kinds, either constructive or degradative. This process is termed metabolism.

The skin, one of the largest organs in the human body, having defensive, excretory and respiratory functions, plays an important role in the metabolism of the human body.

The term "respiration of the skin" may convey an erroneous impression to the layman, who tends to regard it as a kind of breathing in and out, requiring lungs. To the biochemist respiration is the taking up of oxygen or the excretion of carbon dioxide. The outer skin is keratinised and dead material but the lower layers carry on active metabolic functions. The skin must be considered as a complete organ of the body.

The metabolism can be investigated from three different aspects:

(1) Proliferation—the reproduction of the cell.

(2) Glycolysis—the non-oxidative degradation of sugars by the cell.

(3) Respiration—the consumption of oxygen by the cells.

Cells require energy for growth and other functional activities, and usually obtain this when oxygen is available from sugars. If sufficient supplies of carbohydrate are unavailable, proteins and fats may be utilised. In the absence of available oxygen, a non-oxidative degradation of the sugars occurs, termed glycolysis.

Warburg (*J. Cancer Res.*, 1925, **9**, 148) found lowered respiration and active glycolysis in tumour tissue, and advanced the hypothesis that tumour production might result from an oxygen deficiency of normal tissue, and even stated (*The Metabolism of Tumours*, London: Constable, 1930) that interference with the respiration in growing cells is, from the standpoint of the physiology of metabolism, the cause of tumours. E. S. Cook (*Chem. Prod.*, 1939, **2**, 89) has pointed out that " the original concepts of Warburg have been extended and modified, and that although it is frequently incorrect to say that cancer has a lower QO_2 than normal tissue, if certain other factors (e.g. glycolysis) are considered, then, in general, cancer metabolism is characterised by faulty metabolism ". (QO_2 = the oxygen uptake in cubic millimetres per milligram of dry weight of tissue.)

Burke (*Some Fundamental Aspects of the Cancer Problem*, New York: Science Press, 1937) has stated that " the difference between ordered and unordered growth lies in the relation between respiration and glycolysis, in that in unordered tumour growth respiration does not succeed in preventing glycolysis ".

G. P. Sperti, J. R. Loofbourow and C. M. Dwyer (*Stud. Inst. Divi. Thomæ*, 1938, **1**, 163) postulate that in the case of benign and malignant tumours the fundamental mechanism involved is the production in abnormal concentration of metabolic stimulating factors produced by cells as a result of irritation or injury of long standing. (*See* Biodynes.) Long standing injury or irritation is, of course, considered to be a factor in the production of certain cancers.

Biodynes. Selective Agents for the Stimulation of the Respiration, Glycolysis, or Growth of Cells

Carroll (*J. exp. Med.*, 1921, **34**, 425; *J. Amer. med. Assoc.*, 1924, **82**, 255) found that a wound completely free from tissue, debris, and blood clots and absolutely protected from outside irritation, did not heal, and suggested that the injury itself does not bring about the regenerative stimulus but that consequent irritation initiates a mechanism which determines cell proliferation. Fardon, Carroll and Ruddy (*Stud. Inst. Divi. Thomæ*, 1937, **1**, 17), and also Sperti, Loofbourow and Dwyer (*ibid.* 163) have isolated metabolic stimulating factors from

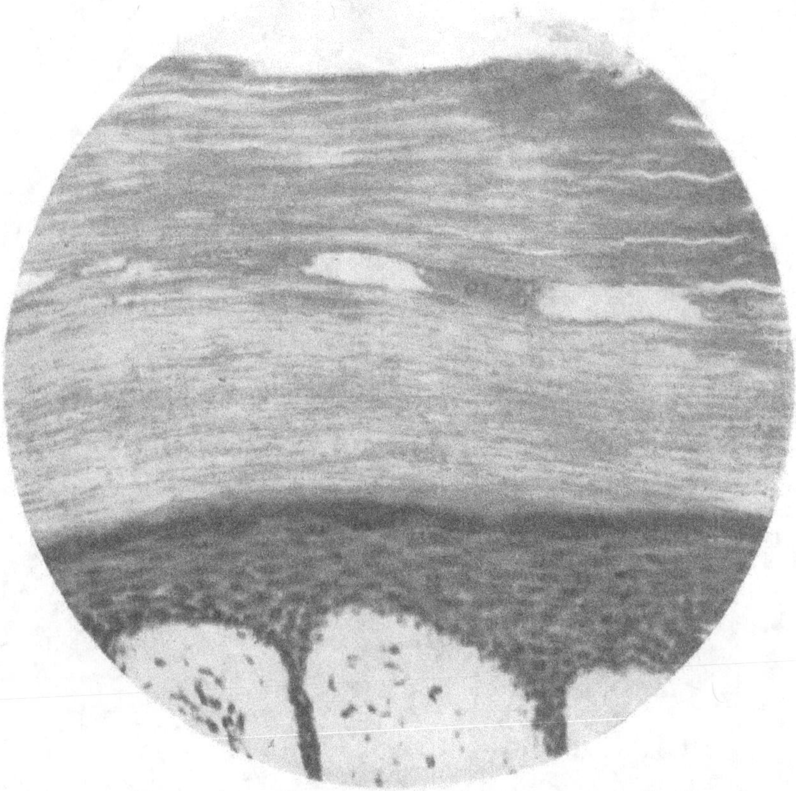

FIG. 5.—Vertical section of skin from palm of hand.
(From the Author's collection. × 300.)

cells and shown that injured cells secrete substances which stimulate growth, respiration, and the utilisation of sugars. (*See also* Fardon and Sullivan, *ibid.*, 1938, **2**, 1, 39.) The production of such wound hormones has been confirmed and a quantitative method established (Loofbourow, Dwyer and Morgan, *ibid.* 1938, **2**, 137).

Some Variable Factors affecting Skin Respiration

S. Bommer ("Haute und Vitamine", *Dtsch. med. Wschr.*, 1934, **60**, 570) has linked the cutaneous symptoms of a vitamin A deficiency with a reduction in cellular oxidation, and P. D. Adams (*J. Biol. Chem.* 1936, **116**, 641) has demonstrated diminution in skin respiration in rats suffering from a deficiency of vitamin B_2. It is also claimed that a vitamin D deficiency lowers skin respiration (A. K. Presnell, *J. biol. Chem.*, 1937, **121**, 5). These results, however, appear to be part of the general deficiency and not specific.

Amersbach, Nutini and Cook (*Arch. Derm. Syph., Chicago*, 1941, **43**, 940) as a result of experiments concluded that soaps, cosmetic creams and lotions depressed the respiration of both rat and human skin. In their studies, the materials were tested by direct addition to the tissue sections in the Warburg vessel and also by direct application to the intact skin after which the skin was excised and the oxygen absorption measured. Killian and Marsh (*Proc. Sci. Sect. T.G.A.*, May, 1946) and Killian and Oclassen (*Proc. Sci. Sect. T.G.A.*, Dec. 1946), however, made a critical study of the methods and conclusions of Amersbach, Nutini and Cook, and came to the conclusion that the application of such cosmetics to intact skin did not depress the respiration. On the contrary, using a plethysmographic technique, Killian *et al.*, found that the addition of petroleum jelly and of cold cream, increased the gaseous exchange through the skin (presumably by altering its permeability.—Author). Adams and Presnell (from "The Gas Exchange of the Skin", P. D. Adams, *Amer. Perfum.*, Feb. 1949, p 134) also made extensive studies and were unable to confirm the conclusions of Amersbach, Nutini and Cook, neither were they able to find any evidence of increased skin respiration through the application of supposedly stimulating substances from yeast (providing the material was thoroughly removed before excision of the skin). Adams (*Amer. Perfum.*, Feb. 1949, p. 134) in summarising the difficulties of these questions states that: "A study of the available literature on the absorption of oxygen by both the intact and excised skin raises more questions than are answered. Apparently much of the oxygen that passes into the skin enters the blood stream. It is not known how much, if any, of this oxygen is utilised directly by the skin. Various factors affect the absorption of oxygen by or through the skin, viz. (*a*) temperature and composition of the gases surrounding the skin; (*b*) gas tension of the blood stream; (*c*) rate of blood flow through the skin; (*d*) dilation of the skin capillaries; (*e*) inflammatory irritation; (*f*) skin diseases; (*g*) external applications such as petrolatum; (*h*) vitamin and perhaps hormone deficiencies; (*i*) age; (*j*) individual characteristics; (*k*) changes in tissue metabolic processes and perhaps many others. . . ."

*p*H Value of the Skin, and its Possible Significance

A number of investigators have reported upon the acidic nature of the aqueous fluid bathing the cells of the skin surface, and have termed it, erroneously, the hydrogen ion concentration of the skin. As Blank (*J. invest. Derm.*, 1939, **2**, 67) has pointed out, it is incorrect to speak of the *p*H of any solid tissue of the body. What is actually meant is the *p*H of the aqueous fluid bathing the skin surface.

Various workers have made determinations of the *p*H of this fluid, and while it is universally conceded that in the normal average healthy person this is acid, there is considerable divergence between the figures actually obtained. Sharlit and Scheer (*Arch. Derm. Syph., Chicago*, 1923, **7**, 592) found an average of 5·5; Schade and Marchionini (*Arch. Derm. Syph., Wien*, 1928, **154**, 690) 3·0–5·0. Lustig and Perutz (*Arch. Derm. Syph., Wien*, 1930–31, **162**, 129) found values of 5·3–6·5, while Levin and Silvers (*Arch. Derm. Syph., Chicago*, 1932, **25**, 825) obtained a value of 5·0–5·3. Blank (*J. invest. Derm.*, 1939, **2**, 67), using a glass electrode with vacuum tube potentiometer in a series of determinations on 100 males and 100 females, found that the *p*H of the exposed areas varied from 4·0–7·0, but that most of the readings lay between 4·2–5·6.

Many of the discrepancies reported in the literature are probably the result of the methods employed. The glass electrode method is the only one which can be relied upon to give accurate results under the conditions prevailing on the surface of the human skin. Owing to the high resistance of such an electrode a vacuum tube (thermionic valve) potentiometer has to be incorporated in the instrument.

Although a reading may be obtained by simply contacting the calomel and glass electrodes with the skin surface, such a reading is variable. In my own investigation (R. G. Harry, *Brit. J. Derm.*, Jan. 1942) therefore, the skin surface was first defatted with a little ethyl ether and moistened with the minimum of distilled water. Readings were then taken and checked after an interval of a couple of minutes to ensure that the results were not due to changes in dilution. To ensure that the potentials were not influenced by muscular reactions or cardiac e.m.f.s, the

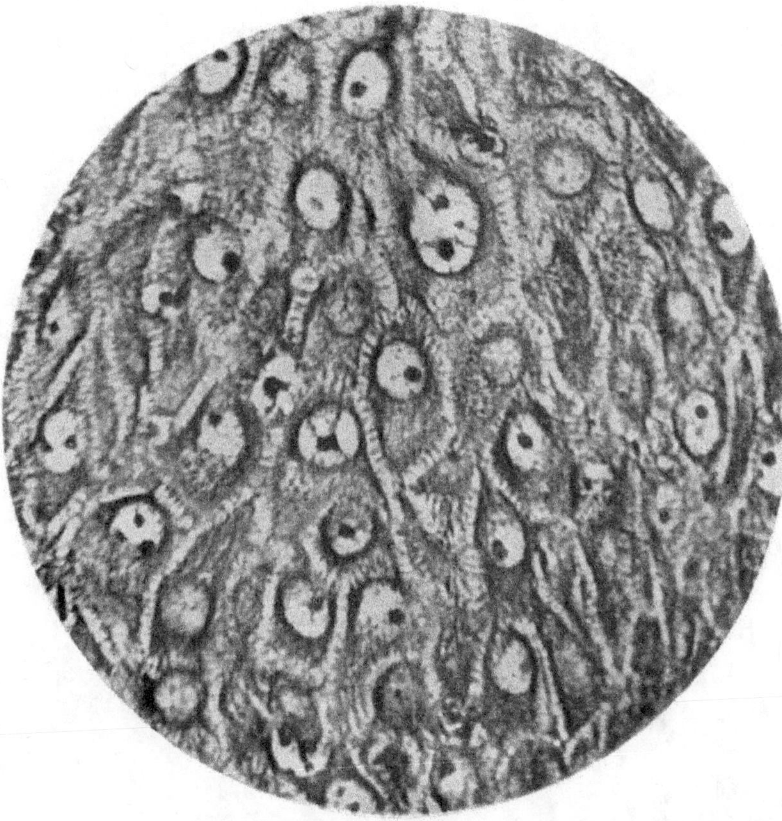

Fig. 6.—Epithelial Fibrils or " Prickles ".

(From a case of an early Epithelioma. Author's collection. × 650.)

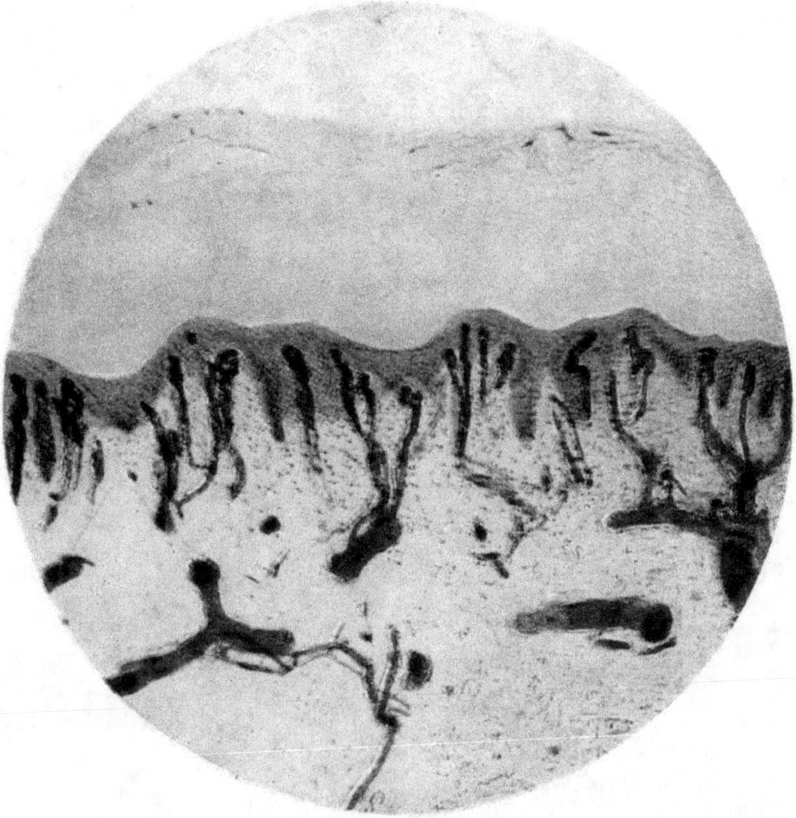

[*Slide by courtesy of Messrs. Flatters & Garnett, Ltd., Manchester.*

FIG. 7.—The blood supply to the skin. Note the absence of blood vessels in the stratum corneum but Sub-Capillary Network of Delicate Anastomising Vessels in Lower Skin layer.

electrodes were placed so as to reduce such possibilities to a minimum, and the readings taken (*a*) after adequate resting, (*b*) after exercise. A further check was made in those cases involving abnormally high or low e.m.f.s by measuring the *p*H of a drop of distilled water (after contacting with as large a skin area as possible), utilising a capillator and bromcresol green (*p*H range 3·6–5·2), bromcresol purple (*p*H range 5·2–6·8) and phenol red (*p*H 6·8–8·4). The temperature adopted was 32° C, based on actual skin surface temperatures measured by means of a special thermocouple. Readings were made on the palm of the hand, the arm and the cheek of the face. Since it was found that the use of a special *micro* sealed glass electrode, fitted with screened cable, yielded results of greater consistency and reproducibility than the standard type, this electrode was adopted for the following tests which were made on 100 patients of both sexes and of ages varying from six months to seventy-six years.

Blank's observations that the majority of readings in exposed areas of the skin lies between *p*H = 4·2 and *p*H = 5·6 was confirmed. The following figures were obtained:

	Highest *p*H	*Lowest* *p*H	*Average* *p*H
Back of Hand			
Females	6·62	4·13	5·53
Males	6·02	4·56	5·40
Palm of Hand			
Females	6·05	4·60	5·51
Males	6·50	4·39	5·33
Arm			
Females	6·0	4·95	5·30
Males	6·1	4·40	5·28
Face (Cheek)			
Females	6·70	5·00	5·58
Males	6·40	5·10	5·50

The *p*H of the skin varies not only with the individual but in different parts of the same individual, and moreover at differing times in the same parts in the same individual. This is not unexpected, when one considers that the skin is a complex conglomeration of inherited tendencies and varying biological and metabolic functions.

Since the skin is generally acid, preparations intended for normal skin should not markedly alter (other possibly than as a transient phenomena) its reaction. In pathological conditions of the skin, it might be, however, that by treatment with buffered solutions of a different *p*H the pathological condition might be inhibited.

J. H. Draize (*J. invest. Derm.*, 1942, p. 77) carried out pH determinations on the skin of 100 white people, on 25 negroes and on animals with the following average results:

White male	4·85	Cat	6·43
Negro	5·21	Rat	6·48
Guinea pig	5·50	Rabbit	6·71
Monkey	6·42	Dog	7·52

More recently Peck (*Proc. Sci. Sect. T.G.A.*, Dec. 1952) has reported the pH values of the skin of the back in the case of 70 individuals. It was found that the skin of the back varied from as low as 3·0, in one individual to a value of 6·6, with an average for all areas of the back of 5·069. It has been the author's experience that occasionally pH readings on the alkaline side are obtained and in a few instances, values of 7·0 and 7·3 have been recorded. These readings were obtained on female subjects and hence attempts were made to determine whether such readings had any correlation with menstrual periods. No such correlation was established, however.

The Role of the Skin's "Acid Mantle"

The role of the skin's "Acid Mantle" has been a matter of controversy. In 1929 Marchionni (*Arch. Derm. Syph.*, *Wien*, 1929, **158**, 290) and others, e.g. Levin and Silvers (*Arch. Derm. Syph.*, *Chicago*, Sept. 1932, **26**, 466) published their theory concerning the acid mantle on the skin as a defence mechanism against infection and against fungi in particular. This theory did not explain the role of the "acidity" in the defence mechanism, apart from the fact that "it was acid", and it was even suggested that dilute hydrochloric acid be used in the treatment of fungus infections. Peck and associates in 1939 became interested in the conception that it was the constituents of sweat which played the chief protective role and were able to demonstrate that a number of the lower fatty acids found in the sweat were fungistatic as well as bacteriostatic (*J. invest. Derm.*, Aug., 1938, **1**, 237; *Arch. Derm. Syph.*, *Chicago*, Jan. 1939, **39**, 126; Nov. 1947, **56**, 601). As Peck (*Proc. Sci. Sect. T.G.A.*, Dec. 1952) states: "It was not the pH *per se* that was important but the factors which go into the formation of the pH value which render the acid cloak a protective film against infection."

In 1942 the author (R. G. Harry, "Hydrogen Ion Concentration in Therapeutic Bases", *Brit. J. Derm.*, Jan. 1942, p. 7) stated: "The normal skin swarms with staphylococci, diphtheroids and often monilia and other organisms, whilst the dermatologist uses Sabouraud's medium (which is acid) to cultivate pathogenic fungi . . ." *the fact that such organisms are normally present without pathogenic effects* would indicate that the skin surface possesses an anti-bacterial activity of some sort which may (1) reduce their pathogenicity without destroying them, or (2) may *preserve certain protective factors in the skin, of which we (at present) know nothing*, whose activity is impaired if an unfavourable *p*H is allowed to develop.

Peck (*Proc. Sci. Sect. T.G.A.*, 1952) has recently shown in another manner the important role of *p*H and records that under adhesive tape the *p*H value slowly rises to the alkaline side and at the same time the bacteria multiply under the adhesive tape.

Titratable Acidity and *p*H

The *p*H determination is of definite value in the study of ointment bases and cosmetic preparations. It gives a measure of their content of alkali or acid and their probable suitability for use on the skin surface, assuming that irritant substances (such as certain perfumes and fatty acids, etc.) are absent.

Like most other scientific measurements, however, it should be used with full consideration of its limitations. For example, it is possible to have a preparation containing a relatively high proportion of alkali in the presence of a large amount of fatty matter and relatively low water content, and such a mixture may give a lower *p*H than would be the case if the water content were increased.

It is advisable, therefore, to consider the *p*H in combination with a determination of free alkali or acid.

Bioelectric Phenomena of the Skin

DONNAN THEORY OF EQUILIBRIUM. It may be asked, " What interest has the cosmetician or dermatologist in skin potentials ? " It appears to me that the external contact of creams, ointments and lotions of varying *p*H and ionic constituents (K, Na, Ca, etc.) and the diffusion of soaps and other wetting agents across the cell membrane probably exerts considerable effect on skin potentials and ultimately (possibly) on skin health though we do not know at present what constituents are helpful to normal metabolic processes. Until recently the only method of studying skin was histologically after biopsy. The bioelectric phenomena of the skin are complex and the subject is only in its infancy ; nevertheless, research on this subject may show it to be valuable in the investigation of the biochemistry of skin, if due allowance is made for its complexities and for certain variable conditions.

Living cells have a potential difference on both sides of the intact cellular membrane in accordance with the Donnan Theory of

Membrane Equilibrium which postulates that if a solution containing diffusible ions is separated by a membrane from another solution containing a salt with a non-diffusible ion, e.g. a protein ion, then a potential difference will exist on the two surfaces of the membrane.

The diffusion and concentration potentials across the cell membranes are largely determined by the concentration and mobility of various organic and inorganic ions.

Apart from such membrane potential differences, considerable potential differences exist along the surface of injured tissue, especially the nervous system.

Over a hundred years ago (*Untersuchungen über tierische Elektrizitat*, Berlin: 1848, E. du Bois-Reymond) it was shown that in injured muscle and nerve a potential difference existed between the injured and uninjured tissue. Since then the electrical changes which accompany the activity of muscle and nerve have been studied in great detail.

H. Burrows, J. Iball and E. M. F. Roe (" Electrical Changes in Wounds and Inflamed Tissues ", Part 1, *Brit. J. exp. Path.*, 1942, **23**, 253) have drawn attention to the fact that exudation oedema, stasis and diapedesis, i.e. the passage of leucocytes through the unruptured walls of vessels, are among the events which seem to demand physical interpretation, and several facts suggest that an important dynamic agent in these phenomena is electricity. These authors point out that so far as the transport of matter through the walls of the blood vessels in regions of inflammation is concerned, it is known that the leucocytes, proteins and most of the other suspended or colloidal components of the blood are negatively charged in that medium. Abramson,[1] who has reviewed the work of earlier observers (1927, 1928, 1934), and has himself investigated some of the physical aspects of the problem (1924, 1925), concluded that " the high gradient of potential existing between injured and uninjured tissues could conceivably account partially for the migration of charged polymorphonuclear leucocytes in a directed fashion towards a point of injury ".

The disposal of foreign particles after their injection into the bloodstream is another event which seems to demonstrate that inflammation is accompanied by local electrical changes, for the distribution of such particles in the body largely depends upon the electrical charges which they carry. In normal conditions, fine suspended particles of colloidal substances carrying a negative electric charge in a watery medium, circulate freely when injected into a vein, until they are arrested and

[1] H. A. Abramson, *Amer. J. med. Sci.*, 1924, **167**, 702; *J. exp. Med.*, 1925, **41**, 445; 1927, **6**, 987; J. Alexander, *Colloid Chemistry*, 2nd edn., New York, 1928, p. 701; *Elektrokinetic Phenomena and their Application to Biology and Medicine*, New York, 1934.

removed from the blood by the reticulo-endothelial organs. If a focus of inflammation is present the substances mentioned adhere to the walls of the small blood-vessels in the region of inflammation, and later traverse them so as to become concentrated in the tissue and tissue spaces outside the vessels; here the extravasated materials are retained, whereas if introduced, e.g. by injection, in the absence of inflammation they drain away.

Various tests with dyes have shown that only those substances which carry an electro-negative charge become abstracted in this way from the blood by the reticulo-endothelial organs and inflamed subcutaneous tissues. An electro-positive dye which is not rapidly reduced in the blood, e.g. night blue, when introduced into the blood-stream does not circulate freely. It adheres to the normal vascular endothelium, and shows relatively little tendency to become arrested by the reticulo-endothelial organs or by the blood-vessels of inflamed tissue (unpublished results). Moreover, electro-positive colloids, when injected beneath the skin, act as inflammatory agents.

A consideration of all the facts mentioned above suggests the desirability of determining the electrical changes which accompany wounds and inflammation, and of correlating them, if possible, with the associated pathological changes.

The first step in this inquiry was to determine the normal variations which may be observed in closely related sites on the normal uninjured skin, and later to note the differences of potential which are shown when a wound is inflicted at one of the chosen sites. In the first instance such observations were made on rats. In nearly all cases wounding caused an increase in potential up to 42 mv., the wound being positive with respect to the uninjured region when the direction of current in the external circuit is considered. (Burrows, Iball and Roe, *Brit. J. exp. Path.*, 1942, 23, 253.)

Apart from the use of potential differences in the skin to determine the period of ovulation in the rabbit and cat and the measurement of electrical changes in wounds and inflamed tissues, attempts have been made to correlate electrical differences of potential in skin and normal basal metabolism.[1]

[1] *Science*, 1931, **73**, 46–49. E. J. Lund, "Relation between Continuous Bioelectric Currents and Cell Respiration: V. The Quantitative Relation between Eh and Cell Oxidation as Shown by the Effects of Cyanide and Oxygen", *J. exp. Zool.*, 1928, **51**, 327–337. E. J. Lund, "Relation between Continuous Bioelectric Currents and Cell Respiration: II A Theory of Continuous Bioelectric Currents and Electric Polarity of Cells", *J. exp. Zool.*, 1928, **51**, 265–290. Charles Sheard and A. Frances Johnson, "Potentiometric and Spectrophotometric Changes in Plants Produced by Infra-red and Ultra-violet Irradiation", *Proc. Soc. exp. Biol., N.Y.*, 1929, **26**, 18–621. W. C. Alvarez, B. L. Freelander and L. B. Clark, "An Electrode for the Measurements of Skin Potentials", *J. Lab. clin. Med.*, 1925–26, **11**, 83–85.

OXIDATION-REDUCTION BALANCE OF SKIN E*h* (rH). Lund (*J. exp. Zool.*, 1928, **51**, 265 and 327) concluded from his investigations on bioelectric currents that the electric polarity of the cell is correlated to the respiratory exchange of the cell and that electric currents produced by cells and tissues are the result of oxidation-reduction potentials developed by the respiratory mechanism of the cell. Most of the investigations on the oxidation-reduction potential of skin have been carried out with dyestuffs, but Kelly and Williams (*J. invest. Derm.*, 1941, p. 274) claimed to have taken several hundred readings of E*h* and *p*H with a standard *p*H meter, using calomel and platinum electrodes and recording the E*h* in millivolts—with satisfactory results.

E*h* is a measure of the oxidation-reduction intensity and not of the capacity of the system to oxidise or to reduce. Just as the potential set up at a hydrogen electrode is a result of the balance between ionised and non-ionised hydrogen and is not directly a function of the total concentration of ionisable hydrogen, so E*h* is a result of the balance between the oxidised and the reduced components of the system and is not dependent upon the total concentration of either.

FACIAL PATTERNS OF ELECTRICAL RESISTANCE. Facial patterns of electrical resistance have been studied by C. P. Richter and B. G. Woodruff[1] of the Johns Hopkins Hospital psychological laboratory, with results of much interest. At ordinary room temperature an oval or shield-shaped area of low resistance (one-fifth of the high-resistance area) was found sharply marked out in forty-two young adults, the area including eyes and eyebrows, nose, contiguous parts of both cheeks and lips, and part of the skin below the lower lip; this area remained the same from day to day. In infants, when awake, the area was of the same kind, but contracted down to one around the mouth only, when asleep. Few such tests could be made in adults without their awakening. The low-resistance area of the face corresponds to the naked facial area of the gorilla, chimpanzee, gibbon, lemur and langur. In bald men it extended up almost to the limit of the hair under the influence of slight excitement or a slightly raised external temperature. In warm external temperature the facial area of low resistance extends widely, while in low external temperature it contracts till it includes only the lips. During sleep the sympathetic nervous system is less active, and the area then becomes restricted to the lips. Warm surroundings cause vasodilatation and sweating, signs of increased sympathetic activity, and the area enlarges. The patterns of low electrical resistance show a close correlation with the patterns of remaining pain and temperature sensitivity found in patients with syringomyelia and syringobulbia, which apparently depend upon the

[1] *Johns Hopkins. Hosp. Bull.*, 1942, **70**, 442.

affected segments of the descending spinal nucleus of the trigeminal nerve. The low-resistance areas show a high metabolic activity and the highest incidence of skin cancer.

THE "NUTRITION INDEX". The exact significance of small differences in electrical potential which may be observed between different areas of the skin, or between an area of skin and some other organ of the body, is at present unknown. From past personal experiences of the difficulties of obtaining *significant and reproducible* skin e.m.f.s, even by the use of modern valve potentiometer equipment, the author is of the opinion that any such results should be interpreted with the greatest reserve until our knowledge of this subject is more complete. It is therefore surprising that Pech (*Soap Perfum. Cosm.*, Nov. and Dec. 1949; Jan. 1950) should propound a so-called "Nutrition Index", based upon such slight differences in e.m.f., as being even of "qualitative value", to the dermatologist or cosmetician.

In setting out his theory, Pech gives the following brief summary of the general biological conclusions which, he states, have so far been arrived at by biophysical research:

(1) All living tissue, animal or vegetable, must be in electrical disequilibrium with the external medium and the humoral media in order to be able to obtain nourishment and live.

(2) To live normally, each tissue must have a determined electrical sign, in relation to the external or internal media in contact with it. If this sign is reversed, the tissue, and quite often the entire individual, will cease to live.

(3) The intensity of the difference in electrical state between a tissue and the media in contact with it bears a direct relationship to its biological activity. The higher this intensity, the greater the biological activity of the tissue.

Pech states that many years ago he suggested giving to this difference in electrical state between a living tissue and an element in contact with it, the name of "Nutrition Index". He determines this index by recording a potential difference (or absence of such a difference) on a galvanometer placed in series with two platinum electrodes, one being inserted into the individual's mouth, and the other placed on top of a film of the cosmetic cream, soap, or other material to be examined, which is spread on the back of the same individual's hand.

In his measurements Pech recognises three qualitative differences, namely, one in which the galvanometer indicates the absence of any electrical current from which he concludes that the paste, cream, or soap, and the individual's skin are in the same electrical state; that the physico-chemical exchange between the preparation and the skin is practically nil and hence that the paste (cream or other preparation applied) merely constitutes a covering matter without any further action on the nutrition of the skin than that of insulating it from the external medium, i.e. air.

In the other two cases, the passage of an electric current is observed through the galvanometer in which the skin is either (*a*) negative to the preparation, or (*b*) positive to the preparation.

Pech sums up his conclusions (*Soap. Perfum. Cosm.*, Jan. 1950, p. 56) thus: "A skin-preserving substance should be electro-positive and its nutrition index should remain less than 1 mv. This figure can only be exceeded for substances that are infrequently used and then for a short period (five to ten minutes contact per twenty-four hours)."

Pech also discusses certain ill-defined, but according to him essential, elements in the skin to which he gives the name of "endocytines". These "endocytines" are considered to provide the tissue which contains them with normal nutrition. It is assumed that the tissue acquires such substances in the course of embryonic life and that they are no longer renewed after actual birth of the individual commences. Their consumption is considered to bring about the ageing of tissues.

The above theories are open to criticism on many grounds: for one thing they are ill-supported by modern authoritative data of statistical significance. As hypothetical conjectures they may be considered, but with reserve.

The method of determining the so-called "Nutritional Index" means that hydrous lanolin, of proven clinical efficacy in dermatological practice (because, as a water-in-oil emulsion it would inhibit the passage of an electric current), would not be considered a "desirable substance". Pech states that certain detergents will give a high nutrition index of 10 mv. and even more. Presumably in diluted solution, they could be adjusted to give the desired, electro-positive index of under 1 mv., and I am certain that application of such a solution to the female breast would not lead to any alteration in its size. Yet the application of certain female sex hormones in a "plain fatty base" (which according to Pech's argument would merely be electrically inert) to such a breast would lead to an increase in its size and in its activity.

The fact that enlargement of the breast by such means is hardly likely to be deemed medically desirable (whilst it most certainly is *not* within the province of cosmetics) is, for the purpose of this discussion beside the point. The fact is that the "*active ingredient*" *in a preparation is important* and one cannot judge a cosmetical product by such a "nutritional index" as that described.

Again, Pech states that the substance should be electro-positive, whereas, as we have already discussed, various tests with dyes have shown that only those substances which carry an electro-negative charge become abstracted from the blood, and, moreover, that electro-positive colloids when introduced beneath the skin, themselves act as inflammatory agents. Burrows, Iball and Roe (*Brit. J. exp. Path.*, 1942, p. 253) showed that in artificial wounding, the *wound* became *positive* with respect to the uninjured portion.

For these and other reasons, I do not consider that the so-called "Nutritional Index" of Pech can—in its present form—be accepted as any kind of guide to either the dermatologist or cosmetician. [*Note:* Skin nutrition is discussed in Chapters 3 (The Role of Diet), 4 (Skin Penetration and Nutrition), and 10 ("Skin Foods" and Lubricating Creams).]

Skin Blemishes

FRECKLES (Ephelides). Freckles are localised collections of pigment forming part of the protective mechanism of the skin. While their cause has not yet been definitely determined, it would appear that in the basal layer of certain susceptible individuals, chiefly those of blonde, red-head, and certain light brunette complexions, the colourless pigment forming material which acts as a protecting mechanism against sunburn by formation of melanin, is not adequately distributed in the basal skin layer but occurs in clumps which on exposure to sunlight form the characteristic markings. At the same time the skin does not tan evenly in the absence of this material, but reddens, or blisters according to the severity of the exposure. Inheritance may play a factor in this clumping of the pigment cells.

Meirowsky considers that a sharp differentiation cannot be made between freckles, flat pigmented moles and lentigines, and that moles, etc. as well as freckles can be increased or made to appear for the first time by infections, trauma or X-rays.

LENTIGINES. Many textbooks have regarded freckles, ephelides and lentigines as synonymous in spite of the differences between them recorded in the literature by many observers. E. E. Brown ("Lentigines and Their Possible Significance", *Arch. Derm. Syph., Chicago*, June 1943, **47**, 804) defines lentigines as brown pigmented flat or raised lesions, darker than freckles, absent at birth but appearing after the second year, often increasing with age and appearing on any part of the body; when these lentigines become papular or raised they are then commonly called moles. Almost every person over two years of age has at least one lentigo, reaching a peak in adolescence, when on an average, more than thirty lesions are present on the whole body—these tend to diminish in number in middle life, and decrease considerably in old age.

Brown considers that lentigines are probably associated with (*a*) acute infections, (*b*) hypoadrenia, i.e. deficiency of adrenal activity. Their relation to infection is suggested by the increase of lentigines in children affected with colds, chronic suppurative sinusitis and bronchietasis, rheumatoid arthritis, diphtheria, typhoid, malaria, poliomyelitis.

The usual appearance of lentigines early in Addison's disease, which is attended by destruction of the adrenal cortex, and their response by depigmentation when such cases are treated with extract of adrenal cortex suggests a relationship between lentigines and deficiency of adrenal activity.

MOLES. While there appear to be some distinct differences between freckles and lentigines, no sharp differentiation between the latter and moles is evident at present, save that moles are usually present in much smaller numbers and, according to Meirowsky, are usually only present on one side of the body. The latter, taking the definition of Unna (1894), broadly considers under the generic designation naevi, "all diffuse or circumscribed anomalies of the skin which are inherited, become visible at various times of life and are distinguishable by their colour or the form of their surface", and considers that man has become prone to such malformations of the skin by the factors of domestication and evolution. His opinion is that naevi are inherited and determined to the extent of 9/10 by the germ plasm, and that their unilateral formation in man is conditioned by the fact that genes can become effective only on one side of the body.

Moles occasionally became malignant. This is a comparatively rare occurrence; but if growth suddenly increases (especially after the age of twenty-five and if the mole is surrounded with a pigmented (red, brown or blue) halo) a dermatologist should be consulted in case it is malignant. For this reason self-treatment or excision of moles should never be carried out.

Summarising the above in the light of our present knowledge, it would appear to me that lentigines (and probably freckles also) are primarily occasioned by an inherited disposition, and that in the event of acute infections such disposition becomes dominant, either by the appearance of lentigines or by an increase in their number. Under suitable conditions not yet fully determined, or by continued infection, lentigines may hypertrophy to form moles. In certain cases these conditions may exist in the germ plasm (or the embryo may be subject to them) and the individual is then born with a mole.

WARTS. A wart is a localised hypertrophy of the Malpighian layer occurring as the result of an infection producing irritation which is not sufficient to cause either degeneration or malignant proliferation. The interpapillary processes become elongated as a result of the increase of the Malpighian layer, and a small characteristic benign growth rises above the skin surface.

According to Osborne and Putnam (*Radiology*, 1931, **16**, 340–345) warts are present in some 1·5–4 per cent. of patients applying for dermatological treatment, and this percentage appears to be increasing.

Warts are caused by a virus (i.e. a living virulent cause of disease of such small size that it can pass the finest filter and cannot in general be seen under a microscope but can be demonstrated by inoculation); they may be produced by inoculation, and are transmissible (U. J. Wile and L. B. Kingery, *J. Amer. med. Assoc.*, 1919, **73**, 970; H. J. Templeton, *Arch. Derm. Syph., Chicago*, 1935, **32**, 102; M. Juliusberg, *Arch. Derm. Syph., Wien*, 1903, **64**, 163).

So far no uniformly successful method of treatment has been elaborated, but there is evidence to show that in many cases they disappear spontaneously, and that a psychological factor may be involved. Bloch (*Klin. Wschr.*, 1927, **6**, 2271) placed patients blindfolded before a pantostat with their hands resting in it and with the motor turned on, but no current being conducted to the patient. The warts were then painted with a coloured fluid and the patients told that the warts would disappear. His results showed that common warts were cured in 44 per cent. of his cases, and in the case of juveniles the percentage was as high as 88 per cent.

Rulison (*Arch. Derm. Syph., Chicago*, 1942, **46**, 1, 75; 78) gives the following tables of results (amongst others) obtained by different (non-medical) treatment of warts.

Burrows, in a more recent paper (*Brit. J. Derm.*, 1943, **55**, 3, 61), states that the psychological aspect of the matter became evident to him when a young hospital resident submitted his wart for treatment to a wart charmer.[1] The latter stroked the growth several times with his finger, became pale and sweated at the forehead. A few days later the wart which Burrows had seen both before and after the seance disappeared.

The confirmatory evidence of reputable dermatologists, and often the apparent success of widely diverse remedies which appear to have no rational pharmacological foundation, makes it evident that psychogenic factors are sometimes involved.

[1] Biberstein (*Arch. Derm. Syph., Chicago*, 1944, **50**, 1, 12) on the basis of experiments, considers that the results he has obtained with *immunisation* therapy are not due to psychotherapeutic effect and rejects the theory that all of the results obtained in the treatment of warts are due to suggestion.

Bloch considers that suggestion provides a stimulus to the vegetative centres which is conducted by the vegetative nerve-channels to the warts, and points out that most of his cures occurred within a month, and nearly all within the second month. Those not cured after this

TABLE 1

EIGHT CASES OF WARTS IN WHICH LAY TREATMENT (NON-TRAUMATIC) WAS USED

Number	Present age	Sex	Age at first attack	Warts, single or multiple	Duration before treatment, Yrs.	Duration of treatment	Number of treatments	Treatment used	Recurrence	New attack	Free period, Yrs.	No more warts
1	33	F	6	M	1/6	?	?	Father spat tobacco juice on warts	0	0	27	+
2	47	F	8	M	7/12	?	?	Mother advised licking warts on rising in morning	0	0	38	+
3	43	F	12	S	1/2	6 wk.	?	Hindu advised sucking wart and touching it with tongue	0	0	30	+
4	29	M	13	M	1	—	1	Rubbed warts with salt pork rind (customary among Swedish people)	0	+	14	—
5	46	F	6	M	?	?	?	Friend of mother suggested the application of axle grease	0	0	40	+
6	39	F	7	M	2	1¾ yr.	—	Dandelion juice applied often	0	0	30	+
7	44	M	8	M	Several weeks	4 days	4	Applied milkweed juice daily at suggestion of playmates	0	0	36	+
8	21	M	9	M	2	2 mo.	2	Soaked hand in lemon juice twice; in later attack used vinegar and water successfully; still has one *verruca vulgaris* on right little finger	0	++	10	—

latter interval did not appear to be susceptible to this treatment. He observed that often after the *suggestion* there was a noticeable swelling of the warts and occasionally slight haemorrhage. W. N. Goldsmith (*Recent Advances in Dermatology*, London: J. and A. Churchill Ltd., 1936) states that the epidermis is so rich in nerve fibrils that there is no great difficulty in accepting the possibility that in this direct way nervous impulses may cause biological changes of a chemico-physical nature which damaged the virus. He points out that, conversely, one must not forget that some of the apparent spontaneous remissions may be the result of emotional experience.

TABLE 2

PSYCHOTHERAPY IN THE TREATMENT OF WARTS (SEVEN CASES)

Number	Present age	Sex	Age at first attack	Duration before treatment, Yrs.	Treatment by relative (R), layman (L), physician (P)	Duration of treatment	Number of treatments	Treatment, failure or success	Means used	Recurrence	New attack	Free Period, Yrs.	No more warts
1	20	M	16	5/12	L	—	1	S	Cord tied around one wart; all warts gone in short time	0	0	3½	+
2	30	M	24	1/2	R	—	1	S	Tied red cotton thread around wart and buried lock of hair under stone in field; wart gone in one week	0	0	5½	+
3	30	F	10	1/2	L	—	1	S	Stole raw beef from butcher; rubbed on warts; buried meat; warts gone in one week	0	0	20	+
4	39	F	12	?	L	—	1	S	Old man passed his hand over wart and then rubbed her head	0	0	27	+
5	45	M	15	?	L	—	1	S	Washed hands in morning dew once; warts gone in a month	0	0	30	+
6	55	M	14	2	P (quack)	—	1	S	"Doctor" rubbed fingers over warts and mumbled a few words; warts gone in one week	0	0	39	+
7	69	M	16	1/2	L	—	1	S	Patient taken to harness-maker by father, who said man had reputation in curing warts; harness-maker knotted a cord over each wart; warts soon gone	0	0	52	+

A study of the literature makes it evident that almost *any* treatment, *may*, in certain cases be successful, due to the psychological effect of mere suggestion. However, a large number of warts do not disappear by such treatment and in such cases X-rays, CO_2 snow, surgical excision, curettage and destruction by various keratolytics (such as glacial acetic acid; salicylic acid and nitric acid), methods based on pressure, desiccation and exclusion of air have been tried, and sometimes such treatment has been effective—but at present—no *infallible* cure for warts in general has been discovered.

Five types of warts are recognised clinically, viz. *Verruca vulgaris, Verruca plantaris, Verruca plana juvenilis, Verruca filiformis,* and *Verruca acuminata,* but whether separate viruses cause these five different forms, or whether the different forms are clinical variations resulting from the same virus is not known. More recently Strauss, Bunting and Melnick (*J. invest. Derm.*, Dec. 1950, p. 433) have reported the presence of spherical virus-like particles which tend to aggregate in regular nets in papillomatous growths of human skin. Based on the clinical characteristics these growths do not appear to differ greatly from *Verruca vulgaris* and *Verruca plantaris.* These particles appear to represent the first crystalline substance isolated from a human growth and the presence of these particles seems to interfere with the orderly process by which epidermal cells develop.

Thomson (*Brit. J. Derm.*, 1943, **55**, 267) has reported good results from the use of 3 per cent. aqueous formaldehyde solution in the removal of plantar warts. The solution is poured into a shallow vessel, such as a saucer, and the foot or hand immersed for ten minutes each night. Particular care must be taken to immerse only the thicker parts of the skin and avoid contact with less highly keratinised skin areas since the application of such a solution involves a real risk of eczematous reactions on all areas, except, according to Thomson, the soles and palms. This type of treatment is *not* applicable to warts on other parts of the body because of severe eczema produced on surrounding skin.

MacGregor (*Brit. med. J.*, 1945, **1**, 293) has confirmed the value of Podophyllum resin in the treatment of soft warts. Using a 25 per cent. suspension of the drug in liquid petroleum oil, applied liberally to the affected area (care being taken that the numerous crevices of the warts are penetrated) MacGregor found the treatment simple and effective. Other investigators have also reported upon the efficacy of this treatment. (See Frank and Cohen, *Arch. Derm. Syph.*, 1947, **56**, 109; Kaplan, *Med. surg. J.*, 1942, p. 338—who originally drew attention to this treatment; Kaplan and co-workers, *J. Urol.*, 1944, **51**, 655; *Ann. Surg.*, 1944, **120**, 251; MacGregor, *Brit. med. J.*, 1945, **1**, 593, etc.)

Sullivan and King (*Arch. Derm. Syph., Chicago*, 1947, **1**, 30), however, have drawn attention to the fact that Podophyllum resin is a sensitiser of the first order and that in using it two precautions should always be observed, namely, (i) it should never be applied in close proximity to the eye, (ii) it should only be used on medical advice and under medical supervision.

As will be seen, apart from " charming " and other psychological factors, the majority of the treatments described above are for use only under medical supervision. A simple method for home use, however, employs elastic adhesive bandage. Attention to the efficacy of this method was drawn by Hope-Simpson (*Lancet*, 28 Feb., 1948), and independently by Fenton (*Brit. med. J.* (Notes and Comments), 14 Feb. 1948). The former recommends that the elastic adhesive bandage be applied and allowed to remain in place for a week or two at a time and removed as it loosens, when the wart will usually be found to peel out with the bandage. Fenton considers such treatment of removal of great use in cases of multiple warts in the knee area so often seen in children, though he suggests that, after removal of the wart, the area at the base of the wart be touched with a simple cauterizing agent.

BOILS. Whilst it is not within the province of this book to discuss diseases of the skin *per se*, two skin conditions are sufficiently common to suggest that some information on them would be of general interest. Boils and so-called " prickly-heat " can be considered in this category.

An epidermological survey of boils carried out over the period 1943–47 by Whitewell and Sutherland (*Brit. J. Derm.*, March 1950, p. 109) showed that the majority of these lesions occur on the head, face and neck, whilst gluteal boils—so prominent in textbooks, occur but rarely. The distribution of the boils was in accord with the hypothesis that the causative agent is staphylococcal and that staphylococcal contamination of the skin is dependent on spread from the nose by the fingers and that boils result mainly from such contamination. It was observed that over the period 1943–47, the incidence of boils appreciably increased in the population and that there was a seasonal incidence with a peak in October or November, and a low incidence in the first three months of the year.

PRICKLY HEAT (*Miliaria*). This may be described as a superficial, non-inflammatory vesicular condition due to sweat retention. O'Brien (*J. invest. Derm.*, Aug. 1950) reported experiments wherein the skin was covered by plain gauze pads, and these experiments suggested that staphylococcal infections of the sweat pores were an important causative factor, and this was supported subsequently by a new technique wherein special nutrient media was inoculated with staphylococcus aureus and then applied to the skin. Biopsies of skin so treated showed lesions which appeared identical with those of the natural disease. Oedema and increased temperature of the stratum corneum were considered to be contributory factors. Lipoid depletion was not considered to be the sole or direct cause of miliaria, nevertheless, a lipoid depletion was considered probably the direct cause of pore closure in many ichthyolic skins and, in a series of five experiments, *excessive* soaping was found to produce pore closure, though this effect was prevented in one experiment in which the skin was treated with a lipoid (lanolin) after each soaping. (No evidence was obtained to indicate that the judicious use of soap was harmful.)

Shelley and Horvath (*J. invest. Derm.*, March 1950, p. 193) distinguished three separate factors in the pathogenesis of experimental miliaria, viz. (i) non-specific minor epidermal injury, (ii) intensive sweating for several hours, and (iii) individual susceptibility. Alone, none of the above three factors was sufficient. These investigators feel that the common denominator is a non-specific injury to the epidermis, resulting usually from maceration due to sweat *per se*. This experimental study therefore supports the hypothesis of Sulzberger and Zimmerman (*J. invest. Derm.*, 1946, **7**, 61).

Shelley and Horvath point out that experiments with atropine point out the essential role of the sweat itself in the pathogenesis since in the absence of sweating no changes could be produced by placing the subjects in a heated atmosphere. They add that it is of interest to note that in *susceptible individuals*, miliaria was produced by the use of aluminium chloride patch tests (an antiperspirant, *see* Chapter 30), which indicated that some of the inflammatory dermatoses seen in the axillae following the use of antiperspirants were miliaria and not contact dermatitis *per se*, and that certain examples of diaper rashes (*see* Baby Preparations, Chapter 35) are probably modifications of miliaria.

There appears to be no specific treatment for " prickly heat ". The best methods would appear to be (*a*) the provision of a suitable antiseptic to kill the pathogenic micro-organisms, and (*b*) the provision of some material which would tend to keep the skin in a dry condition. Emollient substances such as lanolin might be tried but these would probably help to retain moisture in the skin ; alternatively a sterilised absorbent powder, frequently replaced, would assist in keeping the skin urface dry. Further eperiments are necessary to decide whether it is preferable to replace some of the lipoidal components of the skin, e.g. with lanolin—at the expense of reducing loss of perspiration through the fatty layer—or whether it is best to minimise perspiration at the risk of reducing the lipoidal content of the skin ; the latter may prove the more beneficial.

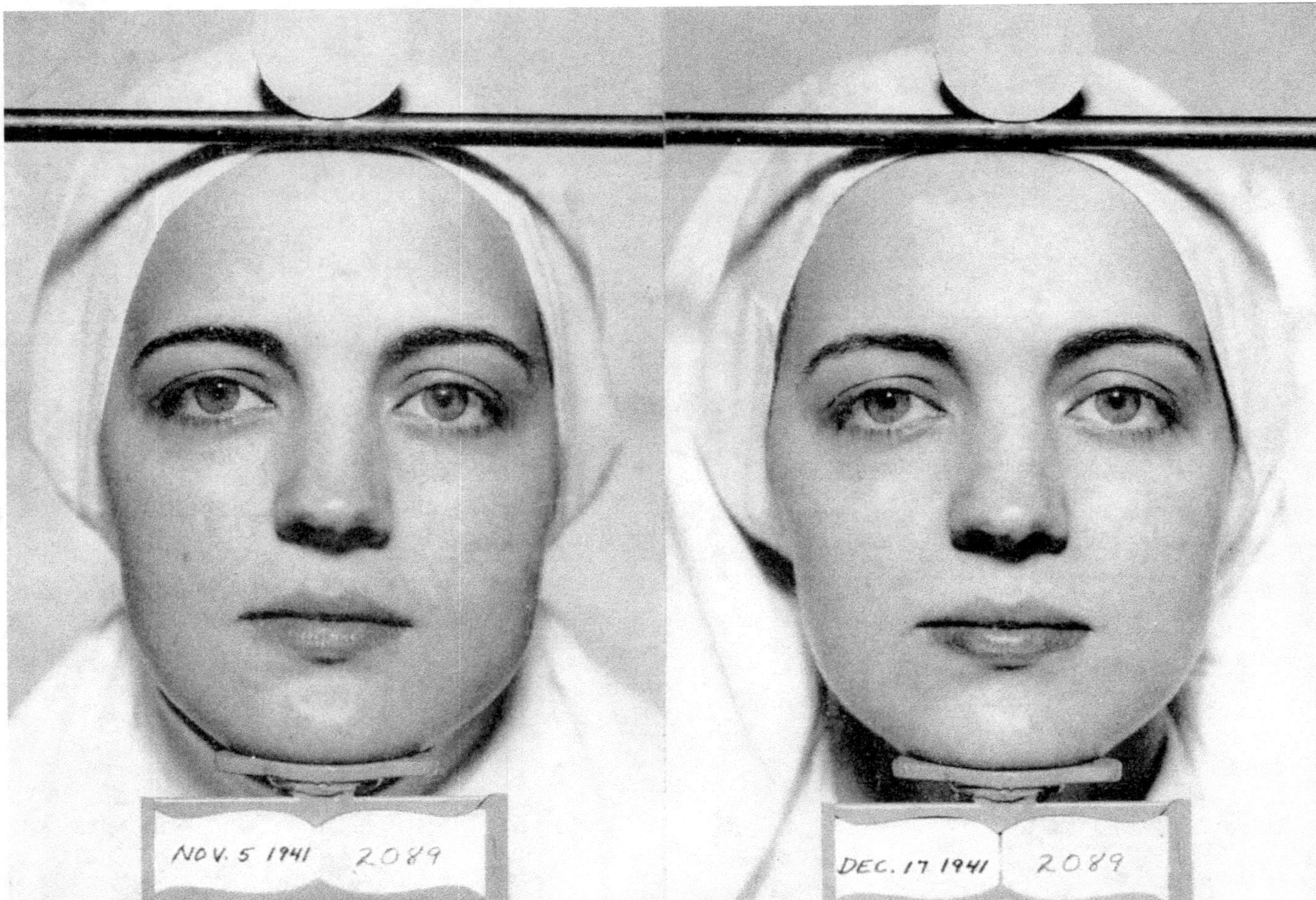

FIG. 8.—Lightening of skin produced by ammoniated mercury.

So far as a suitable antiseptic is concerned, perchloride of mercury or other mercury salts at a level of about 1 : 500 has been recommended (Walton, *Brit. med. J.*, 31 Jan. 1948, p. 228 ; Brown, *Brit. med. J.*, 1950, p. 847). Whilst suitable for medical requirements this is too toxic for cosmeticians and some of the safer antiseptics which are effective against staphylococci, such as G.11, might be tried.

Since boils and miliaria appear to be related to staphylococcal infection, treatment in both instances involves the application of a suitable bactericide. (*See* Chapter 42.)

COSMETIC TREATMENT OF SKIN BLEMISHES

Bleaching Creams. Various substances have been incorporated into "bleaching" creams, designed to remove, or, at least, minimise the appearance of "freckles". Amongst the substances reputed to be useful for this purpose, in the past, were preparations containing either hydrogen peroxide or lemon juice.[1] It has recently been shown, however, that a *general lightening of the skin can be induced* by the use of cosmetic creams containing as little as 1 per cent. of ammoniated mercury.

The following brief account of a study of the skin-lightening effects of ammoniated mercury given by D. F. Nealon (at the Proceedings of the Scientific Section of the Toilet Goods Association, 25 January 1944, New York) is included because of its interest to dermatologists, to students of the mechanism of the skin and to the cosmetic manufacturer.

The Effect of Ammoniated Mercury. The colour of the human skin depends upon : (1) The number of blood vessels present in the tissues and the degree to which they are filled with blood. (2) The natural inherent colour of the materials which compose the skin cells. (3) Carotin. (4) Melanin.

Melanin is the pigment of the skin which causes freckles and tan and is responsible for the colour of negro skin. It is estimated that the entire skin of the blackest adult negro contains not more than 2 g. of melanin.

Reports by Raper (*Biochem. J.*, **20,** 735), Arnow (*J. biol. Chem.*, **118,** 531) and Jones (*Reports to External Products Research Institute*, Vol. 2) have done much to enlighten us on the formation of melanin, and it appears that any one of three amino acids found in the skin may form melanin. These are tyrosine, phenylalanine and tryptophane. The

[1] Some persons claim to have achieved bleaching by the use of mild acids such as citric or lactic acid. These can be applied, if desired, in cream form. (*See* Acid Creams.) There is no published "proof" of the efficacy of such mild acids.

following is a representation of the conversion of tyrosine to melanin :

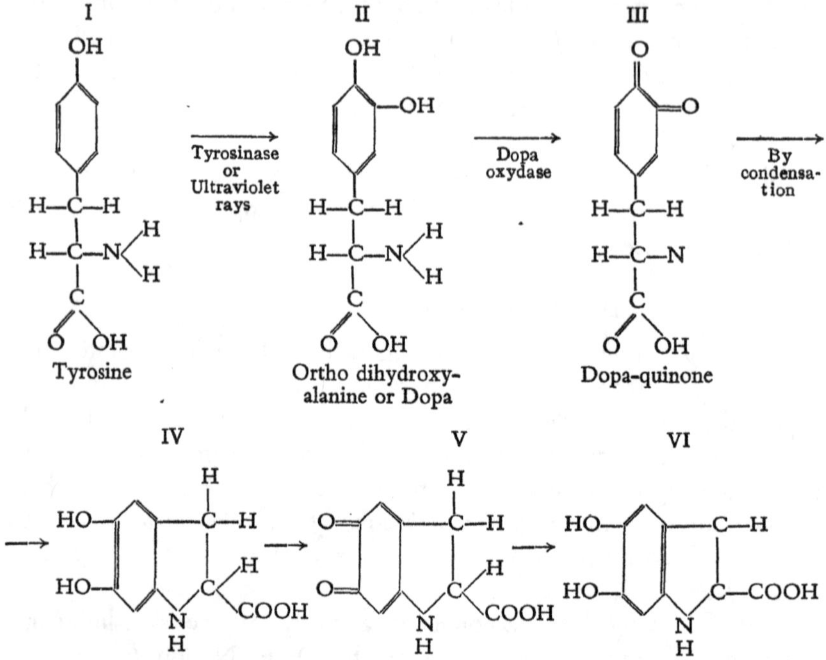

5-6 Dihydroxy-dihydro-indole *a*-Carboxylic acid — Hallochrome — 5-6 Dihydroxyindole *a*-Carboxylic acid

Melanin formed from VI by the polymerisation of two or more molecules

The first step (I) in the above is initiated by tyrosinase, an enzyme, or by ultra-violet light. Stage (II) to (III) is brought by dopa oxydase, an enzyme present in human skin (Bloch, *Arch. Derm. Syph., Wien*, 1917, **124**, 129), the remainder of the changes being brought about by chemical reactions which are always proceeding in the skin.

It is claimed that the action of mercury salts is to interfere with the enzymes in the skin so that the preliminary steps in the above chain of events do not occur. Melanin, is then, it is said, no longer formed and the skin appears lighter.

[A more detailed discussion of the dermatological action and toxicity of such ammoniated mercury creams in cosmetics is given in *Cosmetic Materials*, 1948, pp. 28 ff. by the author. In passing it may, however, be mentioned that over 20,000,000 packages of such preparations have been sold in the United States ; 2,272,380 packages by one company in 1943 with only twenty-five complaints.]

Freckles often show some lightening in winter and in cases where allergy to mercury salts is present, or in cases where it is desired not to use such preparations it is possible to reduce freckle formation by using during the summer months a make-up of high opacity which includes sun-screening compounds and in which the powder base contains a high proportion of zinc oxide. By such means it is possible to minimise their formation during the summer and to some extent, conceal by such make-up the presence of freckles during the winter. Methods for the treatment of warts have already been discussed. Moles should always be left alone, except where medical opinion recommends their removal on the grounds of malignancy. Freckles, lentigines, moles and warts may be " masked " or at least minimised by the use of suitable innocuous make-up of high opacity.

There is no simple, purely cosmetic, method for the removal of lentigines and moles—the most that can be done is concealment by the use of suitably coloured make-up of high covering power (i.e. opacity). Chas. Lázár (*Manual of Cosmetics*, London: Henry Kimpton, 1937) has recommended the intracutaneous injection of 0·3 per cent. hydrogen peroxide, and claims completely scarless results. W. N. Goldsmith (*Recent Advances in Dermatology*, 1936) prefers fulgination with a small high-frequency machine which has the advantage that there is no subsequent inflammatory reaction. If the mole is malignant, surgical treatment is necessary. If surgical excision is made it is imperative that such excision includes a proportion of the surrounding healthy tissue. Goldsmith considers that electro-coagulation is safest as it fixes the cells.

None of these *surgical* treatments should be carried out by anyone save a fully qualified medical practitioner or dermatologist, and the above details are only included to advise any hypersensitive persons that scarless (or almost scarless) treatment is often possible if they will only consult a qualified specialist in the first place.

" Chemical " Components of the Skin

So far we have considered the skin from a histological and dermatological angle; references have also been made to the embryological complications of inheritance factors and the " skin mosaic ". Like all other forms of matter, there is yet a further aspect, that of chemical composition. Whilst a large number of the chemical components of the skin have been identified, isolated and in many cases their approximate amounts determined, yet the difficulties inherent in the supply of material, complexities of analysis—and often the presence of interfering matters on the skin surface [for example, cosmetics, hair creams, etc., on undegreased skin, whilst in degreasing the skin other fatty materials belonging to the skin may be removed]—and biological factors associated with diet, disease and possibly sex and age render an *accurate chemical picture* of the skin impossible in our present state of knowledge.

THE MINERAL AND WATER CONTENT OF THE SKIN. Brown (*J. biol. Chem.* 1927, **75**, 789) has reported data for the moisture, ash, calcium, magnesium, sodium, potassium phosphorous and silicon content of human skin; the data being based upon forty-two cases, twenty white and twenty-two negroes including persons of both sexes and various ages. The following variations were found for moisture, sodium, potassium and phosphorous respectively:

	per cent.
Moisture	56·4–72·1
Sodium	0·118–0·188
Potassium	0·053–0·161
Phosphorous	0·041–0·085

Brown stated that there is a constant changing mineral content of the skin and the assumption of a definite age of chemical maturity for the skin was untenable.

More recently Suntzeff and Carruthers (*J. biol. Chem.*, Oct. 1945, p. 567) have investigated the mineral composition of the human epidermis and reported the average amount of potassium, sodium, calcium and magnesium as:

	per cent.
Potassium	0·322
Sodium	0·122
Magnesium	0·018
Calcium	0·015

These investigators stated that, with the limited amount of material at their disposal, no relationship between the mineral content and the age, sex, or the location of skin was apparent.

Eisele and Eichelberger (*Proc. Soc. exp. Biol., N.Y.*, 1945, **58**, 97) determined the total water, nitrogen, collagen-nitrogen and electrolyte concentrations in human skin which had been removed, at once from portions of the body, surgically amputated. The total skin (corium plus epidermis) gave the following mean average results which are expressed as units per kilo of fat-free skin; total water 717·7 ± 20·1 g.; chloride 79·9 ± 4·8 mM.; sodium 93·0 ± 8·0 mM.; potassium 16·47 ± 3·36 mM.; calcium 2·68 ± 0·52 mM.; magnesium 2·13 ± 0·30 mM.; total nitrogen 45·5 ± 3·8 g.; and collagen nitrogen 33·7 ± 4·5 g. These investigators state that by applying methods now accepted as valid for calculating the weight of connective tissue, the weight of connective tissue in human skin was estimated to be 546±73 g. per kilo of fat-free skin. The calculated 330 g ± 45 g. of water identified with this amount of connective tissue demonstrates that the volume of available water is considerably larger in skin than in any other tissue of the body and that the skin may be regarded as one of the most important water-storage organs of the body.

E. Urbach and E. B. LeWinn (*Skin Diseases, Nutrition and Metabolism*, Wm. Heinemann Medical Books Ltd., 1946, p. 13) gives the following table for the more important constituents of skin :

	Fresh Skin *Normal value in Mg. per cent.*
Water	610–675
Total nitrogen	3500–4000
Non-Protein nitrogen	70–80
Amino acid nitrogen	17–38
Sugar	55–68
Total cholesterol	250–
Cholesterol esters	160–
Chlorides (as NaCl)	200–320
Sodium	95–139
Potassium	60–119
Calcium	9–15
Magnesium	7–12

AMINO ACIDS IN, AND ON, THE SKIN. Hier, Cornbleet and Bergheim (*J. biol. Chem.*, 1946, **166,** 327), using biological methods, identified the following amino acids in sweat : arginine, histidine, threonine, tyrosin, voline, leucine, isoleucine, lysine, phenylalanine, and tryptophane in this order of decreasing concentration.

Rothman and Sullivan (*J. invest. Derm.*, Dec. 1949, p. 319) identified eleven amino acids from skin wipings ; namely, aspartic acid, glutamic acid, serine, glycine, alanine, citrolline, arginine, hydroxyproline, voline, tyrosine and one of the leucines were definitely identified and five more tentatively identified (viz. threonine, proline, lysine, hydroxylysine and ornithine) by paper chromatography in water wipings from dry normal human skin. They state that the presence of arginine and citrolline and the tentatively demonstrated presence of ornithine suggests that in the sweat glands, urea is formed by arginase.

THE COMPOSITION OF THE SURFACE SKIN FAT (SEBUM). The composition of sebum and its possible role in hair affections and infections is discussed in Chapter 20. It may, however, be pointed out that information on this subject is not readily correlated because of different methods of collection employed, and different sources of raw materials. In some cases the sebum has been from the scalp where it may have been contaminated with hair dressings, in others from ovarian dermoid cysts (which appear to be, at least very similar to sebum, if not identical with it) ; and in others by solvent extraction from the skin surface. Jones,

Spencer and Sanchez (*J. invest. Derm.*, Oct. 1951, p. 213) have determined that the amount of fat on the skin of the forearm of a single individual was $45 \cdot 18 \pm 2 \cdot 73 \mu g$. per sq. cm. of skin surface, initially, and that the removal of fat from the skin required repeated washings, the removal following a logarithmic curve. These investigators stated that the interval of time between determinations affects the amount of fat removed and the apparent rate of secretion. Over extended intervals the rate of secretion tends to fall. A hyperbolic curve fitted to these rates indicated that a steady rate of secretion is of the order of $0 \cdot 1 \mu g$. per sq. cm. per min. Skin fat was found to flow with a speed of 3·3 cm. per sec. over a water film and presumably over wet skin. It is stated that it may be considered, therefore, that fat flows from areas of high sebaceous secretion to areas of low secretion and is constantly being removed by objects in contact with the skin. McKenna, Wheatley and Warmell (*Biochem. J.*, 1951, p. 48) found that the unsaponifiable matter of human sebum (32 per cent. of the whole), contains about 46 per cent. hydrocarbons, 14 per cent. cholesterol, and 8 per cent. unsaturated alcohols. (*See* Chapter 20 for further details.)

Functions of the Skin

Besides acting as a covering for the body, and a protection against bacterial invasion, it is, through its blood supply and vast number of sweat glands, very largely concerned in the regulation of body temperature, heat being lost by evaporation of sweat. In a normal healthy person this process is automatic, unless the surrounding air is hot or moist, in which case evaporation may be insufficient to prevent a sharp rise in body temperature and great distress may occur. Perspiration occurs as a colourless opalescent fluid having a peculiar but not unpleasant odour. (The chemistry and histology of the sweat glands and the composition of sweat, etc., is discussed in Chapter 30, Antiperspirants and Deodorants.)

A mixture of perspiration + sebum, the secretion of the sebaceous glands (discussed in detail in Chapter 30), in the presence of bacteria, decomposes, producing the " body odour " commonly ascribed to perspiration. Considerable quantities of water are lost by perspiration, the *insensible* perspiration being from one pint per day and upwards. This is enormously increased by exercise. Emotions, for example, fear or pain, and also certain drugs, such as camphor, ammonium acetate and pilocarpine stimulate the action of the sweat glands whilst atropine depresses them. Heat losses can be rapidly increased, when desired, by bathing the entire skin surface with water.

SELF-DISINFECTING PROPERTIES OF SKIN. Marchionini *et al.* (*Schweiz. med. Wschr.*, 1928, **9**, 1055; *Arch. Derm. Syph., Wien.*, 1929, **158**, 290; *Derm. Z.*, 1934, **68**, 226; *Klin. Wschr.*, 1938, **17**, 1831) adduced evidence to suggest that the bactericidal power of the skin *depends upon or varies with, its degree of acidity*. This aspect of the subject is more fully discussed under that paragraph dealing with the *p*H of the skin. [The author, in 1942 (*Brit. J. Derm.*, Jan. 1942), published the results of an investigation into the *p*H of the skin, using a glass electrode *p*H meter and in discussing the role of the skin's acid mantle, suggested that the bactericidal properties of the skin were due possibly to (i) the direct action of the *p*H *per se* which might reduce pathogenicity without actually destroying the organisms, or (ii) by virtue of the effect of such an acid mantle upon the development or continuance of certain " protective factors " inherent in a normal healthy skin and of which at present we know little or nothing, but whose activity may be impaired if an unfavourable *p*H be allowed to develop. Burtenshaw (*J. Hyg., Camb.*, 1942, **42**, 184; *Brit. med. Bull.*, 1945, **3**, 731) showed the presence of a sterilising substance in hair fat (sebum), soluble in ether but not diffusible in water. On splitting up this fraction, it was found that the portion containing the fatty acids was the only one possessing streptococcidal activity. This streptococcidal activity of the hair fat fraction is of interest in view of Rothman's discovery (*Proc. Soc. exp. Biol.*, 1945, **60**, 394) that adult human hair contains a fatty acid fungistatic to M. audouini in concentrations as low as from 0·0002 per cent. to 0·001 per cent. This fatty acid appears to be from C_7 to C_{11} (in chain length) and affords a rational explanation for the spontaneous cure at puberty, of certain fungal infections of the scalp.

The skin contains a number of ferments, whose exact function is at present not known, but in view of its extensive area the skin probably acts as an important source of body ferments and it may be that one or more of these ferments provide the " certain protective factors ", sensitive to *p*H, postulated by the author in 1942.[1]

The two main classes of skin enzymes are the *hydrolases* which produce hydrolytic dissociation, and the *desmolases* which are involved

[1] It appears probable that a number of factors are operative in maintaining the disinfection of skin: (i) desquamation, (ii) desiccation, (iii) the *p*H of the skin-possibly *per se* in the case of certain organisms, or (iv) as a factor in the role of certain ill-defined though bactericidal substances present in the skin, (v) the presence of certain fatty acids in the skin secretions.

So far as (iii) is concerned Arnold (*J. invest. Derm.*, 1942, **5**, 207) has postulated, as the results of certain experiments, the theory that the horny layer of the skin acts as a protein gel; on acidification it contracts, imprisoning the endogenous bacterial flora, the *p*H destroying any " susceptible bacteria ". On alkalising the skin, the protein gel swells, absorbing water and becomes more porous so that entrapped bacteria can escape to the skin surface.

Bergeim and Cornbleet (*Amer. J. med. Sci.*, 1943, **205**, 785) consider that lactic and the volatile acids of sweat act as mild antiseptics, possibly in view of their *p*H *per se* or possibly due to some specific action.

in the disintegration of intercarbon linkages. The *hydrolases* include (i) esterases, e.g. lipase, cholesterol-esterase, phosphatase, lecithinase, necleotidase, sulphatase, etc., (ii) carbohydrases (which are concerned in the synthesis and/or hydrolysis of carbohydrates) ; diastase is the enzyme which hydrolyses starch, (iii) proteases, including proteinases and peptidases, and (iv) amidases including arginase, histidase and leucinase.

The desmolases include (*a*) heavy metal enzymes, e.g. catalase and phenoloxidases, (*b*) oxyhydrases as for example histaminase, and (*c*) carboxylase. (See Robert and Strahler, *Dermatologica*, 1945, **91**, 1.)

The skin also contains a large amount of sterols, the activation of which by ultra-violet light is an important source of the anti-rachitic vitamin D. (*See* vitamins, Skin Nutrition, Chapter 4.) *It appears to me that the sterols may also, by conferring water-holding capacity upon the skin fats and cells, contribute to the maintenance of the integrity of the skin.*[1] *Cholesterol and cholesterol-containing fats when added to mineral or other oils, greatly increase the capacity of such oils to take up water either in the form of the conventional water-in-oil emulsions or possibly, in conjunction with skin lipoids present, in bimolecular leaflets.* (*See* Emulsions and Dispersions, Chapter 41.)

In discussing skin ferments, etc., mention should be made of a substance described by Fleming as " lysozyme " (*Proc. Roy. Soc. B.*, 1922, **93**, 306 ; *Proc. Roy. Soc. Med.*, 1932, **26**, 1) present in most animal tissues, and also in sebum, sweat, etc. Recent researches suggest that this substance is a protein of low molecular weight having enzymatic properties [Roberts (*Quart. J. exp. Physiol.*, 1937, **27**, 89 ; Abraham and Robinson, *Nature*, London, 1937, **140**, 24 ; Epstein and Chain, *Brit. J. exp. Path.*, 1940, **21**, 324)]. As it is inhibited by traces of acids or alkali, it is almost certain to be inactive when present on the skin surface. [This substance is considered briefly in Chapter 19 dealing with Eye Lotions.]

What part, if any, is played by the skin enzymes in the defensive mechanism of the skin is at present unknown. Tzank (*J. Méd. Chir. prat.*, 1936, **107**, 77) reported a " skin lipase " which was active against tuberculosis and leprosy of the skin. If substantiated, the whole relationship of skin enzymes to skin and bodily health might be affected.

The Ageing of Skin

The biological process of ageing is universal, irresistible, irrevocable, and is therefore a subject of vital importance to all.

The skin, unlike other organs is readily accessible, visible and susceptible to detailed analytical study, a matter of vital importance in the

[1] *See* role of moisture in Skin Nutrition (Chapter 4), and on Skin Foods and Lubricating Creams (Chapter 10).

investigation of a biological process such as ageing, which requires regular detailed scrutiny over a long period of time.

It is appalling to discover the dearth of systematic study on this problem. It is therefore impossible to trace any cogent relationship between the ageing of skin and any measurable biochemical or histological change by which such change could be detected in its infancy and by which the whole process of ageing could be given scientific evaluation.

Apart from hereditary influences which may become dominant in later life and exert a profound influence, the skin from birth is subjected to a common cycle of varying events which, *in toto*, must have considerable effect on the progress of ageing. The cycle includes physical factors, such as heat, light and cold, the humidity of the surrounding air (see Chapters 4 and 10—the role of moisture in skin health), the application of externally applied cosmetic and cleansing preparations, varying activity of the internal endocrine secretions parallel with the sexual function, changes in the diet and in the efficiency of the digestive system, exposure to infections, and finally, psychogenic factors.

The ultimate effect called ageing is not easily defined. I know of no purely specific skin characteristic of old age. In our present state of knowledge, I would place loss of elasticity as the outstanding characteristic, with pruritis (itching) and pigmentation next.

After stretching, senile skin returns to its original position less rapidly than young skin, and in some cases becomes permanently over-stretched.

A *mild* degree of itching (pruritis) is a common physiological phenomenon, and has no pathological significance. In old age, the irritability of skin is very often enhanced. More recently, evidence has accumulated to show that itching, often accompanied by pigmentation, is associated with a malignant disease of internal organs. (W. N. Goldsmith, *Recent Advances in Dermatology*, London : J. & A. Churchill, 1936.) Pruritis may also be associated with glycosuria, i.e. the presence of sugar in normal urine, appendicitis and gout.[1]

Psychogenic factors play an important part (watching other people scratch we feel itchy). It may be that the alteration in the appetite with increasing age and reduced efficiency of the digestive organs results in either the discharge of products into the blood which irritate the skin, or in the non-transference to the blood of factors which in earlier life exerted a protective action. As age increases, the diet is often modified, and the intake of fats or sometimes green foodstuffs, salads, etc., may be

[1] Itching may be associated with an increased non-protein nitrogen content of the skin. In some cases the itching appears to be related to increased uric acid, and the symptoms are relieved by the administration of Cinchophen. Urbach has stated that a prolonged diet poor in protein actually leads to increased uric acid in the skin. (W. N. Goldsmith, *Recent Advances in Dermatology*.)

drastically reduced because of their effect on the individual. This may result in both cases in the reduction of the vitamin A intake, and in the case of the greenstuffs of certain mineral salts. The use of vitamins in skin diseases has proved no panacea, but there are a number of skin conditions which appear to be improved by their administration.[1]

Of the vitamins, vitamin A is worthy of special study. P. A. O'Leary (" Vitamin Therapy in Dermatology and Syphilology ", *Arch. Derm. Syph., Chicago*, 1942, **46**, 5, 628), in a summary of the literature, claimed that in certain skin diseases the response to the administration of vitamin A is so rapid and clearcut that the deduction is warranted that the result is *specific*. These diseases include *Phrynoderma* (toadskin)—a papular dry skin eruption (C. N. Frazier and C. K. Hu, *Arch. intern. Med.*, 1931, **48**, 507), *Pityriasis rubra pilaris*—a disease of the skin characterised by formation of hard elevations around each hair follicle (L. A. Brunsting and C. Sheard, *Arch. Derm. Syph., Chicago*, 1941, **43**, 42), and *Keratosis follicularis*—a papular skin disease characterised by cornification of the epithelial layers of the skin (S. M. Peck, L. Chargin and H. Sobotka) *Arch. Derm. Syph., Chicago*, 1941, **43**, 223). The so-called seborrheids recently described (P. Gross, *Arch. Derm. Syph., Chicago*, 1941, **43**, 504, have been claimed to be due to deficiency of the vitamin B complex.

It is true that these diseases are in many cases due originally to a certain vitamin deficiency, and the administration of the missing vitamin would be expected to cure them. Moreover, they represent a pathological condition. Nevertheless, their connection with the skin and the type of the eruption suggest that milder forms of nutritional deficiencies could produce changes in the skin, and that this possibility should be borne in mind.[1] Deficient intake or absorption of vitamin A may not be a symptom only of ageing. Recently, evidence has been reported which indicates that *Vernix caseosa* is a manifestation of deficiency of vitamin A of new-born infants, and that it represents disturbances in cornification analogous to the dermal changes noted in other manifestations of deficiency of vitamin A. This work has not yet been confirmed (J. V. Straumjord, *West J. Surg.*, 1940, **48**, 341 ; through *J. Amer. med. Ass.*, 1942, **120**, 13, 1032).

In 1911 Luithlen demonstrated that the skin of rabbits fed on a predominating oat diet reacted more markedly to unspecific local irritants than the skin of rabbits fed on predominantly greenstuff diet. J. H. Vogt (*The Influence of Diet on Skin*) has confirmed these results.

The influence of the endocrine glands at puberty on the skin and hair is well known. Recently, H. F. Bullough (" Cyclical Changes in the Skin of the Mouse during the Oestrous Cycle ", *J. Endocrin.*, Aug. 1943,

[1] *See* Diet and Skin Health, Chapter 3.

33, 280) has shown that the mitotic activity and thickness of the epidermis in the mouse varies throughout the oestrous cycle and that there appears to be an increase in the fatty layer during oestrous.

Evidence of the effect of the internal secretions on skin pigmentation is given by the abnormal pigmentation produced by the female genital organs during pregnancy. It is possible that such secretions may be a factor also in maintaining the elasticity of the skin in this condition.

The relationship between internal secretion and pigmentation is further evidenced in Addison's disease.

The irritant effect of *excessive* sunlight and its possible carcinogenic action is discussed in Chapter 13, Sunburn and Sun-tan Preparations. The morphological relationship existing between *Xeroderma pigmentosum* and senile skin raises the question as to whether ageing of the skin is due, at least in part, to its exposure to light or to some photo-sensitising substance discharged into the system during the general metabolic effects accompanying ageing.[1]

A careful spectroscopic study of normal post-mortem skin of infants, adults, and the aged, might reveal differences in their chemical composition, but so far there is no authentic evidence to show that ageing of the skin is associated with any significant changes in its chemical composition. It has been suggested that the moisture content of young skin is a characteristic factor, but Goldsmith (*Recent Advances in Dermatology*, London : J. & A. Churchill, Ltd., 1936) has pointed out that the moisture content of skin is raised not only in infancy but also in old age, obesity, scleroderma, ichthyosis and eczema.

The low nutritional requirements of the skin and its expansive vascular system suggest that ageing is not associated with a diminished blood supply. On the contrary, in cases of arteriosclerosis the face is often flushed and apparently healthy.

In considering the ageing of skin it should be remembered that senile skin still continues its protective, immunological and thermostatic roles.[2]

COSMETICS AND THE AGEING OF SKIN. As already shown, the skin is nourished by a dense network of anastomising blood capillaries in the dermis which is also well supplied with lymph. This is the normal method of nutrition, and in our present state of knowledge we have no evidence that the skin can be nourished by external means. Indeed, as I have discussed in somewhat greater detail under Skin Nutrition, Chapter 4, to *even seek a real skin "food" suggests an ignorance on the part*

[1] For an example of photo-sensitisation, see Allergy and Dermatitis, Chapter 2.

[2] Possibly the thermostatic function is not quite as effective as it is in youth as the aged seem more susceptible to violent changes in temperature.

of the seeker of the biochemistry and functions of the epidermis, and were such a preparation discovered and widely used, its effects might be disastrous.

Researches so far (*see* Skin Nutrition) [1] suggest that skin penetration and absorption occur only in the case of certain selective substances and that in most cases the skin is impervious to externally applied substances. The use of an electric current, however, in some way removes the barriers to penetration normally offered by the intact skin. Abramson and Gorin (*Chemical Products*, 1940, p. 37) have suggested that the epidermis may consist of an inner membrane wetted by the body fluids, and an outer membrane containing air spaces; and that on the application of an electric potential, electro-osmotic forces perhaps cause displacement of air in the pores (whose inner and outer surface will now be in contact with liquid) and ions could thus move through a now unbroken column of conducting liquid.

There is evidence that the moisture content of the skin is important. Emollient creams and lotions keep the outer corneous layer of the skin soft and supple and minimise chapping and windburn (with consequent risk of infection), and in minimising these (and replacing [2] lubricating oils removed from the skin by constant washing with cleansing agents) they do therefore delay the onset of wrinkling and thus delay the premature ageing of normal skin. In aged skin and in facial blemishes their function is decorative and none the less valuable on this account.

[1] *See also* In Favour of Cosmetics, and Cosmetic Facts and Fallacies, *also* Skin Foods.

[2] The term " replacing " is meant to convey that it takes the place of the natural skin oils removed—in a purely *physical* manner—but not that mineral or other oils have exactly the same properties in respect of their *effect upon the skin.* At the moment we have no scientific evidence on this question, apart from clinical observation, that lanolin in a preparation appears to be of value in certain skin conditions. (*See* Lanolin, Chapter 4.)

CHAPTER 2

ALLERGY AND DERMATITIS

To our chemical individualities are due our chemical merits as well as our chemical shortcomings, and it is very nearly true to say that the factors which confer upon us our predisposition to or our immunities from the various mishaps which are spoken of as diseases are inherent in our very structure, and even in the molecular groupings which confer upon us our individualities and which went to the makings of the chromosomes from which we sprang.

[Sir Archibald Garrod, *The Inborn Factors in Disease,* London : Oxford University Press, 1931.]

All cosmetic manufacturers (whose business is of any size) receive complaints from their customers ; some of these refer to an empty package missed on the filling line, or some other packaging complaint ; others refer to the consistency of the product, it is either "too soft and runny" or has "set hard like a brick" but through such complaints runs a small and important thread of "skin irritation" complaints, and few—if any—cosmetic manufacturers have been fortunate to market for long, any cosmetic preparation—of whatever nature—without receiving *some* complaints of irritation.

It may be *the perfume*, it may be *the antioxidant or preservative*, it *may* be the *product per se*, or it may be *the "chemical shortcomings"* of the user ; somehow the user never (or hardly ever) considers the latter possibility, but it is very real. *Hypersensitivity to a product* (as distinct from "sensitisation" discussed below) *may develop as a result of a change in the health of the user, as distinct from the condition of allergy, discussed in this chapter.*

It has been stated (*Lancet*, 27 Sept., 1952, p. 619) that "states of autonomic over-excitability seem to run parallel with an all-round increase of skin sensitivity. This clinical belief has recently been given some scientific backing by the demonstration of increased sensitivity of the skin of guinea pigs to contact irritants applied after a period of interference with the animals' sleep.

Diet may also play an important role in skin irritation, for which cosmetics can quite well be blamed. From personal experience, the author can quote the effect of the ingestion of egg in some individuals—the very ubiquitousness of the allergen renders the identification difficult—eggs are eaten for breakfast, may be included in Yorkshire pudding, or other dish eaten for lunch ; are eaten in cakes, etc., for tea. In fresh or dried form they enter a very wide range of food products in which their presence is often entirely unsuspected by the user. Subsequent to the ingestion of such food, and in a space of time that may vary from fifteen minutes or so, to an hour or more, skin irritation of the *face* may set in, sometimes accompanied by a slight rash or transient pinkness. If following the meal the user has washed with soap, or applied a cosmetic and the procedure happens to have occurred on several other similar occasions, the soap or cosmetic may be blamed ; and if patch tests are applied without a positive response, but the doctor finds that "apparently" the application of the product has again brought up this irritation of the face, the cosmetic or other product may still be subject to suspicion. Here, it is true, we are dealing with a food " allergy ", but on the basis of the complaint, food allergy may not be suspected.

In the following discussion of allergy, it is assumed that the necessary criterion of *specificity* is applied, viz. the exposure to the " allergen " must produce a change which can be shown to be produced *only* by the suspected substance (or by a product, closely related in chemical structure) and the history of the complainant should show no evidence of " allergy " to a wide range of other substances whose presence in the diet, etc., cannot be dismissed at the time that the identification of the offending agent is being made.

Is allergy harmful ? Allergy must always produce some untoward clinical symptom, otherwise it would not be noticed and from this point of view it can be considered harmful. Again, the irritation of the skin produced is psychologically harmful and—if it leads to scratching—may well result in bacterial infections from the fingers and nails. As a secondary effect, the scratching may introduce traces of nail lacquer (to which the user may be sensitive) under the skin. If the face is " blotchy ", this again will cause psychological tension and distress, and, in so doing, " aggravate the condition ".

On the other hand, " allergy " gives the warning signal that the individual concerned is ill-adapted to deal with the offending substance, which should therefore be avoided, or where this is impracticable, dealt with by the process of de-sensitisation. With the increasing armamentarium of synthetic products developed by organic chemistry, to which the human body may not have, as yet, had time to acclimatise itself, the allergic response may be *valuable to the individual concerned.*

In discussing allergy below it is understood that the *toxicological* properties of the preparation are above suspicion and that " true allergy " *per se* is involved.

ALLERGY

The term allergy is derived from the Greek, *ergia* denoting reactivity, and *allos* altered, and is widely used to denote all *altered* conditions of human and animal sensitivity. These conditions are covered more simply (though not quite accurately) in the layman's expression of idiosyncrasy —proverbially expressed in the common expression : " One man's meat another man's poison ".[1]

Some dermatologists have attempted to distinguish between *atopic* allergy in which heredity is the paramount causal factor and in which specific circulating bodies have been demonstrated by their passive transmission to a non-sensitive person's skin,[2] and *non-atopic* allergy.

The term *atopy* was suggested by Coca (*Arch. Path.* (*Lab. Med.*), 1926, **1**, 96), and as examples of atopic allergy he considers asthma, hay-fever, eczema, urticaria and migraine. He drew a number of distinctions between atopic and anaphylactic, between antigens and atopens, and between antibodies and reagins.[3]

W. N. Goldsmith (*Recent Advances in Dermatology*, London : J. and A. Churchill, Ltd., 1936) has stated that in view of our present knowledge it is impossible to make any sharp distinction between antigens and atopens. W. W. C. Topley (*An Outline of Immunity*, London : Arnold, 1933) points out that on the premises of our present knowledge of the influence of genetic factors operating in anaphylaxis and in atopy, there are insufficient grounds for postulating an essential difference between them.

I would define allergy as a condition of altered reactivity. The sufferer reacts abnormally (either in respect of the *nature* of the irritant or in its *concentration*) to (1) substance ingested (eggs, wheat, fish, milk, strawberries, various drugs, etc.), (2) substances inhaled (e.g. plant pollens and dusts of various substances, flour, kapok, silk, wool, powdered drugs), (3) substances in contact with the skin [4] (various chemical substances contacted externally), (4) insect bites.

It is often difficult to differentiate sharply between the above conditions. For example, in any process in which dust is involved, the first three of these factors are operative.

[1] More accurately " Quod aliis cibus est aliis fuit acre venenum " (What is food for some may be fierce poison for others), " De Rerum Natura " (The Nature of Things), Lucretius.

[2] C. Prausnitz and H. Kuestner (*Zbl. Bat.*, 1921, **86**, 160) injected into a normal non-sensitive patient : (1) the serum of a patient who was sensitive to cooked fish, (2) an equivalent amount of serum from a normal person. After twenty-four hours an extract of fish was injected into both of the above sites whereupon the site of serum (1) produced a red weal while that of (2) did not react. This test is called the " P.-K. test " and is often used in dermatological investigation.

[3] The meaning of these terms is given in the discussion on the Ehrlich side-chain theory and allergy.

[4] This must be taken to include also physical agents such as heat, cold and light.

The response of the individual to the inflicted insult may take the form of (1) asthma, hay-fever, etc., in which skin reactions as such give little or no response, or (2) a skin response resulting in erythema, either with or without vesicular eruptions, (3) urticaria (hives), a manifestation characterised by the sudden appearance of smooth elevated weals, markings or patches, usually whiter in colour than the surrounding tissue and attended by severe itching. It is possible that the inhalation of certain powdered cosmetic materials might bring about the first condition. However, the cosmetician is interested only in the second condition.

The term *allergy* should, in its ideal sense, be applied only to those conditions in which an offending substance (the allergen or hapten [1]) can be demonstrated; and when removal of this substance brings relief from the allergic manifestation.

The identification of the offending substance, or substances is usually made by means of a patch and/or user test.

PATCH TESTING. The basis of the patch test, is the application of the substance under test to healthy skin in a dilution such that it is too low to obtain a positive reaction from a normal (non-allergic or non-sensitised) person. In this test the substance is applied directly to the unbroken skin and held in place by means of straps, oiled silk, adhesive tape or by other suitable means. After 24–48 hours the patch is removed and the area examined, immediately after removal of the patch, after 48 hours, and after an interval of between 6 and 10 days. This latter examination should be carried out because patch tests may be complicated by a delayed reaction time, even when there is no question of serum sickness or microbiological multiplication. The application, e.g. of certain plant extracts or of 1,2-dinitrochlorobenzene may produce no erythema after a 24–48 hour patch test, but in certain persons vesiculation may occur about the sixth day and may persist for some three weeks. Once this reaction period has been established, however, it does not require a similar period to react to further applications of the same substance.

The patch test is usually employed to investigate contact dermatitis [2] in which the skin is the host of the hypersensitive state and is thus in a position to react with the substance placed in contact with it. Patch testing, however, may not be suitable for investigating those conditions of allergy which are governed largely by inheritance factors (inheritance

[1] The terms allergen and hapten will be discussed under the theoretical considerations of allergy.

[2] There exists no sharp differentiation between allergy and dermatitis, the difference is mainly one of degree. If a primary irritant is employed, for example, in an industrial process (and by this I mean a substance which in the physical state and concentration employed will produce positive results in a large percentage of those exposed) then the injury sustained may be classed as industrial dermatitis. If, however, the substance in the state and concentration used rarely gives rise to skin reactions, I would class reactions to it as allergic.

probably plays *some* part in all abnormal skin sensitivity) and in which antibodies can be detected in the blood stream and passively transferred by the P.-K. method already mentioned (hay-fever, urticaria, migraine, etc.). In such cases it is more usual to employ the scratch or intracutaneous test, where the offending substance is brought into intimate contact with the blood vessels in the cutis. The reaction is rapid: it may be observed within about half an hour as a maximum. Such tests must *not* be carried out by the cosmetician whose province does not extend beyond patch testing for contact dermatitis.

The *prophetic patch test* was developed some sixteen years ago (L. Schwartz, *J. Soc. cosmet. Chem.*, 1950, p. 321) in the U.S.A., to test the possible irritant properties of the—then new—synthetic fibre, now known as nylon.

Schwartz (*J. Soc. cosmet. Chem.*, 1950, p. 321) states that "... the original prophetic patch test consisted in placing a ½-in. square piece of unprocessed nylon on the skin of 200 subjects, covering it with a piece of cellophane 1 in. square and sealing this on the skin with a piece of adhesive plaster 3 in. square. A piece of unbleached unprocessed cotton fabric of similar size was fastened on the skin of the opposite side of the body to act as control. The patches remained on for forty-eight hours, then were removed and the reactions read and recorded. The sites of the patches were examined for three consecutive days for delayed reactions. Ten days after last reading, the patch testing was repeated, on the same 200 subjects and on approximately the same skin areas. The patches were removed after forty-eight hours and the sites examined for signs of reactions for three consecutive days. The second series of patch tests were done to see if any of the subjects were sensitised by the first test...

Schwartz adds that "... realising that no reactions to patch tests on 200 subjects is not sufficient to be statistically safe, undergarments were made of nylon and were worn for several months by more than a thousand subjects without any signs of irritation before nylon was placed on sale to the public". He gives the following table of the likely maximum percentage rate of positive reactions in a sample of infinite size when the subjects tested number from 100 to 10,000.

Subjects Tested	*No Reactions*	*One Reaction*	*Two Reactions*
100	3·00	4·40	5·80
200	1·50	2·20	2·90
300	0·99	1·50	2·00
500	0·60	0·90	1·20
1000	0·30	0·45	0·60
2000	0·15	0·23	0·30
5000	0·06	0·09	0·12
10000	0·03	0·05	0·06

In the case of cosmetics certain differences are apparent. In the first place, many cosmetic preparations have volatile components such as water, which evaporates when applied to the skin. If the above "closed" patch test is performed, the skin may be irritated because the cosmetic is being used under conditions widely differing from those that would be encountered in practice; for example, in aqueous media, sealed in contact with the skin, *p*H becomes very important and contact even with dilute alkali under such conditions would lead to alteration in the usually almost impervious layer of the keratin of the stratum corneum.

If *closed* patch tests are to be employed they should be employed for the purpose of *comparison*, a control test being carried out alongside on an old and well tested cosmetic formulation, and the behaviour of the new formulation on the skin compared with that of the control.

Where information is required as to whether a substance or formulation is a "primary irritant" or not (and in those cases in which the answer cannot readily be obtained by a study of the literature or a close knowledge of the components of the formulation) then short-duration patch tests on between twenty to thirty persons, preferably of both sexes and mixing blondes, brunettes and red-heads, should suffice to give an answer. But in seeking further dermatological data, the best test is to ensure that the cosmetic is used under the normal conditions by a mixed group of at least 200 persons for a period of from three to four weeks to cover the usual period of sensitisation. The statement "used under normal conditions" means just what it says and if the product is one which is usually applied once or twice *every day*, then during the test described steps should be taken to see that the individuals tested do, in fact, apply it with such regularity.

The patch test may be used to study problems of sensitisation by repeating such tests on the same subjects, at intervals of ten days. *In such testing care must be taken to ensure that the formulation contains no well-known or suspected, sensitising agents.*

Patch tests should never be left on for long periods as they may lead to sensitisation. Schwartz, Tulipan and Peck (*Occupational Diseases of the Skin*, London, 1939) have pointed out that a patch test left on longer than five days may sensitise the patient to subsequent application of the substance tested. Ritter (*Brit. J. Derm.*, May 1948) records an example of the abuse of the patch test by a hairdresser who patch-tested a client with a popular proprietary paraphenylenediamine hair dye and left the patch on for a *week*. At the end of this time there was no visible reaction and the hair was dyed forthwith. Three days layer acute typical dermatitis developed.

A method of patch-testing where it is desired to investigate the efficacy of remedial measures has been reported by Anderson (*Arch. Derm. Syph., Chicago*, 1944, **49**, p. 181) who describes Parkhurst's modification which consists of the simultaneous application of two or more patches of a known irritant. One site is allowed to remain "as is" for a positive control, whilst the other sites are allowed to remain for varying periods before a known neutralising substance is applied, in order to ascertain how long a period may elapse before neutralisation is no longer effective.

In carrying out patch tests, care should be taken, so far as is possible, to employ normal and not sunburnt skin. Colebatch (*Med. J. Aust.*, 1941, **2**, 23, 640 through *Bull. Hyg.*, June 1942, p. 400) found that in three cases in which simultaneous patches were applied to sunburnt and to normal skin, reactions were three times as great in the normal as in the sunburnt areas.

Various methods of obtaining adhesion of the patch to the skin and in carrying out the tests have been described in the literature. Sterner (*Arch. Derm. Syph., Chicago*, April 1942, p. 761) has, for example, described the use of small cups of Pyrex glass of 15 mm. diameter and 5 mm. depth (the glass being 1 mm. thick), into which a 10 mm. ball of cotton-wool moistened with the test solution is inserted. The cup is held in firm contact with the skin by means of adhesive tape, which if desired, may be perforated in order to show the contents of the cup. R. R. Schwartz and E. J. Marcus (*Proc. Sci. Sect. T.G.A.*, Dec. 1946, p. 10) have described special problems arising in the multiple patch testing of soaps. In testing of soaps and detergent solutions, in addition to comparative patch tests for determining the relative mildness of soaps, immersion tests several times a day have been found very useful by the author. (Somewhat similar tests have been described by J. A. Killian and M. E. Marsh, *Proc. Sci. Sect. T.G.A.*, May 1949, p. 32.)

Even though the actual procedure is simple, patch tests should not be carried out by beauty parlour operators, as in unskilled hands very disastrous results may accrue. On the manufacturing side these tests are often conducted by qualified specialists in the biochemistry of skin, who are intimately acquainted with the chemical constitution of the substance being tested, its *p*H, titratable alkalinity (or acidity), toxicity and its chemical and structural relationships to substances already known to be irritant. Untoward results in such cases are rare, and even when they do occur can usually be treated by soothing lotions. No valid objection exists to patch tests by such investigators. Apart from such specialised research work, however, patch testing is definitely the province of the dermatologist to whom all such tests should be referred.

Having found the offending agent (or a product with similar allergenic properties), at least in theory, one should ascertain whether the sufferer has had the opportunity of contact at any time with this substance, and then for conclusive proof the offending substance should be removed from all possibility of contact with the affected person and observation made as to whether the condition disappears permanently in the absence of the suspected substance.

Actually this is, in practice, almost if not entirely impossible, except in those cases of susceptibility to pollen as in hay-fever, where nature by means of seasonal variations insures an absence of the pollen at certain periods of the year, or in the case of susceptibility to an individual drug or article of food which can readily be omitted from the diet. In most cases our life has become too complicated to readily identify and omit the offending substance. I cannot do better than quote Dr. H. E. Cox's description of the modern girl (" Chemicals in Fabrics as Potential Skin Irritants ", *Proc. Roy. Soc. Med.*, 1941, **35** 1, 27) : ' . . who may have as eyelashes the product of the grease pencil, whose lips and cheeks may derive their beauty not from oxyhaemoglobin but from eosin or ponceau, whose teeth—natural or artificial—may be brushed with a waterproof synthetic fibre, and her fingers adorned with nitrocellulose dissolved in complex solvents and plasticised with still more complex chemicals. Perhaps she has applied chloramine-T or oxyquinoline derivative to her axillae or even used mercapto-glycollic acid as a depilatory, perhaps she has a corset made of latex rubber with fillers and antioxidants in it, a bleached woollen vest impregnated with synthetic finishes, other intimate garments made of cotton with synthetic resins as anti-crease, stockings of delustered viscose, a frock of rayon containing perhaps regenerated cellulose or cellulose ethers impregnated with quaternary ammonium compounds to render them water-resisting ; shoes of new plastics resembling snake skin and fur cape of leopard skin in which the familiar spots have been produced by mating a polyphenol with a diamine. Probably she has spectacles of synthetic glass with sides of plastic resin, a handbag of suede leather compounded of cotton and rubber and an orchid made from doped and dyed cellulose in her buttonhole, perfumed with otto of the laboratory, not attar of rose.'

Hypersensitivity to a substance may include sensitivity not only to that particular substance but to other substances closely related to it allergenically. This relationship may be entirely different from that expressed by their chemical constitution or pharmacological action. Hypersensitivity may not even be confined to a single substance but may extend to a group of apparently unrelated substances. Baer, Leider and Mayer (*Proc. Soc. exp. Biol., N.Y.*, 1948, **67**, 489 ; *vide also J. invest.*

Derm., Nov. 1949, **13**, 223) have pointed out that skin tests with certain certified food dyes in patients sensitive to *p*-phenylenediamine *suggest* that eczematous hypersensitivity to *p*-phenylenediamine may not only cross over to azo dyes used for dyeing leather and fabrics, or in ointments, but also to certain azo dyes certified under the U.S. Food and Drug and Cosmetic Act of 1938, for use in foods, drugs and cosmetics. It will be seen, therefore, that proof of prior contact with an offending substance and its subsequent elimination is, to say the least, a matter of very great difficulty, and this fact has probably led to some of the disappointing results obtained in practice even where it is believed that the offending substance has been identified and then omitted from all possibility of contact.

Before considering, briefly, some explanations which have been advanced to account for allergic response and for anaphylaxis it will be as well to discuss the meaning of this latter term.

ANAPHYLAXIS. This condition was discovered by Richet (1898), who injected a dog with doses of sea anemone poison. He found that a second dose given a few days after the first, exerted a far more toxic effect. In 1903 Arthus showed that similar effects were obtained with non-toxic proteins.

The introduction of a foreign body into the blood stream of an animal (the foreign body being termed the antigen) results in the elaboration of a substance in that animal to specifically combat the invader or precipitate it, thus making it harmless (this defence factor being termed the antibody). If the injections continue, however, succeeding doses may produce a toxic effect greater than the primary injection when no antibody was present. This effect is termed anaphylaxis, and although numerous theories have been elaborated which explain some phases, the complete explanation is still obscure. From the above it will be readily seen that anaphylaxis is a specific form of allergy applied to hypersensitiveness due to antigenic substances.

THEORETICAL CONSIDERATION OF ALLERGY

Ehrlich's Side-chain Theory. The condition of allergy has been explained on the basis of Ehrlich's side-chain theory, which postulates that body cells consist of complex organic molecules having a stable central group attached to labile chains, i.e. receptors. These receptors enter into reactions in the body, the central stable group of the molecule under ordinary conditions remaining unaffected.

On this basis Warren T. Vaughan (*Allergy—Strangest of all Maladies*, London : Hutchinson, 1942) has summarised in a series of simple illustrations the generally accepted view of antibody production, immunity and the explanation of anaphylaxis, in which it is considered that combination occurs between a foreign protein and " receptors " which are presumably part of the human protein molecule in all living cells. This combination in some way injures or interferes with the integrity of the cell. To protect itself the cell sheds the receptor which (presumably) remains attached to the foreign protein. The injured cell then produces many more receptors to take the place of the shed receptor and in order to protect it from further injury (in a somewhat analogous manner to the way in which a gardener produces dense foliage by clipping the ends of branches, or to the way in which biodynes stimulate fresh cell production in injured tissue ; see the paragraph on biodynes and skin respiration). These receptors are termed antibodies and circulate freely in the body fluids. If the same foreign protein again enters the blood it meets these circulating antibodies which combine with it and neutralise its action, thus protecting the cell, viz. :

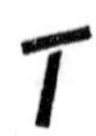

Foreign protein.

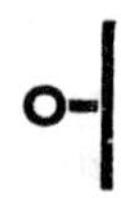

Receptive part of human protein molecule.

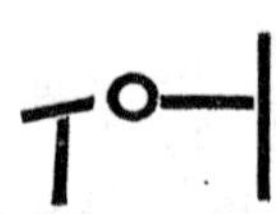

Combination of foreign protein and human protein molecule.

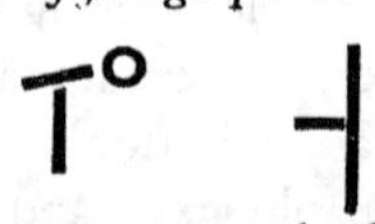

Human protein molecule sheds receptor link.

Injured human protein molecule then produces many more receptors (antibodies) for its subsequent protection.

The final stage graphically represented is that condition we term immunity. To explain anaphylaxis the author postulates that normally the amount of foreign protein with which an immunised person comes into contact is small ; for example, in human immunisation against typhoid fever three injections at weekly intervals of increasing quantities of typhoid protein stimulate the cells to produce increasing quantities of protective antibodies, which are well able to cope with the few living typhoid germs which would pass through the walls of the intestine into the blood.

It is known that the combination of foreign protein and antibody results in the release of histamine from the injured cell, and that the histamine renders the membrane lining of the capillary blood vessels permeable. Leakage occurs through them ; the blood pressure falls and collapse of the individual ensues.

It appears to me that in anaphylactic shock we have a preliminary period during which protective antibodies are formed, then if the second dose of foreign protein is relatively large, the large amount of histamine produced by the *antigen-antibody* combination will produce the symptoms of anaphylactic shock.

In desensitisation the second dose given is less than the dose necessary to produce shock ; this removes most of the antibodies, but the amount of histamine released by the antigen-antibody combination *may be just too small to produce anaphylaxis.* Most of the antibodies have now been removed and therefore a third injection will not produce this condition.

So far we have considered the introduction of a foreign *protein* and in this case the offending substance is termed an antigen. But similar effects can be produced by substances which are definitely not proteins. In this case it has been shown that the offending substance, though not a protein itself, can combine with a protein which is dissolved in blood (not the protein of the human cell already discussed) and this new *combination* then acts as a *foreign protein.* In such cases, where the offending substance is not itself a protein but combines with a protein constituent of the blood to form a combination which acts as a foreign protein, the offending substance is termed a *hapten.*

The above explanation has dealt with the protective mechanism of the normal body. In an allergic person it is assumed that the antibodies formed for protection for some reason remain attached instead of being shed, and the offending substance (protein or hapten) combines with these antibodies still attached to the original cell, with the result that the cell becomes damaged.

MCDONAGH THEORY. McDonagh (*The Nature of Disease*, 3 vols., London : Wm. Heinemann Ltd.) has propounded a dictum that there is but *one* disease, that of *colloidal disequilibrium*, and that the action of different invading substances whether they be chemicals or micro-organisms is to disturb this equilibrium. This disturbance will vary with the particular invader but always follows, so McDonagh states, the chemico-physical laws of matter in the colloidal state.

At one time it was thought that in every infection there was a corresponding specific reaction and that in order to combat successfully any disease by inoculation the corresponding specific serum or vaccine must be employed. In modern treatment, however, many proteins which are not connected with the disease in question are introduced into the body, for example, bee stings for rheumatism, bacterial proteins prepared from their *dead* bodies, serums, or, for example, the artificial induction of malaria in the treatment of general paralysis of the insane. Such treatment suggests the possibility that some general physical-chemical reaction may be responsible for the results obtained.

According to McDonagh's theory *immunity* depends upon the state of the protein particles of the plasma at the moment of infection.

If the conditions are such that the plasma particles can abstract electrons from the invading organisms and drive them into solution, the patient will be immune. The final result will be a hydration of the plasma particles resulting in the dissemination of the particles, leaving a highly disseminated mass of colloid particles well supplied with electrons and able to drive the micro-organisms of any second invasion into bacteriolysis (i.e. destruction or solution of bacteria), thus rendering the patient immune.

If the result of the first invasion was instead of dissemination a permanent and stable hydration of the protein particles, a second invasion will produce still further hydration of these—and they will pass into coarse dispersion and ultimately be precipitated in some organ resulting in symptoms which we call allergy. If this second invasion be sufficiently concentrated and sudden, a large precipitation of the hydrated particles will suddenly occur with all the symptoms of shock —the symptoms differing according to the site of the precipitation.

Of these two theories, the former is generally accepted and to my mind more nearly represents the prevailing conditions, though in a few respects neither of them is entirely irreconcilable. There are, e.g. some similarities between McDonagh's disseminated mass of colloid particles and the circulating antibodies postulated on the side-chain theory of Ehrlich. The release of histamine might be tied up with cell damage occasioned by a sudden precipitation of coarsely hydrated protein particles.

While I do not subscribe to McDonagh's present conception of the nature of all diseases, I believe future research will demonstrate the paramount importance of physico-chemical (as opposed to purely chemical) changes in the body. Such studies will necessarily be complex. They will involve not only the effects of pH, hydration, dehydration, dispersion and coagulation of proteins, but also the normal resting electromotive forces existing across cellular membranes and the effect of currents, released by muscular exercise, as well as cardiac currents on the integrity of the cellular membrane (since generated e.m.f.s may affect permeability of the involved membranes), surface adsorption, and osmosis. The determination of these single effects is, in all probability, masked in many cases by the simultaneous presence of other ones.

PHOTO-DERMATITIS. The absorption of certain pigments and drugs (lipstick containing eosin), acriflavine, sulphonamide, and external contact with certain plants (bergamot, lime, wild parsley, milfoil, buttercup, mustard, figs, angelica), may render the human skin *photo-sensitive*, i.e. on subsequent exposure to sunlight eruptions occur which differ from those normally produced by sunlight. These eruptions do not occur on exposure to sunlight or ultra-violet light in the absence of a sensitising agent.

The sensitiser itself is inert, and it is the absorption of light of certain wave-lengths by the sensitiser that produces the photo-chemical reaction. Only the wave-lengths absorbed are effective in producing a chemical change (Draper's Law), hence a determination of the absorption spectra of the suspected photo-sensitising substance and the exposure of the individual after contact with this suspected substance to filtered light of the requisite wave-length will provide evidence of the truth of the supposition.

A. C. G. Guillaume (*Les Radiations Lumineuses*, Paris : Masson, 1927), using eosin, erythrosine, methyl-violet and acridine, obtained photo-sensitisation only by scarifying the horny layer and thus allowing the dyestuff to reach the Malpighian layer. Otherwise the dye only functioned as a protective filter. On the other hand, the presence of fatty materials, wetting agents, friction or perspiration may facilitate absorption. Experiments carried out by Klaber (*Brit. J. Derm.*, 1942, **7**, 208) suggest that at least in the case of sap from the fig tree penetration may occur under the influence of heat without the necessity of any friction. (*See also* Chapter 4, Skin Penetration.)

PHOTO-DYNAMIC ACTION. H. F. Blum (*Photo-Dynamic Action and Diseases caused by Light*, New York : Reinhold, 1941) has further classified certain substances as photo-dynamic. These substances all *fluoresce in ultra-violet light.* They exhibit a latent period prior to the photo-chemical reaction and cause organisms and tissues to exhibit abnormal reactivity to light. He describes photo-dynamic action as " the sensitisation of a biological system to light by a substance which serves as a light absorber for photo-chemical reactions *in which molecular oxygen takes part* ".

PHYTO-PHOTO-DERMATITIS. Klaber (*Brit. J. Derm.*, 1942, **7**, 193) suggested that the term *phyto-photo-dermatitis* be adopted as a generic title to cover every variant of those eruptions produced by external contact with *plants* and their extracts after subsequent exposure to light. It is therefore (as its name suggests) a subdivision of photo-dermatitis. Klaber states in his paper that cases described as phyto-photo-dermatitis may not be examples of photo-dynamic action, and to settle this question it would be necessary to see whether the pure substances exhibited the properties of fluorescence.

Phyto-photo-dermatitis produced by oil of bergamot and by lime oil are of interest to the cosmetician, and it may be found that many more perfume constituents will require classification under this heading.

It should be noted that true photo-sensitivity (including phyto-photo-dermatitis) *differs from allergy or idiosyncrasy in that, although some variations in individual sensitiveness occur, the eruptions are encountered in the majority of persons if the necessary conditions governing photo-sensitivity* (*i.e. contact penetration, and exposure to light of the required wave-length*) *are fulfilled.*

DERMATITIS. Dermatitis is a term of wide connotation signifying *any* inflammatory disease of the skin, and for this reason this term is usually qualified with an objective relating the source of such inflammation, for example:

Actinic dermatitis, produced by exposure to sunlight or ultra-violet light; dermatitis *Artefacta*, produced intentionally by the sufferer by means of scratching; *Berlock* dermatitis, produced by exposure to light after application of eau-de-Cologne (*see* phyto-photo-dermatitis); dermatitis *calorica*, produced by heat or cold; dermatitis *medicamentosa*, produced by medicines, drugs, etc.; *mycotic* dermatitis, caused by yeast infections; *occupational* or *industrial* dermatitis; *photo*-dermatitis, dermatitis *venenata* (contact dermatitis); dermatitis *vegetans*, due to secondary contamination of lesions with staphylococci, etc.

The forms of dermatitis of interest to the cosmetician and manufacturing chemist (and also the general public) are dermatitis *venenata* and *photo*-dermatitis.

Dermatitis venenata, contact dermatitis, comprises a group of inflammatory skin affections due to external irritants, no matter whether of animal, vegetable or mineral origin. The term covers occupational or industrial dermatitis, though this latter designation is more correctly reserved for processes in which the percentage of employees affected is sufficiently high for the question of allergy to be ruled out and for the offending substance to be definitely classed either as a primary irritant or as a sensitiser.

Prejudice against cosmetics on the grounds of either allergy or dermatitis is unfounded. Except in the case of a very small number of cosmetic and toilet preparations, the percentage of complaints *proved to be genuinely due* to such preparations is infinitesimally small compared to the amount of these preparations sold.

At the same time both cosmetician and dermatologist should realise that there is probably no material to which somebody is not allergic. The literature records cases due to such innocuous substances as :

Acacia gum (*Canad. med. Ass. J.*, 1942, **3**, 253), *boric acid* (A. Rothberg and G. A. Merrill, *N.Y. St. J. Med.*, 1938, **38**, 1284), Cholesterol esters (S. J. Fanburg, *Arch. Derm. Syph., Chicago*, 1940, **42**, 479), *cod-liver oil* (*Arch.* Derm. *Syph., Chicago*, 1942, 140), *dextrins* (J. D. Walters and E. C. Stern, *J. Amer. med. Assoc.*, 1941, **116**, 1518), *karaya gum* (R. Bowen, *Arch. Derm. Syph., Chicago*, March 1939, **39**, 506), *magnesium hydroxide* (E. W. Abramowitz, J. J. Rosso, *Arch. Derm. Syph., Chicago*, 1940, **41**, 707), *olive oil* (R. L. Sutton, Jr., *J. Amer. med. Assoc.*, 1943, **122**, 34), *petrolatum, liquid* (H. S. Niles, *Arch. Derm. Syph., Chicago*, 1941, 689), *soya bean and petroleum* (*Jap. J. Derm. Urol.*, 1940, **48**, 1). (For a more detailed literature on the subject of allergic reactions to materials employed in toilet preparations, reference should be made to R. G. Harry, *Cosmetic Materials*, London : Leonard Hill Ltd., 1948.)

Obviously cases such as these are allergic. If the list was extended to cover the *majority of substances* used in *everyday life* the list of recorded cases would be legion.

Indeed the American Medical Association reported (through *Amer. Perfum.*, 1937, p. 41) that " . . . *no cosmetic preparation can be strictly* ' *non-allergic* ' and that such designation will no longer be permitted in cosmetic advertising in publications associated with it ".

ANTIHISTAMINICS IN COSMETICS. The production of histamine, or histamine-like substances, in the body by a combination of antigen, or hapten, and antibody has already been discussed earlier in this chapter.

Whereas in many infections of the body, repeated attacks lead to the development of immunity either partial or more or less complete, unfortunately this is not the case with histamine as Feinberg (*J. Amer. med. Assoc.*, 1946, **132**, 702) has pointed out. Experiments on animals and man have shown that an increase in tolerance to histamine cannot be expected through repeated injections of histamine itself.

Since 1942, when Antergan was introduced in France and found effective clinically in relieving various allergic conditions, thousands of potential antihistaminics have been examined and a number have been found useful in the treatment of allergic urticaria, rhinitis, and many other allergic reactions, including those to drugs and serums. These antihistamines include such well known drugs as " Benadryl ", " Antistin ", etc.

Solutions of histamine are readily absorbed through the skin ; in fact such solutions have been employed to act as a pharmacologic tracer permitting observation of the pathway of absorption through the skin (Shelley and Melton, *J. invest. Dermat.*, 1949, **2**, 61). In view of the action of such substances in allergic conditions, deNavarre (*Amer. Perfum.*, Nov. 1949, p. 369), suggested that these substances might be considered for use in cosmetic preparations on the grounds that " the inclusion of such a material in cosmetics could conceivably render them more non-allergic than they have ever been ". The writer has criticised strongly (*Cosmetic Materials*, London : Leonard Hill Ltd., 1948) suggestions that penicillin, sulphathiazole and sodium fluoride respectively should be incorporated into toilet preparations, has seen many of his criticisms justified, and would now criticise similarly the use of antihistamines for *general* " *cosmetic* " use.

There is, of course, evidence that antihistaminics in ointments may relieve certain types of itching (A. J. Philips, *N.Y. St. J. Med.*, 1949, **47**, 1179) and it is possible that a case could well be made out for the use of such preparations to relieve the irritation and any allergic reaction, following insect bites and stings, but for *cosmetics*, I consider their use unnecessary and not altogether free from risk. For one thing the use of these preparations is still too recent to be sure that the *long-term results*, of repeated and indiscriminate application, involve no potential hazard.

Moynahan (*Practitioner*, March, 1950, p. 218) in discussing the use of the antihistamine drugs in dermatology, points out that the way in which these drugs inhibit the action of histamine has not yet been determined with certainty. Moynahan points out that :

(i) they may prevent the liberation of histamine from the hypothetical protein-histamine complex in the cell ;

(ii) they may actually destroy histamine as it is formed or released, in much the same way that the enzyme histaminase behaves ;

(iii) they may combine with histamine after its release from the cell and thereby inactivate it by forming a pharmacologically inert compound with it, or

(iv) they may act as competitors with histamine for attachment to the cell receptor.

It is stated that the bulk of the evidence is in favour of the last view, and that it is probable that they exert their action by preventing its access to the receptor in the cell.

It must be remembered that histamine is destroyed rapidly in the living animal by an enzyme histaminase, which is identical with, or closely allied to, diamine oxidase. Moynahan states that the intestinal epithelium has a high content of this enzyme which may be regarded as a natural antihistaminic.

In his tests Philips (*N.Y. St. J. Med.*, 1949, **47,** 1179) reported that eighty-five unselected types of itching dermatoses were treated with an ointment containing 2 per cent. diphenylhydramine hydrochloride, an antihistaminic. Fifteen control cases were treated with a similar ointment but containing no antihistaminic. None of the controls received complete relief. Of the treated cases 51·8 per cent. obtained complete and lasting relief, 21·1 per cent. received partial (less than 50 per cent.) relief and 27·1 per cent. had little or no relief. No irritation or sensitivity was observed.

In a therapeutic trial on ninety persons with pyribenzamine ointment, Sulzberger, Baer and Lewin (*J. invest. Derm.*, 1948, **10,** 41) reported in two of their cases an eczematoid dermatitis from the ointment. Strauss (*J. invest. Derm.*, 1948, **11,** 55) also reported an eczematous contact-dermatitis from pyribenzamine.

Because antihistaminics are potent drugs, themselves of *very complex organic nature,* the possibilities of skin sensitisation and of cross-sensitisation when used over a long period of time must be very carefully evaluated before they can be used indiscriminately in cosmetics. Not only this, but also what is their long term effect, if any, on the other natural enzymes and biochemical components of the skin ?

CHAPTER 3

DIET AND SKIN HEALTH

Definition of " Vitamin "—Vitamin A—The Vitamin B Complex, Vitamin B_1, B_2, B_6, B_{12}, Pantothenic acid, Choline, Biotin, Inositol, Folic acid, Para-aminobenzoic acid, Nicotinic acid, Niacin—Vitamin C—Vitamin D—Vitamers—Vitamin E—Recommendations for Daily Allowances—Vitamins in adaptation to stress—Mineral Salts in Food—What Diet ?—Vegetarianism—Alcohol and Skin Health—Role of Sugar in Skin Diseases—Constipation Fallacies—Obesity and the Ideal Weight—Dieting.

THE relationship existing between diet and skin health and appearance is well exemplified by the urticarial eruptions which occur through the circulation of a foreign or toxic protein in the blood stream. Among foods particularly associated with uticaria, in susceptible individuals, are shellfish, strawberries, eggs, game, etc., and their toxicity may be due to decomposition or putrefaction, or if the food itself is healthy, to the penetration of protein material into the blood stream without proper digestion, or to allergy on the part of the individual concerned.

Here the skin has been the first indicator, sometimes the only one, that all is not well with the proper functioning of the body.

Similarly, the skin can be, and often is the first (and in the absence of a serious deficiency, possibly, the only) indicator of a deficiency in the diet. Much has been written concerning the role of the vitamins and other food factors in skin health. In the following brief notes, these are considered from the angle of their oral administration and not from any external application.

THE VITAMINS

A brief discussion of the various vitamins is given in this chapter, together with a note concerning the various foodstuffs in which they occur. (For a more detailed discussion of the role of vitamins applied externally in relation to skin conditions, reference should be made to the paragraph entitled Vitamins in the chapter on Skin Nutrition, Chapter 4.)

DEFINITION OF " VITAMINS ". H. R. Rosenberg (*Chemistry and Physiology of the Vitamins*, New York : Interscience Publishers, 1945) has defined the vitamins as . . . *organic compounds which are required for the normal growth and maintenance of life of animals, including man, who, as a rule, are unable to synthesise these compounds by anabolic processes that are independent of environment other than air, and which compounds are effective in small amounts, do not furnish energy, and are not utilised as building units for the structure of the organism but are essential for the transformation of energy and for the regulation of the metabolism of structural units.*

VITAMIN A. The relationship of an adequate vitamin A intake to proper keratinisation of the skin appears fairly well proven. Hyperkeratosis involving deposition of keratinous material in the hair follicle has been proved to be symptomatic of a vitamin A deficiency in laboratory animals, and there is evidence also to show that this applies to man. Lehman and Rappaporti (*J. Amer. med. Assoc.*, 1940, **114**, 386) concluded that vitamin A avitaminosis is much more common than is supposed, and that various skin lesions classified under hyperkeratosis are inextricably associated with a sub-optimum supply of vitamin A. Swift concluded as a result of a large series of investigations involving cases with pruritis vulvae and kraurosis that " Leukoplakia, kraurosis, neurotic pruritis and atrophic vulvitis are varying names which have been given to conditions resulting from the same deficiency, i.e. lack of absorption of vitamin A caused by achlorhydria ".

Occurrence. Fish-liver oils,[1] escarole,[1] kale,[1] parsley,[1] turnip greens, [1] apricots, bananas (also plantain), butter, cantaloupe, carrots, cheese (whole milk), cherries, cream, crude yellow vegetable oils, egg-yolk, green vegetables, liver, cow's milk (fresh, dried, evaporated), oysters, prunes, salmon, spinach, tomatoes, yellow vegetables.

Stability. Practically no loss occurs in canning of foodstuffs owing to absence of oxygen. In ordinary cooking, where oxygen is present, some loss occurs.

Clinical aspects. An early clinical symptom of vitamin A deficiency is night blindness or nyctalopia. Vitamin A is an aid towards establishing the resistance of the body to infections in general ; it is not a specific in preventing infections. Xerophthalmia, a characteristic eye disease, may result from marked deficiency of this vitamin. Clinical diagnosis of vitamin A deficiency may be aided by bio-photometer tests of dark adaptation.

THE VITAMIN B COMPLEX

The " vitamin B complex " contains a number of nutritional factors including vitamins B_1, B_2, B_6 and B_{12}, pantothenic acid, choline, biotin, inositol, folic acid, nicotinic acid, niacin, etc., which are briefly described below :

VITAMIN B_1 (thiamine chloride, aneurine chloride) is essentially associated with the metabolism of carbohydrates. In its absence pyruvic acid accumulates in the tissue which then loses its power of oxygen absorption. The first and most serious symptoms of vitamin B_1 deficiency

[1] Outstanding source.

occur in the heart and nervous system. Vitamin B_1 is rapidly lost in the tissues and since it is not stored in, nor synthesised by, the body, normal health cannot be maintained unless the diet, *regularly contains a sufficiency of this vitamin.* [It should be mentioned that *excessive* doses of vitamin B_1 *concentrates* may interfere with the bodily metabolism of other members of the vitamin B complex.] Apart from its implication in the maintenance of normal health there is at present no evidence connecting this vitamin with cosmetic appearance. Bodily requirements of vitamin B_1 can be met by the intake of a well-balanced diet.

Occurrence. Rice polishings, dried yeast, peas, beans, oatmeal, wholewheat, lean pork; appreciable sources are contributed by such foods in the diet as milk, fruit and vegetables.

Stability. Fairly stable to heat in an acid medium, but rapidly destroyed in an alkaline medium (e.g. use of $NaCHO_3$ in cooking). About half of the vitamin is lost in cooking, due to its water solubility.

Clinical aspects. Vitamin B_1 is of value in healing and preventing beri-beri. It is also of value in correcting and preventing anorexia of dietary origin. It has been used with beneficial results in the treatment of neuritis of many kinds. Clinical diagnosis of vitamin B_1 deficiency may be aided by biological assay of the urinary excretion test.

VITAMIN B_2 (Riboflavin, Lactoflavin). This vitamin has been shown to be necessary for the growth of animals. Landor and Pallister (*Trans. R. Soc. Trop. Med. Hyg.*, 1935, **2**, 133) stated that it had been found of value in the treatment of avitaminosis B_2 involving eczema of the scrotum and of the angles of the mouth. Sebrell and Butler (*Pub. Hlth. Rep., Wash.*, 1939, **54**, 2, 121) claim that reddened lesions of the lips and fissures in the angles of the mouth are symptoms of ariboflavinosis or vitamin B_2 deficiency.

There is evidence to show that vitamin B_2 can be synthesised in the intestinal tract and (except in the treatment of vitamin B_2 deficiency states) there is little evidence to indicate that this vitamin is of therapeutic value.

Occurrence. Milk, Malted Barley, Green vegetables. Reasonably substantia amounts of riboflavine have been found to occur in certain beers (*See* paragraph on " What Diet? ")

Stability. Vitamin B_2 resists heat and alkalis at ordinary cooking temperatures; but considerable loss occurs due to its solubility in water.

Clinical aspects. Vitamin B_2, as first isolated, was thought to be a single entity. and, as such, was found to prevent pellagra. It has since been found to be a complex of many factors.

VITAMIN B_6 (Pyridoxine Hydrochloride). Smith and Martin (*Proc. Soc. exp. Biol.*, 1940, **43**, 660) have stated Vitamin B_6 to be useful in the treatment of lip lesions (cheilitis). It has also been claimed to be a necessary factor for the utilisation of unsaturated fatty acids.

C. S. Wright, M. H. Samitz and H. Brown (*Arch. Derm. Syph., Chicago*, 1943, **47**, 651) gave pyridoxine (vitamin B_6) to a group of patients with seborrhoeic dermatitis, atopic eczema with seborrhoeic features and eczematous eruptions of unknown etiology. The immediate response in a great many patients following injections of pyridoxine was indeed striking, many of the patients expressing amazement at the results. Other patients with identically similar appearance clinically, showed little or no response. From these results the authors suggest that if vitamin B complex therapy is to be of definite value in the treatment of dermatoses of the seborrhoeic or eczematous type, the pyridoxine content must be adequate.

The exact role of vitamin B_6 in human nutrition has not been established. If it *is* essential it would appear that the daily requirement is met by means of an ordinary mixed diet, as there is no evidence of any dietary deficiency of this vitamin. Vitamin B_6 may be of importance in reaction to stress. (*See* Vitamins and Stress.)

Occurrence. Yeast, liver, cereals. Also prepared synthetically.

VITAMIN B_{12} (Cyanocobalaminum). This is the essential anti-pernicious anaemia factor of liver. Supplementary human feeding may be an advantage and assist growth. It may also be of interest in relation to stress. (*See* Vitamins and Stress.)

Occurrence. The richest sources are the livers of ruminant animals. According to Wakelam (*Manufacturing Chemist*, 1952) there is no evidence that any of the higher animals are able to synthesise this vitamin.

PANTOTHENIC ACID. Pantothenic acid (Chick anti-dermatitis factor), is present in all living tissues, and is considered to be a member of the vitamin B complex. It came into " cosmetical " prominence on account of its claimed properties as an " anti-grey hair " vitamin. It appears to be true that either pantothenic acid or para-amino-benzoic acid can cure achromotrichia produced by artificial feeding of certain animals, such as rats or mice on a diet deficient in these elements. So far there is no evidence that such conditions bear any relationship to the condition known as grey hair in human beings.

Certain members of the vitamin B complex are also components of certain enzymes. The name vitazyme was suggested by von Euler and Zondek (*Skand. Arch. Physiol.*, 1934, **68**, 232) for vitamins which function in the organism by combining with a colloidal carrier (protein) to form an enzyme (e.g. riboflavin is a constituent of Warburg's yellow enzyme, thiamin of carboxylase, and nicotinic of certain dehydrogenases). Thus their relationship to the skin and mucous membranes is not surprising. Gross (*Arch. Derm. Syph., Chicago*, March 1941, **43**, 504) has presented a series of cases involving non-pellagrous eruptions due to a deficiency of the vitamin B complex.

Occurrence. Meat, Milk, Cereals. Also prepared synthetically.

No specific human conditions have been correlated with a pantothenic acid deficiency and little is known regarding its role in human nutrition.

CHOLINE. This is considered to be an important member of the vitamin B complex, its function having been correlated with the utilisation of fatty acids in the body. It is believed that a normal mixed diet contains an adequate amount for ordinary human needs.

Occurrence. The best dietary source of choline is egg yolk[1] though liver,[1] dried yeast,[1] brain,[1] kidney,[1] etc., can all be considered good sources.

BIOTIN (vitamin H). It is believed that a normal mixed diet (together with a certain amount of intestinal bacterial synthesis) ensures an adequate supply of this substance.

Occurrence. Liver,[1] yeast,[1] and egg yolk.[1] (The human body also synthesises a part of its biotin requirements by means of intestinal bacteria.)

INOSITOL. The role of this member of the vitamin B complex in human nutrition is not known.

Occurrence. Present in animal tissue, plant cereals, plant brans and seeds.

FOLIC ACID (Pteroylglutamic acid). Occurs in nature in the form of a peptide linkage. Folic acid has been shown to be essential for the production of red cells, white cells and platelets, in various animals, and appears to be essential for normal blood production in man. It may be of interest in relation to stress. (*See* Vitamins and Stress.)

Occurrence. Liver,[1] yeast,[1] etc. (Also synthesised to a considerable extent by intestinal bacteria.)

PARA-AMINO-BENZOIC ACID. Para-amino-benzoic acid is usually included as a member of the vitamin B group, but its exact role and necessity in human nutrition has not been established.

NICOTINIC ACID. NIACIN (Nicotinic acid amide). These are essential to human nutrition but the bodily requirements for these substances appear to be met by a normal mixed diet.

Occurrence. Rice polishings,[1] liver,[1] and lean meat[1], yeast, potatoes, and vegetables.

[1] Outstanding source.

VITAMIN C (Ascorbic Acid). This vitamin regulates the processes of oxidation-reduction in the living cell. Its deficiency results in increased capillary fragility, and appears to be bound up with dental caries and gingivitis. Apart then from its necessity in order to maintain bodily health and prevent scurvy, it is also a factor in the health of the gums. There is evidence that vitamin C is a clinical necessity for the rapid and healthy healing of wounds.

Occurrence. Citrus fruits,[1] parsley,[1] peppers (green or red),[1] raw new cabbage,[1] tomato juice,[1] watercress,[1] cranberries, cucumbers, fresh fruits, fresh raw vegetables, fresh raw liver, pimentos, potatoes, tomatoes.

Stability. Vitamin C is readily affected by heat, by washing and by storage. It is rapidly destroyed in the preparation of foodstuffs by heating; less rapidly on storage.

Clinical aspects. Vitamin C prevents and cures scurvy and is of value in early and latent scurvy characterised by haemorrhages, sore and swollen joints, bleeding gums and asthenia. Dental caries, pyorrhoea, certain gum infections, anorexia, anaemia, under-nutrition and infection may be benefited by vitamin C, but only when it is definitely shown that these symptoms are the result of a deficiency or sub-optimal supply of the vitamin.

VITAMIN D OR D_2.[2] Several substances capable of preventing and curing rickets are included under this term. Originally the term D_1 was applied to a mixture believed to be pure vitamin D. D_2 denotes calciferol.

The difference between D_2 and D_3 is that while man, and usually rats, respond equally well to vitamin D_2 and D_3, chickens are *relatively* insensitive to D_2 and require very much greater amounts of D_2 than D_3 to get similar results.

Vitamin D_3 is 7-dehydrocholesterol and is the form of vitamin that occurs in fish liver oils.

Vitamin D is intimately bound up with the deposition of calcium and phosphorous in the body and the formation of healthy bones and teeth. In its absence rickets is produced. So far no changes in the health of the skin have been linked primarily with a deficiency of vitamin D, though recently vitamin D has given dramatically favourable results in the treatment of cutaneous tuberculosis and hence demonstrated, for the first time, that vitamin therapy may cure a condition which is not due to a vitamin deficiency. (*See* Chapter 4; Vitamin D in Skin Nutrition.)

[1] Outstanding source.

[2] *Vitamers.* This new term was coined at Gibson Island Vitamin Conference, July 1942, *to describe and identify vitamin factors that produce similar effects in different species of plants or animals but which may be different chemical substances.* Importance is attached to the principle that animal tests are indispensable to determine symptoms of vitamin deficiency, but are worthless to determine what will cure those symptoms when observed in humans (*Science*, 15 Jan., 1943, p. 57).

Occurrence Fish-liver oils[1] (Ling, European), butter (variable), clams, cream, egg-yolk, haddock, halibut, herring, oysters, salmon, sardines.

Stability. Vitamin D has a high stability to heat, and is consequently retained in canned and cooked foods.

Clinical aspects. Vitamin D is recognised as a specific medicament in the treatment of infantile rickets, osteomalacia and spasmophilia (infantile tetany); diseases which are the manifestations of defective calcium and phosphorus metabolism. Clinical diagnosis of vitamin D deficiency may be aided by X-ray examinations and blood phosphatase tests.

VITAMIN E (the tocopherols possess the same physiological effects as vitamin E). Vitamin E has been used in the past for the treatment of sterility and habitual abortion. However, it has proved disappointing in use and as Meiklejohn puts it (*Practitioner*, Dec. 1949, p. 359), "It is one of those embarrassing vitamins that has been offered to us in synthetic form before there is any real certainty that it is necessary for man"; or even more strongly as F. J. Stare and G. V. Mann (Dept. Nutrition, Harvard School of Public Health) state: "First let us dispose of vitamin E or the tocopherols. These are interesting antioxidants . . . they play a role in experimental nutrition. They have no known function in human health or disease; let us not imply (at least till facts are available) that the dietician, nutritionist, and physician should further complicate practical human nutrition with a consideration of the vitamin E content of the diet. . . ." (*J. Amer. Oil. Chem. Soc.*, June 1951, p. 232.)

Occurrence. Wheat germ,[1] butter (pasture-fed cows), cereal seeds, eggs, leafy vegetables, legumes, meat, milk, molasses, peanuts, vegetable oils.

VITAMIN F. The so-called "vitamin F" is discussed in Chapter 4 (under the paragraph entitled Unsaturated Fatty Acids).

RECOMMENDATIONS FOR DAILY ALLOWANCES

The following amounts of nutrients have been suggested as being desirable to maintain normal health:

	U.S. National Research Council Recommendations Daily Allowances (1945)	*British Medical Association. Recommendation* (1949)
Calories	2564	2554
Protein (g.)	65	71
Calcium (mgm.)	917	917

[1] Outstanding source.

	U.S. National Research Council Recommendations Daily Allowances (1945)	*British Medical Association. Recommendation* (1949)
Iron (mgm.)	11·8	11·8
Vitamin A (mixed diet (I.U.)) .	4460	4570
Thiamine (mg.)	1·27	1·02
Riboflavine (mg.)	1·74	1·53
Niacine (mgm.)	12·7	10·2
Vitamin C (mgm.)	71	20–30
Vitamin D (I.U.)	130	150

[*Report of the Committee on Nutrition*, British Medical Association, 1950.]

Fat

So far as fat is concerned the B.M.A. Committee on Nutrition states : " Whilst the Committee is unaware of any evidence that there is a minimum daily intake of fat required to maintain the health and well-being of the human body, it finds ample support for the opinion that fat (visible and invisible) should provide at least 25 per cent. of the calorie value of the diet in order to maintain the general character and food habits of the people of the U.K. If the diet is not to become bulky and unsatisfying it is appropriate to increase this to 35 per cent., as the energy demands of the body rise with increasing physical effort."

VITAMINS AND STRESS. R. S. Goodhart [1] and N. Joliffe [2] (*The Merck Report*, Oct. 1952, p. 7) have pointed out that the general adaptation syndrome as defined by Selye (*J. Clin. Endocrin.*, 1946, **6**, 117) is "the sum of all non-specific systematic reactions of the body which ensue upon a long-continued exposure to stress. This is distinct from specific adaptive reactions which endow the body with resistance to the particular agent to which it has been previously exposed. . . ." In discussing vitamins and other nutrients in adaptation to stress, these authors state : " Among the known B vitamins which seem likely to prove to be the most directly involved in reactions to stress include vitamin B_6, pantothenic acid, folic acid and vitamin B_{12}. In addition there are one or more unknown substances present in liver and yeast which appear to have considerable bearing on the nature of the organisms' reaction to stress." They conclude : " It would be premature at this time to predict

[1] Scientific Director of the National Vitamin Foundation Inc.

[2] Director, Bureau of Nutrition, Dept. of Health, New York City ; President, National Vitamin Foundation Inc.

which vitamin(s) will prove to be of the most practical importance in enabling humans to withstand acute and chronic stress. . . . What can be said without fear of contradiction is that optimal nutrition with vitamins and the other necessary nutrients helps to maintain the organisms' resistance to stress at its maximum. As stated by the Committee on Therapeutic Nutrition of the Food and Nutrition Board, National Research Council (Committee on Therapeutic Nutrition, Food and Nutrition Board, Therapeutic Nutrition with special reference to military situations, Washington, D.C. National Research Council, 1951) "Adequate nutrition is prerequisite for the maintenance of good health and optimum efficiency. . . ."

It must always be remembered that vitamins are *accessory* food factors essential to health, and that, though important, they are not the only factors involved. To maintain bodily health, proteins, carbohydrates and fats and a number of mineral salts are necessary.

Calcium is necessary for the teeth and bones, and a deficiency is also believed to be associated with certain forms of urticaria.

CALCIUM IN FOOD

Daily amount required for an adult, 917 mgm.

Food	*Customary portions*	*Calcium, mgm.*	*Food*	*Customary portions*	*Calcium, mgm.*
Milk	½ pt.	332	Bread, whole wheat	2 oz.	28
Buttermilk	½ pt.	298	String beans	2 oz.	28
Cheese, cheddar	1 oz.	281	Carrots	2 oz.	26
Cauliflower	4 oz.	139	Cabbage, white, raw	2 oz.	26
Molasses	1½ oz.	110	Bread, white	2 oz.	18
Figs, dried	2 oz.	92	Oatmeal, uncooked	1 oz.	18
Spinach	4 oz.	87	Wheat bran	½ oz.	17
Beans, kidney, dried	2 oz.	75	Wheat, entire	1 oz.	15
Bread, brown	2 oz.	73	Peas, green, fresh	2 oz.	14
Dandelion	4 oz.	72	Tomatoes	1 (4 oz.)	13
Maple syrup	1½ oz.	46	Potatoes	3 oz.	12
Orange	1 (6 oz.)	44	Bread, white, salt-free	2 oz.	9
Rutabaga	2 oz.	42	Cornflakes	1 oz.	4
Celery	2 oz.	39			
Egg	2 oz.	39			

Phosphorous and magnesium are necessary for the same reason as calcium.

Kruse, McCollum and co-workers have shown that a deficiency of magnesium in the rat produces vasodilation and hyperaemia of exposed skin areas.

IRON. The value of iron in the formation of red blood cells is well known, but it has been shown that iron acts only in the presence of traces of copper.

Iron in Food

Daily amount required for an adult, 11·8 mgm.

Food	*Customary portions*	*Iron, mgm.*	*Food*	*Customary portions*	*Iron, mgm.*
Liver, calves' . .	4 oz.	6·13	Peas, green . .	2 oz.	0·94
Spinach	4 oz.	4·54	Bread, whole wheat	2 oz.	0·89
Beef, loin . . .	4 oz.	4·20	Cornflakes . .	1 oz.	0·82
Molasses	1½ oz.	3·40	Sweet potatoes .	3 oz.	0·78
Oysters	½ doz.	3·12	Potatoes . . .	3 oz.	0·72
	(3½ oz.)		Bananas . . .	1 (4 oz.)	0·68
Raisins	1 oz.	1·99	Milk, whole . .	½ pt.	0·66
Bread, brown .	2 oz.	1·70	Bread, white .	2 oz.	0·59
Dates	1 oz.	1·44	Almonds . . .	½ oz	0·58
Egg	2 oz.	1·43	String beans . .	2 oz	0·54
Bread, Graham .	2 oz.	1·42	Onions . . .	4 oz.	0·51
Beets, root . . .	2 oz.	1·34	Tomatoes . .	1 (4 oz.)	0·50
Fish, fried . . .	4 oz.	1·25	Apples, fresh .	1 (4 oz.)	0·43
Strawberries . .	6 oz.	1·22	Turnips . . .	2 oz.	0·40
Wheat bran . .	½ oz.	1·21	Pineapple . . .	4 oz.	0·36
Prunes, dried . .	1 oz.	1·08	Carrots . . .	2 oz.	0·34
Oatmeal, uncooked	1 oz.	1·08	Peanuts . . .	½ oz.	0·32
Lettuce, leaf . .	2 oz.	1·00	Cabbage, white, raw	2 oz.	0·28

The following tables give the uses of various mineral salts in the body and the foods in which they are found :

Mineral Salts

Substance	*Occurrence in the body*	*Function in the body*
Sodium	Blood and other fluids.	Regulates osmotic pressure, assists in regulation of heart beat.
Potassium	Constituent of cells, pericardial fluids	Helps to maintain normal alkalinity and regulates osmotic pressure ; assists in regulating normal contraction and relaxation of muscles.
Calcium	In bones and teeth.	Builds bones and teeth ; essential for coagulation of blood ; regulates contraction and relaxation of heart muscle ; assists in regulation of mineral metabolism.

Substance	*Occurrence in the body*	*Function in the body*
Magnesium	In muscle tissue, blood and lymph.	Preservation of mineral balance; antagonistic to calcium in body.
Phosphorus	Constituent of bones and teeth; constituent of every cell, muscle, nerve and brain. Constituent of lecithin, blood and glandular tissue.	Builds bones and teeth; essential to all cellular activity; as lecithin, assists cell to connect with its environment; assists in maintaining normal reaction of body.
Chlorine	Chiefly present as sodium chloride, essential constituent of hydrochloric acid in gastric juice.	Assists in digestion of protein as part of hydrochloric acid; assists in regulating osmotic pressure as sodium chloride.
Iodine	Part of thyroxin, an essential element in the structure of the thyroid gland.	Essential constituent of the thyroid gland; an important regulator of the basal metabolism; an essential part of thyroxin, stimulating development, indispensable to growth; preventive in the development of simple goitre.
Iron	Essential constituent of haemoglobin; constituent of chromatin substances.	As part of haemoglobin carries oxygen to the tissues; assists in the elimination of carbon dioxide.
Sulphur	Constituent of protein, e.g. cystine, partly as a constituent of the chemical regulator glutathione, partly as conjugated sulphates.	Essential to growth. Regulation of oxidation processes.
Water	Fluid medium in all body fluids, blood, lymph, digestive juices, secretions of body; contained in all cells.	Furnishes fluid medium for all body excretions and secretions, prevents friction; assists in elimination, digestion, metabolism.

Substance	*Source in Food*	*Daily requirements*
Sodium	As sodium chloride (NaCl) in all foods except pure fats and carbohydrates.	Average diet sufficient. Requirements from 1½ to 2 g. a day.
Potassium	Lean meat, milk, most plants.	Average diet sufficient.
Calcium	Milk, Cheese, nuts, cereals, vegetables.	Adults, 0·917 g.
Magnesium	Cereals, potatoes, most plants.	Adequate in average diet.
Phosphorus	Milk, meat, egg yolk, nuts, vegetables, fruits.	Adults, 1·32 g. Children 1 g. or more.

Substance	*Source in Food*	*Daily requirements*
Chlorine	As sodium chloride in all foods except pure fats, pure carbohydrates.	Intake sufficient in average diet.
Iodine	Sea food, marine algae, certain plants.	About 5 mg. a year for adults.
Iron	Glandular organs: liver, kidney; gizzard; egg yolk; green vegetables, spinach in particular; fruits: dried apricots, peaches, raisins, etc. Whole grain cereals.	Adults, 11·8 mg.; during pregnancy and lactation, 22 mg. Children, 7½ to 10½ mg. per 1000 calories.
Sulphur	Chiefly protein foods.	Diet adequate in protein is adequate in sulphur.
Water	As water, fruit juices, milk; all fruits except those dehydrated or artificially dried.	6 to 8 glasses daily in addition to that supplied in food.

What Diet?

It is necessary to choose a diet which is *as mixed and as well balanced as possible*. Many foods and drinks [1] formerly despised have been found to contain valuable factors. *In general, if the diet includes meat, fish, butter, eggs, fresh green vegetables, wholemeal bread (or other cereal foods), a plentiful supply of milk, and fresh fruits in variety there is little reason to suppose that any deficiency in diet will occur*. In those cases in which the individual is allergic to some particular constituent of the above, e.g. eggs, or cannot digest wholemeal bread, then recourse to any standard work on dietetics will soon demonstrate how any deficiency that may occur can be made up.

Above all, one should avoid fancy diets designed to slim. *Never slim without medical advice* but only under medical instruction. Some people are just naturally fat and attempts to slim may lead to serious consequences. Some few years ago there was a craze for certain diets, in particular the Hay diet, which was extremely well debunked in the *Lancet*, 26 June, 1937. Hay's idea that carbohydrates and protein should not be eaten at the same time was shown to be a fallacy, and Dr. Eugene Foldes showed how completely experience and experiment contradicted this theory in that the amount of acid secreted after

[1] For example it has been shown that two important members of the vitamin B complex, namely riboflavine and nicotinic occur in various beers. The amounts of these substances occurring in different beers have been estimated at the School of Malting and Brewing, Birmingham, and at the Central Research Station of the Ministry of Food and it has been found (Drummond and Moran, *Nature*, London, 1944, **153**, 99; *Lancet*, 12 Feb. 1944, p. 220) that a pint of "even the British beer of that period" may add 283 to 962 μg. of riboflavine together with some 400 μg. of nicotinic acid. Drummond and Moran also point out that it is a reasonable assumption that beer also contains appreciable amounts of biotin, pantothenic acid and inositol. Tea also provides a small amount of riboflavine; a breakfast cup may contain 10 μg.

taking carbohydrates was not very different from that after taking protein. Even if there were, it would not wholly interrupt starch digestion, and even if it did so, fermentation in the stomach would not follow. Against this theory also is the intimate admixture of protein and carbohydrate in many natural foods, and the fact that the contents of the stomach ferment only when there is an *absence* of hydrochloric acid in the gastric secretion.

VEGETARIANISM. Vegetable foods provide a valuable and comparatively inexpensive supply of carbohydrate, fat, protein, mineral salts and vitamins. Unfortunately a purely vegetarian diet may be deficient, because such foods are less digestible by the gastric juice, and owing to their bulk, fermentation and cellulose content produce acceleration of peristalsis with reduced protein absorption. In addition, it is believed that animal protein contains nutrients other than protein whose presence in this diet is of great value; for example, Meiklejohn (Dept. of Medicine, University of Edinburgh, *Practitioner*, Oct. 1949, p. 357) drew attention to the "animal protein" factor, pointing out that *evidence from various animal feeding experiments had recently brought to light the fact that there may be some virtue in animal protein that is not present in vegetable protein.* This factor in animal protein was found to occur in good amounts in dried cow dung, and was later identified as vitamin B_{12}—cyanocobalaminum, the anti-pernicious anaemia principle.

These deficiencies in vegetable protein may result in impaired development of growing children and in diminished power of resistance to certain acute diseases, particularly in the convalescent stages. It has been noted that persons on a minimum protein diet make but slow recovery from such illnesses.

A wide gap separates *optimum* health and *actual disease*, and in between there are many persons on a diet deficient in some respect who may only exhibit such general symptoms as lassitude, irritability, neurasthenia and various neuroses, indigestion, sore or inflamed gums or skin irritability and lesions. Others may feel quite fit and then suddenly succumb to a minor illness from which the majority of persons would speedily recover. For this reason *individual cases cannot* be used as arguments in assessing the relative merits of animal and vegetable diets. *Strict vegetarianism*, however, is nothing more than *a fallacy*. This appears to be recognised by the so-called vegetarians themselves who usually include foods of animal origin such as eggs, butter, cheese, milk and even fish.

Animal proteins (meat, eggs, fish, butter, cheese and milk) are good sources of protein of biological value and of certain of the vitamins, and such a modification is quite satisfactory to establish and maintain bodily health and fitness. It cannot be too strongly urged that, in the absence of special therapeutic conditions which may involve a special diet, the best thing to do is to mix the diet, including a sufficiency of the foods which modern science has shown to possess value in virtue of the quality of their protein and their content of mineral salts and vitamins.

Alcohol and Skin Health

Consumption of alcohol increases perspiration and heat loss through the skin, and causes dilation of the blood vessels. *Constant* dilation of these vessels produces the red nose sometimes associated with chronic alcoholism, though alcohol is not the only aggravating factor in all such cases. In *skin diseases*, therefore, alcoholic beverages are better avoided and also strong tea and coffee in excess.

In normal skin health the position is radically different, and it is sheer unadulterated nonsense to suggest that the ordinary moderate consumption of alcoholic beverages is deleterious to bodily health or to natural beauty. Wines and spirits have a definite psychological and social value and are considered a token of hospitality. They repress psychological inhibitions, promote a general feeling of comfort and well-being the value of which, in the strain and stress of modern life, should not be under-estimated. By stimulation of the gastric juices, they improve the appetite and in *moderation* may thus improve the digestion. Spirits, however, should be taken well diluted to avoid gastric irritation.

The above are impartial scientific facts. One's reaction to them on ethical grounds depends on prejudice, either for or against. Prohibition in other countries has led to worse addictions (W. E. Dixon, *Brit. med. J.*, 11/21, 822). Sir J. Barre (*Brit. med. J.*, 11/22, 199) attributed unrest to the expensiveness of alcohol and stated he would be sorry to see the moderate use of alcohol abolished, and the eminent physiologist, Professor Starling, maintained that, in moderation, alcohol does not shorten life as compared with total abstinence. (*Lancet*, 1/13, 705.)

The Role of Sugar in Skin Diseases

CARBOHYDRATE INTOLERANCE. *Those who associate dilated blood vessels in the nose and face with the consumption of alcohol may be surprised to learn that sugar (and stimulants such as tea and coffee) may produce similar results.* The necessity for reducing the intake of sugar and sweets in certain skin diseases is well known, and Stokes, Beerman and Ingraham (*Amer. J. med. Sci.*, 1938, **195**, 562) have shown that intestinal carbohydrate intolerance produces local vasodilation in the skin. This facilitates the taking root of infection, because of its effect on the water retention and the formation of lactic acid which changes the pH and affects the local cellular and leucocytic reactions. Pillsbury and Kulchar (*Amer. J. med. Sci.*, 1935, **190**, 169) showed that intraperitoneal injections of hypertonic glucose solution in rabbits increased experimental staphylococcal infections of the skin.

On the other hand, sugar has many medicinal virtues, particularly in preventing liver damage and shock. Restriction of intake is usually necessary only in those cases in which there is intolerance to sugar or a skin disease is present. This exemplifies once again the value of *moderation in everything*.

Constipation Fallacies

The majority of beauty experts, and many dermatologists, have stressed the importance of *inner cleanliness* and skin health. To a certain extent this is true although " constipation ", which is so heavily condemned, is not so readily " defined ". *In the first place outward beauty is not always associated with perfect health.* One has only to compare the blotchy face of the adolescent with the delicate milk and roses complexion of many consumptives to realise this. It is, however, intimately built up with *general bodily metabolism*, and a vitamin or other deficiency, or an urticarial sensitivity is often demonstrated in the skin when a proof in other bodily organs is lacking. In fact, in the case quoted, the blotchy condition is evidence of changes in metabolism though these may be quite natural and not pathological.

Constipation is a much used but little understood word, and the condition arises not only from the lack of bulk or roughage in the diet—as a student of modern advertising might suppose—but from other and more important causes, e.g. excess or lack of muscular tone, nervous and other psychological causes, colonic irritation with production of periodic constrictions, obstruction due to intestinal kinking or displacement and tumours. Obviously administration of purgatives in a case of obstruction may prove dangerous, but even in normal cases, except where all other means have failed, the routine administration of aperients is to be deplored. Not only do they lead to looseness of the stools with consequent lack of muscûlar effect and tone but also there may be a deficiency of residual matter which aggravates the very condition which it is desired to cure. Many laxatives widely sold and used are of the *salts* type which produce a watery stool and in which there is a danger of loss of valuable nutrients from the body.

Healthy evacuation should be mildly firm, and *slight constipation is preferable to looseness.* If this fact is remembered a lot of damage may be avoided. Today, it is believed that little absorption of poisonous toxin occurs if the bowel contents are solid, but that unhealthy absorption of such contents occurs when they are rendered fluid; moreover, bacterial decomposition is facilitated. Witt (*Lancet*, 1937, **1**, 427) has pointed out that the ill effects of constipation are almost entirely psychogenic and due to worry over disturbance of *habit*. Linnell and Thompson (" Some Therapeutic Fallacies ", *Brit. med. J.*, 1943, p. 572) have drawn attention to the fact that there is seldom any urgency to open the bowels in acute infections under four or five days and then this should be done by enemata and not by purgatives.

Liquid paraffin is a mild and gentle lubricant and laxative and is especially valuable where there are haemorrhoids (so-called " piles "), or where there is present any lesion or soreness in the anal canal. Nevertheless, it is now known that the *regular* administration of liquid paraffin may lead to a deficiency of the fat-soluble vitamins in the body, which become dissolved in, and removed with, the paraffin. To obviate this it is suggested that medicinal paraffin should be saturated with the fat-soluble vitamins so that, at body temperatures, it will not rob the body of these factors. Mineral oils sometimes used in salad dressings may produce similar effects and it is considered that the presence of mineral oil in such a dressing should be declared to the purchaser. Whilst it is true that, in a fat-reducing diet some authorities recommend the avoidance of salad dressings unless made with mineral oils, the writer does not consider that such dressings should be sold without adequate labelling. There is good evidence that mineral oils can interfere not only with the absorption and retention of the fat-soluble vitamins but also with the carotene reserves of the body and with the absorption of calcium, phosphorous and vitamin K. It has been pointed out (*Brit. med. J.*, Aug. 1944, p. 199) that there is some evidence that the *prolonged administration* of mineral oils may cause gastro-intestinal symptoms accompanied by loss of weight, though this does not contra-indicate its *use as a laxative when given under medical supervision*. Similar warnings have appeared in the *Journal of the American Medical Association* (Dec. 1943, **123**, 15, 967).

In view of the oft repeated injunction to increase the roughage in the diet it may be remarked that bran, like most other remedies may be *valuable* in certain individuals who appear to possess a sluggish motion, and a lack of health which is alleviated by the consumption of some form of roughage.

Roughage, bran or other patented cereals (or their ilk) are not well tolerated in cases of hyper-irritability (which they aggravate) nor in gastritis or gastric hyperacidity. Many persons find such roughage irritant and painful and its use should be based upon one's individual reaction to the food in question and not taken blindly as a routine panacea.

The Ideal Weight

The tables given below for average weights and heights are those generally used; they must, however, be accepted with reserve. Free ("Mid-Year Scientific Section of the U.S. Proprietary Association", through *Drug All. Ind.*, Dec. 1949, p. 15) has questioned height-weight tables as a means of measuring obesity, pointing out that many athletes are (according to such tables) overweight; that such tables are more than thirty years old and that at best they were intended to be averages rather than optimum. Such tables pay no attention to differences in bone structure and the different build of individuals. Free pointed out that physical exercise as a means of reducing weight has been overemphasised since it would take the equivalent of a *thirty-six mile hike to reduce ONE pound*, and in most cases the exercises increase appetite to a point such that intake offsets output.

THE "OLD FASHIONED", IDEAL WEIGHT. [For every inch in height above 5 ft add $5\frac{1}{2}$ lb. to 110, which is the normal weight at 5 ft. For instance: a person 66 in. tall should weigh approximately 110 lb., plus six times $5\frac{1}{2}$ = 143 lb.]

AVERAGE HEIGHTS AND WEIGHTS. The weights are for persons with shoes on, and without coat and vest (which weigh from 3 to 7 lb., depending on height of individual and season of the year).

(*Weight in lb.*)

MEN

Height	15–19 *years*	20–24 *years*	25–29 *years*	30–34 *years*	35–39 *years*	40–44 *years*	45–49 *years*	50–54 *years*
5 ft. 0 in.	113	119	124	127	129	132	134	135
5 ft. 1 in.	115	121	126	129	131	134	136	137
5 ft. 2 in.	118	124	128	131	133	136	138	139
5 ft. 3 in.	121	127	131	134	136	139	141	142
5 ft. 4 in.	124	131	134	137	140	142	144	145
5 ft. 5 in.	128	135	138	141	144	146	148	149
5 ft. 6 in.	132	139	142	145	148	150	152	153
5 ft. 7 in.	136	142	146	149	152	154	156	157
5 ft. 8 in.	140	146	150	154	157	159	161	162
5 ft. 9 in.	144	150	154	158	162	164	166	167
5 ft. 10 in.	148	154	158	163	167	169	171	172
5 ft. 11 in.	153	158	163	168	172	175	177	178
6 ft. 0 in.	158	163	169	174	178	181	183	184
6 ft. 1 in.	163	168	175	180	184	187	190	191
6 ft. 2 in.	168	173	181	186	191	194	197	198
6 ft. 3 in.	173	178	187	192	197	201	204	205

(*Weight in lb.*)

WOMEN

Height	15–19 *years*	20–24 *years*	25–29 *years*	30–34 *years*	35–39 *years*	40–44 *years*	45–49 *years*	50–54 *years*
4 ft. 11 in.	110	113	116	119	122	126	129	131
5 ft. 0 in.	112	115	118	121	124	128	131	133
5 ft. 1 in.	114	117	129	123	126	130	133	135
5 ft. 2 in.	117	120	122	125	129	133	136	138
5 ft. 3 in.	120	123	125	128	132	136	139	141
5 ft. 4 in.	123	126	129	132	136	139	142	144
5 ft. 5 in.	126	129	132	136	140	143	146	148
5 ft. 6 in.	130	133	136	140	144	147	151	152
5 ft. 7 in.	134	137	140	144	148	151	157	157
5 ft. 8 in.	138	141	144	148	152	155	162	162
5 ft. 9 in.	141	145	148	152	156	159	166	166
5 ft. 10 in.	145	149	152	155	159	162	170	170
5 ft. 11 in.	150	153	155	158	162	166	171	174
6 ft. 0 in.	155	157	159	162	165	169	173	177

For the reasons stated below, any such average weight tables must be accepted with considerable scepticism.

OBESITY. If many of the articles which have appeared in both the medical and the lay press *were* to be believed the problem of obesity is very simple, viz. excess of calorific intake (in the form of food), over calorific expenditure (in the form of energy), results in the production of fat. Such writers usually advise one to " take more exercise " or " eat less fattening foods ", or both!

Anybody who takes the trouble to observe the, often, surprisingly large amounts of fattening foods eaten by supposedly small and wiry men (and, very often, the complete lack of exercise taken by such people), in comparison with comparatively small helpings of food, and often quite vigorous exercises (taken in the hope of reducing), by obese people *knows* the above argument to be fallacious.

The fallacy of this argument is even more evident when one often tries to fatten the naturally thin person by " feeding up ".

The first erroneous supposition made in the above argument concerns the supposedly slimming effects of exercise, the second—an even more serious one—is the supposition that obesity is due to fat, whereas it is usually due to excessive retention of water by the tissues.

So far as the role of exercise is concerned, medical opinion has undergone considerable revision in recent years as a result of realising just how much work *is* required in order to dispose of some " superfluous calories ". Professor C. E. Dodds * (" Discussion on Obesity ", *Proc. R. Soc. Med.*,

* Now *Sir* Charles Edward Dodds (Courtauld Professor of Biochemistry, University of London).

May 1950, p. 339) points out that: "Every pint of beer requires half an hour of Squash, or if the person is not capable of expending energy at this rate the equivalent of a five mile walk would just about equal it. . . . An even more depressing calculation is that during an average dinner in pre-war days something between 700–800 calories could be consumed in the form of alcohol. In order to work this off it would be necessary to play Squash for five and a half hours or alternatively to climb Ben Nevis several times."

Millman (*Today's Health*, May 1951, **29**, 14) has pointed out that to lose a pound of body fat by physical activity a person would have to saw wood for ten and a half hours, lay 14,731 bricks, or shovel 114,000 pounds of sand. Moreover weight reduction through exercise is not a "loss in fat" but is fluid loss in perspiration and weight so arduously lost is, as Allweiss points out (*Industr. Med.*, 1949, **1**, 63) quickly regained by drinking water. A similar lack of efficacy accompanies massage, steam baths and similar treatments though it is not denied that as pointed out by Douthwaite (*Brit. med. J.*, 1951, **1**, 291) exercise can be of value to tone up muscles.

In discussing obesity Professor Dodds (*Proc. R. Soc. Med.*, May 1950, p. 339) states: ". . . the real problem is that we do not really understand the mechanism of weight regulation. General experience shows very clearly that subjects fall under two headings. (A) People who maintain a constant weight over many years despite excessive intake of food and (B) the second group who respond immediately to an increase in calorie intake by putting on weight." Professor Dodd continued: "I think very few people realise that an astonishing mechanism must be in constant operation. If one weighs the subject, at the same time of day, say on rising in the morning, the weight of the individual is astonishingly constant, assuming that the subject is neither gaining nor losing weight, the weight remains constant to within roughly one pound and this means in the person of average weight, a reproducibility of between 0·5 per cent. and 1·0 per cent. on a weight of over 1 cwt. This is astonishing when one considers to what influences the body weight might be subjected in twenty-four hours, such as varying degrees of exposure, output of fluid, perspiration and so forth."

During the subsequent discussion Dr. Raymond Green (*Proc. R. Soc. Med.*, May 1950) stated that ". . . much of the speculation and experiment about the origin of obesity was misdirected owing to its emphasis on fat instead of water. If we believed that people were overweight because of an excessive deposit of fat we were confronted by a series of insoluble dilemmas, because fat people do not eat more than their fellows and their absorption, their metabolism and their specific dynamic action are normal. Clinical and experimental evidence suggested that adiposity may be caused by damage to the hypothalamus, in which lies the central control station of water metabolism. Dr. Raymond Green concluded that a fat person is one whose adipose tissue is overhydrated rather than overfatted.

Mitchell (*J. clin. Nutr.*, Sept.-Oct. 1952, p. 70) has pointed out that the term " obesity " defies precise definition.

The dominance of hereditary factors in human obesity has been emphasised by Davenport (Carnegie Institution of Washington Publ. 1923, p. 176, through Mitchell, *J. clin. Nutr.*, Sept.-Oct. 1952), Gurney (" The Hereditary Factor in Obesity ", *Arch. int. Med.*, 1936, **57**, 557), and Angel (" Constitution in Female Obesity ", *Amer. J. Phys. Anthrop.*, 1949, **7**, 433).

Armstrong, Dublin, Wheatley and Marks (" Obesity and its Relation to Health and Disease ", *J. Amer. med. Ass.*, 1951, **147**, 1007) point out that " . . . In spite of the evidence that has accumulated on the serious effects of overweight on health and longevity . . . there is surprisingly little information available on the long-term results of weight reduction. Adequate long-term studies of weight reduction are few and indicate that only a minority of overweight persons persist in their effort long enough to reap the greatest potential benefit. Beyond that, we lack properly controlled studies to show whether or not the benefits of weight reduction in terms of health and longevity are as real and substantial as they are assumed to be. . . ."

It has long appeared evident to the author that the tacit assumption that, because many pathological conditions and diseases are *associated* with obesity, that they are the *causative* factors is a most unwarranted and unscientific conclusion. The mere fact that obesity has been blamed for so many bodily ailments is, in itself, suggestive that obesity is far more likely to be a common effect than the " cause ".

Dieting

Dieting should be carried out only on medical advice and under medical supervision. Where dieting *has been medically advised*, the following diets for reducing (or increasing) weights may be of interest in any case in which the patient appears doubtful, or has forgotten whether she should, or should not, eat a particular item of food.

Fat-Reducing Diet

Soups. Clear soups and broths, unsalted soup, made with little fat.
Cereals. Occasionally, the coarse kind, served with skimmed milk.
Bread. One slice at a meal.

Eggs. Boiled or poached, not fried or prepared with butter, cream or fat.

Dairy Products. Cheese made with skimmed milk.

Fish and Meats. Lean beef and pork, roasted or boiled. Lean chicken and turkey, roasted or boiled. Lamb chops. Boiled fish. Small portions only.

Vegetables. Greens, asparagus, beans, green peas, cabbage, cauliflower, brussels sprouts, onions, turnips, spinach, parsnips, carrots, mushrooms, watercress, green olives. Potatoes once or twice a week. Only enough butter for seasoning. No sauces.

Desserts. Fresh fruits only. Ices sweetened with saccharin or very little sugar.

Fruits. All raw fruits, except bananas.

Beverages. Buttermilk, skimmed milk, coffee or tea without sugar or cream. Since obesity is often related to *excess hydration* rather than to *excess fat*, in dieting to reduce weight, the intake of beverages —including water—(and particularly of salt in any form) should be curtailed.

To be avoided. Butter, cream, oily salad dressings, unless made with mineral oil.[1] Fats of all kinds, cereal foods, potatoes, sweets of all kinds. All of these must be taken very sparingly.

FOODS THAT INCREASE WEIGHT

	Portions giving 100 *calories*		*Portions giving* 100 *calories*
Bacon, fat	1 tablespoonful	Nuts	About 12
Butter	1 tablespoonful	Honey	1 tablespoonful
Cheese	1⅛ in. cube	Margarine	1 tablespoonful
Cream, thick	1⅓ tablespoonfuls	Olive oil or other vegetable oil	1 tablespoonful
Cream, thin	¼ cup	Raisins	¼ cup
Cream, whipped	2 tablespoonfuls	Rice, steamed	¾ cup
Dates	3 or 4	Sugar, brown	2 tablespoonfuls
Eggs	1⅓ small—1 large	Sugar, white	2 tablespoonfuls
Walnuts	About 12 medium size	Milk	⅝ cup
Figs	2 medium size		

Finally, always remember that " true beauty " is *not* just a matter of heights and weights but that it also involves, besides artificially added " make-up ", *a happy and pleasant expression.* Mere slimming for reasons of vanity will detract from, rather than add to, the latter characteristics.

[1] Salad dressings made with mineral oil, unless labelled either as drugs as " for special dietary uses only ", are in violation of the United States Food Drug and Cosmetic Act.

Mineral oil internally may be deleterious to health since among other things it prevents the utilisation of oil-soluble vitamins. [See discussion on mineral oils under " Constipation ", above.]

CHAPTER 4

SKIN PENETRATION AND SKIN NUTRITION

Skin Absorption and Penetration—Local Cosmetic Action—Vitamins and Hormones in Cosmetics—Unsaturated Fatty Acids—Lanolin—Protein Hydrolysates—Massage—The Hydration of Skin

THE claims advanced for the supposed nutritional benefits of nourishing creams are based upon the assumption that the underlying cause of wrinkles, i.e. slackness of the skin produced by atrophy of the subcutaneous tissue, can be remedied by the percutaneous introduction of suitable rejuvenating substances.

In assessing the credence to be accorded to these claims it is first necessary to consider impartially

(1) Whether absorption *can* occur through the normal healthy unbroken skin.
(2) If such absorption occurs, what is the influence, if any, of the cream base employed.
(3) Can products locally applied by such means possibly exert any purely local effect.
(4) The toxicity and general metabolic effect on the human organism.
(5) The cosmetic value of the ingredients employed.

As discussed more fully under " Skin Foods " (Chapter 10), though it can now be shown that the cells of the skin can be influenced by the external application of certain substances, it by no means follows that such substances feed the skin. Indeed, even to seek a skin food betrays an ignorance—on the part of the seeker—of the true function of the human epidermis.

SKIN ABSORPTION AND PENETRATION

Although the skin is, in general, impervious to normal aqueous preparations, investigations have now definitely proved that absorption can and does occur in the case of certain drugs, vitamins and hormone preparations.

Until quite recently it was universally considered that bases consisting of natural animal and vegetable fats, e.g. lard, goose fat, lanolin, almond and olive oils, etc., were readily absorbed, while mineral oils and greases, such as liquid paraffin, petroleum jelly, etc., were either unabsorbed or any absorption was negligible. Lanolin was considered particularly efficacious, and earlier skin foods were based almost entirely upon w/o emulsions, in which the emulsifying agent was lanolin. Consequently animal and vegetable fats, lanolin and similar natural products were extensively used in the formulation of ointments and creams containing other substances of therapeutic value.

This theory was apparently refuted by the experiments of Dr. A. R. Bliss, a member of the U.S. Pharmacopoeia Committee on Revision 1934–40 (*Drug Cosmet. Ind.*, Sept. 1934, p. 247). Using methyl salicylate, and testing the absorption from various bases (lanolin, lard, petroleum jelly) by clinical quantitative analysis after inunction over a definite skin area, Dr. Bliss found that lard gave the best results, then petroleum jelly, and finally, contrary to popular belief, lanolin, and concluded that "absorption was a function of the drug itself and not of the vehicle containing it".

The position has been somewhat complicated by certain other investigators, in particular the experiments of D. I. Macht (*J. Amer. med. Ass.*, 1938, **110**, 409), who tested a number of emollients and found that none was apparently effective in promoting drug absorption, but of those tested lanolin was probably the most efficient.

The fact that none was particularly effective would appear to support the fact that the ointment base exerts but little influence, and that it is possible for the discrepancy in the relative value of the emollients tested to be due to experimental difficulties, which in tests of this type are bound to be relatively large. Moreover, the very careful experiments on the absorption of salicylic acid by the human skin (H. Leslie-Roberts, *Brit. J. Derm.*, 1928, **40**, 325) have shown that pure synthetic salicylic acid can be transported through the epidermis into the connective tissue and then into the blood stream, and that absorption can occur not only from an emollient base, and from alcohol, but *also from water*. Since, in general, aqueous preparations are not absorbed by the skin, this clearly demonstrates that in this case absorption is a function of the *drug* and not of the base. *Experiments so far carried out deal with the application of an active therapeutic agent whose presence is detectable in the urine by chemical examination, and unfortunately this is of little guide to the cosmetician who may desire information on the absorption of the ointment base itself.*

J. J. Seelman (*J. Amer. med. Ass.*, 1938, **110**, 1127) considers that the term "absorption" should only be used when absorption of agents into the blood stream is meant, and that the term "penetration" should be used to indicate the penetration of medicaments into, or through, the skin.

It was possible that developments in textile and leather chemistry might provide a basic reasoning for experiments in skin penetration. Dr. J. B. Speakman, in experiments on textiles, had shown that a molecule has penetrating properties conferred on it only if the molecule is of the polar type. Hydrocarbons are not of this type, their molecules at both ends are of non-polar types such as CH_3. The most highly penetrating materials are straight chain aliphatic compounds which at one end have a non-polar group, and at the other end a polar group, such as OH, COOH, or the salt or ester form of these groups.

In the filling of animal skins and tanned leathers, it had been found impossible to oil or fill such skins with mineral oils because they would not penetrate the interspaces. However, fatty alcohols and sulphonated fatty alcohols, and sulphonated oils did so, and if a mineral oil was emulsified with one of these polar compounds, the resulting emulsions would enable a certain amount of mineral oil to penetrate into the interspaces.

How far such facts coincided with those of penetration of the human skin by ordinary emollient substances was unknown. Methods so far used to determine the efficacy of an emollient by the incorporation in it of a suitable drug which could be chemically determined in the urine were open to grave criticism. *All such experiments measured the absorption and excretion of the active drug and did not express the penetrating properties of the vehicle itself.*

In 1941, the author published the results of an extensive investigation into the above problems on human post-mortem material of both sexes and varying ages, ranging from eighteen months to sixty-five years of age. Experiments were also conducted on live guinea-pigs, rabbits and rats. Some of the composite conclusions were then checked in the case of a human amputation (R. G. Harry, " Skin Penetration ", *Brit. J. Derm.*, March 1941). A specialised histological technique was employed and the methods of examination included :

(*a*) Application of suitable dyes in the emollient base, and microscopical examination of the section in visible light.

(*b*) Application of therapeutic chemical agents, and development on the slide of their image by chemical means.

(*c*) The use of special dyes, and examination in infra-red rays.

(*d*) Fluorescence examination in ultra-violet rays.

The above methods were employed to determine the skin penetration of :

(1) Simple animal and vegetable oils and fats, essential oils, etc.

(2) Mineral oils and greases.

(3) Hydrogenated oils.
(4) Emulsions of the water-in-oil type.
(5) Emulsions of the oil-in-water type.
(6) Vehicles of varying *p*H.
(7) Fat molecules of varying molecular chain length.
(8) Aqueous solutions.
(9) An applied galvanic current.

The composite conclusions of this investigation were as follows: " Oils, fats, and aqueous substances in general do not penetrate the intact epidermis to any appreciable extent. A certain amount of surface diffusion occurs but in no case did this amount to greater than about one-third of the depth of the corneous layer. Since, however, the thickness of the latter varies in differing parts of the body, being thinnest on the face, such slight penetration may exert, temporarily, a counteracting influence upon skin surface dryness and thus help to prevent premature skin surface flaking.

" *The path by which absorption occurs, is in the case of oils, fats (and emollients containing a polar group) down the aperture of the hair shaft and also through the sebaceous glands. The results confirmed the excellent penetrating properties of the essential oils (clove, eucalyptus and turpentine) and of oleic acid.*

" Good penetrant properties were exemplified by cod-liver oil, lanolin, lanolin absorption bases, lard, goose grease, vitamin F (so-called) and oleyl alcohol.

" Penetration was also observed in the case of the following oils: arachis, avocado pear, castor, grape-seed, hydrogenated arachis, olive, and turtle oil, but was negligible in the case of liquid paraffin and petroleum jelly. There was no evidence to suggest that avocado pear oil or turtle oil were superior to other vegetable oils. Hydrogenation did not (in the case of arachis oil) inhibit its absorption. In this connection it must be remembered that one of the first effects in hydrogenation is to reduce any highly unsaturated oils to olein, and if this process is stopped sufficiently early to leave a product with comparatively low melting point, it is possible to harden an oil without seriously affecting its power of penetration.

" The presence of polar groups, either with, or without, water was found to confer penetrant properties upon mineral oils and greases otherwise impermeable and to improve their adherence along the skin surface, but no evidence was obtained to confirm the theory that molecular chain length of the fat molecule was of major importance in skin penetration. . . ."

Criticisms which might be made against the above investigation

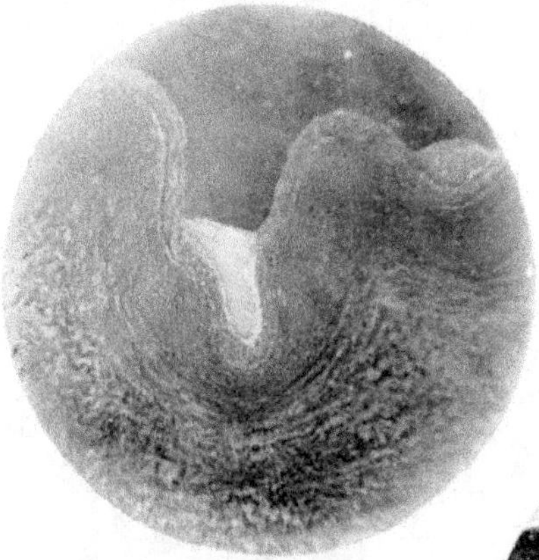

Fluorescence of liquid paraffin containing a trace of anthracene, under U.V.R. The oil has simply collected in a depression. There is no penetration.

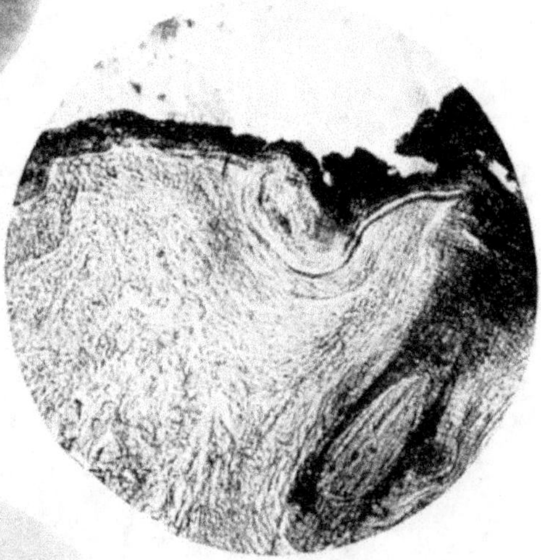

Absorption of lard containing Scarlet R, down human hair follicle (human leg amputation). Some absorption in sebaceous gland is visible, but in relatively thick "frozen" sections the focus of follicle and gland is in different fields. (Visual red dye photographs black.)

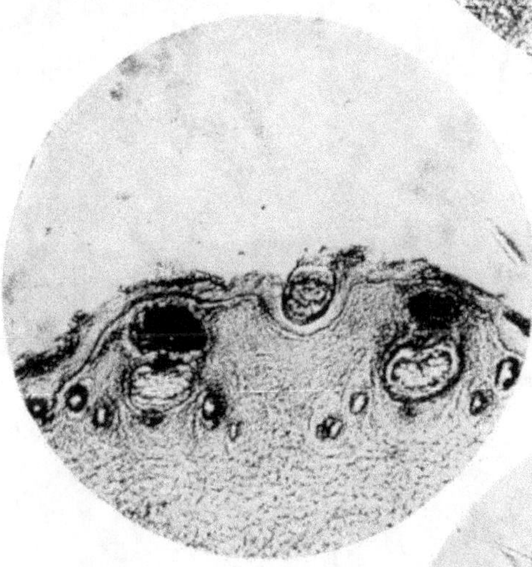

Absorption of lard containing Scarlet R (in guineapig). (The visual red dye deposits photograph black.)

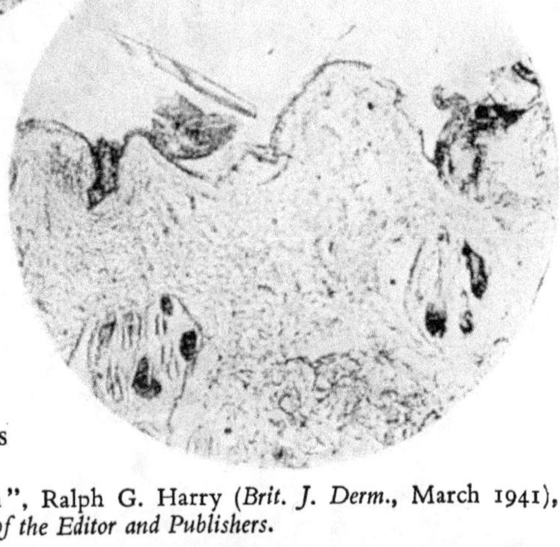

Absorption of mercuric oxide from a lard base (in a rat). Mounted in dilute sodium sulphide solution. Mercury deposits are blackened.

FIG. 9.

Comparison of human and animal s

Reproduced from "Skin Penetration", Ralph G. Harry (*Brit. J. Derm.*, March 1941), *by courtesy of the Editor and Publishers.*

are that in the first place method (*a*) above, does not indicate absorption of the oil vehicle but only of the dissolved dye in the sebaceous secretion. But this would ignore the fact that the absorption of the dye by the gland was greatest from *animal and vegetable oils*, in which the dye is comparatively strongly held, while it is least from mineral oils in which it is least strongly held. Method (*b*) *provides a chemical check in those cases in which it is desired to show the absorption of heavy metals, while the fluorescence method,* (d), *measures the extent of the penetration by the oil itself.* Hence I consider that a *combination of all of these methods* and the conclusions derived from the *composite* results thereby, offered the best approach to this question in our state of knowledge at that time.

Questions of variation in the method and results owing to the different viscosity of the oils and fats are not admissible, and any attempt to explain results on these grounds is excluded by the fact that vegetable and animal oils were compared with paraffins and medicinal paraffin of different viscosities ; and lanolin, lard and goose grease with petroleum jelly.

In considering some of the conflicting statements on the penetration of various substances into the skin which various writers have reported, it must be remembered that the skin is not a continuous surface but contains many " pockets " or apertures, as for example, hair follicles, sweat and sebaceous glands, into which—on massaging a cream or ointment—that preparation may be forced and *enmeshed,* though not necessarily absorbed. Hence any inferences reached as a result of superficial observation (or even of applying small weighed portions of a vehicle to the skin and removing and re-weighing the amounts which do not appear to be absorbed) are fallacious.

Some very interesting results appertaining to the permeability of animal skin to mercury, have been reached more recently by Laug [of the Divison of Pharmacology, U.S. Food and Drug Administration, Washington] (*J. Soc. cosmet. Chem.*, March 1948, **1**, 2, 81) ; *these results are, in many cases, in such good agreement with my own tentative deductions, made seven years earlier, that it is considered of interest to devote some little space to them.* Laug's broad conclusions were that the sex, litter and weight of the animal had no significant influence on penetration and that the location of the inunction site appeared to have no effect on penetration. The vehicle was found, in these experiments to have the greatest influence on penetration, the compound of mercury less and the concentration of mercury least. The method of assessing penetration of mercury depended upon the principle that the quantity of mercury which accumulates in the kidney during a twenty-four hour cutaneous exposure to mercury is a measure of the penetration of this metal through the skin (E. P. Laug, E. A. Vos, E. J. Umberger and F. Kunze, *J. Amer. pharm. Ass., Sci. edn.*, Jan. 1947, p. 14).

In Table I below is shown the striking superiority of lard, and propylene glycol and—in particular—oleic acid as a vehicle for absorption. (It is of interest to note that in my studies of skin penetration in 1941 excellent penetrant properties were assigned to oleic acid and to certain essential oils, whilst lard, goose grease and oleyl alcohol were found to be somewhat inferior to oleic acid. I found penetration from petroleum oils and jelly to be negligible.)

TABLE 1

THE CUTANEOUS PENETRATION OF MERCURY WHEN APPLIED AS A 30 PER CENT. SUSPENSION OF CALOMEL IN A NUMBER OF SINGLE COMPONENT VEHICLES

The measure of penetration is the storage of mercury in the kidneys of the rat

Micrograms Mercury per Gram Wet Kidney									
Control	*Water*	*Petrolatum*	*Mineral oil*	*Anhydrous lanolin*	*Hydrous lanolin*	*Corn oil*	*Lard*	*Propylene glycol*	*Oleic acid*
Series A, Females [1]									
0·07	4·4	6·0	5·6	6·0	5·9	13	11	19	26
Series B, Males [1]									
0·17	4·1	5·6	5·2	5·6	—	11	10	16	—

After Laug

Laug draws attention to the fact that, from the above table, it is apparent that, in the case of the absorption of mercury, the vehicle exerts a profound influence and he adds that one of the most striking facts is that petroleum jelly, lanolin and mineral oil, which have been used so extensively in many ointment bases provide a penetration of mercury which is so low.

Laug adds that it had been suspected for some time that the presence of petroleum jelly in large proportions in many vehicles was not conducive to good penetration of mercury, and to confirm this, four different mercurials, ammoniated mercury, metallic mercury, yellow oxide of mercury and calomel were suspended respectively, in each of two double component bases consisting of equal parts of lard and lanolin, and equal parts of petroleum jelly and lanolin. In Table 2 below is shown the marked superiority of the lard component vehicle over the petrolatum component vehicle.

MacKee, Sulzberger, Hermann and Baer (*J. invest. Derm.*, 1945, p. 43), as a result of their histological studies on percutaneous penetration, confirmed that penetration occurred through the follicles and that these and not the sweat glands, were decisive for penetration. As compared

[1] Average of six animals on each treatment.

with the follicles, the sweat glands were found to play a negligible role in absorption.

G. W. Johnston and C. O. Lee (*J. Amer. pharm. Ass.*, 1943, **32**, 278) used radio-active sodium chloride as a tracer and for the detection of the radio-active substance, a Geiger counter. Five typical ointment bases were selected for tests, anhydrous lanolin, white petroleum jelly, lard, a cetyl

TABLE 2

COMPARISON BETWEEN TWO TYPES OF VEHICLES CONSISTING OF LARD AND PETROLATUM WITH LANOLIN AS COMMON CONSTITUENT ON THE PENETRATION OF FOUR DIFFERENT MERCURIALS

The concentration of mercury in all ointments is 25 per cent. The measure of penetration is the storage of mercury in the kidneys of the rat

	Micrograms Mercury per Gram Wet Kidney			
Vehicle	*Calomel*	*Ammoniated mercury*	*Metallic mercury*	*Yellow oxide mercury*
E 50 per cent. Petrolatum 50 per cent. Lanolin	4·2	5·5	7·9	11
A 50 per cent. Lard 50 per cent. Lanolin	8·8	19	14	23

After Laug

The results are averages of six animals on each treatment.

alcohol cream of the " washable " type and a cholesterol cream of the water-in-oil type. After absorption had occurred urine samples were collected and measured for radio-activity. Anhydrous lanolin gave the best and most consistent results, followed by lard. The cholesterol and cetyl alcohol creams gave slightly lower and very similar results, while petroleum jelly gave slightly lower still. In these experiments the substance tested for skin penetration was the " salt ", sodium chloride, and not the base in which it was contained.

More recently L. C. Barail and J. J. Pescatore ("Introduction to Testing Cosmetics containing Radioisotopes", *J. Soc. Cosmet. Chem.*, Dec. 1951, **5**, 277) have shown that cold cream made with synthetic cetyl palmitate (tagged by means of the radioisotopic element carbon 14) does not penetrate the skin ; thus indicating that spermaceti, as part of a cold cream does not penetrate the skin under normal conditions of use nor after periods of massage and application as long as seven hours.

Summarising the position in respect of skin penetration it can be stated that the normal intact skin is not permeable, so far as we can tell, to aqueous solutions in general though exceptions to this statement do occur, e.g. salicylic acid, etc., or to fatty or oily substances. The resistance to aqueous solutions is not due to its covering of skin lubricant (sebum) but is believed to lie in the stratum lucidum and stratum granulosum due to an electrical layer which they present (with positively charged Hydrogen ions and negatively charged Hydroxyl ions orientated to provide an electrical barrier). *The apertures of sweat ducts and hair follicles, however, afford a break in this barrier and materials may penetrate the sebaceous glands via the hair follicles and thus circumvent the electrical barrier to absorption.*[1]

[1] ". . . All living organs are enclosed in a membrane and the properties of the membrane largely govern the action of a particular organ. The membrane to which reference is made must not be confused with the fibrous tissue which may merely act as a physical support for an organ, without displaying any specific chemical role. The term 'membrane' refers rather to that very thin interface between the internal and external contents of a cell; such an interface being only a few molecules in thickness and, of course, invisible to the eye even when aided by a microscope. Nevertheless, these membranes control the passage of substances into and out of the various living cells. A full account of membrane function must include a study of the membranes of the intestine, of the nerve fibres, of muscles, of blood cells, of bacteria, and of the brain, etc. The complete story will not, of course, be told for generations to come.

"In view of the importance of the surface charges of colloidal systems much attention has been given to this aspect of the subject in order to define the role that surface charges play in controlling membrane permeability.

"The charge on colloidal particles is due to an asymmetry in the distribution of positively and negatively charged portions of the system. No flow of current takes place between the positive and negative centres of a colloidal system.

"Particles having more positive charges at the surface than negative are said to have (in colloid science terminology) a positive *zeta* potential, and the *zeta* potential may be regarded as the potential between the surface of the particle or membrane and the surrounding media. The basic idea of the charge distribution around colloidal particles is illustrated in simple fashion below.

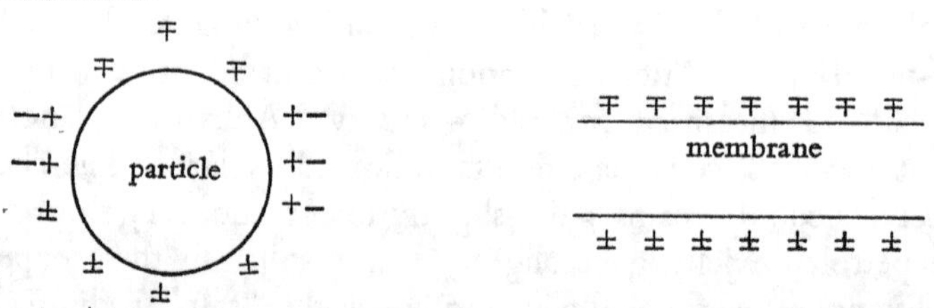

"It is possible to impart positive or negative charges to surfaces by use of certain substances which 'anchor' the charges to the surface. Common 'charge anchoring' substances are soap and detergent molecules. . ."

Schulman and Hocking,* using an oil membrane which was permeable to ions and controlling the surface properties of this membrane by the addition of detergent molecules to the oil, studied (with an extremely simple apparatus) the potentials across such membranes when dividing various combinations of simple salts and at the same time established the *zeta* potentials at the membrane surface by measurement in an electrophoresis apparatus. *The experiments demonstrated unequivocally that the charge of the membrane surface is of prime concern in controlling the migration of ions.* The use of detergent molecules to control permeability has not previously been demonstrated.

In a further study of the factors controlling the passage of colloidal particles through porous membranes (regarded as of direct importance in solving the passage of fat particles across the intestinal wall) it was established that the amount of colloidal material which

* In Press—Personal communication from Professor J. H. Schulman, O.B.E., Sc.D., F.R.S., Ernest Oppenheimer Laboratory, Department of Colloidal Science, The University Cambridge.

Calvary, Draize and Laug (*Physiological Reviews*, 1946, 4, 495 ff.) drew attention to the fact that " lipoid solubility " is probably one of the most important factors governing penetration since the presence of lipoid material (sebum, etc.), either surrounding the individual cell or within the openings of the appendages of the skin, determines to an extent what shall pass, and hence the distribution coefficient Lipoid Solubility/Water Solubility of a substance is probably an extremely important factor. [This is in line with the statement (R. G. Harry, " Skin Penetration ", *Brit. J. Derm.*, March 1941) that " it is a remarkable fact that nearly every substance known to be absorbed is oil-soluble, whilst mercury can combine with fatty acids to produce oil-soluble salts. . . ."][1]

Possibility of Local Cosmetic Effect

Until recently the possibility of a local cosmetic effect from externally applied cosmetic preparations had been denied rather too readily. It is true, for example, that if vitamin D be administered to a rachitic person, i.e. one suffering from rickets due to a vitamin D deficiency, the condition will disappear, resulting in improvement in general bodily health, which in turn will naturally be reflected in the improvement in tone of the whole skin surface. For similar reasons, it was argued that since the skin is nourished from the blood and lymphatic vessels traversing it, any absorption which might possibly result would affect the whole metabolism of the body, and not the particular site of application, e.g. if methyl salicylate is applied externally to any part of the body, salicylic acid is detected in the urine shortly afterwards.

Against this supposition, it must be remembered that, in the process of absorption, the substance must pass through the skin in a relatively concentrated state, in the region in which it is applied, and therefore the possibility of some local action on the cells through which it passes

migrates across the membrane is controlled by the *membrane* potential and the *zeta* potential of the particles. (A membrane potential may be regarded as a difference in electrical pressure across a membrane and such potentials can be produced by the diffusion of simple salts and are known to exist across the membranes of living organisms.)

From these studies it can be seen by what manner a relatively large electrically charged fat particle can be induced to cross the intestinal wall and clearly demonstrates the role and importance of membrane potentials in controlling fat transport.

To summarise it has been demonstrated that a Membrane Potential can induce the transport of otherwise extremely slow moving substances. Living organisms utilise the energy of those ions which do diffuse rapidly with consequent production of an electrical membrane potential. The potential, in turn, induces the permeability of the membranes.

[1] In this brief review of skin penetration discussion has been limited to the more modern views on this subject and in particular those having a bearing on the influence of the base since this aspect of the subject is the one that primarily concerns the cosmetician. For a more detailed study of the metabolism and permeability of the skin those interested are recommended to study the review by Calvary, Draize and Laug quoted above, and subsequent papers which have appeared in the *Journal of Investigative Dermatology*.

cannot be entirely ruled out. [While aspirin might be taken orally for rheumatism in any part of the body with *general* benefit, one would not apply synthetic oil of wintergreen to one's little toe, in case of rheumatism of the shoulder.]

Furthermore, any local erythema produced by the use of such a substance would be particularly evident at the *site* of application.

The action of massage in stimulating the blood supply to the region so treated also assists in improving its tone.

For the above reasons I have always stated that there is a distinct possibility of some local *cosmetic effect* quite apart from any general effect which may, or may not, be produced. Indeed, MacBryde (*J. Amer. med. Ass.*, 1939, **112**, 1045) provided proof of this fact (consistently enunciated by the writer), in that he produced clinically, definite enlargement of the breasts to a considerable degree by the application of an ointment containing 5000 units of oestradiol benzoate. MacBryde found that when breast growth was produced by injections of oestrogenic hormones there was diminishing effectiveness of the injected hormone but that when the hormones were applied to the skin there was steady progressive growth. I do not, however, consider that the skin can be "fed" by such means (*see* Skin Foods), though its condition can be improved.

General Metabolic Effect and Possible Toxicity of Certain Skin Foods

In general, such products are emollient, and are physiologically inactive, therefore the question of toxicity or derangements of metabolic function does not arise.

Unfortunately this has not always been the case. Animal extracts have been exploited on the ground that they exerted a favourable physiological action. Such *cutaneous* or *skin hormones* were added to a suitable base, these being obtained from the subcutaneous tissue of certain animals, notably the lizard, tortoise, salamander, and frog, since these animals possess a long life.

No one desired to possess skins such as these animals have, *even* if such an effect were possible. Their use was without proper scientific foundation and savoured more of the practice of uncivilised witch-doctors than of modern scientific research.

Fortunately this practice has now fallen into disrepute, probably on account of the difficulties of adequate preservation and of the possibility of their decomposition.

Today, the fashion is to use vitamins and sex hormones in such preparations. The vitamins are discussed more fully at a later stage in this chapter.

Hormones

Hormones may be regarded as substances produced by internal glandular secretions which act as accelerating or retarding catalysts in metabolism, or in simple words as *substances produced internally by gland secretion, which in small quantities are capable of affecting the entire mental and bodily health.*

The Use of Hormones in Cosmetics

In general, the sex hormones are increasingly recommended by some cosmeticians for inclusion in cosmetic creams and lotions.

Objections which have been made in the medical press as to the possibility that these substances might produce cancer appear to be based upon the following observations.

In a healthy body the production of normal cells is limited. In the case of malignant cells, however, for some reason, *uncontrolled proliferation* occurs, the cells migrate to set up fresh growths in different parts of the body. Ultimately a vital organ becomes involved with fatal results.

In 1933 Cook, Hewitt and Hieger (*J. chem. Soc.*, 1933, p. 395) isolated an active cancer-producing agent from coal tar, the structure of which was found to be 1,2-benzpyrene. This substance possesses a structure similar to the sterols and bile acids, and has been shown to have " estrogenic " as well as malignant properties (W. O. Kernack, *Sci. Prog.*, 1933, **28**, 117). Cell proliferation is a characteristic of both oestrus and the early stages of malignant growth, and it is assumed that carcinogenic agents of the benzanthrene type may be derived in the body from sterols by dehydration.

Lacassagne (*Comp. Rend.*, 1932, **195**, 630; Lacassagne and Nykta, *C. R. Soc. Biol.*, 1934, **116**, 844) succeeded in producing a mammary cancer in male mice, in which it does not normally appear, by injections of oestrone benzoate in sesame oil. Burrows (*Brit. J. Surg.*, 1935, **23**, 191) observed that *cystic mastopathy* (regarded as a preparatory stage to cancer) frequently followed the administration of oestrone to male and female mice.

The above observations may be taken as the basis upon which the supposition that sexual hormones may produce cancer is founded.

An imposing array of specialists, however, refute this suggestion *clinically*, and it would appear that the use of oestrin in therapeutic doses does not, in practice, afford any support for the above suggestion.

Professor Sir E. C. Dodds in a discussion on the position of hormones in obstetrics and gynaecology at a meeting of the Royal Society of Medicine (*Lancet*, 1936, p. 1269), declared that the conclusions on these points should only be based upon definite evidence, and that *oestrone and its derivatives had absolutely no carcinogenic activity when tested in the same way as the carcinogenic hydrocarbons.*

W. Cramer and W. E. Gye (of the Imperial Cancer Research Fund) have drawn attention to the fact that the carcinogenic changes described by D. E. Horning (*Lancet*, 1936, **1**, 247) were attained only by the continuous administration of oestrone over a considerable period of the mouse's life, corresponding in man to a period of from seven to ten years, while therapeutically their use is limited to a period of a few weeks or months. Burrows (*Lancet*, 1936, p. 1544) has also drawn attention to the fact that there is no comparison between such prolonged experimental investigation and its use in clinical practice.

A. S. Parkes (National Institute of Medical Research, Hampstead), M. P. Bishops (Dept. of Endocrinology, Guy's Hospital), and Sir E. C. Dodds (Courtauld Institute of Biochemistry, The Middlesex Hospital) conclude that oestrin and its derivatives show no signs of carcinogenic properties when tested by the classical method of Kennaway and collaborators, although this was the method originally employed to demonstrate the carcinogenicity of the synthetic hydrocarbons. Moreover, they add that oestrone only produces an increase in the incidence of mammary and other cancer when injected from birth onwards into *susceptible mice*, and that even in massive doses it does not produce cancer in a non-susceptible strain (*Lancet*, 1936, p. 1366).

In the report on the State of Cancer Research (" 34th Annual Report of the Imperial Cancer Research Fund ", *Lancet*, 1936, p. 1483) attention is drawn to the *difference* between the cancer produced in mice by the chemical carcinogens and that of the oestrogenic hormones. The former always produce cancer at the site of application, and there are no marked changes in the internal organs, while the carcinogenic effects of the oestrogenic hormones appear not at the site of application, i.e. the skin, but in one specific organ remote from it (the mamma), and the general condition resembles that observed after surgical removal of the pituitary gland. They conclude with the statement that there are no grounds for the fear that the therapeutic application of oestrin in skilled hands may induce cancer. (*See also* Sunburn and Cancer.)

Recent work has shown that oestrogenic activity is not confined to sterols or phenanthrene derivatives, and that even such simple compounds as *p*-hydrophenylethly alcohol and para-hydroxy-propenyl-benzene exhibit such properties.

Essential for the effect of an estrogenic molecule appears to be a *p*-hydroxy (or methoxy) phenyl group attached to an unsaturated chain of two or three carbon atoms.

It is well known that in pregnancy the skin of the expectant mother often improves to a remarkable degree and the remark is often made that the mother-to-be has never " looked so young " or " so beautiful ". Undoubtedly this effect is due to hormonal influences. When applied percutaneously as in a cosmetic cream, it has been established that hormones are absorbed and, moreover, there is evidence that suggests that the external application of hormones produces, at least in some cases, a marked effect upon the condition of the skin, giving it a more youthful appearance. As discussed later in this chapter, it appears that this effect is maintained so long as the application of the cosmetic cream is continued; on cessation of the treatment the skin reverts to its original condition.

It is suggested that such external application satisfies a local need of the skin which cannot—particularly in the normal ageing woman—be satisfied because of the avidity with which the female genital organs " seize " for their own use any oestrogen circulating in the body. The amounts used in cosmetic creams are considered to be so small as merely to satisfy such skin requirements leaving little or none for any systemic effect. (Dr. E. G. Klarmann, " The Cosmetic Aspects of Estrogenic Hormones ", *J. Soc. cosmet. Chem.*, Dec. 1949, p. 406.)

There is evidence in support of the above contention. Eidersberg (*Amer. J. med. Sci.*, 1947, **214**, 630) carried out an investigation as to whether or not the amount of oestrogen present in a hormone cream is capable of producing *systemic* effects on the user, and his results suggest that they are not. In his work a cream containing 7500 International Units (I.U.) of natural oestrogenic hormone (essentially oestrone and oestradiol) per ounce of base was used. Using urinary oestrogen output and vaginal smears as indices of systemic effects a total of fourteen patients were studied, their ages ranging from eighteen to fifty-six years. In addition four women were used as untreated controls. Eidersberg found that the fluctuations in oestrogen excretion in the four untreated controls and in the fourteen patients before and during the use of the oestrogen cream by facial inunction were similar in pattern and not significantly different in amount. Likewise their vaginal smears appeared to show no significant alteration in cytological cycles. Therefore he concluded that, in the amounts applied and the methods used (3750 I.U. per week or 535 I.U. daily) the oestrogen cream did not appear to produce any systemic effect.

Klarmann (*J. Soc. cosmet. Chem.*, Dec. 1949, p. 406), states : " . . . Most cosmetic hormone creams, available on the market today contain from 7500 to 10,000 I.U. of oestrogenic substance per ounce of vehicle. This substance is usually of natural origin and consists essentially of oestrone ; smaller proportions of alpha-estradiol, equiline, and equilinin may be present in extracts from the urine of gravid mares which constitutes one of the most important sources of this material.

"When applied in a cosmetic cream, this hormone potency may be safely regarded as being well below the threshold value for any systemic action. Assuming that a 2-oz. jar of hormone cream with a total potency of 20,000 I.U. is used up over a period of one month, the individual daily application would contain 666 I.U. It is known, however, that absorption from an externally applied ointment does not take place to the extent of 100 per cent.; at best, it is not greater than 40 per cent., and usually considerably less. Therefore, a maximum absorption of 290 I.U. should be taken into account, which certainly is far less than required for any systemic effect. According to the *New and Nonofficial Remedies* (a publication of The American Medical Association), the therapeutic dose is 2000 to 10,000 I.U., by intramuscular injection, depending on the patient's response. As much as 50,000 I.U. per week may be required in certain cases. Of course, intramuscular injection results in a practically complete absorption, in contradistinction to percutaneous application.

"An experiment with a cosmetic hormone cream (containing 7500 I.U. per ounce) was conducted by Curth (personal communication), on women ranging in age from 26 to 65 years. For a period of four weeks the hormone cream was applied to one thigh, and the cream without the hormone to the other thigh every day, preceded by cleansing with soap and water. The subjects did not know which cream contained the hormone principle. At the end of the four-week period, biopsies were performed on each of the areas treated.

"The most constant finding was a succulence of the epidermal cells in the biopsies of the skin treated with the active cream."

Klarmann continues ". . . Another experiment with the same cream formula was carried out by Traub and co-workers (Hearing before the Louisiana State Board of Health, 2 April 1946); as a control, the cream vehicle which did not contain the hormonal substances was used on the opposite side of each subject. Twenty-five women, ranging between the ages of 35 and 55 were selected for this experiment. They were given the hormone cream to use on the right side of the face, neck and the right hand. The control cream was used on the left side of the face, neck and back of the left hand. The subjects used the creams for a period of more than six months continuously. They were under the observation of a number of physicians, and a nurse was in constant charge of the experiment. None of the subjects confused the cream by using it on the wrong side. At the conclusion of the experiment, twenty-four of the patients showed a greater improvement on the hormone-treated right hand, as compared with that on the left. In one of the cases, no difference could be noted between the two sides. Twenty-three of the women appeared to have improved more decidedly on the hormone-treated right side of the face and neck than on the left. In one, the opposite side appeared to be better. In one case no appreciable difference could be noted between the two sides. There were no untoward local effects whatever observed on the skin, or complained of during the course of the experiment, nor was there any evidence of systemic action, although no special study was undertaken to verify this point.

"A comparative histologic study was undertaken using the original sections of skin, one from each hand, removed from the subjects prior to the onset of the experiments, and those from the same subjects at its conclusion. The dermatological interpretation of these findings may be summarised as follows :

(1) The original section conformed to the histologic picture of the skin of the back of women's hands ranging between the ages of 35 and 55.
(2) The final sections, both from the hormone-treated side and the control side showed that the use of the creams did not effect the epidermis.
(3) It was possible from the histologic sections to differentiate between the active and the control sides.
(4) The active side was recognised by observing various degrees of dilatation of the blood vessels, an increase in simple cellular elements, a greater succulence of the derma, as well as a betterment of the elastic tissue. There appeared to be no essential changes in the basophilic strands when the final sections removed at the conclusion of the experiment were compared with the original sections of the skin."

Gross examination indicated also a tendency toward the diminution of senile pigmentation or freckling.

Moreover, it could be shown by a comparatively simple experiment that skin areas treated with the hormone cream developed a greater avidity for taking up fluids (physiological saline) than the control areas.

In two more recent publications, Goldzieher (*Geriatrics*, 1946, 1, 226 ; *J. Geront.*, 1946, 1, 196) reported upon the topical application of hormone cream to senile skin. He used one preparation assayed at 10,000 I.U. to the ounce, and another one containing the synthetic estrogen, diethylstilbestrol (1 mgm. per oz.).

With biopsies taken from both the treated and untreated areas (of the inner surfaces of the thighs and forearms) he found striking changes following a daily application of the hormone-bearing ointments over a period of six weeks. There was evidence of a regeneration of the surface epithelium. There were also significant changes in the mesoderm; thus the water content of the oestrogen-treated site was greater, the number and size of the capillaries seemed increased, the bundles of collagenous fibres appeared less fragmented, and the elastic fibrils were more numerous. No such changes were elicited with the hormone-free ointment base.

It is argued that topical application of oestrogens affects the skin to a much greater degree than oral or parenteral administration because by the latter modes of administration substantial amounts are lost for the skin through excretion, through inactivation by the liver, through attraction to the genital and mammary tissues, and through dilution by body fluids. In Goldzieher's opinion, the demonstrated absorption and utilisation by the skin of topically applied oestrogens opens a new field of therapy applicable to skin conditions not only induced by a hormone deficiency, but also to those involving other pathologic changes.

Eller and Eller (*Arch. Derm. Syph., Chicago*, 1949, **59**, 449) have carried out an extensive investigation of hormone creams and found that oestrogenic hormone ointments (with 7500 to 15,000 I.U. per ounce of excipient) produced consistent proliferative effects upon the skin epithelium (Fig. 10), the response varying with the age of the subject, the concentration of the oestrogen, the duration of the individual application, and the total duration of the treatment; no epithelial response was obtained in the case of young women (twenty to thirty years of age) who were free of any symptoms of endocrine dysfunction and who exhibited a fully developed epidermis of normal thickness (Fig. 12).

Definite histological changes were observed in all nineteen post-menopausal subjects (aged fifty-one to seventy-nine) whose control biopsies showed senile atrophy with thinning of the epithelium. These changes were:

(*a*) The cytoplasm tended to increase in volume,
(*b*) the nuclei increased in size and assumed a rounded rather than ovoid form,
(*c*) the basal cell layer increased in waviness indicating proliferative activity,
(*d*) the epidermis gradually increased in thickness, and the epidermal pegs reappeared,
(*e*) the capillary blood supply became more prominent,
(*f*) the supportive elastic fibrillar structures became more pronounced,
(*g*) the elastic tissue and collagen (of the underlying corium) was affected only to a minimal degree.

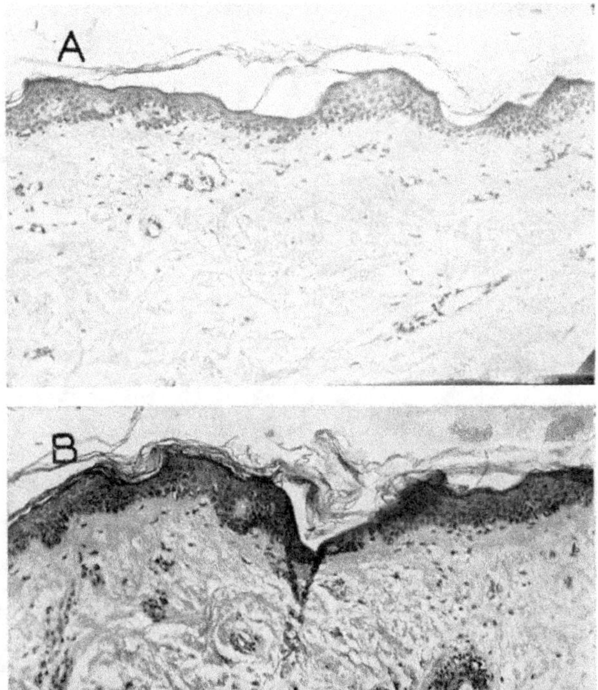

A. Biopsy specimen of the skin of the back before treatment. Note the thin epidermis, the absence of pegs and the cuboidal cells of the basal cell layer.

B. Biopsy specimen of the skin of the back after application of an estrogen-free ointment for thirty days. There are thickening of the epidermis, greater cellularity and slight waviness of the basal cell layer.

C. Biopsy specimen after application of estrogenic ointment for thirty days. Note the increased sizes of the epidermal cells and the pronounced waviness of the basal cell layer, indicating proliferative activity.

[*By courtesy of the American Medical Association.*

FIG. 10.—Average response of senile female skin to continuous application of ointment containing 242 international units of estrogen per gram (7500 international units per ounce).

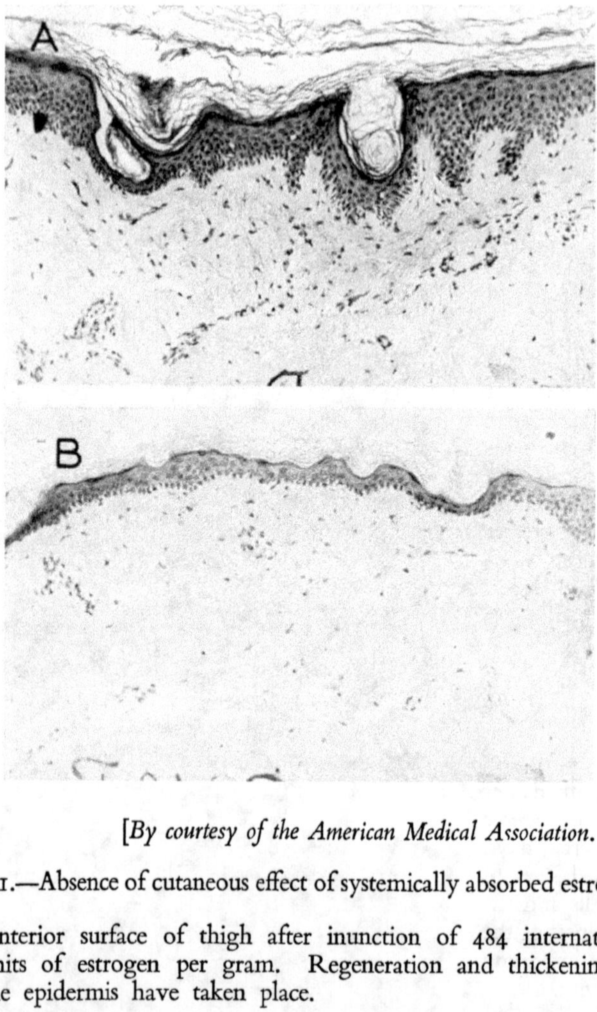

[By courtesy of the American Medical Association.

FIG. 11.—Absence of cutaneous effect of systemically absorbed estrogen.

A. Anterior surface of thigh after inunction of 484 international units of estrogen per gram. Regeneration and thickening of the epidermis have taken place.

B. Skin of opposite thigh after inunction with estrogen-free ointment only. There is no perceptible change, showing that neither estrogen-free ointment nor systemically absorbed estrogen has any cutaneous effect.

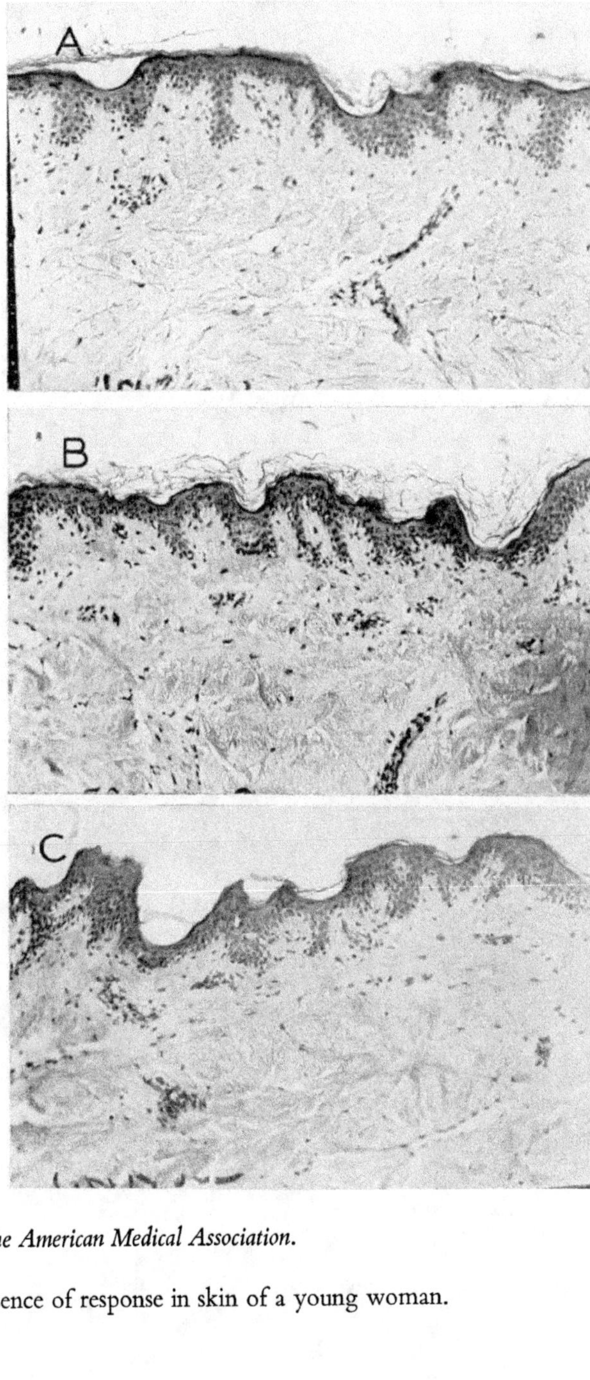

A. Biopsy specimen from the skin of the back before treatment. Note the essentially normal epidermis with large, well-developed pegs and vasicular cells.

B. Biopsy specimen taken after inunction of estrogen-free ointment for sixty days. There is no perceptible change.

C. Biopsy specimen taken after inunction of ointment containing 242 international units of estrogen per gram. There is no difference between this and the control specimen.

[*By courtesy of the American Medical Association.*

FIG. 12.—Absence of response in skin of a young woman.

The changes in the skin's epithelium reached a maximum at some time between thirty and fifty days ; this maximum was attained more promptly with the large doses, and with the more prolonged periods of contact with the oestrogenic material. They were maintained as long as the application was continued ; omission of treatment caused reversion to the original atrophic condition.

There was a latent period of ten to twenty days before the appearance of a demonstrable effect.

These investigators also reported insignificant variations in the appearance of the vaginal smears of their subjects ; from this they drew the conclusion that under the conditions of their procedure the absorbed oestrogen affected the cutaneous epithelium directly, rather than via the systemic route. The postulate as to a direct, local action was borne out also by an *ad hoc* experiment, in which the hormone cream was applied to one thigh, and the hormone-free excipient to the other ; regeneration and thickening of the epidermis took place only in the former instance (Fig. 12).

What are the Hazards of Hormonal Cosmetics ?

A realistic view of the situation is most necessary. Practically all useful cosmetic or medical preparations involve *some* potential hazard. One cannot travel, one cannot even cross the street without potential hazard. All that can be reasonably expected is that the potential hazard should be slight. Hormones have the advantage that, unlike many other cosmetics and medical ingredients, they *are not " foreign "* to the body. Viewed in the cold light of scientific reason, modern hormone creams have achieved a very favourable cosmetic record in respect of absence of consumer complaints. These creams have reached wide sales in the United States, running into millions of jars over a period of more than thirteen years, without ill-effects having been reported. During that time they have, on various occasions from the very beginning, been under " fire " by State (and occasionally Medical) bodies who—in the interest of safety—went " gunning " for them. Their best testimony is that in spite of such " gunning " they may still be sold quite freely in the United States, and that States who originally banned the sale of such preparations have, upon investigation of the pertinent evidence, either dropped directly their ban or amended it merely to ensure that the label on the product bore adequate directions for use. In the United States, the " official " position of the Federal Security Agency (Food and Drug Administration) is given in a letter dated 26 October 1949, addressed to deNavarre (*Amer. Perfum.*,

April 1950, p. 289) from which it appears that the Food and Drug Administration:

(1) whilst they were sceptical of the ability of these creams to accomplish the results promised, were not in a position to disprove their claims;
(2) did not look favourably upon the distribution of these creams for lay use (because of the lack of definite information concerning the ultimate effect of the continued use of these creams), but possessed no conclusive evidence that harm had resulted from the use of creams containing the amounts of oestrogens found in those creams then on the market.

[In this respect it must be remembered that toilet and cosmetic preparations both in the respect of composition and of labelling are under much more stringent regulations in the United States than they are in this country.]

Dr. Schwartz (" Hearing before the Louisiana State Board of Health ", 2 April 1946) stated that the Section of Dermatoses Investigations of the U.S. Public Health Service had no record of skin damage resulting from the use of hormone creams.

Eller and Eller paid particular attention to the cytologic character of the epidermal cells of the patients showing a response to oestrogen aud state: " It can be stated unequivocally that no abnormalities were observed. There was no increase in the number of mitoses, or any suggestion of changes other than those of simple regeneration. . . ."

Klarmann points out that no quantity of oestrogen administered for therapeutic purposes can produce a concentration in the blood stream comparable to that during the second half of gestation. As shown by Salter, Humm, and Oesterling (*J. clin Endocrin.*, 1948, **8**, 295), also by Jailer (*J. clin. Endrocin.*, 1948, **8**, 564), the excretion of natural oestrogen in the urine of the normal female, at its peak, amounts to an oestrone equivalent of 600 to 1000 I.U. daily [between the peaks the variation is from 50 to 200 I.U. daily] nevertheless, the uterine and mammary carcinomas do not occur in child-bearing women more often than in nulliparous women of the same age and hereditary background.

The remarks so far made concern the use of hormones in the amount normally recommended for use in cosmetic preparations, viz. 7500 to 10,000 I.U. per ounce of product. When more concentrated preparations of hormones are applied the situation is entirely different.

Barber (*Modern Trends in Dermatology*, edited by R. M. B. MacKenna, p. 106 ff., London: Butterworth & Co. 1948) has pointed out that two essential facts about hormones have been established:

(*a*) that androgens stimulate the surface epithelium and the sebaceous glands tending to produce hyperkeratosis and seborrhoea,

(*b*) that oestrogens have a contrary action in that they diminish keratinisation and the activity of the sebaceous glands.

Hodgson (*Practitioner*, 1948, p. 373) quotes from a personal communication from Dr. Barber, that " . . . Barber has seen cases of uterine bleeding and swelling of the breasts following the inunction of 5 per cent. and 2 per cent. dienoestrol *even to quite small areas of the skin* . . ." and adds " the indiscriminate use of oestrogens in cosmetic creams can only be strongly disapproved of by medical men at present. . . ."

Williams (*Practitioner*, 1948, p. 367) points out that whilst the obvious association between conditions and texture of the skin—as well as certain specific conditions of the skin—with these hormones should, by now, have led (it might be thought) to clear-cut indications for their use : so far from being the case, the story, with few exceptions is one of increasing confusion and bewilderment in that clinical trials have, only too often, been on but few cases and these inadequately controlled. In discussing the use of hormones for the treatment of acne, he adds : " . . . It is probably never wise to use them at all in women under the age of 20. . . ."

deNavarre (*Amer. Perfum.*, Dec. 1952, p. 423) has referred to, and criticised a short article by Goldberg and Harris (*J. Amer. med. Ass.*, 1952, **150**, 790) which claims to show that oestrogen cosmetics were harmful in *one* case. In my opinion the use of a hormone cream involving the external application to the face and/or body of a total of 20,000, or less, I.U. oestrogenic hormones per month involves no risk to the user, and such creams may be of value to the older woman.[1]

I would, however, deprecate their use locally to the breasts by young women aiming at a specific degree of enlargement.

The Percutaneous Administration of Vitamin Preparations

There is evidence not only that the hormones may exert a *local* effect apart from a general systemic effect but that, in many cases, the percutaneous application of them is far more effective than merely giving them by the mouth. (*See* discussion on hormones in cosmetics earlier in this chapter.) Moreover, owing to metabolism being faulty, it may

[1] *See also* " Hearings before the House Select Committee to Investigate the use of Chemicals in Foods and Cosmetics", Part 3, p. 1066. Washington. Sulzberger (*Jour. Amer. Med. Ass. May* 1954) ; Peck and Klarman, " Practitioner ", August, 1954.

be that ingestion of the vitamin by the mouth may not lead to its proper distribution throughout the body whereas by inunction an effective concentration, at the desired location, may be attained. In certain cases percutaneous application may be the only alternative to injection in those cases where the active material is hydrolysed or otherwise acted upon by the acid of the mouth and/or the ferments, etc., of the digestive system.

I consider that the proper way to treat a vitamin A deficiency (when proven) is not by creams but by the administration of suitable amounts, under medical supervision, in the normal manner; at the same time there is a possibility that the percutaneous application of vitamin A may have some uses not hitherto established.

(The above reasons, advanced in connection with percutaneous administration of certain substances, refer to the vitamins as a whole.)

Vitamins in Cosmetics

VITAMIN A. The relationship of an adequate vitamin A intake to proper keratinisation of the skin appears fairly well proven. Hyperkeratosis involving deposition of keratinous material in the hair follicle has been proved to be symptomatic of a vitamin A deficiency in laboratory animals and there is evidence to show that this applies to man. Lehman and Rappaport (*J. Amer. med. Ass.*, 1940, **114**, 386) concluded that vitamin A avitaminosis is much more common than is supposed and that various skin lesions classified under hyperkeratosis are inextricably associated with less than the optimum requirement of vitamin A.

O'Leary (*Arch. Derm. Syph., Chicago*, 1942, **46**, 5, 628), in a summary of the literature, has pointed out that in certain skin diseases the response to the administration of vitamin A is so rapid and clear-cut that the deduction is warranted that the result is " specific ". These diseases include phrynoderma (toadskin),[1] a papular dry skin eruption (C. N. Frazier and C. K. Hu, *Arch. intern. Med.*, 1931, **48**, 507); pityriasis rubra pilaris, a disease of the skin characterised by formation of hard elevations around each hair follicle (L. A. Brunsting and C. Sheard, *Arch. Derm. Syph., Chicago*, 1941, **43**, 42); and keratosis follicularis, a papular disease characterised by cornification of the epithelial layers of the skin (S. M. Peck, L. Chargin and H. Sobotka, *Arch. Derm. Syph., Chicago*, 1941, **43**, 223). It is true that these diseases are in many cases due originally to a certain deficiency, and the administration of the missing deficiency would be expected to cure them. Moreover, they represent a pathological

[1] It is not yet clear whether toadskin (phrynoderma) is due only to vitamin A deficiency or whether some other factor is involved. Vitamin A deficiency alone can cause this condition but often there is also some other factor involved, something which may decrease the vitality of the skin.

condition which is probably abnormal under ordinary nutritional conditions in man. Nevertheless, their connection with the skin and the type of the eruption suggests that milder forms of nutritional deficiencies could produce changes in the skin, and this possibility must be borne in mind.

The close connection between the skin and vitamin A is shown by the fact that changes in the skin occur before changes in the eye. (Frazier and Hu, *Arch. Derm. Syph., Chicago*, 1936, **33**, 825; Corlette, *et al.*, *Amer. J. med. Sci.*, 1938, **195**, 54; Aykroyd and Rajagopal, *Indian J. med. Res.*, 1936–37, **24**, 419, and 707; Pemberton, *Lancet*, 1940, **1**, 285.)

It appears that blackheads are common in such conditions, though apart from this the face is not usually involved,[1] the nails may be ridged and the hair may be dry. In general, however, the hair and nails are normal.

In view of the above relationship between the skin and vitamin A, the incorporation of this vitamin into toilet creams has been suggested, and as a matter of fact at least one well-known firm of manufacturers incorporating this vitamin as the " skin vitamin ". There is no doubt that vitamin A can be absorbed through the skin. It is generally assumed that any effect it exerts must be synthetic and that therefore it is illogical to give vitamin A except through the mouth. It is by no means proven that the effect of such preparations is *only* systemic or indeed, even if systemic, that no advantage may accrue from percutaneous administration.

VITAMIN B_1 (Thiamine Hydrochloride). Bicknell and Prescott (*The Vitamins in Medicine*, London: Wm. Heinemann, 1942) have pointed out that although vitamin B_1 has been given in alopecia, pruritis and pyodermatoses due to streptococcal and staphylococcal infections, no controls were used and the results of these tests should be accepted with reserve.[2] There is evidence that an adequate intake of vitamin B_1 is essential to normal health and that in its absence pyruvic acid accumulates in the tissue which then loses its power of oxygen absorption. The first and most serious symptoms of vitamin B_1 deficiency occur in the heart and nervous system. There is no evidence that it has outstanding properties

[1] Vitamin A and acne. *See*, however, a paper by J. V. Straumfjiord (*Northwest Med.*, 1943, **42**, 219; also G. Bamber, *Brit. J. Derm.*, June 1942, p. 163).

[2] Experiments by Najjar and Holt (*J. Amer. med. Ass.*, 1943, **123**, 683) suggest that vitamin B_1 can be synthesised in the human bowel. A striking factor is the variability of biosynthesis in different people even on the same diet and a lot more information will be required before any general conclusions can be reached.

These results revolutionise our outlook on vitamins and suggest answers for the fact that some people can remain healthy on diets which are low in vitamin B. It would appear that the vitamin B content of the diet is sometimes of less consequence than a diet capable of maintaining adequate vitamin syntheses by the intestinal flora (*Lancet*, 30 Dec. 1944, p. 854).

in connection with the health of the skin[1] apart from the fact that what interferes with bodily health must affect the health of the skin to some extent. It is not a constituent of toilet preparations.

VITAMIN B_2 (*d*-Riboflavine; Lactoflavine; formerly called by some writers "Vitamin G"). Vitamin B_2 is not yet a constituent of toilet preparations nor has its role, if any, in dermatology been elucidated up to the present. Lander and Pallister (*Trans. R. Soc. Trop. med. Hyg.*, 1935, **2**, 133) stated that it has been found of value in the treatment of avitaminosis B_2 involving eczema of the scrotum and of the angles of the mouth. More recently Sebrell and Butler (*Publ. Hlth. Rep., Wash.*, 1939, 54, **2**, 121) claimed that reddened lesions of the lips and fissures in the angles of the mouth were symptoms of vitamin B_2 deficiency. It is of course quite possible that vitamin B_2 functions as a "link" in the vitamin B-complex (or other vitamin complex) chain. In such an event it would not be surprising to have difficulty in demonstrating any *particular* lesion as specifically due to lack of this vitamin. Machella and MacDonald (*Amer. J. med. Sci.*, 1943, **205**, 214) reported cases of cheilosis which did not respond to treatment with riboflavine but were healed with brewers yeast.

Certain members of the vitamin B complex are components of certain enzymes (riboflavine is a constituent of Warburg's yellow enzyme, thiamin of carboxylase, etc.) which are concerned in the oxidation-reduction reactions of living cells and thus their relationship to local skin conditions would not be surprising. (*See* Skin Enzymes, etc., Chapter 1.)

In other words, whilst we have no definite evidence of its value, we have no reason to suppose that it is valueless. For a considered opinion we must await the results of further research.

VITAMIN B_6 (Pyridoxine). Smith and Martin (*Proc. Soc. exp. Biol., N.Y.*, 1940, **43**, 660) stated that this substance (a member of the vitamin B complex), was useful in lip lesions (cheilosis). Gyorgy (*J. clin. Nutr.*, 1938, **16**, 69) stated that there is a striking similarity between chilblains and the dermatitis induced in rats by a vitamin B_6 deficiency and that a vitamin B_6 deficiency in man may predispose to chilblains. Bicknell and Prescott (*The Vitamins in Medicine*, London: Heinemann, 1942) consider it possible that both vitamin B_2 and vitamin B_6 may be essential for the nutrition of the lips at the mucotaneous junction and that a deficiency of either of them may precipitate lip lesions. Samitz and Brown (*Arch.*

[1] Large doses of vitamin B_1 have been given internally in cases of itching affections of the skin, mostly in children and infants. The conditions treated included chilblains, urticaria, eczema, pityriasis, scabies, measles and chicken-pox. In some cases the relief was immediate —e.g. measles and chicken-pox; in others a varied response was obtained, these were cases of urticaria and eczema. Sixty-two per cent. of the cases were completely relieved of itching within a short time after the institution of treatment (*Urol. cutan. Rev.*, Dec. 1942, **46**, 786). Whether local applications to localised areas of irritation may exert a sedative effect has yet to be determined.

Derm. Syph., Chicago, 1943, **47**, 651) gave vitamin B_6 to a group of patients with seborrhoeic dermatitis, atopic eczema with seborrhoeic features and eczematous eruptions of unknown etiology. Some of the patients showed amazingly good results; others showed little or no response.

In short, it is now believed that pyridoxine may be one of the more active substances in liver and yeast. Its *exact* function in respect of the skin is unknown. It has been claimed that it is a necessary factor for the utilisation of unsaturated fatty acids; if this is correct and if the value and *specific role* of the unsaturated fatty acids can be established it *may* have uses in percutaneously applied creams and ointments.

VITAMIN C (Ascorbic Acid). Vitamin C is not, to my knowledge, employed in cosmetic preparations though it *may* be present in certain high-priced cosmetic lotions containing fruit juices obtainable in the more exotic regions of the world. The amounts present in such preparations would, however, be small since in aqueous solution ascorbic acid rapidly deteriorates in the presence of air. Pharmacologically ascorbic acid regulates the processes of oxidation-reduction in the living cell. Its deficiency results in increased capillary fragility and appears to be bound up in part with *some* cases of gingivitis. Vitamin C is of particular value in the prevention and treatment of scurvy and it is claimed (*Practitioner*, 1937, **2**, 418) to be of value in cases of exfoliating dermatitis. It is generally agreed that an adequate intake of vitamin C is essential to proper tooth health but, to date, there is no conclusive evidence which would associate vitamin C with dental caries. On the contrary, dental caries occurs not only in Scotland but also in Hawaii, the land of fruit (and sunshine).

Evidence has recently been accumulating to show that vitamin C is a clinical necessity for the rapid and healthy healing of wounds. (Bartlett *et al.*, *New England J. Med.*, 1942, **226**, 474; *Ann. Surg.*, 1940, **111**, 1; Lund, *New England J. Med.*, 1939, **221**, 123; Crandon, *J. Amer. med. Ass.*, 1941, **116**, 669.) Kashara and Kawashina (" The Resorption of Vitamin C through the Skin ", *Klin. Wschr.*, 23 Jan. 1937, **16**, 135) reported that vitamin C was absorbed through the skin, this fact being evidenced by the increase in vitamin C content of mothers' milk following application of a 30 per cent. solution of ascorbic acid to the surface of the skin of the mammae. Little work appears to have been carried out on the absorption of vitamin C through the intact epidermis. Although the usual method of vitamin administration is by ingestion, it is by no means certain that the external application of vitamin C may not have value in the local treatment of certain skin conditions, though at present this is merely conjecture. Should this be demonstrated clinically then presumably vitamin C—or fruit juices—will become part of the toilet advertising campaign.

VITAMIN D. Several substances capable of preventing or curing rickets are included under this term. Originally the term vitamin D was applied to a mixture believed to be pure vitamin D, but today when the terms vitamin D and D_2 are used it is understood that they refer to calciferol. Calciferol (vitamin D_2) is produced by activating ergosterol and has not been found to occur in nature. The designation vitamin D_3 is applied to activated 7-dehydrocholesterol and is the form of vitamin that occurs in fish liver oils. Chickens are insensitive to calciferol but cured by D_3. The rat is sensitive to, and cured by both D or D_3; and man similarly does not distinguish between them so far as curing rickets is concerned. Vitamin D_2 (calciferol) is the form in which vitamin D is the most readily incorporated into creams. So far as man is concerned, it would appear that this form has the same properties and uses as fish oils and, from the aesthetic standpoint is preferable to the fish oils but, in the writer's opinion, it is by no means certain that the unsaturated fatty acids in fish oils may not have valuable properties of their own, quite distinct from any vitamin D activity which they may possess. (*See* Unsaturated Fatty Acids, etc.)

An adequate intake of vitamin D is essential for the proper formation of bones and teeth but so far no changes in the health of the skin have been linked *primarily* with a deficiency of vitamin D, although it is possible that the integrity of the skin may be affected by such deficiencies in a way not yet recognised.

VITAMIN D HAS PROVIDED, HOWEVER, THE MOST DRAMATIC ADVANCE IN THE TREATMENT OF CUTANEOUS TUBERCULOSIS. In 1943 Charpy (*Ann. Derm. Syph., Paris,* 1943, **3**, 331 and 340; 1944, **4**, 110; 1946, **6**, 310) and shortly afterwards but independently, Dowling and Thomas (*Brit. J. Derm.,* 1946, **58**, 45) achieved dramatic results in the treatment of cutaneous tuberculosis by the administration through the mouth of massive doses of Vitamin D_2. *Though these results are not, of course, applicable to cosmetic preparations in any way, they do demonstrate* (1) *that vitamin therapy can, in some cases apparently, cure a condition which is not due to a vitamin deficiency.* (Previously it had always been assumed that there was no point in giving vitamins to anybody unless it could be shown that a vitamin deficiency existed.) The implications of the above work in other fields may well be enormous, and, (2) it illustrates a tie-up between vitamin D and conditions in the skin. Charpy (*Ann. Derm. Syph., Paris,* 1946, **3**, 310) suggested that a local tissue acidosis was produced by the administration of the vitamin D and that the aim of the treatment should be the maintenance of this condition.

At the moment *there appears to be no valid argument for the inclusion of vitamin D in cosmetic or other creams* but in view of the recent results obtained with this vitamin in the investigations reported above it would be foolish to assert dogmatically that, when locally applied, this vitamin is devoid of value, and before passing judgement one must await the result of further research.

Unsaturated Fatty Acids

The term " essential fatty acids " is loosely used to designate a group of unsaturated fatty acids that will restore growth in the case of rats which have stopped growing on a low fat diet. Linoleic acid appears to be the only essential one, but—like certain amino acids—some fatty acids may, more or less, completely replace one another although there are differences in their effect.

Linoleic acid, linoleyl alcohol, linolenic, arachidonic, docosanhexenoic and hexahydroxystearic acids give a positive response in restoring growth in fat deficiency, but only linoleic and arachidonic also cure the skin effects occurring in rats on a fat-deficient diet (G. O. Burr, *Federation Proc., Baltimore*, 1 June, 1942, no. 2, p. 224).

Vitamin F was introduced to the toilet industry for its supposed cosmetic effect. After Burr and co-workers had demonstrated that when rats were placed on a diet from which certain neutral fats were excluded, the animals failed to grow properly and developed symptoms resembling those of eczema and dermatitis—even if compensating amounts of the fat-soluble vitamins already known were administered, Shepherd (*Drug Cosmet. Ind.*, March, 1936) claimed not only to have substantiated these results but also to have isolated an isomeric form of linoleic acid which would prevent or cure the Burr fat deficiency syndrome. Following the nomenclature of Evans, Lepkovsky and Murphy (*J. Biol. Chem.*, 1934, **106**, 431, 441 and 445) she gave this isomeric form the title vitamin F, and with E. R. Linn suggested a method for its evaluation and quantitative estimation in terms of a suitable unit (*Drug Cosmet. Ind.*, May 1936). The following were considered by these investigators to be characteristic of a vitamin F deficiency, viz. dryness or roughness of the skin and a tendency to develop sores and ultimate eczema. Brittleness of the hair, thinning and eventually alopecia ; brittleness of the nails with tendency to ridging. (In fact, if it were all it was claimed to be, the majority of cosmetic ills would be cured.) As usual there was a mass of conflicting evidence regarding its supposed efficacy. The most comprehensive bibliography on the evolution of vitamin F, with a considerable reference to the scientific facts upon which this supposition was based appeared in the *Amer. Perfum.*, March 1937, pp. 18–24 (Advertisement section).

Whilst not denying the results quoted in the bibliography, the main body of expert opinion in this country considered that such claims as were advanced for vitamin F, in cosmetics, had not been substantiated ("Vitamin F. Symposium", *Mfg. Perfum.*, March and April 1937). Reports from abroad indicated that the considered opinion of United States experts was the same ("Summary of the Board of Standards of the U.S. Toilet Goods Association", *Amer. Perfum.*, May 1937).

The arguments advanced against such claims were based in general upon the following facts:

(*a*) There was no evidence of any deficiency of vitamin F in normal healthy human beings on an average diet. (The experiments on vitamin F had been carried out upon rats who were fed upon an abnormal diet, in that all the ordinary saponifiable fats had been removed from it.) Moreover, experiments on rats and other animals do not necessarily coincide with human requirements.

(*b*) To term a chemical substance a "vitamin" was to place the cart before the horse. The term vitamin is only given to substances of unknown composition, usually necessary for human nutrition. Unless such a definition is observed there will be no limit to what might be called a vitamin.

More recently, Hume, Nunn, Smedley-MacLean and Smith (*Biochem. J.*, 1938, **32**, 2162) and other investigators have confirmed the general applicability of linoleic acid in rats fed upon a diet from which saponifiable fats were removed (but all the fat-soluble vitamins added) which developed skin dryness, scurfiness and thinness of hair.

At present there is no evidence to suggest that the normal diet of man is deficient in such unsaturated fatty acids or that upon a normal diet skin lesions or dryness develop which can be cured by the external application of vitamin F. At the same time the unsaturated fatty acids of fish oils (e.g. "Cod-liver Oil")—which differ from vitamin F—are believed to have useful dermatological properties. The action of these unsaturated fatty acids is not yet understood although there is evidence that the fatty acids and lipoids of skin, hair and nails possess bactericidal properties. (Burtenshaw, "The Mechanism of Self-Disinfection of the Human Skin and Its Appendages", *J. Hyg., Camb.*, 1942, **42**, 184.) Such bactericidal action would account—at least in part—for the value of unsaturated fatty acids in cleaning up unhealthy wounds. (*See* Chapter 1).

Bodman and Felix (*Med. Pr.*, 1943, **105**, 331) claim that insufficiency of unsaturated fatty acids in the diets plus strain may be frequently a cause of industrial dermatitis. They claim that in almost all of sixty-seven cases, the skin condition was improved or cured by treatment with an ointment rich in these unsaturated fatty acids.

It is interesting to note the discovery by Rothman (*Proc. Soc. exp. Biol., N.Y.*, 1945, **60**, 394) that adult human hair contains a fatty acid of chain length C_9 approximately (in the C_7 to C_{11} chain range) which is fungistatic for M. audouini in concentrations of from 0·0002 per cent. to 0·001 per cent., as this affords a logical explanation for the spontaneous cure of certain microsporon infections of the scalp after the sufferer has arrived at the age of puberty.

Also interesting is the development in recent years of the use of naturally occurring fatty acids as fungicides in certain skin affections. Peck and Rosenfeld (*J. invest. Derm.*, 1938, **1**, 237) first drew attention to the use of caprylic, propionic and undecylenic acids in the treatment of dermatophytic conditions. Keeney *et al.* (*Johns Hopk. Hosp. Bull.*, 1946, **78**, 33) and Shapiro and Rothman (*Arch. Derm. Syph., Chicago*, 1945, **52**, 166) have further studied this problem and suggested the uses of propionate-propionic acid, undecylenate-undecylenic acid, and zinc undecylenate-undecylenic acid respectively in the treatment of fungus infections of the feet.

To sum up, we are becoming increasingly aware of the uses of certain unsaturated fatty acids in the local treatment of certain skin conditions although their exact mode of action is not fully understood. *There may well be valid reasons for the use of some unsaturated fats or fatty acids in certain skin conditions*, but at the time of writing no dogmatic statements can be made, apart from the fact that, no matter what value such fatty acids may possess, there is no justification for calling them " vitamin F " or any other " vitamin ".

Lanolin

All the available evidence at present suggests that lanolin, of all the various cosmetic materials available, is the one most closely akin to sebum —the natural skin lubricant. Indeed this is not surprising since it is the natural skin lubricant of the skin and wool of the sheep which has been suitably cleansed and purified. Modern research into the structure of the amino acids and X-ray diffraction patterns of the molecular structure of the keratins of skin, hair and feathers (*Brit. J. Derm.*, 1950, Jan., **62**, 1–15) have indicated that Nature is sparing in her use of fundamental materials and that she tends to build apparently dissimilar structures and compounds from a few fundamental and comparatively simple " bricks ". Over very many years, lanolin has proved very efficacious in the treatment of chapped skin surfaces and in the prevention of industrial dermatitis. It has been shown that the addition of saponifiable oils to mineral lubricating oils has consistently led to a reduction in the number of experimental tumours produced in animals and *no oil has been found so far which surpasses lanolin in this respect.* It is also remarkable for the manner in which it preserves the skin smooth and soft. (*See* Report of the Manchester Committee on Cancer, 1923–34; and also C. C. Twort and J. M. Twort, "The Utility of Lanolin as a Protective Measure against Mineral Oil and Tar Dermatitis and Cancer", *J. Hyg.*, 4 March, 1935, **35**, no. 1).

Simpson and Cramer (*Cancer Res.*, 1945, **5**, 1–4) have also drawn attention to the fact that lanolin has some action in preventing skin cancer from the application of chemical carcinogens pointing out that *it is known that methylcholanthrene suffers a considerable reduction in its capacity to produce cancer when it is dissolved in lanolin.*

Whilst too much should not be read into the above facts, in our present state of knowledge, the evidence does suggest that lanolin is a desirable ingredient of cosmetic and toilet preparations. It should be noticed that the emphasis is on "lanolin" *per se* and that no evidence is available to show that lanolin derivatives possess the same properties as lanolin. As Malmstrom (*J. Soc. cosmet. Chem.*, June 1949, 1, **4**, 244) has pointed out ". . . contrary to popular belief the benefits derived from lanolin are not centred about the properties of the individual fatty acids or alcohols present. . . . This mixture which we call lanolin is essentially a chemical combination of fatty acids and alcohol in ester form. No evidence has been published to show that any individual chemical contained in the mixture is entirely, or partly, responsible for the properties of lanolin. . . ." (*See also* possible Role of Sebum (and Lanolin) in the "Hydration of the Skin" below.)

Proteins and Protein Hydrolysates

There is evidence that small amounts of protein may, under suitable conditions, penetrate the skin, and also circulate in the blood. (Walzer, *et al. Arch. Derm. Syph., Chicago*, 1940, **41**, 692; 1944, **49**, 427.) Recently deNavarre (*Amer. Perfum.* 1949, p. 205) has drawn attention to the introduction of a new material containing cystine and methionine in a hydrolysate, presumably derived from hair. Pointing out that Wiesenfeld had recently reported the value of an ointment containing a protein hydrolysate in the treatment of anterior poliomyelitis, in that on massaging this ointment over a portion of the limbs in twelve children there had been an increase in the circumference of the thigh so treated and an improvement in the muscular tone and colour, deNavarre suggested that such protein hydrolysates might be considered for inclusion in cosmetic preparations pointing out that milk had often been recommended for use, in the past, in toilet preparations.

In my opinion the possible introduction of foreign proteins directly into the blood instead of through the stomach *always involves a risk of allergic shock* ; for this reason I do not favour the use of proteins or hydrolysed proteins externally as a cosmetic means of treating the skin.

The Value of Massage

F. H. Krusen (*Physical Medicine*, p. 527, Philadelphia : W. B. Saunders and Co.), 1941, states that experiments on the capillary circulation in the ear of the rabbit lead to the conclusion that massage of the skin is accompanied, or followed by, an increased interchange of substances between the blood stream and tissue cells, with an altered and presumably improved metabolism of the tissues.

Kovacs (*A Manual of Physical Therapy*, p. 226, Philadelphia : Lee and Febiger, 1946), confirms that massage exerts a mechanical stimulation on the skin, its immediate effect being a dilation of the capillaries accompanied by a feeling of warmth ; massage also promotes the movement of fluids, and loosens the elastic layer in the subcutaneous tissue.

The " Hydration of the Skin "

The skin is a " protein-gel " hydrated in its innermost layers and largely dehydrated in its surface layer. The proportion of water in the outer corneous layer of the skin is obviously of great physiological importance in that (1) a certain amount of desiccation of the skin surface minimises bacterial multiplication on the skin surface, and assists in maintaining its integrity ; (2) the continual desquammation of the skin is Nature's method of removing debris and foreign matter which have become mechanically embedded in the skin apertures.

At the same time it is not desirable that drying of this layer should proceed to such an extent that the corneous layer prematurely " flakes away ", and cracks develop in the skin surface (often followed by bacterial invasion)—a phenomenon which we often term " skin chapping ", intermediate phases being classified as " dry skin ", etc.

For many years my conception of the moisture-regulating mechanism whereby the skin is kept in a smooth, healthy condition has been as follows :

(i) A continual transference of moisture occurs from the lower skin layers to the skin surface where it is lost by the process of evaporation. In addition, if the temperature is sufficiently high, sensible perspiration is supplied to the skin surface from the sweat glands,

(ii) the rate of evaporation of moisture from the skin surface will be governed by:

(*a*) the "drying character" of the surrounding atmosphere which will depend upon the temperature and humidity of the air and presence or absence of air currents.

(*b*) the presence of fatty material (sebum) on the skin surface which may assist the retention of water in the skin in two ways: firstly because *any* layer of "fatty" matter will tend to reduce moisture evaporation from a film of water beneath it; secondly because the fatty material (sebum) possesses hydrophilic properties which tend to hold the water *within the fatty phase*, either emulsified as a water-in-oil emulsion, or as bimolecular leaflets. (*See* Chapter 41, Emulsions and Dispersions.)

(*c*) the fact that if the aqueous matter in the sebum film is held in the form of bimolecular leaflets then there is the *possibility*, though it may appear remote, that quite a complex phenomenon is involved. It is pointed out (Chapter 41) that the water-holding capacities of such leaflets is considerably influenced and diminished by the presence of electrolytes (e.g. perspiration) and thus the "sebum-electrolyte balance" of the skin may be of great importance.

The above conception also provides an explanation of why both aqueous preparations (based on glycerin, glycerin and rose water, "mucilaginous" glycerin preparations, etc.), and fatty and emulsified preparations, prove beneficial for chapped hands. At first sight the actions of these two types of preparations seem diametrically opposed. An explanation can be given along the lines that the non-fatty preparations (which are effective) contain a fair proportion of glycerin, or other humectant. In drying they leave a film on the skin which, in the case of glycerin, consists of a film of glycerin together with an approximately similar weight of water held by the hygroscopicity of the glycerin. Because of its hygroscopicity the glycerin will obtain this amount of water either from the preparation itself (if aqueous) from the air, or—if there is no water in the preparation and the humidity of the air is too low—from the lower layer skin layers. Having obtained such an "equilibrium moisture" content it will *retain* it (within certain limits).

On the other hand the purely fatty or emulsified creams, in drying, leave a fatty layer deposited on the skin surface which reduces moisture loss by hindering evaporation.

The general correctness of my tentative hypothesis has recently been confirmed by the publication of two papers by I. H. Blank ("Factors which influence the water content of the Stratum Corneum ", *J. invest. Derm.*, June 1952, **18**, 433), and L. E. Gaul and G. B. Underwood (" Relation of Dew Point and Barometric Pressure to Chapping of Normal Skin ", *J. invest. Derm.*, July 1952, **19**, 9).

Blank found that a piece of cornified epithelium, when allowed to dry out, became hard and brittle, and that any attempt to soften this cornified epithelium by the application of petroleum jelly, lanolin, or olive oil met with complete failure. If, on the other hand, similar pieces of cornified epithelium were allowed to absorb a little moisture they became soft and pliable. It was therefore considered apparent that the water content was of paramount importance in maintaining the flexibility of the stratum corneum.

Blank considered that if the skin sebum provided a natural barrier at the skin surface (in a manner similar to an artificial barrier such as petroleum jelly which leads to the corneous layer becoming macerated) then the corneous layer would normally have the characteristics usually associated with maceration. In my opinion, based upon experience with protective creams, the explanation of why the skin does not become macerated under a layer of sebum lies in the fact that lanolin and related compounds (and presumably sebum) are not impervious to a film of water, but allow transfer of such moisture, slowly, *through the lanolin ;* thus they hinder but do not prevent evaporation in the way in which a layer of petroleum jelly prevents evaporation. Blank pointed out that under most climatic conditions the stratum corneum would dry out and become brittle if it were not for the fact that for relative humidities of about 60 per cent. and higher an equilibrium state exists which does not permit the mositure content to drop below 10 mg. per 100 mg. dry weight ; at this moisture content the stratum corneum remains soft and pliable. Under the relatively low humidity of winter weather, heated houses, or the rapid air currents of windy conditions, the stratum corneum does dry out and the fissures of chapped skin and scaling of windburn can develop because of the brittleness of the stratum corneum.

L. E. Gaul and G. B. Underwood have also drawn attention to the remarkable action of rising dew points on chapped skin, and state that this strongly suggests that the degree of air moisture is directly associated with softness, smoothness and suppleness of the skin. These investigators were unable to correlate " complexion " with chapping ; the " dark " chapped as much as the " light ", the obese as much as the lean, the skin of negroes was as susceptible as that of white patients. The presence or absence of an oily skin did not affect susceptibility. An oily type acne chapped as much as the fair dry skin. Occupation played no part except where it led to " wetting " of the skin. Inheritance seemed important ;

where a mother or father chapped severely, often the children resembling the parent were affected.

Whilst inheritance would be expected to play a role in skin chapping, it must be remembered that families living together are subjected to a number of conditions not directly related to inheritance. These include the type and quantity of food eaten, the climatic condition of the area in which the family is dwelling, the temperature and humidity of their rooms; even the type of soap used for washing the skin. Again although these investigators state that the "presence or absence of an oily skin did not affect susceptibility", in an earlier part of the same paper they state that ". . . any cleaning or treatment procedure which immediately or later enhances desiccation can predispose to a dermatitis . . ." and later state: "Occupation played no part except where it led to *wetting* the skin". From what has been said already about skin hydration (and from what we know as a result of the treatment of chapped hands with aqueous preparations containing humectants) it is obvious that wetting alone cannot predispose to skin dryness *unless at the same time—in the process of cleansing the skin—some other protective factors (which could well be sebum) are removed.* The statement regarding the role of an oily skin and the influence of sebum on chapping hence requires further elucidation.

Dr. Powers [*Amer. Perfum.*, Nov. 1952, p. 372] points out that "indoor humidity" frequently drops to 20–25 per cent. and that under these conditions the rate of moisture loss from a sorbitol solution is markedly less than from solutions containing the same amounts of either glycerin or propylene glycol. (*See* Chapter 44, Humectants.) Dr. Powers refers to the fact that the outer layer of the skin contains from 65 per cent. to 80 per cent. water.

The importance of maintaining an adequate moisture level in the skin is therefore obvious.

CHAPTER 5

COLD AND CLEANSING CREAMS, CLEANSING MILKS AND LOTIONS

To Claudius-Galenus—a physician in Rome in the second century—is attributed the invention of cold cream, though many persons feel he may have obtained it in turn from Hippocrates, who was the source of much of Galen's inspiration and the "Father of Modern Medicine".

In his "Methodus Medendi vel de Morbis Curandis" (10th Book), Galen directs that one part of purified wax be carefully liquefied in a mortar together with three or four parts of olive oil (in which rose petals have been macerated) and then allowed to cool, whereupon as much water as can be incorporated into the above mass is added.

As "Unguentum Refrigerans", a cold cream formula was included in the "Pharmacopoeia Collegii Regalis Medicorum Londinensis" of 1618 and, under the title "Unguentum Aqua Rosae", in the *British Pharmacopoeia* of 1898.

Numerous different cold cream formulae are in existence, and even the "official" pharmacopoeial formulae of different countries show wide variation, ranging from 5–37 per cent. water, 70–50 per cent. almond oil, and from 12 per cent. beeswax to 24 per cent. mixed beeswax and spermaceti.

The characteristic feature of a true cold cream is the presence of a relatively large amount of water, loosely held in the wax mixture. On application to the skin, such water-in-oil emulsions (or possibly bi-molecular leaflets) [1] *break and, in the majority of cases, water separates. The evaporation of this water produces a very cooling sensation on the skin.*

An example of such a cold cream is given under the designation "Ceratum Galeni" in the French Codex, viz.:

	Parts
(*a*) White wax (i.e. beeswax)	12·0
(*b*) Almond oil	50·0
(*c*) Rosewater	37·50

Procedure

Melt (*a*) in (*b*) and slowly incorporate (*c*) with constant trituration.

[1] *See* Emulsions and Dispersions.

Almond oil is expensive and develops a very slightly fatty odour unless very carefully preserved with a suitable antioxidant. A more modern variety of such a "cold" cream is given by:

	per cent.
(*a*) Mineral oil	48·0
(*b*) Beeswax	6·0
(*c*) Spermaceti	6·0
(*d*) Cetyl alcohol	1·0
(*e*) Lanolin	1·0
(*f*) Water	38·0
(*g*) Preservative	*q.s.*
(*h*) Perfume	*q.s.*

Procedure

(1) Melt together (*a*), (*b*), (*c*), (*d*) and (*e*), to a clear homogeneous liquid.
(2) Dissolve the preservative (*g*) in (*f*) (if water-soluble; if not, dissolve it in the melted oils and fats) and when the mixture of oils and fats (1) has cooled to 45°–50° C., add, slowly with continual stirring (2) at the same temperature. Stir to 40° C., incorporate the perfume and stir down to 25°–30° C.

According to Mendelsohn (*Mfg. Chem.*, Dec. 1951, p. 474), it is believed that V. C. Daggett prior to 1900 initiated the use of mineral oil to replace vegetable oils in the manufacture of cosmetic creams, the primary object of the substitution being to ensure whiteness, inhibition of rancidity and uniformity of the finished product.

Because of the characteristic feature of *water separation* on rubbing out cold creams of the above type, these creams were rendered more stable by the inclusion of some borax which reacted with the free fatty acids present in the beeswax to form the sodium soap, this soap contributing to the stability of the cream. For example, the composition of "Unguentum Aqua Rosae" of the British Pharmaceutical Codex of 1934 is given as:

	per cent.
(*a*) White beeswax	18·0
(*b*) Almond oil	61·0
(*c*) Borax	1·0
(*d*) Rose water	20·0
(*e*) Oil of rose (additional)	0·1

Procedure

(1) Melt (*a*) in (*b*).
(2) Dissolve (*c*) in (*d*). Add with constant stirring (2) to (1). Add the oil of rose and continue to stir till cold.

Ratios of Beeswax, Oil, Water and Borax

The optimum ratios of beeswax, water, oil and borax, have been determined by Marsek to be as follows:

		per cent. approx.
Beeswax	1 part by weight	= 16
Water	2 parts by weight	= 33
Oil	3 parts by weight	= 50
Borax	5 per cent. to 6 per cent. of the beeswax used.	

deNavarre (*The Chemistry and Manufacture of Cosmetics*, p. 214, D. Van Nostrand Co. Inc., 1941) quotes the following formula which is identical with these ratios, viz. :

	per cent.
(*a*) Beeswax	16·0
(*b*) Mineral oil	50·0
(*c*) Water	33·0
(*d*) Borax	1·0

Procedure

(1) Heat (*a*) and (*b*) to 70°–75° C. until a clear homogeneous liquid is obtained.

(2) Dissolve (*d*) in (*c*) by gentle heat and adjust the temperature of this solution to 75° C. Slowly add this latter mixture to the melted fats at about 75° C. Stir down to 45° C. and add the perfume. At 42° C. pour into jars. Alternatively this cream may be either passed through a colloid mill at 45° C. or allowed to stand overnight and passed through a colloid mill, a homogeniser or through a triple-roll mill and packed cold. Such a processing gives a softer product.

deNavarre (*The Chemistry and Manufacture of Cosmetics*) gives the reaction occurring between the beeswax fatty acids and the borax as :

$$C_{25}H_{51}COOH + Na_2B_4O_7 = C_{25}H_{51}COONa + H_3BO_3 + H_2O$$

(Beeswax Fatty Acids) + (Borax) = Sodium Cerotate + Boric Acid + Water.

[This is in fact the usual statement given in the literature, as almost all the published literature on beeswax refers to its content of cerotic and melissic acids—about 15 per cent. It is also stated to contain some 80 per cent. ceryl myristate. Hilditch, however (*The Chemical Constitution of Natural Fats*, London : Chapman & Hall) has pointed out that cerotic acid does not exist and is now recognised to be a mixture of several *n*-aliphatic acids and is not solely *n*-hexacosanoic. Similarly Chibnall, Piper, Pollard, Williams and Sahai (*Biochem J.*, 1934, **28**, 2189) state that the use of such terms as ceryl, or melissyl alcohol for, respectively, the alcohols $C_{26}H_{53}(OH)$ and $C_{30}H_{61}(OH)$ is misleading since these are almost invariably mixtures of the even numbered homologues.]

The actual amount of borax required to neutralise the free fatty acids present in the beeswax is calculated from the " Acid Value " of the beeswax which is obtained by a simple titration experiment (details for carrying out this procedure will be found in the British Pharmacopoeia or in any book dealing with the analysis of oils, fats and waxes). The British

Pharmacopoeia 1953 requires that beeswax shall have an acid value (as determined by the B.P. Method) of 17 to 24. The higher the acid number of a sample the greater amount of borax will it require.

However, no correlation has been established between the emulsifying characteristics of a particular sample of beeswax and its acid value. Indeed, the Board of Standards of the U.S. Toilet Goods Association have realised this and have inserted into their specifications a test for emulsifying properties in which they state: "Owing to lack of a satisfactory method for determining emulsifying properties, it is suggested that the individual purchaser specify in all contracts of purchase that the wax purchased under this specification must produce a satisfactory emulsion."

A figure of about "6 per cent. of the beeswax employed", is often suggested as a suitable proportion of borax to employ in a cold cream. This is derived from the U.S.P. acid values for beeswax (18–24 g.), which means that 1 g. of beeswax will be neutralised exactly by 18–24 mg. of potassium hydroxide; this corresponds to about 16 parts of beeswax to 1 part of borax, i.e. about 6 per cent.

Determination of the Continuous Phase of a "Cold Cream"

There has been considerable controversy as to whether cold cream is a water-in-oil or oil-in-water emulsion and considerable discrepancy is to be found in the literature, due in many instances to the methods used for determining the continuous phase of the emulsion. Methods based on the miscibility of the cream with (*a*) oil or (*b*) water, or methods based upon mixing the cream with (i) oil-soluble or (ii) water-soluble dyestuffs are inaccurate since phase inversion may occur. *p*H determinations by means of the glass electrode, or electrical methods of measuring the resistance of the cream appear to be satisfactory. In the case of oil-in-water emulsions, a *p*H reading (or comparatively low resistance reading) will readily be obtained. Where the emulsion is of the water-in-oil type, it will be found impossible to obtain a reproducible *p*H reading owing to the high internal resistance of the oil phase; similarly the electrical resistance will be high.

Using the above methods it will be found that *the majority of cold creams are of the oil-in-water type.*

It is my experience that a number of factors influence the continuous phase of the emulsion; these include:

(i) the ratio of oil to water;
(ii) the emulsifying agent;
(iii) the process of manufacture.

Of paramount importance is the influence of the emulsifying agent, although the ratio of oil to water, the presence of other substances and the conditions of processing all have an influence on the final cream.

The influence of the emulsifying agent may readily be observed by adding a metal soap, such as zinc stearate to an oil-in-water cold cream; inversion to the water-in-oil state readily occurs. In the case of the borax-beeswax fatty acid soap, it would appear that reduction in the amount of soap formed, caused by reducing the amount of borax in the formula, favours water-in-oil emulsions; conversely when the borax is present in amounts of 5-6 per cent. and upwards, the tendency is for the resultant cream to be of the oil-in-water type.

The ratio of oil to water also affects the type of emulsion (providing the amount of emulsifying agent is not such as to override its influence). For example, an excess of 15-20 per cent. of oil over the amount of water favours emulsions of the water-in-oil type; for greater safety in preparing this type of emulsion it would be advisable to increase even further the preponderance of oil over the water in the formula. Conversely, a preponderance of water favours emulsions of the oil-in-water type.

Apart from the influence of processing, such as milling or homogenisation, upon the resultant product, the temperatures at which the aqueous and oily phases are mixed is important. Here again, the final product will be influenced by the factors of ratios of oil to water, borax to beeswax, etc., as discussed above.

It has been stated (*Soap Perfum. Cosm.*, 1938, **11**, 625) that mixing the aqueous and oily solutions, both at a temperature of 70° C., produces a medium heavy cream which will easily liquefy on application. If the aqueous solution, at a temperature of 55° C., is added to the melted oil and beeswax, and heated to 90° C., the resultant cream is said to be a very glossy, medium heavy cream which liquefies slowly. If the oily and aqueous portions, both at a temperature of 55° C., are mixed together, it is stated that the cream obtained is soft, slightly grainy and easily liquefies.

An example of a modern cold cream of the orthodox beeswax-borax type is given by:

	per cent.
(*a*) Beeswax	12·0
(*b*) Mineral oil (low viscosity)	55·0
(*c*) Borax	1·0
(*d*) Water	32·0
(*e*) Perfume	*q.s.*

Procedure

(1) Heat (*a*) and (*b*) at 70° C. until a clear homogeneous liquid.
(2) Dissolve (*c*) in (*d*) and bring to 70° C.

Add (2) to (1), both solutions being at 70° C., with continuous but gentle stirring. Continue stirring at a lower speed, and when the temperature falls to 45°–50° C. add the perfume. Product may be "hot poured", or processed by homogenisation as desired.

The above cream is softer than the usual types of cold cream, and more in line with a cleansing cream. It may be stiffened, if desired, by incorporating a small proportion of other waxes, or by increasing the content of beeswax.

Even the beeswax-borax type of cold cream has undergone modifications in formulation and complexity, varying from the incorporation of hydrophilic lanolin derivatives into an "orthodox" cold cream formula to beeswax "soap-free" formulations based upon non-ionic emulsifiers, for example the two formulations set out below (W. C. Griffin, P. J. Carter, R. W. Behrens, *Drug Cosmet. Ind.*, Sept. 1948):

	per cent.
(*a*) Beeswax	15·0
(*b*) Mineral oil	50·0
(*c*) G-1431 (Atlas Co.) (Polyoxyethylene sorbitol-lanolin)	3·0
(*d*) Borax	1·0
(*e*) Water	31·0

Procedure

(1) Heat (*a*), (*b*) and (*c*), to 80° C.
(2) Dissolve (*d*) in (*e*) and heat to 85° C.
Add (2) to (1), with gentle agitation. Pour at 40°–50° C.

	per cent.
(*a*) Mineral oil 65/75	50·0
(*b*) Beeswax	15·0
(*c*) Spermaceti	2·0
(*d*) Lanolin (anhydrous)	0·5
(*e*) G-1441 (Atlas Co.) (Polyoxyethylene sorbitol-lanolin)	4·0
(*f*) Arlacel 60 (Atlas Co.) (Sorbitan monostearate)	4·0
(*g*) Arlacel 83 (Atlas Co.) (Sorbitan sesquioleate)	0·5
(*h*) Veegum Gel (Vanderbilt) (magnesium aluminium silicate)	0·5
(*i*) Water	23·5
(*j*) Preservative	*q.s.*
(*k*) Perfume	*q.s.*

Procedure

(1) Mix (*h*), (*i*) and (*j*), heat to 70° C.
(2) Mix (*a*), (*b*), (*c*), (*d*), (*e*), (*f*) and (*g*) and heat to 70° C.
Add (1) to (2) at 70° C. with moderate agitation. Continue agitation during cooling. Perfume at 45° C. and pour at 40° C.

Apart from such complex formulations as the above, modifications in the structure of beeswax itself have more recently come into vogue.

In U.S.P. 2,361,477, it is claimed that by submitting beeswax to low pressure distillation, within the range 1·0 to 0·001 mm. of mercury, a product is obtained which has an acid number greater than 35, an ester number less than 35, and which possesses improved emulsifying properties.

In the United States, the Atlas Powder Co. have developed a series of hydrophilic beeswax derivatives; chemically, these are polyoxyethylene sorbitol beeswax derivatives. There are seven principal emulsifiers in this group, all of which are more hydrophilic than beeswax itself. For convenience, they are grouped as follows:

More Hydrophilic: G-1725, G-1726, G-1727, and G-1734.

More Lipophilic: G-1702, G-1704, and G-1706.

All of these beeswax derivatives are light tan in colour and have a consistency and odour similar to beeswax. It is claimed that cold creams made with such derivatives show several advantages over ordinary cold creams, in that they are softer in consistency, liquefy readily and allow the incorporation of larger amounts of water in the formulation; moreover, they are neutral in reaction (whereas most commercial cold creams have an alkaline *p*H), and are stable at 50° C. When a heavy textured cream is desired, the more lipophilic products (those more closely resembling beeswax) give best results. If a thinner consistency is desired, it is desirable to include in the formulation one of the "Tween" (Atlas Co.) emulsifiers.[1]

The following formula (*Hydrophilic Beeswax Derivative Emulsifiers for Cosmetics*, Atlas Powder Co., Wilmington, Jan. 1950), illustrates the use of such hydrophilic beeswax derivatives in combination with a "Tween" and with beeswax; the second formulation illustrates the use of such derivatives alone:

	per cent.
(*a*) Mineral oil	50·0
(*b*) Beeswax	7·0
(*c*) Tween 40 (Polyoxyethylene sorbitan monopalmitate)	2·0
(*d*) G-1726	8·0
(*e*) Water	33·0
(*f*) Preservative	*q.s.*
(*g*) Perfume	*q.s.*

Procedure

(1) Heat (*a*), (*b*), (*c*) and (*d*) at 70° C. until clear.

(2) Heat (*e*) and (*f*) until (*f*) (if water soluble), is dissolved.

Add (2) at 70° C. to (1) at the same temperature, slowly, and with thorough agitation. Perfume at 50° C. and pour at 45°–50° C.

[1] These are essentially polyoxyethylene derivatives of the "Spans", which in turn are essentially partial esters of the common fatty acids—lauric, palmitic, stearic, oleic—and hexitol anhydrides derived from sorbitol.

	per cent.
(*a*) Mineral oil	50·0
(*b*) G-1704	12·0
(*c*) G-1726	3·0
(*d*) Water	35·0
(*e*) Preservative	*q.s.*
(*f*) Perfume	*q.s.*

Procedure

(1) Heat (*a*), (*b*) and (*c*) to 70° C.
(2) Dissolve (*e*) in (*d*) and heat to 70° C.

Add (2) to (1) slowly, with thorough agitation. Continue stirring while cooling. Perfume at 50° C. and then pour.

In general beeswax creams possess a characteristic odour which is not very easy to disguise except by means of the usual " rosaceous " type of odour. Such defects may be overcome by the use of comparatively simple formulations based on " Lanette Wax SX ", or self-emulsifying Glyceryl Monostearates [available as such and under proprietary designations such as Abracol G.M.S. (A. Boake Roberts Ltd.), " Tegin " (Goldschmidt Corporation)]. For example :

	per cent.
(*a*) Lanette wax (cetyl/stearyl alcohols, c. 10 per cent. sulphated)	16·0
(*b*) Mineral oil	20·0
(*c*) Ozokerite	3·0
(*d*) Glycerin	5·0
(*e*) Water	56·0
(*f*) Preservative	*q.s.*
(*g*) Perfume	*q.s.*

Procedure

(1) Heat (*a*), (*b*). (*c*) to 70° C. and maintain at this temperature until homogeneous.
(2) Heat (*d*), (*e*) and (*f*) to 70° C.

Add (2) to (1) with continuous stirring. Continue stirring, perfume at 45° C. and stir down to 25°–30° C. Homogenise.

The following formula illustrates the use of Glyceryl Monostearate (" Tegin ") and is quoted from *Emulsifiers*, Goldschmidt Chemical Corporation, New York, 1951 :

	per cent.
(*a*) " Tegin "	15·0
(*b*) Mineral oil	18·0
(*c*) Spermaceti	5·0
(*d*) Cetyl alcohol	2·0
(*e*) Water	54·9
(*f*) Glycerin	5·0
(*g*) Preservative—" Tegosept P " (ester of *p*-hydroxybenzoic acid)	0·1

Procedure

Heat all the above ingredients in a single container to 90°–100° C. (whilst agitating) until dissolved. Continue agitation (with heating discontinued), until cool. Perfume at lowest convenient temperature, usually about 45° C.

It is the author's experience that the inclusion of cetyl alcohol in certain formulations has an effect greater than that which might be predicted, merely on the basis of "fatty matter". For example, in certain cold cream formulations having resistances of the order of 10,000 ohms (o/w type), the introduction of cetyl alcohol increased the resistance to about 100,000 ohms (whereas the resistance of similar water-in-oil formulations was greater than 1,000,000 ohms). The cream containing the cetyl alcohol appeared to be of a complex emulsion type, possibly "(water-in-oil)"-in-water.

It is possible to build up cold cream formulations without beeswax, without soap, and without proprietary emulsifying agents along the following lines:

	per cent.
(*a*) Cetyl alcohol	4·0
(*b*) Ceresin	4·0
(*c*) Lanolin	3·0
(*d*) Sodium cetyl/stearyl sulphates [1]	2·0
(*e*) Mineral oil (low viscosity)	50·0
(*f*) Water	37·0
(*g*) Preservative	*q.s.*
(*h*) Perfume	*q.s.*

Procedure

(1) Heat (*a*), (*b*), (*c*) and (*e*) at 70° C. until clear and homogeneous.
(2) Dissolve (*d*) and (*g*) in (*f*) and heat to 70° C.

Add (2) to (1) in a slow stream with fairly high speed agitation. Perfume at 45° C. After perfuming, the product may be homogenised and filled either hot or after cooling. A firmer preparation may be obtained by including higher melting waxes and/or by increasing the proportion of cetyl alcohol or ceresin.

In addition to the oil-in-water types of cold creams discussed, a number of creams of the water-in-oil type are sold for this purpose. Although these may not feel quite as cooling on the skin as those of the oil-in-water type (or as the older type of cold cream in which the water content is but loosely held and separates on application to the skin) nevertheless, because such creams contain both fatty materials and water, they probably contribute to keeping the skin in a soft and pliable condition. As mentioned

[1] Commercial cut of cetyl/stearyl sulphated alcohols, extracted to free from sodium sulphate. Cetyl/stearyl alcohols used in preference to lauryl alcohol on grounds of skin irritation. See note on Sulphated Fatty Alcohols. R. G. Harry, *Cosmetic Materials*, London: Leonard Hill Ltd.

under Hand Creams (Chapter 38) and discussed more fully under Skin Foods (Chapter 10), loss of moisture from the skin surface is certainly a major factor in dryness of the skin, though it is probable that emollient fatty materials also have an important role to play.

In addition, water-in-oil creams tend to dry out less when stored under tropical conditions; that is, assuming the cream has been formulated so that separation of the emulsion does not occur.

Janowitz (*Soap Perfum. Cosm.*, Oct. 1944, p. 750), gives a simple formulation of the water-in-oil type in which zinc stearate, in conjunction with beeswax-soap, is the water-in-oil stabiliser, viz.:

	per cent.
(*a*) Beeswax	14·0
(*b*) Mineral oil	59·3
(*c*) Borax	0·7
(*d*) Water	25·0
(*e*) Zinc stearate	1·0
(*f*) Perfume	*q.s.*

Procedure

Prepare the cold cream base in the normal way by heating the fatty materials to 75° C., the aqueous materials to 75° C. and then mixing, with agitation. The perfume is then added and the mass milled in an ointment mill with the zinc stearate.

Lanolin absorption bases may also be used to formulate water-in-oil cold creams. The following two formulae exemplify some basic formulations which lend themselves to further experiment:

	per cent.
(*a*) Protegin X (Goldschmidt Corp.)	22·0
(*b*) Lanolin	3·0
(*c*) Mineral oil	25·0
(*d*) Beeswax	7·0
(*e*) Water	43·0

Procedure

(1) Melt (*a*), (*b*), (*c*) and (*d*) by steam heat maintaining as low a temperature as possible. Adjust temperature of the mixture to 40°–50° C.

(2) Slowly add (*e*) at 40°–50° C., to (1), each addition being stirred in completely before more of (*e*) is added. Perfume (not included in the above formula) may be added, with continuous agitation until the temperature has fallen to about 25° C. The product may be milled, if desired.

(From: *Emulsifiers*, Goldschmidt Chemical Corporation, New York.)

	per cent.
(*a*) " Cremba " absorption base (Croda)	20·0
(*b*) Lanolin	3·0
(*c*) Beeswax	4·0

	per cent.
(*d*) Ceresin	10·0
(*e*) Liquid paraffin oil	10·0
(*f*) Glycerin	5·0
(*g*) Water	48·0

Procedure

(1) Melt (*a*), (*b*), (*c*), (*d*) and (*e*) by steam heat maintaining as low a temperature as possible. Adjust temperature to about 50° C.

(2) Mix (*f*) with (*g*) and raise the temperature to 50° C.

Add slowly (2) to (1), each addition being stirred in completely before adding further amounts of (2). Perfume and continue stirring until the temperature has fallen to about 25° C.

(Formula from : *Lanolin Absorption Bases*, Croda Ltd.)

It should be noted that small amounts of lanolin, and often glycerin, assist the stability of absorption base emulsions. Small amounts of magnesium salts, particularly the sulphate, and also of the metallic soaps, magnesium and zinc stearates, also assist stability.

A modern, emollient, water-in-oil cold cream of the more complex type is quoted by Griffin, Carter and Behrens (*Drug Cosmet. Ind.*, Sept. 1948) and is given below :

	per cent.
(*a*) Petrolatum	35·0
(*b*) Mineral oil 65/75	15·0
(*c*) Paraffin wax	5·0
(*d*) Ceresin wax	5·0
(*e*) Lanolin	1·0
(*f*) Arlacel 83 (sorbitan sesquioleate)	2·0
(*g*) G-1425 (polyoxyalkylene sorbitol-lanolin)	4·0
(*h*) Water	30·8
(*i*) Arlex (commercial sorbitol solution)	2·0
(*j*) Magnesium sulphate	0·2
(*k*) Preservative	*q.s.*
(*l*) Perfume	*q.s.*

Procedure

(1) Heat together (*a*), (*b*), (*c*), (*d*), (*e*), (*f*) and (*g*) and adjust the temperature to 70°–75° C.

(2) Heat together (*h*), (*i*), (*j*) and (*k*), and adjust the temperature to 70°–75° C

Add (2) to (1) gradually, whilst stirring. Add (*l*) at 55°–60° C. Homogenise at 55°–60° C., and fill directly into jars.

Cleansing Creams

As their name implies, cleansing creams are used for the purpose of cleansing the skin, either in place of, or sometimes in conjunction with, the (subsequent) application of water.

The usual pigments used in face "make-up", particularly rouge, are hydrophobic and lipophilic, that is to say, they are more readily wetted by oil than they are by water. In the presence of a surface active agent such as soap, such make-up may, by vigorous rubbing, be removed. However, as discussed under emulsions and dispersions (Chapter 41), soap, when dissolved or dispersed in water produces colloidal aggregates termed micelles. These micelles have considerable affinity for absorbing oil and in so doing, do not distinguish between surface "soil" and the natural oils of the skin; hence to some persons, soap is "drying", or perhaps more correctly "defatting". (*See also* Skin Nutrition, Chapter 4.)

By the use of a cleansing cream, make-up is removed from the skin more readily and it is likely that less degreasing of the skin occurs.

Cleansing creams are of three types: (*a*) liquefying cleansing creams consisting of oily materials only and containing no water; (*b*) emulsified creams of the water-in-oil, or "reverse" type; and (*c*) emulsified creams in which water is the continuous phase. In general classes (*a*) and (*c*) are of the greatest interest.

Creams of type (*a*) contain no soap and may be classed as emollient, although it is possible that the "excessive use" of such preparations containing saturated mineral oils only, may "flush away" the natural unsaturates present on the skin surface. Evidence of any harmful effects of such preparations is, however, lacking. In the case of creams of type (*c*), whilst it is true that they contain, in many instances as emulsifier, small amounts of soap or other surface active agents, nevertheless, the amount of oil present in the emulsion appears to be sufficient to reduce, or even saturate, the capacity of the detergent micelles to absorb further fatty matter. In this latter instance it might be questioned as to whether such a preparation could have any "cleansing" action.

Under Shampoos and Detergents (Chapter 22), will be found a brief note of the mechanism of detergent action. In general, detergency involves the ability of the detergent to wet both the dirt and the structure of the material upon which it is deposited, in this case the skin. Secondly, oriented adsorption causes the formation of a protective film around the dirt particles and thirdly, the particles must be kept dispersed in order that they may be washed away.

It is not difficult to assume the oily portion of the cleansing cream wetting both the skin and also lipophilic dirt, or of the mechanical application of a cleansing cream of suitable viscosity resulting in the dirt particles being broken up and suspended in the cleansing cream. What is perhaps surprising is that some experiments carried out by the author give no support for the assumption, often made in the technical literature, that an emulsion of the oil-in-water type is more effective as a cosmetic cleansing agent than a simple mixture of oils and waxes containing no water and no detergent material.

These experiments were carried out to assess the relative cleansing properties of (*a*) a simple liquefying cleansing cream containing no water, (*b*) a cleansing cream of the oil-in-water type, and (*c*) a cream of the water-in-oil type.

Three types of surface dirt were investigated, namely (i) aqueous dirt, (ii) suspended " particulate " dirt, and (iii) oily dirt.

To assess the efficacy of the removal of such dirt by the cleansing creams, fluorescent dyes were incorporated into the soiling medium, in the case of " aqueous dirt ", water-soluble fluorescein was dissolved in the aqueous portion of an ordinary vanishing cream. In the case of particulate dirt, finely divided bromo-acid in excess was ground into a lipstick base, whilst in the case of greasy dirt the natural bluish fluorescence of the hydrocarbon base was increased by the addition of a small quantity of a highly fluorescent perfume.

The above three types of dirt were applied to the skin, well rubbed in and allowed to remain for thirty minutes after which, each of the cleansing creams was applied, separately, to an area of the skin so treated, the excess cream being removed with tissue. These operations were carried out in normal daylight so that the efficacy of the cleansing could not be fully assessed until the skin area was re-examined in ultra-violet light.

Surprisingly, it was found that irrespective of which of the cleansing creams was employed, all traces of the fluorescent materials had in fact been removed, whereas, if the skin area was simply wiped with tissue without creaming, fluorescent areas remained visible on the skin.

It is possible that, in the case of the cleansing cream containing only oily materials, the minute amount of skin lipoids which are oil-miscible, taken up by the cream, is sufficient to allow of the small amounts of aqueous matter (perspiration, etc.) on the skin surface being taken up by the mixture of " oily-cleanser + lipoids ", in the form either of bi-molecular leaflets (*see* Chapter 41), or as a water-in-oil emulsion. In the case of the cleansing cream of the oil-in-water type (or of the water-in-oil type) the aqueous dirt may be absorbed into the continuous phase in the case of the former (providing it *remains* as an oil-in-water cream, on application to the skin) and into the dispersed phase in the case of the latter.

[It is of interest to note that some oil-in-water creams, when applied to the skin surface and then carefully scraped off, appear to have inverted to the water-in-oil phase; this is probably due to the influence of skin lipoids, which, though small in amount, may be relatively high in their ratio to the amount of cream spread as a surface film on the skin. It is also of interest that, in the author's experience, the influence of adding lanolin to otherwise hydrophobic fatty matters is to *reduce* the water-repellency of the fatty film, though it still remains water-repellent to some degree. Both of these factors may play a role in explaining the behaviour of cleansing creams on the skin.]

That cleansing creams and lotions *cleanse the skin* is evidenced by the fact that the application of a cleansing cream to a skin already cleansed by means of soap and water, will almost always, if not invariably, remove further dirt as evidenced by the appearance of the tissue or towel used finally to remove it. The user has thus the *evidence of her own eyes that such a preparation does cleanse.*

Properties Desirable in a Cleansing Cream, Milk or Loton

As with all cosmetical preparations, it is a *sine qua non* that such preparations should be dermatologically innocuous and stable under all the varying temperature conditions likely to be encountered in practice. In addition, such preparations should:

(i) leave the skin feeling "smooth" and preferably, non-greasy;
(ii) readily cleanse stale "make-up" and other dirt from the skin;
(iii) either be in liquid form or should readily liquefy or soften at that temperature at which it is used (body temperature), in order not to exert any undue "drag" on the skin.

Apart from "liquefying cleansing creams", which will be discussed first, no sharp line of demarcation occurs between cold creams and cleansing creams. Indeed, cold creams have been widely used for this purpose. Modern cleansing creams are perhaps in general softer in consistency than the old-fashioned cold creams, but hardly less so than some of the more modern types of creams. The use of surface-active emulsifiers (other than borax-beeswax soap) in both types of preparations, in any case now renders any distinction artificial.

Liquefying Cleansing Creams

These consist of simple mixtures of mineral oils, or synthetic fatty materials, with hydrocarbon waxes, ceresin, ozokerite, paraffin wax, etc. In more modern formulations cetyl or stearyl alcohols are often included.

The following may be taken as a typical example :

	per cent.
(*a*) White Mineral oil	42·0
(*b*) White petroleum jelly	18·0
(*c*) Spermaceti	12·0
(*d*) Ozokerite	14·0
(*e*) Cetyl alcohol	14·0
(*f*) Perfume	*q.s.*

Procedure

Melt by steam heat, without overheating, mix and pour into jars. Consistency of product may be adjusted within reason as desired, by adjusting the ratio of hydrocarbon waxes to mineral oil.

Isopropyl myristate has found increasing use in the cosmetic industry as it is of very low viscosity, is not prone to rancidity and gives an almost greaseless film on the skin. The following formulation exemplifies its use in a liquefying cleansing cream :

	per cent.
(*a*) Isopropyl myristate	25·0
(*b*) Mineral oil	25·0
(*c*) Petroleum jelly	30·0
(*d*) Paraffin wax	20·0

Procedure

(1) Melt and mix together all the above ingredients at about 65° C.
(2) Cool, with constant stirring until the mixture is a little over solidifying point. Pour into jars.

(From : *The Use of Isopropyl Myristate in Cosmetics*, A. Boake Roberts Ltd., London.)

Emulsified Creams

The following formula for a " Quick Melting " Cleansing Cream (" Readers' Questions ", *Drug Cosm. Ind.*, May 1936, p. 393) is stated to produce a white cream of fine texture which liquefies readily :

	per cent.
(*a*) Paraffin wax	6·0
(*b*) White beeswax	12·0
(*c*) Mineral oil	54·0
(*d*) Stearic acid	1·0
(*e*) Borax	1·0
(*f*) Water	25·5
(*g*) Perfume	0·5

Procedure

(1) Heat (*a*), (*b*), (*c*) and (*d*) at 70° C. till dissolved.
(2) Dissolve (*e*) in (*f*) and heat to 70° C.

Add (2) to (1) at 70° C. Stir down to 45°–50° C., perfume and pour as the mixture begins to thicken.

The following is an example of a cleansing cream of the water-in-oil type made with Sorbitan sesquioleate (Arlacel 83) ("Drug and Cosmetic Emulsion Formulation, etc.", Atlas Powder Co., Wilmington, U.S.A.). It must be remembered that products such as Arlacel 83 are non-ionic emulsifiers of complex composition, and bear the chemical designation of the simple ester or esters to which they most nearly correspond in respect of analytical constants:

	per cent.
(*a*) Arlacel 83	4·0
(*b*) Petroleum jelly (medium or long fibre)	31·0
(*c*) Mineral oil 65/75	20·0
(*d*) Paraffin wax (or microcrystalline wax)	7·0
(*e*) Lanolin	3·0
(*f*) Water	32·3
(*g*) Sorbitol 70 per cent. soln. (Sorbo)	2·5
(*h*) Magnesium sulphate U.S.P.	0·2
(*i*) Preservative	*q.s.*
(*j*) Perfume	*q.s.*

Procedure

(1) Heat (*a*), (*b*), (*c*), (*d*) and (*e*) to 70°–75° C.
(2) Heat (*f*), (*g*), (*h*) and (*i*) to 70°–75° C.

Add (2) to (1) gradually, whilst stirring. Add perfume at 55°–60° C. Homogenise at 55°–60° C., filling directly into jars.

The following cleansing creams are of the oil-in-water type:

	per cent.
(*a*) Stearic acid	8·0
(*b*) Mineral oil	35·0
(*c*) Petroleum jelly	10·0
(*d*) 2-amino-2-methyl-1,3-propanediol (amino glycol)	3·0
(*e*) Glycerin	5·0
(*f*) Water	39·0
(*g*) Preservative	*q.s.*

Procedure

(1) Heat (*a*), (*b*) and (*c*), to 75° C.
(2) Heat (*d*), (*e*), (*f*) and (*g*) to 75° C.

Add (2) to (1), with gentle stirring. Perfume at 45°–50° C. and stir (avoiding aeration) down to 25° C.

(From: *Amino Glycol for Cosmetic Formulation.*)

	per cent.
(*a*) Stearic acid	13·5
(*b*) Liquid paraffin	29·0
(*c*) Triethanolamine	1·8
(*d*) Sodium alginate (Manutex SA/KP)	1·8

	per cent.
(e) Glycerin	2·0
(f) Water	51·9
(g) Preservative	q.s.
(h) Perfume	q.s.

Procedure

(1) Mix (*d*) with (*e*); add (*f*), (*c*) and (*g*) and stir till dissolved. Heat to 70° C.

(2) Mix (*a*) with (*b*) and dissolve by heating to 70° C.

Add (1) to (2) at 70° C. and stir. Continue to stir, avoiding aeration. Perfume at 45° C. and stir down to 25°–30° C.

[*Note.*—Manutex SA/KP is a sodium alginate of high viscosity.]

(From: *Alginates in Pharmaceuticals and Cosmetics*, Alginate Industries Ltd., London.)

Apart from formulations such as the above, cleansing creams may be made along the lines of foundation creams, employing, however, rather a larger amount of oil phase; if desired, some free detergent may also be included, for example:

	per cent.
(a) Diglycol stearate	20·0
(b) Detergent	5·0
(c) Glycerin	5·0
(d) Water	70·0

Procedure

(1) Heat all the above ingredients together, by steam heat until dissolved.

(2) Cool whilst stirring. Perfume at 45° C. and stir down to 25°–30° C.

(*Note.*—The detergent employed should be innocuous at the concentration employed, to the skin.)

	per cent.
(a) Lanette wax (cetyl/stearyl alcohols, approx. 10 per cent. sulphated)	16·0
(b) Water	74·0
(c) Propylene glycol	5·0
(d) Detergent	5·0
(e) Preservative	q.s.
(f) Perfume	q.s.

Procedure

(1) Heat together, at 70°–75° C., until dissolved, (*a*), (*b*), (*c*), (*d*) and (*e*).

(2) Cool whilst stirring. Add (*f*) at 45° C. and stir down to 25°–30° C.

Cleansing (Complexion) Milks

Complexion milks have been employed for many years under such titles as "laits virginals", "laits de beauté", "laits de toilette", etc. These older preparations consisted of an aqueous solution of soap, with such additions as glycerin, distilled extract of witch hazel, or rosewater to which were added alcoholic tinctures of gums such as gum benzoin, or of resinous substances such as styrax, myrrh, etc.

On addition of the alcoholic tincture to the aqueous phase, the benzoin, styrax, etc., were precipitated in the form of an extremely fine dispersion, thus giving the solution the "appearance" of a milk.

Subsequently preparations involving the use of soap, water and oils produced the forerunners of the modern complexion milks. Modern preparations are largely based on amino soaps produced *in situ* or upon the use of certain proprietary emulsifiers.

Such milks are essentially diluted cleansing creams, and are applied to the face by means of a small sponge or by cotton wool, etc.

Triethanolamine combines with free fatty acids, such as stearic acid with the formation of soaps which are characterised by their low alkalinity and freedom from skin irritation and toxicity, when applied externally. Triethanolamine stearate is an excellent emulsifying agent for use in the preparation of complexion milks, e.g.:

	per cent.
(*a*) Mineral oil	10·0
(*b*) Cetyl alcohol	0·5
(*c*) Stearic acid	3·0
(*d*) Triethanolamine	1·8
(*e*) Preservative	*q.s.*
(*f*) Water	84·7
(*g*) Perfume	*q.s.*

Procedure

(1) Heat (*a*), (*b*) and (*c*) until dissolved and adjust the temperature to 70° C.
(2) Dissolve (*d*) and (*e*) in (*f*) and raise the temperature to 70° C.

Add (2) to (1) with gentle stirring. Continue to stir whilst cooling and perfume at 40°–45° C. Continue stirring to 25° C. The product may be homogenised if desired.

By adjusting the ratio of oil and water, and the amount of stearate soap formed, or by using mixtures of stearic-oleic acids in replacement of the stearic acid, the viscosity of the milk may be varied widely. Such milks tend to thicken on storage, equilibrium being attained most rapidly in the case of the unhomogenised milks.

Complexion milks may also be prepared, in the cold, by the use of diglycol laurate, for example:

	per cent.
(*a*) Diglycol laurate (Glyco Products)	14·0
(*b*) Liquid paraffin	40·0
(*c*) Water	46·0
(*d*) Preservative	*q.s.*
(*e*) Perfume	*q.s.*

Procedure

(1) Dissolve (*d*) in (*c*); heat may be required at this stage unless the preservative is readily soluble.

(2) Mix (*a*) with (*c*), fairly rapid agitation is desirable.

(3) Add (*b*) with rapid stirring; then add (*e*).

In some instances it may be found preferable to mix (*b*) and (*e*) and add this mixture in (3).

Of rather a different type is the following formula by Kalish (*Drug Cosmet. Ind.*, Aug. 1938):

	per cent.
(*a*) Stearic acid	0·8
(*b*) Beeswax	1·0
(*c*) Triethanolamine	0·2
(*d*) Borax	0·1
(*e*) Cocoa butter	1·5
(*f*) Lanolin	0·8
(*g*) Glycerin	5·0
(*h*) Perfume	0·6
(*i*) Preservative	0·1
(*j*) Water	89·9

Procedure

(1) Heat (*a*), (*b*), (*e*) and (*f*), at 70°–75° C. until dissolved.

(2) Heat (*c*), (*d*), (*g*), (*i*) and (*j*) at 70°–75° C. until dissolved.

Add (2) to (1), both solutions being between 70°–75° C., with thorough mixing; as the temperature falls mix slowly to avoid aeration. Perfume at 40°–45° C.

The following example of a liquid cleansing milk also based on the use of triethanolamine stearate, but with the addition of "Carbitol" and propylene glycol as cleansing agents and containing quince seed mucilage, is quoted from *Emulsions*, 7th edn. (Carbide and Carbon Chemicals Corporation, New York):

	per cent.
(*a*) Lanolin	6·35
(*b*) White mineral oil	10·66
(*c*) Stearic acid	4·68
(*d*) Quince seed mucilage	3·55
(*e*) Carbitol (diethylene glycol mono ethyl ether)	4·67
(*f*) Propylene glycol	9·35
(*g*) Triethanolamine	1·78
(*h*) Perfume	0·06
(*i*) Water	58·90

Procedure

(1) Melt (*a*), (*b*) and (*c*) and adjust temperature to 70° C.

(2) Heat (*g*) and (*i*) to 70° C.

Add (1) to (2) and stir to form a good emulsion.

(3) Prepare the quince seed mucilage (*d*), by adding 9½ oz. of quince seed to 20 lb. water at 80° C., soaking overnight and then straining through a cloth.

[Suitable preservative needed if a bulk of this mucilage is to be retained.]

(4) To the emulsion formed above, add (*e*) followed by (*d*).

(5) Mix (*h*) in (*f*) and stir this into the cream when it has cooled to 50° C.

(6) Continue stirring at slow speed until the emulsion has cooled to room temperature.

(The original gives " Terpineol " as the " perfume ".)

Cleansing Lotions

In the treatment of very greasy skins, the use of cleansing lotions may be helpful, such as those given below :

	per cent.
(*a*) Triethanolamine lauryl sulphate, liquid	5·0
(*b*) Water	95·0
(*c*) Perfume (if desired)	*q.s.*
(*d*) Preservative	*q.s.*

	per cent.
(*a*) Sulphonated olive oil	10·0
(*b*) Water	90·0
(*c*) Preservative	*q.s.*

	per cent.
(*a*) Propylene glycol	10·0
(*b*) Triethanolamine lauryl sulphate, liquid	5·0
(*c*) Water	85·0
(*d*) Preservative	*q.s.*

These above preparations are made by simple solution, mixing and filtration.

Winter (*Soap Perfum. Cosm.*, 1947, **20**, 359) suggested the use of pepsin lotions for digesting accumulations of kerato-albuminous matters and clarifying the skin, for example :

	per cent.
(*a*) Pepsin	1·0
(*b*) Boric acid	2·0
(*c*) Water	97·0

Preparation is by simple solution.

[Care would have to be taken to ensure that the Pepsin did not decompose and the addition of an *effective* preservative would seem to the author highly desirable. (*See* Chapter 42, Antiseptics and Preservatives.)]

Other "cleansing" lotions may contain borax, together with a little alcohol and witch hazel (menthol may be included as a cooling and freshening agent):

	per cent.
(a) Borax	1·0
(b) Water	69·0
(c) Witch hazel (Distl. Extract)	10·0
(d) Alcohol	20·0

Procedure

Dissolve (a) in (b) with the aid of heat. Cool.
Add (d) and then (c). Filter if necessary.

Sulphonated Oils as Skin Cleansers

Within recent years interest has been shown by dermatologists in the use of sulphonated oils as substitutes for soap, in cleansing the skin, particularly in those persons suffering from eczema and in those idiosyncratic to soap. Blank (*Arch. Derm. Syph., Chicago*, 1939, **39**, 811) showed that the presence of alkalis and saturated fatty acids of low molecular weight in some soaps caused irritation in certain persons.

In these experiments a sulphonated oil mixture containing 25 per cent. sulphonated "olive and linseed oils", 25 per cent. liquid petroleum oil and 50 per cent. water was found satisfactory in 150 cases of contact and atopic dermatitis. Irritation, redness or itching was found in only a small percentage of the cases in which it was used, and this preparation was suggested as a substitute for soap when the latter was contra-indicated. (It is understood that such a preparation has been marketed in the United States under a proprietary name.)

The choice of sulphonated oil as a cleanser would appear to be due to its good cleansing action (though its lack of foaming properties may be a psychological disadvantage), its "acid" character, and its small content of fatty acids of low molecular weight. The sulphonated oil should be chosen with care, since different products may vary in their action on the skin, and, in fact, some sulphonated oils have been reported as an irritant to the skin of textile workers (*Publ. Hlth. Rep., Wash.*, 1934, **40**, 1176; *J. Amer. med. Ass.*, 1932, **99**, 972).

CHAPTER 6

ACID CREAMS, MILKS AND LOTIONS

IN the formation of bleaching creams and lotions based on lemon juice or other fruit juices, or their acid equivalents, either alone or in conjunction with hydrogen peroxide (which is only stable in acid media), it is necessary for the base in which they are incorporated to have an acid reaction. In the formulation of creams containing certain plant and animal extracts also, it is necessary that the base should—at least—not be " alkaline ".

Creams having a reaction slightly on the acid side are also helpful when applied following contact of the skin with rather alkaline solutions or substances, in that they assist the skin keratin to regain its normal reaction.

Today, with all the various emulsifiers derived from surface active materials and with non-ionic emulsifiers available, the cosmetic chemist and dermatologist is faced with a very large array of materials from which he may make his choice.

The use of neutral and " acidic " creams is, however, by no means such an innovation as a perusal of the older cosmetic literature and technical journals would suggest.

It does not appear to be so widely known as one might expect, that ordinary co-called stearate-soap vanishing creams are almost invariably *acid* in reaction, due to the formation of " acid soap ". (*See* " acid soaps " in Chapter 9, Vanishing, Foundation and Powder Creams.)

*p*H VALUE

It is highly desirable that the cosmetician should be conversant with the measurement of the acidity of a solution or cream, and hence what is meant by the term " *p*H value ", and how it is determined. In certain cosmetic processes such as chemical depilation and hair waving, the *p*H value of the preparation used is of great importance.

Acidic substances, such as hydrochloric acid, ionise in solution according to the following equation, liberating hydrogen ions :

$$HA \rightarrow H^+ + A^-$$

Basic substances ionise, liberating hydroxyl ions :

$$BOH \rightarrow B^+ + OH^-$$

Water which has the formula H — O — H, can be considered as a combination of hydrogen and hydroxyl ions with corresponding acidic and basic characteristics combined. It therefore ionises to give both H and OH ions in solution

$$H - O - H \rightleftarrows H^+ + OH^-$$

The double arrow indicates that the reaction is reversible and that a rapid interchange is going on in which the H and OH ions are always combining to give water, whilst other water molecules are breaking up to give ions. With pure water, at ordinary temperatures, a balance is obtained in which on an average there are 0·0000001 g. equivalents hydrogen ions per litre with the same number of gram equivalents of hydroxyl ions per litre :

$$H_2O \rightarrow 0{\cdot}0000001 \text{ H ion} + 0{\cdot}0000001 \text{ OH ion.}$$

It follows from the law of mass action that if the hydrogen ions in solution are increased or decreased, a new balance between the ions is obtained in which the concentration of gram equivalents of hydrogen ion (H) multiplied by the concentration of hydroxyl ion (OH), is always 0·00000000000001 at 20° C.

This expression is rather cumbersome so recourse is taken to the mathematical device of expressing this in the form $\frac{1}{10^{14}}$ or 10^{-14}. Thus we have the expression :

$$(H) \times (OH) = \frac{1}{10^{14}}.$$

In pure water (H) and (OH) are present in equal concentrations, i.e.

$$(H) = \frac{1}{10^7} \text{ and } (OH) = \frac{1}{10^7}.$$

Let us see what happens when the hydrogen ion concentration is increased from 0·0000001, $\frac{1}{10^7}$ gram equivalents perlitre, to 0·000001, $\frac{1}{10^6}$ gram equivalents per litre. In this case, by the ordinary laws of adding and subtracting indices during multiplication and division,

$$(H)\,(OH) = \frac{1}{10^{14}}, \text{ therefore } (OH) = \frac{1}{10^{14}} \div \frac{1}{10^6} = \frac{1}{10^8}.$$

Thus if the (H) is known, (OH) may easily be found, and if (OH) is known (H) may be found.

If a solution or cream contains acid there will be, as we have seen above, an excess of (H) ions whilst if it contains alkali there will be an excess of (OH) ions. The (H) and (OH) ions are interdependent in that if we give the one, the other may be calculated.

It follows that instead of giving two scales, one for acidity and one for alkalinity, it is better to have one scale from which the other may be calculated at will. The scale chosen is the hydrogen ion concentration, and in order to shorten the mathematical expression, such as $\frac{1}{10^7}$, i.e. 10^{-7} to denote neutrality this was replaced by an expression which is the logarithm of the reciprocal of the hydrogen ion concentration, termed the *p*H value, in which the above expression became, simply, *p*H = 7·0.

For some years the above definition was adopted for the expression *p*H. However, more recently it became realised that, as thus defined, *p*H was not measurable. Bates (*Chem. Rev.*, 1948, **42**, 1) showed that *if in fact* pH *is to be a measurable quantity it cannot possess any simple exact fundamental significance.* As a result of recommendations made at a conference called at the request of the Royal Society of London, to discuss the need for a standard *p*H scale, the British Standards Institution issued in 1950, "British Standard 1647", dealing with the *p*H scale in which the quantity "*p*H" has a *practical* but *not a precise simple fundamental meaning.*

THE MODERN DEFINITION, AND METHOD OF MEASUREMENT OF, *p*H. In British Standard 1647, the "difference in *p*H between two solutions, X and S at the same temperature is *defined* as follows:

The electromotive force E_x of the cell

Pt,H_2/solution X/3·5 MKCl/Reference electrode

and the electromotive force E_s of the cell

Pt,H_2/Solution S/3·5 MKCl/Reference electrode

shall be measured, both cells being at the same temperature throughout and the reference electrodes being identical in the two cells.

The *p*H of the Solution X, denoted by *p*H(X), is then related to the *p*H of the Solution S, denoted by *p*H(S), by the definition:

$$pH\,(X) - pH\,(S) = \frac{E_x - E_s}{2{\cdot}3026RT/F}$$

where R denotes the gas content, T the absolute temperature and F the Faraday.

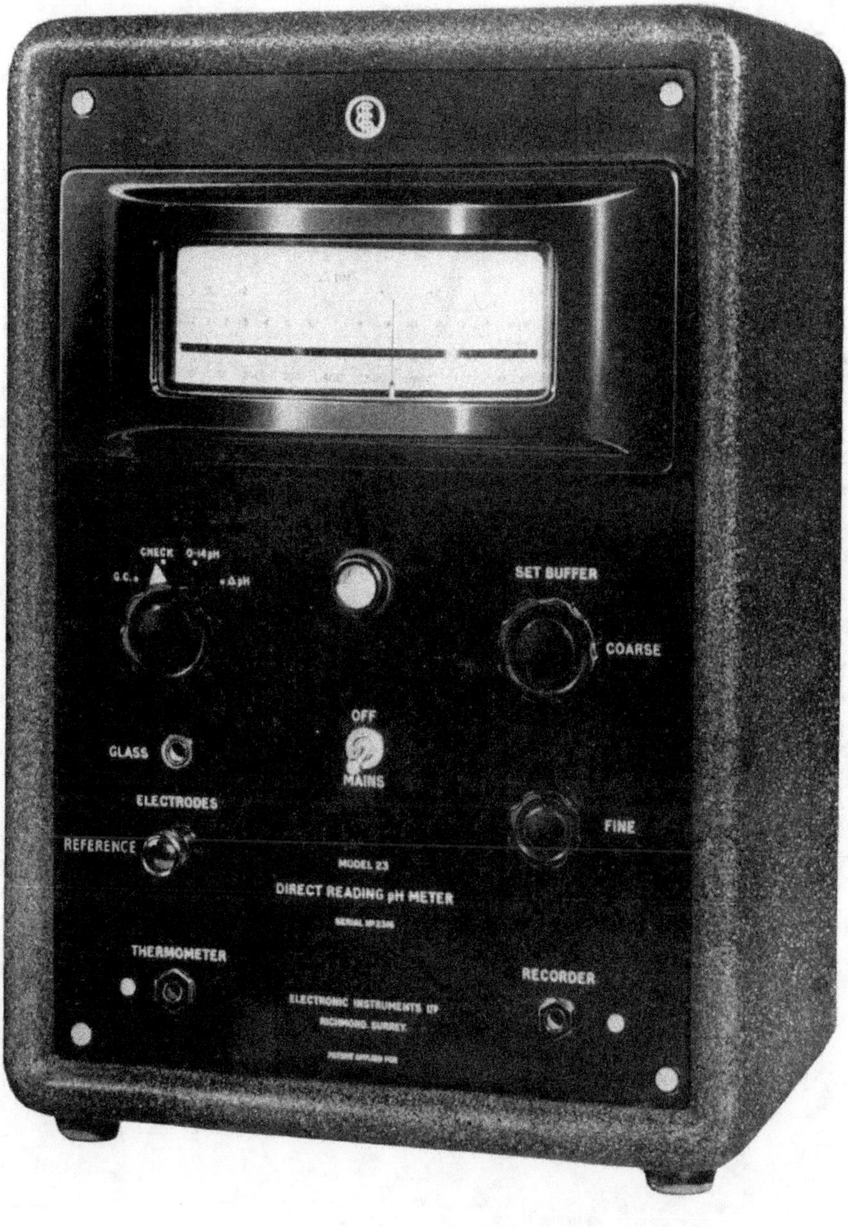

[*By courtesy of Electronic Instruments Ltd.*

FIG. 13.—Direct reading *p*H meter. A good example of a modern instrument.

Primary Standard

The difference between the *p*H of two solutions having been defined as above, the definition of *p*H is completed by assigning a value of *p*H at each temperature to one chosen solution called the *primary standard.* The primary standard specified is a 1/20 molar solution of pure potassium hydrogen phthalate. The *p*H of this solution is *defined* as having the value 4 exactly at 15° C. At any other temperature *t*° C. between 0° C. and 60° C. its *p*H is defined by the formula :

$$pH = 4{\cdot}00 + \frac{1}{2}\left(\frac{t - 15}{100}\right)^2.$$

[*Note* : For full details of the values of the primary standard at different temperatures, specifications of the standard solutions, and use and calibration of the glass electrode, consult B.S.1647, issued by the British Standards Institution, 2 Park Street, W.1.][1]

The object of the above standard is to ensure that, when different workers refer to a stated measured value of *p*H, they mean the same thing within $\pm$ 0·005. The standard makes it quite clear that this degree of accuracy is only attainable with *aqueous* solutions at temperatures between 0° C. and 60° C. and that oxidising agents or other highly reactive materials tend to reduce this accuracy.

Acid Creams, Milks and Lotions

It is essential that, whatever emulsifying agent is used, it be chemically compatible with all of the ingredients of the emulsion and dermatologically innocuous. Because of recent experiences in the United States in connection with shampoos, it is highly desirable that such products should also involve no potential hazard to sight should the final product come into contact with the eyeball, though it is not very likely that normal cosmetic formulations of such creams, milks or lotions, would be in any way comparable with a detergent shampoo formulation. [In this respect it should be noted that Dr. Lehman, Chief of the Division of Pharmacology of the Food and Drug Administration, Washington, has warned manufacturers of the possibility that mixtures of surface-active agents (and presumably emulsifiers—*Author*), may be more irritating to the eyes than could be predicted from the ocular toxicity of the individual constituents. (*See* Chapter 22, Hair Shampoo, etc.).]

[1] Extracts from B.S. 1647 : 1950—*p*H scale—are reproduced by permission of the British Standards Institution, British Standards House, 2 Park Street, London, W.1, from whom official copies of the Standard can be obtained.

One of the earliest successful emulsifiers for use with acid creams in this country was Lanette Wax [which consists essentially of cetyl-stearyl alcohols (90 per cent. unsulphated), 10 per cent. sulphated]. An example of its use in a "genuine" lemon juice cream is given below:

	per cent.
(*a*) Lanette wax SX	12·0
(*b*) Myristyl alcohol	5·0
(*c*) Water	57·0
(*d*) Glycerin	6·0
(*e*) Lemon juice	20·0
(*f*) Oil of lemon	*q.s.*
(*g*) Preservative	*q.s.*

Procedure

(1) Heat (*a*) and (*b*) at 75° C. till homogeneous. Adjust to 75° C.
(2) Heat (*c*), (*d*) and (*g*) at 75° C. till homogeneous. Adjust to 75° C.

Add (2) to (1) with stirring. As soon as a good emulsion has formed, stir in (*e*) which may either be added at room temperature, a little at a time (in order to preserve the natural characteristics of the juice), or may be previously warmed prior to mixing in. When the temperature has fallen to about 45° C. add the oil of lemon.

A cheaper "synthetic" product may be obtained by replacing the lemon juice by an equivalent amount of aqueous 7 per cent. citric acid and the oil of lemon by a trace of citral, but such a cream, whilst it may be of the "lemon type", can hardly be described with any honesty as a "lemon" cream.

Lactic acid has also been employed in so-called butter-milk lotions and creams, and in bleaching creams presumably as a relic of the days when "soured milk" may have been employed for this purpose. (So far as "bleaching creams" are concerned there is little doubt that one of the few, apparently, *effective* skin bleaches is "ammoniated mercury", this substance must, however, only be incorporated in creams with due regard to its toxicity. [*See* R. G. Harry, *Cosmetic Materials*, London, 1948, pp. 28–32.]

The following is an example of a lactic acid cream based on Lanette Wax SX:

	per cent.
(*a*) Lanette wax SX	10·0
(*b*) Cetyl alcohol	4·0
(*c*) Mineral oil	4·0
(*d*) Glycerin	6·0
(*e*) Water	75·0
(*f*) Lactic acid B.P.	1·0
(*g*) Preservative	*q.s.*
(*h*) Perfume	*q.s.*

Procedure

(1) Heat (*a*), (*b*) and (*c*) to 75° C., until clear solution obtained.
(2) Heat (*d*), half of (*e*), and (*g*) to 75° C.

Add (2) to (1) at 75° C. whilst stirring.

(3) Add (*f*) to remaining half of (*e*), warm this solution to about 60°–65° C. and add to the Lanette wax emulsion formed above. Perfume at 45° C. and continue stirring to 25°–30° C. Homogenise if desired.

By the use of "buffer solutions", and the use of a suitable emulsifier, especially a non-ionic emulsifier, creams of any particular pH (within the capabilities of the emulsifier) may be prepared.

The following examples (from R. G. Harry, "Hydrogen Ion Concentration in Therapeutic Bases", *Brit. J. Derm.*, Jan. 1942) illustrate the use of Lanette wax SX (an "anionic" emulsifier), for this purpose.

For "buffered" creams, more emulsifier is often required owing to the effect of the dissolved salts. To obtain the requisite buffering effect, the following two solutions may be mixed *in the proportions* stated below: (1) 2·101 per cent. citric acid solution, and (2) 7·165 per cent. sodium phosphate solution viz.:

Approximate pH of Cream (Glass electrode at 20° C.)	6·4	5·4	4·6
	per cent.	*per cent.*	*per cent.*
(*a*) Lanette wax SX	20·0	20·0	20·0
(*b*) Mineral oil	5·0	5·0	5·0
(*c*) Glycerin	5·0	5·0	5·0
(*d*) Sodium phosphate solution	48·5	38·7	31·2
(*e*) Citric acid solution	18·2	28·0	35·5
(*f*) Water	3·3	3·3	3·3
(*g*) Preservative	*q.s.*	*q.s.*	*q.s.*

Procedure

(1) Heat (*a*) and (*b*) to 75° C.
(2) Warm (*c*), (*d*), (*e*), (*f*) and (*g*), to 70°–75° C.

Add (2) to (1).

The above creams, it should be noted are *very heavily buffered* and in most instances, providing the ratio of buffer solutions is kept the same, the amounts of each can be considerably reduced, the difference being made up with water. By so doing, the ease of emulsification (and stability) can be greatly improved.

Except where a "buffered" cream is desired (either for a certain salt effect at a particular pH, or for the inclusion of some active ingredient which is more stable at a particular pH) the use of buffer solutions is unnecessary, and an approximate pH can be attained by the inclusion of a small amount of a mild organic acid such as citric acid.

For example, the pH of a normal "Lanette Wax SX" cream is slightly on the acid side, say between 6·7 and 7·0, but can be sharply reduced by a trace of acid. If in the above three creams, the buffer solutions are replaced by water and about 0·1 g. of citric acid added, the *p*H may be reduced to just under 3·0.

Fruit Juice Creams

Although the use of fruit juices appeals to feminine psychology, the expense of such juices militates against their employment in ordinary commercial preparations. Perhaps the most popular of the more expensive fruits is the strawberry, references to which may be found in the *Medicina Britannica* of Short (1746) [R. G. Harry, "Herbals", *Cosmetic Materials*, London, 1948, p. 139]. Although freshly gathered strawberries are a very good source of vitamin C (containing up to 260 mg. of ascorbic acid per 100 g. substance, like other fruits, on keeping their vitamin C content markedly decreases and may fall to 20 mg. per 100 g.) Moreover, the *value* of such "fruit juice preparations" is problematical. (*See* Chapter 4, Skin Nutrition.)

Where it is desired to prepare a "genuine" (or synthetic) fruit juice cream, the non-ionic emulsifying agents are of particular interest. An example of this class of emulsifier—in this case a condensation product of stearyl alcohol and ethylene oxide reaction products—is "Polawax" (Croda Ltd.). The following has been found to produce a satisfactory basic cream, which may be modified by replacing part of the water, as desired, by fruit juices, or other water-soluble materials.

	per cent.
(*a*) "Polawax" (Croda)	16·0
(*b*) Mineral oil	5·0
(*c*) Glycerin	5·0
(*d*) Water	74·0
(*e*) Preservative	*q.s.*
(*f*) Perfume	*q.s.*

Procedure

(1) Heat (*a*) and (*b*) to 75° C., till homogeneous.
(2) Heat (*c*), (*d*) and (*e*), to 75° C., till homogeneous.

Add (2) to (1) with stirring. Perfume at 45° C. Stir down to 25°–30° C.

[An economy may be effected by reducing the proportion of Polawax in the above formula to 10 per cent. If desired, the consistency of the product may be adjusted by the inclusion of fatty alcohols and/or waxes.]

Although the usual oil-in-water emulsifiers based upon glyceryl monostearate contain a small amount of soap and are thus incompatible with acid solutions, several proprietary glyceryl monostearates especially designed for the production of creams on the acid side are available.

These include "Tegacid" (Goldschmidt Corporation, New York, U.S.A.), "Abracol G.S.P." (A. Boake Roberts Ltd., London).

The following is an example of the use of "Tegacid" in a "Peroxide Cream".

	per cent.
(*a*) "Tegacid"	12·0
(*b*) Glycerin	4·0
(*c*) Spermaceti	3·0
(*d*) Mineral oil	5·0
(*e*) Lanolin	2·0
(*f*) Salicylic acid	0·5
(*g*) Citric acid	0·2
(*h*) Lactic acid	0·1
(*i*) Water	70·1
(*j*) Preservative ("Tegosept")	0·1
(*k*) Hydrogen peroxide	3·0

Procedure

(1) Heat (*a*), (*b*), (*c*), (*d*), (*e*), (*f*), (*g*), (*h*), (*i*) and (*j*) together to 90°–100° C. whilst stirring until dissolved.

(2) Cool to about 30° C. whilst stirring. Add (*k*).

To list in this chapter all the various formulations given in this book and suitable for use as acid creams would involve unnecessary repetition. Many of the formulae quoted under cold and cleansing creams and milks, and, in particular, under "Antiperspirants and Deodorants" (*see* Chapter 30), lend themselves readily to adaptation for other purposes. It should be remembered in particular that the "non-ionic" emulsifying agents are not sensitive to the acidic substances normally employed in cosmetic and toilet preparations. As an example of adaptation, the following formula for an oil-in-water "hand cream" (*Drug and Cosmetic Emulsions*, Atlas Powder Co., Wilmington, U.S.A.) may be quoted. This cream, whilst retaining cosmetic elegance, is compatible with lemon juice, citric acid or other similar acidic substances:

	per cent.
(*a*) Stearic acid	10·0
(*b*) Span 60 (Sorbitan monostearate)	5·2
(*c*) Span 80 (Sorbitan monooleate)	1·0
(*d*) Tween 60 (Polyoxyethylene sorbitan monostearate)	2·8
(*e*) Water	81·0
(*f*) Preservative	*q.s.*
(*g*) Perfume	*q.s.*

Procedure

(1) Heat (*a*), (*b*), (*c*) and (*d*) to 80° C. until homogeneous.

(2) Heat (*e*) and (*f*) to 85° C.

Add (1) at 80° C. to (2) at 85° C. with rapid stirring.

Perfume at 50° C. Pour at 45° C.

Acid Lotions

There is little if any demand for acid lotions as such. The majority of cosmetic lotions are of the astringent or of the skin tonic type (*see* Chapter 7) sometimes sold as " skin freshener ", etc.

It is true that acid lotions containing up to about 4 per cent. boric acid can be prepared and that by the addition of citric or tartaric acids the solubility of the boric acid in water can be increased. Such solutions can be tinted and perfumed. Such solutions are " very mildly " antiseptic, and by the incorporation of other antiseptics this effect could be increased. It should be realised, however, that boric acid is very toxic and when taken internally can produce serious poisoning. (The lack of odour and colour makes boric acid an insidious poison.)

Genuine " glycerin and lemon ", pineapple, lettuce and cucumber extracts, etc., may be formulated along various lines such as:

	per cent.
(*a*) Fresh lemon juice	10·0
(*b*) Glycerin	10·0
(*c*) Water	77·0
(*d*) Pectin (100 grade)	3·0
(*e*) Yellow dye	*q.s.*
(*f*) Oil of lemon or citral	*q.s.*
(*g*) Preservative	*q.s.*

Procedure

(1) Mix (*b*), (*d*) and (*g*), add (*c*) and (*e*), and heat to dissolve.
(2) Cool, add (*a*) and (*f*).
(3) Filter through talc.

(7 per cent. aqueous citric acid may replace lemon juice; the lotion is no longer a " lemon " lotion, however, though it might be considered of the " synthetic lemon " type.)

The inclusion of a little gum tragacanth, or other mucilaginous substances, in an acid lotion will yield a product having a higher viscosity and a pleasant velvet-like feel on the skin.

CHAPTER 7

ASTRINGENT (" PORE ") LOTIONS AND SKIN " TONICS "

Astringent Lotions

These are usually advised by " beauty experts " for the correction of an oily skin or for the removal of wrinkles. Since wrinkles are caused by the skin losing its elasticity, probably through degeneration of its fibres, no " astringent " (or any other agent at present known) can cure this condition, although by preventing drying and cracking of the skin the use of emollient creams may delay its onset. (*See* Chapters 4 and 10, Skin Nutrition and Lubricating Creams, respectively.)

Astringent lotions are sometimes recommended to " close the pores " (prior to applying " make-up " to the face) following the application of cleansing creams and lotions. They are also used in the treatment of enlarged pores, or " orange-peel skin ". Their application appears to make such " pore " openings *less readily visible. Actually these so-called " pores " are not pores at all but are the openings of hair follicles.*

Astringent lotions are in fact *mild* " antiperspirant " preparations and their mode of action will be found discussed in Chapter 30 (Antiperspirants and Deodorants).

In general, astringent lotions contain the milder aluminium salts, such as potassium aluminium and/or zinc salts such as the phenosulphonate or sulphate. Some alcohol is often present though if this exceeds 20 per cent. the solution may " smart " or sting when first applied to the face. Aromatic waters such as rose and orange flower waters are often employed for their odour value. Other substances sometimes included are camphor water, tincture of benzoin, tincture of sage and distilled extract of witch hazel.[1]

[1] Whilst tincture of witch hazel, a dark reddish brown liquid is a powerful astringent, the distilled extract of witch hazel commonly employed as a mild astringent in cosmetic preparations probably possesses little if any astringency due to " witch hazel ". The action of the distilled extract is probably due to the alcohol subsequently added to prevent decomposition of the solution, since on distillation, the tannin remains in the residue and is absent from the distilled extract (*Yosida. Chem. Abst.*, **34,** 1130). However, because of its wide use in the toilet industry, distilled extract of witch hazel has been included in some of the formulations given below.

	per cent.
Potassium aluminium sulphate	1·0
Zinc sulphate	0·3
Glycerin	5·0
Rose water	50·0
Water	43·7
Preservative	*q.s.*
Colouring matter	*q.s.*

	per cent.
Zinc phenolsulphonate	2·0
Zinc sulphate	1·0
Rose water	57·0
Water	40·0
Preservative	*q.s.*
Colouring matter	*q.s.*

A somewhat stronger " pore " lotion may be made as follows :

	per cent.
Potassium aluminium sulphate	4·0
Glycerin	6·0
Orange flower water	35·0
Rose water	35·0
Water	20·0
Preservative	*q.s.*

Procedure

In preparing the above solutions, the aluminium or zinc salts are dissolved (together with the preservative) in the water, by the aid of gentle heat. The solution is cooled and then the aromatic " flower " waters added. The colouring of these solutions is most readily effected by the addition of a few ml. of a strong aqueous solution of the colouring matter to be employed. The solutions should be stood for several weeks to achieve clarity and filtered through paper, or talc. Alternatively the mixtures may be gently chilled and the preliminary period of storage shortened somewhat.

Astringent Creams

The use of astringent creams for " curing a *greasy skin* " appears to me to be illogical. However, if an astringent cream or lotion is desired, these may be formulated along the lines given for antiperspirants (*see* Chapter 30), due regard being given to the fact that astringent preparations for use on the face should be very much milder than the usual antiperspirants. This may be achieved by use of a milder astringent material, or by a very considerable reduction in the amount of one of the stronger astringent substances. Before adopting the latter course, very careful skin tests should be conducted to ensure that the preparation is not too harsh.

Very mild so-called astringent creams may be obtained by the replacement of part of the water in an ordinary vanishing cream by distilled extract of witch hazel, or alternatively using one of the non-ionic emulsifiers in a foundation or cleansing cream, part of the aqueous phase of which is replaced by a dilute solution of zinc phenolsulphonate, or possibly even potassium aluminium sulphate.

Statements have appeared in the literature claiming that " turtle oil " is one of the most powerful natural astringents known. It is difficult to see how this can be substantiated since it possesses none of the properties which are usually associated with " astringency ". On the other hand, because it is emollient, it may (like other emollient matters) help to *delay* the onset of premature wrinkles due to such factors as dry skin or windburn.

No externally applied preparation can actually " remove wrinkles " nor delay the ageing (so far as we know) or wrinkling of the skin due to advancing years or to disease.

The use of mechanical methods, slapping, friction, etc., and/or steam heat to produce temporary inflammation of the surrounding tissue and thus give the " appearance of pore shrinkage ", need not be considered here. However much used by certain beauty salons, the effect achieved is not astringency.

Skin Tonics

These preparations are cooling and freshening to the skin, for this reason the term " skin freshener " describes these lotions more accurately than skin tonics.

These preparations may be diluted " astringent lotions ", or freshening lotions based essentially on alcohol, or eau-de-cologne, with witch hazel. A little borax or other mild alkali may be included. Camphor water is sometimes included in such products because at a strength of about 1 : 1000 it is stated to dilate the vessels of the skin (in much higher concentrations it is rubefacient) and to possess stimulating properties. If desired, and if costs permit, fruit juices may be included. In the latter instance special care is necessary to ensure adequate preservation of the juices both prior and subsequent to incorporation. Tincture of sage is reputed to have a freshening action ; tincture of arnica is also suggested in the technical literature to exert a pleasant feel on the skin. I know of no evidence to support, scientifically, the claims for either of these substances ; in particular, solutions of arnica have been known to produce dermatitis and must never be employed if the skin is broken. In my opinion arnica is better avoided.

The following exemplify some of these preparations :

	per cent.
Zinc phenolsulphonate	1·0
Glycerin	10·0
Camphor water	20·0
Alcohol	10·0
Rose water	40·0
Water	19·0
Preservative	*q.s.*

	per cent.
Alcohol	20·0
Orange flower water	30·0
Rose water	30·0
Potassium aluminium sulphate	0·5
Water	19·5
Preservative	*q.s.*

If desired a " trace " of menthol may be added, to produce a cooling effect; the amount should not be sufficient to give " burn ".

Skin " tonics " are often recommended for the purpose of removing cleansing cream. This is illogical, unless the product has been formulated with such a use in mind, since many of them contain zinc or aluminium salts and are acid in reaction. A mildly alkaline skin freshener which might be used for such a purpose is exemplified below :

	per cent.
Borax	2·0
Alcohol	10·0
Rose water	40·0
Water	48·0
Preservative	*q.s.*
Colouring matter	*q.s.*

If a " herbal " note is desired, lotions may be built up on herbal infusions or tinctures. [A short collection of herbal notes of substances which might be of interest to the cosmetic chemist, in which the evidence, both old and new, has been sifted, from the " Greek Herbal of Dioscorides "—compiled in the first century—through Short's *Medicina Britannica*, 1746, to the present day, appears in R. G. Harry, *Cosmetic Materials*, London, 1948, pp. 139–147.]

CHAPTER 8

FACE PACKS AND MASKS

(*Masques de Beauté*)

SUCH preparations are truly an example of history repeating itself, since mud packs have been used by women from earliest antiquity. As Searle (*Mfg. Chem.*, Sept. 1933, p. 261) has stated, certain earths were, in ancient times, credited with almost miraculous powers, some of them being regarded as under the trusteeship of certain priests and priestesses, the "terra sigillata" of the ancient Greeks being of this class.

Their present vogue may be ascribed to their combined psychological and cleansing effects. The warmth and sense of tightening gives a feeling that "something is being done to this face of mine", whilst the presence of colloidal and adsorptive clays and earths, helps to adsorb grease and dirt from the skin. In the course of their removal, surface skin debris is removed at the same time.

Such preparations may possess one or more of the following properties, according to the formulation employed :

(i) softening ;
(ii) cleansing ;
(iii) diaphoretic ;
(iv) astringent ;
(v) stimulating and refreshing.

At least four general types of preparations are recognised :

(*a*) Essentially *diaphoretic*, and consisting of wax preparations—a little rubber latex may also be included to assist in the ease of removal. These may be melted and "brushed-on", hot. They produce profuse perspiration and help to flush dirt and impurities from the follicular openings in the skin surface.

(*b*) *Gelanthum* masks, consisting of solid gels based on gelatin, glycerin ; and a mucilage such as gum tragacanth. These are melted by immersion in hot water before application to the face ; the face may then be covered with warm cloths. These masks produce a feeling of tightening of the skin and are softening and cleansing.

(*c*) *Albuminous and casein masks.* These are considered to have softening and cleansing properties but are very liable to decomposition. Great care must be taken in the choice of preservatives, etc.

(*d*) *Argillaceous*, based on clays and earths. These have adsorbent and cleansing properties. These preparations may be modified by the addition of other materials, " astringents ", skin-softening, or bleaching agents to suit any particular purpose.

[In addition the the above packs, " face masks " cut from absorbent material, impregnated with warm oils, skin fresheners (see Chapter 7), or with astringent solutions are often applied to the face in beauty salons. Such preparations should be distinguished from the beauty packs and masks described above.]

(*a*) *Diaphoretic masks.* These may consist merely of paraffin wax of a suitable melting-point, or may be mixtures of wax with the addition of a little petroleum jelly and polar materials such as cetyl and stearyl alcohols ; the use of microcrystalline waxes may assist the continuity of a suitable " wax mask ".

(*b*) *Gelanthum masks.* Janistyn (*Soap Perfum. Cosm.*, May 1937, p. 405), gave the following formula for a " gelanthum " mask, containing gelatin and tragacanth :

	per cent.
Gum tragacanth (best)	2·2
Glycerin	2·5
Gelatin (white)	2·3
Water	90·5
Zinc oxide	2·5

For a " gelanthum mask with honey ", Janistyn suggested the replacement of about 4·5 parts of the water in the above formula by honey.

Winter (*Alchemist*, Sept. 1947, p. 228) suggested :

	parts
Gelatin	10·00
Water	50·00
Camphor (dissolved in a little alcohol)	0·05
Zinc oxide	3·00
Kaolin	5·00
Titanium dioxide	2·00

Procedure

It is suggested that preparations along the above lines are best prepared by first moistening the gum when present with glycerin, then adding the gelatin and water and raising the temperature. (Solids should be mixed in the hot solution and their dispersion is facilitated by first moistening them with a drop of glycerin, or with a drop of a surface-active agent.)

Both of the above preparations are heated before use and applied in the warm state.

(*c*) *Albuminous and Casein masks.* Janistyn (*Soap Perfum. Cosm.*) points out that these preparations are popular in France and suggests amongst others, the following basic formula :

	parts
Casein (best quality)	20·0
Borax (powdered)	0·5
Glycerin	5·0
Water (distilled)	100·0
p-hydroxybenzoic acid propyl ester	0·1

Procedure

It is suggested that the casein be moistened with the glycerin and dissolved in the aqueous borax solution (containing also the preservative) with the aid of heat.

(*d*) *Argillaceous masks.* These offer considerable scope for formulation. China clay, colloidal kaolin, fuller's earth, bentonite, etc., may be used as the " argillaceous " material, the choice depending in part on the criteria which it is proposed to apply to the finished product.

If the colour of fuller's earth or bentonite is considered objectionable, this difficulty may be met by blending with kaolin, and/or the addition of zinc oxide or titanium dioxide.

Bentonite is a colloidal clay derived from volcanic ash found in certain parts of the United States, which is characterised by its strong affinity for water and its thixotropic properties. Certain bentonites will absorb up to fifteen times their volume of water, this property being greatly increased by the addition of a small quantity of magnesium oxide, or some other substance possessing a similar *p*H. There are considerable variations in different beds in the Benton formation, and even in different strata in the same beds, which has resulted in wide variations in the analyses of bentonites reported in the literature by competent authorities (Ewing, Polite and Shackelford, *J. Amer. pharm. Ass., Sci. ed.*, May, 1945, No. 5).

As a guide to the consistency of bentonite gels, it may be noted that Griffon (*J. Pharm. Chim., Paris*, **27**, 159) states that a gel containing 6 per cent. bentonite has the consistency of glycerin, whilst a 20 per cent. gel has the consistency of lanolin. (These consistencies will be considerably influenced by the *p*H of the gels.—*Author.*)

Bentonite gels are soothing to the skin (Kulchar, *Arch. Derm. Syph., Chicago*, 1941, **44**, i, 43), and have been claimed to be of value in the treatment of eczema, abscesses, sores and wounds (Davis, Vacher and Conley, *Bentonite, Its Properties, Mining, Preparation,* *and Utilisation*, U.S. Dept. Interior, Bureau of Mines, Washington, D.C., 1940). They have been used in a number of dermatological preparations (Fantus and Dyniewicz, *J. Amer. pharm. Ass., Sci. ed.*, 1938, **27**, 878; 1939, **28**, 548; Hubbard and Freeman, *ibid.* 1941, **2**, 78).

Kaolin and Colloidal Kaolin. Halpern, Powers and Bradney (*Proc. Sci. Sect. T.G.A.*, Dec. 1950, p. 4) point out that "... kaolin is not a primary mineral but is a generic term applied to several hydrated aluminium silicates. Not all aluminium silicates, however, may be called kaolin. On the basis of X-ray and physical studies, Ross and Kerr (U.S. Geol. Surv. Prof. Paper, No. 165E; 151 (1934)), established that three different groups of clay are classified as kaolin. These clays (kaolinite, nacrite, and dickite) have essentially the same formula ($Al_2O_2 . 2SiO_2 . 2H_2O$). It is generally regarded that the best sources for the pharmaceutical kaolins are England and the United States. These writers point out that the method of manufacture of the kaolin is an important factor in determining the properties of the resultant product; ordinary china clay is obtained by elutriation and on microscopic examination, mica, quartz and felspar are readily discernible. Pharmaceutical grades of kaolin are obtained by a peptising process in which the clay is suspended in water containing a suitable electrolyte (e.g. sodium pyrophosphate) which confers an electrical charge upon the clay and keeps the finer particles in suspension. Removal of the suspension of fine particles, followed by removal of the electric charge (by addition of another electrolyte or by means of an electric field), yields the finest forms of kaolin.

Searle (*Mfg. Chem.*) quotes the following recipe for an argillaceous pack:

	parts by weight
Kaolin (or other prepared earth)	100·0
Ground alum	10·0
Hydrogen peroxide	10·0
Epsom salt	15·0
Citric acid	10·0
Glycerin	15·0
Water	50·0

Procedure

All the ingredients except the kaolin, or other earth, are dissolved in the water and the kaolin is then added and mixed thoroughly to produce a smooth paste.

Winter (*Alchemist*) gives the following two formulations for face packs for (*a*) a dry skin, and (*b*) a greasy skin respectively:

Face Pack for Dry Skin

	parts by weight
Kaolin	80·0
Starch	10·0
Cold cream	20·0
Cetyl alcohol	2·0
Hydrophilic oil	5·0
Water, boric water or infusions	*q.s.*

Procedure

Melt the cold cream and the cetyl alcohol in warm water. Next add the oil, the powders and then the water or other aqueous matter.

Face Pack for Greasy Skin

	parts by weight
Kaolin	80·0
Magnesium carbonate	15·0
Starch	5·0
Tragacanth gum (powdered)	1·0
Water	*q.s.*

Winter adds that by the inclusion of 5 g. of triethanolamine one obtains a mask with a very pronounced degreasing action. (This proportion of free triethanolamine is considered by the Author to be too high.)

The following formulation illustrates the use of triethanolamine alginate with china clay, mild astringents and rubefacients (in very low concentration):

	parts by weight
Triethanolamine alginate TS/RE	12·0
"Nipagin" M (preservative)	0·1
China clay	10·0
Menthol	0·05
Camphor	0·1
Witch hazel extract	5·0
Orange flower water	0·5
Glycerin	10·0
Zinc carbonate	2·0
Perfume (rosaceous)	0·2
Distilled water to	100·0

Procedure

Dry mix the triethanolamine alginate and "Nipagin" M; disperse in glycerin stirring in water until dissolved. Dry mix china clay and zinc carbonate and add to the solution. Add witch hazel extract; then dissolve menthol and camphor in the perfume and orange water, stirring into mix until uniform.

(*Courtesy Alginate Industries Ltd.*)

Qualities Desirable in a Face Pack or Mask

The following characteristics are very desirable in a face pack or mask. The qualities listed apply to the finished preparation if sold as such or, if the pack is sold as a powder to be prepared at home, the powder should readily disperse in water to produce a preparation possessing similar qualities:

(i) It should be a smooth paste without gritty particles and without an "earthy" or other objectionable odour.

(ii) Applied to the face it should dry out rapidly to form an adherent coating on the skin, but this coating should be capable of subsequently being removed by peeling off the face without producing any pain; any residual matter should be capable of being readily removed with cotton wool and warm water.

(iii) If packaged in a tube, it must extrude without undue pressure being exerted, under all climatic conditions likely to be encountered in practice but must not show signs of separation.

(iv) It must be dermatologically innocuous and non-toxic.

(v) Although it must dry rapidly on the face, it must not dry out readily if the tube container is left uncapped for a while.

Probably the greatest difficulty which the cosmetic manufacturer has to face is that of obtaining a product which will combine the diametrically opposed qualities outlined in (ii) and (v) above.

CHAPTER 9

VANISHING, POWDER AND ALL-PURPOSE CREAMS; FOUNDATION CREAMS AND FOUNDATION MAKE-UP PREPARATIONS

Vanishing Creams

Vanishing creams were, some twenty years ago, defined by the Author "as suspensions of stearic acid in a stearate soap". Because of developments in the supply of emulsifying agents available to the cosmetic industry, the above definition requires amendment to the following modified form: "Vanishing creams consist of suspensions of crystalline, free fatty acid—usually stearic acid—in a non-alkaline suspending medium of suitable viscosity."

As mentioned in Chapter 6, the use of non-alkaline (and even "acid-reacting" cosmetic) creams is not such an innovation as a perusal of the technical literature would suggest. It appears to have been tacitly assumed in the industry and amongst dermatologists, that vanishing creams, because they contained soap, were alkaline. The fallacy of this has been evident to me for some years since numerous *p*H measurements which I have recorded on such creams using a glass electrode *p*H meter, have consistently given readings on the acid side, usually between *p*H 6·0 and *p*H 6·9. The explanation for such readings evidently lies in the existence of "acid soaps", viz. compounds of alkali-stearate with stearic acid, in very definite proportions.

[Ryer (*Oil and Soap*, 1946, **23**, 310), prepared a number of acid soaps, intermediate in composition between neutral sodium stearate and stearic acid and succeeded in obtaining acid soaps of well defined composition corresponding to the formulae 1 . NaST : 1 . HSt; 2 . NaST; 3 . HSt, and 1 . NaSt : 2 . HSt but obtained no evidence of the existence of a soap corresponding to 2 . NaSt; 1 . HSt.]

A typical example of a "simple" vanishing cream is:

	per cent.
(*a*) Stearic acid	15·0
(*b*) Potassium hydroxide	0·7
(*c*) Glycerin	8·0
(*d*) Water	76·3
(*e*) Preservative	*q.s.*
(*f*) Perfume	*q.s.*

Procedure

(1) Heat (*a*) to 75° C.

(2) Dissolve (*b*), (*c*) and (*e*) in (*d*) and raise the temperature of this solution to 75° C.

Add (2) at 75° C. to (1), also at 75° C., with gentle but thorough agitation. Continue stirring until the temperature of the mixture falls to about 40° C. Add the perfume, stir and allow the cream to stand for 24-48 hours, occasionally turning over the top crust of cream that forms. At the end of this time, pass the product through a triple-roll mill or, if preferred, homogenise.

At first sight the *composition* of the cream resulting from the above mixture seems to be very simple indeed, but this is far from being the case. Commercial stearic acid is not pure stearic acid but is a mixture of stearic and palmitic, together with a small quantity of oleic, acids. Only a portion of this commercial stearic acid *is saponified*, so that the cream will contain, in addition to the soaps of the fatty acids mentioned, free stearic, free palmitic and free oleic acids in the ratio in which they were present in the commercial stearic acids used. These " free " fatty acids can then form complexes, e.g. " acid soaps ", with some of the neutral soaps already formed in the cream. Thus, so far, our " simple " cream may contain any or all of the following :

potassium stearate,
potassium palmitate,
potassium oleate
stearic acid,
palmitic acid,
oleic acid,
stearic acid-potassium stearate acid soap,
stearic acid-potassium palmitate acid soap,
stearic acid-potassium oleate acid soap,
palmitic acid-potassium stearate acid soap,
palmitic acid-potassium palmitate acid soap,
palmitic acid-potassium oleate acid soap,
oleic acid-potassium stearate acid soap,
oleic acid-potassium palmitate acid soap, etc.

and so on. If, instead of using only potassium hydroxide in the above formula, we use a mixture of potassium and sodium hydroxides, then we shall, at least, double the above number of possible combinations, since we shall have the potassium and sodium salt of each one. If we use a mixture of " triethanolamine " and sodium hydroxide (since triethanolamine is not a pure compound but contains other " ethanolamine " derivatives) the complexity of the mixture extends even further. If boric acid is included, in the presence of glycerin, the glyceroboric acid—which is a strong acid—thus formed will react with and split some of the soaps formed, the amount of such splitting depending upon the proportions of the ingredients in the formula.

If the above facts are taken into consideration, and also the fact that very many of the auxiliary emulsifiers sold for cosmetic purposes are "polyhydric alcohol esters of fatty acids", for example, glycerin monostearate, diethylene glycol stearates, etc., which (as discussed in R. G. Harry, *Cosmetic Materials*, 1948, Leonard Hill Ltd., pp 244-255) are "extremely complicated and complex mixtures"—not simple products—the complexity of the "average" cosmetic preparation in terms of pure "chemistry" will be realised.

The following are other examples of slightly more complex formulations for vanishing creams:

	per cent.
(*a*) Stearic acid	15·00
(*b*) Potassium hydroxide	0·50
(*c*) Sodium hydroxide	0·18
(*d*) Cetyl alcohol	0·50
(*e*) Isopropyl myristate	3·00
(*f*) Glycerin	5·00
(*g*) Water	75·82
(*h*) Preservative	*q.s.*
(*i*) Perfume	*q.s.*

Procedure

(1) Heat (*a*), (*d*) and (*e*) at 75° C. until homogeneous.

(2) Heat (*b*), (*c*), (*f*), (*g*) and (*h*), until a clear solution is obtained. Adjust temperature to 75° C.

Add (2) to (1) with gentle but continuous agitation. Stir down to 45° C. Perfume, allow to stand 24-48 hours. Mill or homogenise.

	per cent.
(*a*) Stearic acid	20·00
(*b*) Cetyl alcohol	0·50
(*c*) Triethanolamine	1·20
(*d*) Sodium hydroxide	0·36
(*e*) Glycerin	8·00
(*f*) Water	69·94
(*g*) Preservative	*q.s.*
(*h*) Perfume	*q.s.*

Procedure

(1) Heat (*a*) and (*b*) at 75° C. until homogeneous.

(2) Dissolve (*c*), (*d*) and (*g*) in (*e*) and (*f*) and raise temperature to 75° C.

Add (2) to (1) with gentle but continuous agitation. Stir down to 45° C., add perfume, allow to stand 24-48 hours and mill, or homogenise.

	per cent.
(*a*) Stearic acid	23·00
(*b*) Cetyl alcohol	0·50
(*c*) Spermaceti	3·00
(*d*) Glycerin	8·00
(*e*) 2-amino-2-methyl-1, 3-propanediol (" Aminoglycol ") [Commercial Solvents Corp.]	1·50
(*f*) Water	64·00
(*g*) Preservative	*q.s.*
(*h*) Perfume	*q.s.*

Procedure

(1) Heat (*a*), (*b*) and (*c*) at 75° C. until homogeneous.

(2) Dissolve (*d*), (*e*) and (*g*) in (*f*) and raise the temperature to 75° C.

Add (2) to (1) with gentle but continuous agitation. Stir down to 45° C., add perfume; allow to stand 24-48 hours. Mill or homogenise.

	per cent.
(*a*) Stearic acid	20·00
(*b*) Diglycol stearate	4·00
(*c*) Propylene glycol	5·00
(*d*) Isopropanolamines	0·80
(*e*) Potassium hydroxide	0·33
(*f*) Sodium hydroxide	0·24
(*g*) Water	69·63
(*h*) Preservative	*q.s.*
(*i*) Perfume	*q.s.*

Procedure

(1) Heat (*a*) and (*b*) at 75° C. until homogeneous.

(2) Dissolve (*c*), (*d*), (*e*), (*f*) and (*h*) in (*g*) and raise the temperature to 75° C.

Add (2) to (1) with gentle but continuous stirring. Stir down to 45° C. Perfume and allow to stand for 24-48 hours. Mill or homogenise.

	per cent.
(*a*) Diglycol stearate	3·00
(*b*) Cetyl alcohol	0·50
(*c*) Stearic acid	10·00
(*d*) Potassium hydroxide	0·40
(*e*) Propylene glycol	8·00
(*f*) Water	78·10
(*g*) Preservative	*q.s.*
(*h*) Perfume	*q.s.*

Procedure

(1) Heat (*a*), (*b*) and (*c*) at 75° C. until homogeneous.

(2) Dissolve (*d*), (*e*) and (*g*) in (*f*) and raise the temperature of the mixture to 75° C.

Add (2) to (1) with gentle but thorough agitation. Stir down to 45° C. Add perfume; allow to stand 24-48 hours, then mill or homogenise.

CONSISTENCY AND MANIPULATION

The consistency of a vanishing cream depends upon :

(*a*) the amount of stearic acid saponified ;
(*b*) the type of alkali used to effect saponification ;
(*c*) the proportion of water ;
(*d*) the percentage of auxiliary substances introduced ;
(*e*) manipulation, including the degree of aeration.

The quantity of stearic acid may vary widely. Usually it is about 20 per cent., although it may vary from 10-30 per cent. or more. The amount of this to be saponified may vary from 20-30 per cent., according to the cream desired. The consistency depends, as has been shown, on the type of alkali used ; potash, triethanolamine, isopropanolamines giving soft creams, sodium hydroxide harder ones. Obviously the proportion of water also affects the consistency of the finished product, but even after allowing for all these variants, the *question of manipulation is of outstanding importance.*

Improper mixing can, with the identical cream, produce in one case a lumpy cream, hard and difficult to apply smoothly, or, in the other case, a cream so liquid that it would not be policy to pack it in jars. This applies in particular to those cases where stearic acid is saponified *in situ* and auxiliary stabilising agents are not present. The temperature of mixing, stirring and setting are of great importance, as is also the exact method of *beating*, and having once determined these conditions, they should be rigidly adhered to.

ALKALI REQUIRED TO OBTAIN SPECIFIC RESULTS

From the following equivalent weights it is possible to calculate readily the amount of alkali required to saponify any required proportion of stearic acid :

Table of Equivalent Weights

Potassium hydroxide	56·0
Sodium hydroxide	40·0
Ammonia	35·0
Borax	190·6
Triethanolamine	approx. 142·0
Isopropanolamines	approx. 140·0
Stearic acid	284·0

For example, if the cream contains 20 lb. of stearic acid and it is desired to saponify 25 per cent. of it (i.e. 5 lb.) then

$$\frac{\text{equivalent weight alkali}}{\text{equivalent weight stearic acid}} = \text{lb. alkali}$$

necessary to neutralise 1 lb. stearic acid, from which the necessary amount is readily obtained. The above figures for equivalent weights refer to the pure 100 per cent. substance, and must be *corrected for the percentage strength of the alkali which is to be used, and for the acid value of the stearic acid.*

SHEEN. Sheen in a vanishing cream is due to the crystalline laminae of stearic acid (or possibly " stearate-acid soap ") reflecting incident light. The best method of producing such sheen was in the past a matter of controversy but with the availability of high quality grades of stearic acid, and by the use of potassium hydroxide—or better, one of the newer amino emulsifying agents—there should be no difficulty in obtaining the sheen desired, though a little " ageing " of the cream may be necessary to obtain the best results.

CHOICE OF ALKALI. Sodium and potassium hydroxides are both good; the former alone yielding a rather hard cream while the latter will produce a much softer product with plenty of sheen. The use of carbonates may result in the finished product sinking badly, due to the gradual release of carbon dioxide entrained physically in the cream during the saponification process. Borax gives a white cream, is easy to work with, but the product tends to grain. Ammonium hydroxide is unpleasant for the employees and is considered to produce, under ordinary conditions of manufacture, discoloration of the finished product. The writer *has* produced creams from absolutely pure chemical products which, if protected from light and air and in the absence of perfume, were satisfactory in this respect, but it appears almost impossible under the normal conditions of cream production and perfuming to obtain a first-class product by its use.

Triethanolamine produces on combination with fatty acids, soaps which are only very slightly alkaline and vanishing creams prepared with this alkali develop excellent sheen but are rather soft. This defect may be remedied by incorporating a proportion of sodium hydroxide. Triethanolamine products also tend to discolour somewhat, and recently mixed isopropanolamines have been introduced to obviate this. It is claimed, however, that if strict attention is paid to the absence of metallic contamination, especially iron, and if suitable perfumes are chosen and the cream protected from excessive exposure to light, discoloration in triethanolamine vanishing creams may be prevented. It is also claimed that amino glycol soaps do not darken on ageing. [J. Kalish, *Drug Cosmet. Ind.*, Jan. 1941.]

Wolff (*Fette u. Seif.*, March 1952, p. 142) has pointed out that by the inclusion of small amounts (1-2 per cent.) of sulphurous acid into triethanolamine at room temperature, part of the triethanolamine is converted to sulphite. This salt is so weak, however, that in ensuing reactions with fatty acids, a small amount of sulphurous acid is liberated, which keeps the cream white—providing a temperature of 70° C. during the process of manufacture has not been exceeded. When preparing triethanolamine stearate from such triethanolamine containing sulphurous acid, it is pointed out that the reaction is exothermic. For the preparation of salts, Wolff recommends a stoichiometric quantity of 149 for the triethanolamine.

INCLUSION OF CETYL ALCOHOL. Experiments have shown that the inclusion of a small amount of cetyl alcohol in a vanishing cream is beneficial in two ways. It improves the texture of the cream and also improves its stability at low temperatures. From 0·5-1·0 per cent. is considered adequate.

CHOICE OF HUMECTANT. The choice of humectant (glycerin, propylene glycol or sorbitol) may influence the characteristics of the cream in several ways. (*See* Humectants, Chapter 44.)

CHOICE OF PLANT. The best material to use for the mixing vessels are stainless steel steam-heated pans; alternatively, aluminium may be used for the fats and for the finished cream, but in this case the solution of the alkali must be heated in a vessel of suitable material.

So far as the fatty acids are concerned, aluminium appears to be harmless under normal conditions of usage; moreover, its salts are colourless and aluminium stearate, if formed in very small amounts, would not be detrimental to the cream.

Iron and copper must, however, *not* be used and tinned copper is risky since the tinning may wear off.

It should be noted that fatty acids of a high degree of purity are now available; for example, from the Armour Company (the Neo-Fats), from Atlas Powder Company (Hystrenes), from Hess Products in the United Kingdom (the Distec range of fatty acids), etc. In some cases interesting variations on current formulae may be obtained by their use; in other cases a fair degree of re-formulation may be necessary as the small amounts of other fatty acids, such as oleic, commonly present in normal commercial stearic acid, considerably help the plasticity of the product.

As mentioned in Chapter 41, the "Spans" and "Tweens" are complex emulsifying agents, especially "tailored" to have the requisite balance of H.L.B. (hydrophilic-lipophilic balance) for the particular job in hand. Their constitution is such that they are referred to under the particular heading of "Span 'so and so'"; and "Tween 'so and so'"; Hystyrene, as mentioned above, is a high purity stearic acid; "Arlex" is a special grade of commercial sorbitol solution. The following is a modernised version of a vanishing cream:

	per cent.
(*a*) Hystyrene T-70 (70 per cent. stearic acid)	15·0
(*b*) Isopropyl palmitate	1·0
(*c*) Arlacel 60	2·0
(*d*) Tween 60	1·5
(*e*) Arlex (Atlas commercial sorbitol solution)	2·5
(*f*) Water	78·0
(*g*) Preservative	*q.s.*
(*h*) Perfume	*q.s.*

Procedure

(1) Heat together (*a*), (*b*), (*c*) and (*d*) until dissolved.

(2) Heat together (*f*), (*g*) and (*e*) and raise temperature of the solution to 95° C.

Add (1) at 90° C. to (2) at 95° C. with thorough agitation.

Add perfume at 50° C. Hand work (i.e. give a hand stir) occasionally, until the temperature falls to 25° C. Re-work and pack the following day.

(Atlas Powder Co.)

It is claimed that the combination of Arlacel and Tween emulsifiers prevents the formation of "top crust" when the cap of the jar is left off for some time.

Foundation Creams

In the province of vanishing creams, but differing from them in that they possess greater "holding" properties for "make-up" and in that they may, or may not, possess a crystalline sheen, are a number of types of preparation. In the past these were obtained termed "foundation creams". The difference between a vanishing cream and a foundation cream is open to argument; at some ill-defined stage, the one passes into the other. With the popularity of the heavier coloured types of skin "make-up" to which the term "foundation" has become attached, even the term foundation cream hardly applies at present to the creams under discussion.

An example of the "vanishing cream type" which, because of its content of glycerin, has a greater aptitude for holding "make-up" than the usual vanishing cream, is given by the following:

	per cent.
(*a*) Stearic acid	18·00
(*b*) Potassium hydroxide	0·52

	per cent.
(c) Sodium hydroxide	0·18
(d) Cetyl alcohol	0·50
(e) Glycerin	18·00
(f) Titanium dioxide	3·00
(g) Preservative	q.s.
(h) Water	59·20
(i) Colour	q.s.
(j) Perfume	0·60

Procedure

(1) Heat together (*a*) and (*d*) at 75° C. till homogeneous.

(2) Heat together (*b*), (*c*), (*e*), (*g*) and (*h*) at 75° C. till dissolved.

Add (2) to (1), continue to stir until the temperature falls to 50° C., when (*f*) [milled with any insoluble colours (*i*)] is stirred into the mixture. Add perfume at 40° C. and allow cream to stand. On the following day mill or homogenise.

Glyceryl monostearate and diglycol stearate, when stirred in hot water and cooled whilst stirring, form neutral creams. These stearates are marketed in emulsifying and non-self-emulsifying grades; the former contains a trace of soap or soapless surface-active agent, whilst the latter grade is free from soap, etc. The following formulae exemplify their use:

	per cent.
(a) Glyceryl monostearate (self-emulsifying)	12·0
(b) Spermaceti	5·0
(c) Glycerin	5·0
(d) Titanium dioxide	2·0
(e) Water	76·0
(f) Preservative	q.s.
(g) Perfume	q.s.

Procedure

This cream may be made in the conventional two-phase manner by melting the oil-soluble ingredients and the water-soluble ingredients separately, mixing them at 75° C. and as the emulsion begins to form, the titanium dioxide may be wetted by grinding with some of the emulsion and the "wetted" mass then stirred into the main bulk. Alternatively it may be made as follows:

(1) Heat (*a*), (*b*), (*c*), (*e*) and (*f*) together at 90° C. until homogeneous then continue to stir whilst cooling.

(2) Wet the titanium dioxide (*d*) by grinding with a small amount of the emulsion (1), and stir the "wetted" titanium dioxide into the main bulk. Continue stirring until the paste becomes a smooth cream. Perfume at about 50° C.

(Formula by courtesy Rex Campbell & Co. Ltd.)

	per cent.
(*a*) Diglycol stearate	18·0
(*b*) Cetyl alcohol	1·0
(*c*) Lanolin	2·0
(*d*) Titanium dioxide	2·0
(*e*) Glycerin	8·0
(*f*) Water	69·0
(*g*) Preservative	*q.s.*
(*h*) Colouring matter	*q.s.*
(*i*) Perfume	*q.s.*

Procedure

(1) Heat (*a*), (*b*) and (*c*) at about 90° C. till homogeneous.

(2) Heat (*e*), (*f*) and (*g*) till dissolved and raise temperature of the solution to about 90° C.

Add (2) to (1) with stirring; continue to stir. When the temperature has fallen to about 60° C. (and a stable emulsion is forming) "*wet*" (*d*) with some of this emulsion and stir it into the main bulk of cream. Continue to stir whilst cooling. Perfume at 45° C. Allow to stand 24-48 hours and mill.

(*Note.* If a coloured cream is desired (*d*) should be milled with the insoluble colouring matter (*h*), prior to being wetted with the emulsion.)

	per cent.
(*a*) Lanette wax SX	15·0
(*b*) Butyl stearate	3·0
(*c*) Lanolin	3·0
(*d*) Sorbitol syrup	7·0
(*e*) Water	72·0
(*f*) Preservative	*q.s.*
(*g*) Perfume	*q.s.*

Procedure

(1) Heat (*a*), (*b*) and (*c*) at 75° C. until dissolved.

(2) Dissolve (*f*) in the mixture of (*e*) and (*d*) and raise the temperature of this mixture to 75° C.

Add (2) to (1) with stirring; perfume at 45° C.; stir down to about 25°-30° C. and allow to stand overnight.

[If desired a little coloured titanium dioxide may be incorporated along the lines of the examples of other formulae given above.]

"Polawax" (Croda Ltd.), a non-ionic reaction product of stearyl alcohol and ethylene oxide reaction products, may also be used as a basis for a foundation type cream, viz.:

	per cent.
(*a*) Polawax	14·0
(*b*) Lanolin	2·0
(*c*) Petroleum jelly (white)	2·0
(*d*) Glycerin	8·0
(*e*) Titanium dioxide	3·0

	per cent.
(*f*) Water	71·0
(*g*) Preservative	*q.s.*
(*h*) Colouring matter	*q.s.*
(*i*) Perfume	*q.s.*

Procedure

(1) Heat (*a*), (*b*) and (*c*) at 75° C. until homogeneous.
(2) Heat (*d*), (*f*) and (*g*) until homogeneous and adjust temperature to 75° C. Add (2) to (1) whilst stirring.
(3) Wet the " milled (*e*) and (*h*) mixture " with a little of the emulsion and then stir the wetted mixture into the bulk of the cream. Stir down to 45° C., perfume and continue to stir until the temperature falls to about 30° C.

Colloidal aluminium silicate, available in the United States under the trade name of " Veegum " (R. T. Vanderbilt & Co.), has many interesting properties. This material forms high viscosity, white, gels at low solids content due to its colloidal and thixotropic properties. (This material differs from bentonite in several respects, one of them being the fact that " Veegum " crystals are rods whilst bentonite crystals are plate-like.)

The following formulation by J. C. Kern and R. T. Stetson (*Amer. Perfum.*, Aug. 1950, p. 140) illustrates the use of " Veegum " in a foundation cream :

	parts
(*a*) Glyceryl monostereate (self-emulsifying grade)	4·50
(*b*) Lanolin	2·48
(*c*) Cetyl alcohol	4·95
(*d*) Light mineral oil	18·60
(*e*) Colloidal magnesium aluminium silicate (" Veegum ")	1·65
(*f*) Glycerin	5·80
(*g*) Triethanolamine	0·52
(*h*) Water	64·35
(*i*) Preservative	*q.s.*
(*j*) Perfume	*q.s.*

Procedure

(1) Mix (*a*), (*b*), (*c*) and (*d*) and heat at 70° C. until homogeneous.
(2) Add (*e*) slowly to (*h*), continually agitating until smooth.
(3) Add (*f*) and (*g*) to (2) and heat to 70° C. Add (1) to (2) and stir until smooth and cool.

Powder Creams

Many of the above creams contain a small amount of powder, and thus in considering foundation and other creams, it is logical to discuss creams formulated with an " increased powder content ".

A powder cream has been defined (R. G. Harry, *Modern Cosmeticology*, 1944, London: Leonard Hill Ltd.) as a "suspension of a *suitable* face powder in a vanishing cream base, the functions of which are:

(*a*) reduction of creaming and powdering to one operation;

(*b*) adhesion of powder to skins which appear to lack adhesive power."

It was pointed out, that although powder creams are occasionally used with a view to carrying out (*a*) above, this does not appear to be the main function of such creams and that powder creams are used in a great many cases by persons who find that they appear more effective in covering a shiny nose or skin.

This was largely due to the choice of constituents employed in making the powder portion of the cream. Such creams therefore—from the point of view of appearance—appeared to have better "foundation properties" for any subsequent make-up, and as will be seen subsequently the development of modern pigmented make-up has developed from a combination of experiences gained with powder creams and with "all-purpose" creams.

PROPORTION OF POWDER IN A POWDER CREAM. Recommendations of about 5 per cent. powder in a cream base are too low to produce what the public have learnt to expect from such a cream, and amounts of from 10–20 per cent. give much better results depending upon the type of base employed; several successful creams have considerably higher proportions of powder than the amounts mentioned; such powder is often in a "non-fatty" base.

Whilst a number of the normal face powder constituents such as titanium dioxide, zinc oxide, colloidal kaolin, magnesium stearate, etc., can be included, it is usual to confine choice to the use of titanium dioxide and/or zinc oxide, because of their superior covering properties (*see* Chapter 11, Face powders, etc.). Because of the incompatibility of zinc salts with certain emulsifiers, titanium dioxide was in the past very often employed; it is claimed also that this material is less drying on the skin. With the infinite number of emulsifiers now coming on the market, many of them "non-ionic", the question of the incompatibility of zinc oxide with the emulsifier is of very much less importance.

Many of the cosmetic cream bases described under different chapters in this book will serve, with some modification, as starting points for laboratory experiments; information on the properties of the powder components can be obtained from Chapter 11 and adapted where necessary, to suit individual needs. The following, however, give some illustrative examples :

	per cent.
(*a*) Glyceryl monostearate (self-emulsifying)	16·0
(*b*) Water	44·0
(*c*) Preservative	*q.s.*
(*d*) Glycerin	25·0
(*e*) Powder base	15·0
(*f*) Colour	*q.s.*
(*g*) Perfume	*q.s.*

Procedure

(1) Heat (*a*), (*b*) and (*c*) to 85°-90° C. until homogeneous.

(2) Continue to stir (1) whilst cooling.

(3) Grind (*e*) and (*f*) and when thoroughly dispersed, wet the mixture by thoroughly dispersing in (*d*).

(4) Add (3) to (2) ; to ensure adequate removal of (3) from its container wipe round the container several times with further amounts of (2) and add to main bulk.

	per cent.
(*a*) Lanette Wax SX	8·0
(*b*) Stearic acid	8·0
(*c*) Water	64·0
(*d*) Preservative	*q.s.*
(*e*) Glycerin	10·0
(*f*) Powder base	10·0
(*g*) Colour	*q.s.*
(*h*) Perfume	*q.s.*

Procedure

(1) Heat (*a*), (*b*), (*c*) and (*d*) to 85°-90° C. until homogeneous.

(2) Continue to stir (1) whilst cooling.

(3) Grind (*g*) with (*f*) until thoroughly dispersed, then wet the mixture by dispersing in (*e*).

(4) Add (3) to (2) and stir down to about 30° C.

During recent years there has been a swing-away from the ordinary, slightly tinted powder cream, to the more heavily pigmented types in which the pigment material is chiefly titanium dioxide which has been coloured by grinding with certain coloured oxides of iron, or coloured lakes. Such preparations are very often found to produce instability in ordinary vanishing and foundation cream formulae because they are preferentially " wetted " by " oil " rather than water, and may therefore tend to invert the emulsified phase. By the use of some of the non-ionic agents this difficulty may be overcome ; this point is illustrated in dealing with " foundation make-up ", later in this chapter.

"All-Purpose Creams" (Sports Creams)

Because some persons found the usual vanishing and foundation creams not sufficiently emollient for their skins (if these skins tended to be on the "dry" side), there arose a vogue for a more emollient type of preparation which, if used correctly, would not be too greasy to be used as a foundation cream. On the Continent the development of "All-Purpose" creams based on lanolin, cholesterol and cholesterol esters, had achieved popularity, and the use of these creams became popular in this country under the title "Sports Creams", All-Purpose Creams, etc.

The title "All-Purpose", although popular, is something of a misnomer. To be really an "All-Purpose" cream, such a preparation should comply with the following requirements:

(i) As a *foundation* cream for general use it must provide a satisfactory foundation base for make-up without being too greasy.

(ii) As a *cleansing* cream, it should liquefy readily, be of an oily nature but should be free from "drag". It should not be readily absorbed by the skin.

(iii) As a *massage* cream it should possess sufficient "drag" to facilitate facial massage.

(iv) As a *lubricating* cream (or so-called "skin-food"), it should be emollient, but not excessively greasy.

Obviously no "one" preparation can satisfy each of the above conflicting requirements, and hence any such one preparation must be, of necessity, a compromise. In general, such creams fulfil their purpose fairly well. From the sales angle, the position is not quite so advantageous, since one must first convince a woman that her face is of no greater cosmetic importance—so far as quality of product and of "perfume" is concerned—than various other "portions of her anatomy" for which she might wish to use an all-purpose cream; secondly, if one succeeds in doing this successfully, one sells *one* product instead of four which were previously sold, each for a specific purpose. The writer's experience is that comparison of "all-purpose" creams on all counts, against a specialised cream for each particular purpose, gives a higher credit vote to the specialised creams, though in several of the specified uses, the "all-purpose" cream may run the specialised product pretty closely!

The following formula was suggested by Pfaff (*Soap Perfum. Cosm.*, July 1939, p. 604):

	per cent.
(*a*) Protegin	25·0
(*b*) Protegin X	5·0
(*c*) Wool wax	1·0

	per cent.
(*d*) Glycerin	3·0
(*e*) Petroleum oil	6·0
(*f*) Water	60·0

[Protegin X is an oxycholesterin absorption base whose active ingredients are the cholesterols and cholesterol esters extracted from lanolin. Other U.S. absorption bases are "Falba" and "Isco" (Morningstar Nicol Inc.); in this country "Cremba" and Isocreme bases (Croda Ltd.) are available, together with a number of the "Abracol" Absorption Bases (A. Boake Roberts Ltd.). Such replacement bases may be utilised for experimental investigation where desired.]

Procedure

(1) Melt (*a*), (*b*), (*c*) and (*e*), keeping as low a melting temperature as possible.
(2) Mix (*d*) and (*f*); warm to 45°–50° C.
(3) Add a little of (2) to (1), both solutions being between 40°–50° C. Stir to thoroughly incorporate before adding more of (2). Add perfume, then agitate gradually but continuously, keeping the water phase incorporated within the oil phase until the temperature falls to about 25° C.

The following exemplifies the use of one of the "Abracols" in such creams (courtesy A. Boake Roberts Ltd.):

	per cent.
(*a*) Abracol V.P.X.	20·0
(*b*) Petroleum jelly (white)	4·0
(*c*) White mineral oil	10·0
(*d*) Lanolin (anhydrous)	3·0
(*e*) Beeswax	4·0
(*f*) Glycerin	3·0
(*g*) White ceresin	8·0
(*h*) Water	48·0

Procedure

(1) Heat (*a*), (*b*), (*c*), (*d*), (*e*) and (*g*) until dissolved, keeping the temperature as low as possible. Adjust temperature to 45°–50° C.
(2) Mix (*f*) and (*h*). Warm to 50° C.
Add (2) to (1), a little at a time, making sure that all of (2) added has been incorporated thoroughly before adding more. Mixing is continued, whilst cooling, to 25° C. Homogenise.

E. S. Lower (*Soap Perfum. Cosm.*, 1945, **18**, 299) gives the following:

	Parts (by weight)
(*a*) Absorption base (semi-fluid type)[1]	4·0
(*b*) Petroleum jelly	7·7
(*c*) Lanolin	4·0
(*d*) Liquid paraffin	1·5
(*e*) Water	20·0

Procedure

As above. (Homogenisation is recommended.)

[1] Such as Isocreme Base (Croda).

The formulation for a "dry skin" cream of the absorption cream base type is reproduced below (by courtesy Goldschmidt Chemical Corporation, New York):

	per cent.
(*a*) Protegin X	26·0
(*b*) Tegin (glyceryl monostearate self-emulsifying)	1·0
(*c*) Spermaceti	5·0
(*d*) Lanolin	5·0
(*e*) Cetyl alcohol	2·0
(*f*) Vegetable oil	8·0
(*g*) Glycerin	3·0
(*h*) Mineral oil	5·0
(*i*) Tegosept P (ester *p*-hydroxybenzoic acid)	0·15
(*j*) Water	44·85

Procedure

(1) Heat (*a*), (*b*), (*c*), (*d*), (*e*), (*f*) and (*h*) at as low a temperature as possible; adjust to 40°–50° C.

(2) Heat (*g*), (*i*) and (*j*) to clear solution and adjust temperature to 40°–50° C.

Add (2) to (1), a little at a time, ensuring that all of (2) has been absorbed before making any fresh addition. Perfume and stir down to 25° C. Milling is optional.

Thorpe Deakers (Pfaff, *Soap Perfum. Cosm.*, July 1939) found that small proportions of magnesium salts, such as magnesium sulphate, assist very considerably in the stabilisation of water-in-oil creams. The following formula illustrates such usage:

	per cent.
(*a*) Mineral oil 65/75	5·0
(*b*) Atlas G.1500	4·0
(*c*) Petroleum jelly (short fibre)	40·0
(*d*) Lanolin (anhydrous)	4·0
(*e*) Paraffin (or micro-crystalline) wax	12·0
(*f*) Water	32·8
(*g*) Magnesium sulphate U.S.P.	0·2
(*h*) Arlex (sorbitol syrup)	2·0
(*i*) Preservative	*q.s.*
(*j*) Perfume	*q.s.*

Procedure

(1) Heat (*a*), (*b*), (*c*), (*d*) and (*e*) to 70°–75° C.

(2) Heat (*f*), (*g*), (*h*) and (*i*) to 70°–75° C.

Add (2) to (1) gradually at 70°–75° C., with stirring. Perfume at 55°–60° C. It is stated that this product may be filled directly into jars at 55°–60° C., or homogenised in the cold and filled.

[From *Drug and Cosmetic Emulsions*, Atlas Powder Co., U.S.A.]

[Atlas G. 1500 is described as a blend of polyoxyalkylene stearate with polyoxyalkylene (propylene glycol glucoside) tetraoleate.]

An alternative formula, based upon the use of the more recently developed hydrophilic lanolin derivatives, is given below. [W. C. Griffin, P. J. Carter and R. W. Behrens, *Drug Cosmet. Ind.*, Sept. 1948.] In this formula two hydrophilic lanolin derivatives are used as the emulsifiers :

	per cent.
(*a*) Stearic acid (best)	15·0
(*b*) Beeswax (white)	2·0
(*c*) Lanolin (anhydrous)	1·0
(*d*) Mineral oil 65/75	23·0
(*e*) G-1425 (polyoxyalkylene sorbitol-lanolin)	5·0
(*f*) G-1441 (polyoxyalkylene sorbitol-lanolin)	1·0
(*g*) Arlex (commercial sorbitol solution)	10·0
(*h*) Water	43·0
(*i*) Preservative	*q.s.*
(*j*) Perfume	*q.s.*

Procedure

(1) Heat (*a*), (*b*), (*c*), (*d*), (*e*) and (*f*) to 70° C.

(2) Heat (*g*), (*h*) and (*i*) to 72° C.

Add (2) to (1) slowly and under continuous agitation. Perfume at 45° C. and pour just before setting point.

Foundation Make-Up Creams

Although persons with dry skins have for some time used either a cold cream or a so-called " all-purpose " cream as a foundation base, it was only just prior to the last war that a demand developed in Hollywood for a new type of " oily " make-up base. As deNavarre (*Amer. Perfum.*, Sept. 1938, p. 25) has pointed out, these newer creams give a *glow* to the skin—an *irridescence* not possible to obtain in any other way.

Several different types of preparation have been developed, all of which had their devotees. Some of these foundations consisted of anhydrous fatty bases, or mixtures of oils, fats and waxes with heavily pigmented powders. Such powders usually consisted of zinc oxide and/or titanium dioxide, and these foundations possessed a relatively high covering power which disguised minor skin blemishes and acted as a base for face powder, giving the skin a smooth matt tinted surface, for example :

	per cent.
Petroleum jelly (low melting-point)	85·0
Zinc oxide	15·0
Pigments	*q.s.*
Perfume	*q.s.*

Procedure

Grind the pigment colouring matters with the zinc oxide and when these are properly dispersed, mix with the melted petroleum jelly, then add the perfume. The mass may then be milled several times through a steel roller mill. If greater covering power is required, the zinc oxide may be replaced, either wholly or in part by titanium dioxide. Wetting agents may be incorporated in order to assist the spreading properties on the face, but if too high a proportion is included they are likely to detract from the water-proofness of the make-up, though in point of fact this is not in any way a serious defect except for those who wish to use the make-up prior to, and during, bathing and swimming.

For those who may wish to use water in the formulation of their products, experiments may be carried out on water-in-oil creams similar to those discussed in All-Purpose Creams (this Chapter) and also under Cold and Cleansing Creams (Chapter 5), the pigments and powder being first ground together in the presence of a suitable surface-active material to render the pigment mixture hydrophilic or lipophilic as required, the mass then "wetted" with the continuous phase of the cream and mixed into the main bulk of cream.

Liquid "Oil" Make-Up

The "House of Westmore", Hollywood, U.S.A., have patented (Brit. Patent No. 577,040, 1946), an improvement in liquid cosmetic make-up foundation, employing an oily foundation which, in the preamble to the patent, includes the following statements of interest:

". . . the main object of the invention is to provide an improved liquid cosmetic make-up which overcomes all of the objectionable features of the prior 'grease paint' type of make-up bases and which is compounded that it may quickly and uniformly spread over the skin to produce a non-drying thin film thereon on which cosmetics usually employed by women in everyday use can be readily applied. A further object of the invention is to provide a free flowing liquid cosmetic make-up foundation for the skin including a vegetable oil which (it is stated) has a beneficial effect on the skin and which does not leave a greasy feeling in use.

"The free flowing liquid composition is composed of:

Vegetable oil. Preferably sesame. However, it is stated, cottonseed peach kernel, peanut, corn and other vegetable oils may be used.

Pulverant Texture Ingredients. Preferably zinc or titanium oxide although other oxides, clays, stearates and talcs may also be used.

Skin Penetrant. Oxycholesterol.

Dispersing Agent. Triglyceryl stearate.

Preservative. May be para hydroxybenzoate.

" The specific proportions claimed in the example are :

	per cent.
Sesame oil	64·0
Zinc oxide	11·0
Oxycholesterol	2·0
Triglyceryl stearate	1·0
Perfume and colouring	6·0
Titanium dioxide	16·0
Preservative	*q.s.*

" It is stated that the percentage of liquid ingredients, however, may vary between 55–65 per cent. and percentages of solids from 32–42 per cent., and it adds that the triglyceryl stearate is intended to be used for the specific purpose of changing the composition into a free flowing liquid by reducing the surface tension of the oil contained therein and not for the purpose of making the product water washable. It is claimed that vegetable oil comprises at least 55 per cent. of the mixture and that this preparation contains a larger proportion of oils and less solids than previous liquid cosmetics because the foundation is designed to be a non-drying one and more solids would tend to cause the composition to dry after application to the skin. . . ."

Discussing liquid make-up bases, Hilfer (*Drug Cosmet. Ind.*, April 1944, **54**, 401) suggested the following formula :

	per cent.
Olive oil	75·0
Oil-soluble preservative	0·1
Titanium dioxide	24·6
Octyl alcohol [1]	0·1
Perfume	0·2

Hilfer points out that in any product of this type the incorporation of air should be carefully avoided, as such an inclusion tends to thicken the product, making it difficult to pour and handle and further, the gradual rise of air bubbles to the surface, bringing with them particles of powder, detracts from the appearance of the preparation.

Air may already be adsorbed on the surface of the powder and is difficult to remove by ordinary means, but the addition of a wetting agent such as octyl alcohol to the vehicle before grinding reduces the surface tension of the powder-air phases and allows the escape of the air. It is added that if the odour of octyl alcohol is considered objectionable, other suitable wetting agents may be considered.

[1] Octyl alcohol is employed in the above as a wetting agent.

As in the case of liquid powders, and liquid "cosmetic stockings", it is difficult if not impossible to prevent settling of the powder suspension, but by using a bulky filler (i.e. low unit weight per volume) and/or colouring, both the suspension of powder and the oily phase, this effect may be minimised.

Probably stimulated by developments along the lines discussed above, advances have been made in the development of coloured oil-in-water cream bases, having a high covering power.

For the purpose of emulsifying the cream base, one of the more recently developed non-ionic emulsifying agents may be used; if soap is used in any form then zinc salts should be avoided and titanium dioxide may be used instead. The following formulae provide a "basis for experiment" though it may well be found that the use of a *non-ionic emulsifying* agent, as exemplified later will prove more satisfactory:

	per cent.
Cetyl alcohol	2·0
Glyceryl monostearate (self-emulsifying)	10·0
Mineral oil	10·0
Titanium dioxide	6·0
Talc	6·0
Glycerin	6·0
Water	60·0
Preservative	*q.s.*
Colouring matters	*q.s.*
Perfume	*q.s.*

	per cent.
Lanette wax SX	12·0
Mineral oil	14·0
Glycerin	5·0
Titanium dioxide	8·0
Zinc stearate	8·0
Stearic acid	3·0
Water	50·0
Preservative	*q.s.*
Colouring matters	*q.s.*
Perfume	*q.s.*

The colours may consist of a mixture of pigments which are given a preliminary grinding with the titanium dioxide, and any other powder constituents prior to incorporating the coloured powder into the emulsion base. In addition, if desired, some oil, or water soluble colours may also be included, these being dissolved in the oil, or water, prior to emulsification.

Manufacture of the emulsion base is accomplished in the usual manner, the oil-soluble components being heated together and the temperature adjusted to 75° C. and the water-soluble components heated with the water and their temperature adjusted to 75° C. Both these phases are then mixed, whilst stirring ; some of the " emulsion "/or the glycerin, being used to " wet-out " the pigments before incorporating into the bulk of the cream.

As mentioned in an earlier part of this chapter, due to the fact that the colours and pigments used in such preparations are preferentially wetted by oils and fats, they cannot be added to ordinary vanishing creams without breaking the emulsion. By careful choice of emulsifier this difficulty may be overcome. The following formulation is from *Drug and Cosmetic Emulsions*. Atlas Powder Co., U.S.A.

	per cent.
(*a*) Isopropyl palmitate	1·0
(*b*) Stearic acid	12·0
(*c*) Span 60 (Sorbitan monostearate)	2·0
(*d*) Tween 60 (Polyoxyethylene sorbitan monostearate)	1·0
(*e*) Arlex (commercial sorbitol solution)	2·5
(*f*) Propylene glycol	12·0
(*g*) Titanium dioxide : Talc mixture (1 : 5)	10·0
(*h*) Iron oxide	1·0
(*i*) Water	58·5
(*j*) Preservative	*q.s.*
(*k*) Perfume	*q.s.*

Procedure

(1) Heat (*a*), (*b*), (*c*) and (*d*) to 90° C.

(2) Heat (*e*), (*f*), (*g*), (*h*), (*i*) and (*j*) to 95° C.

Add (2) to (1) slowly and with constant stirring. Perfume at 45° C. If not smooth and uniformly dispersed, pass through a homogeniser or ointment mill.

It is stated that this cream goes through several stages during the mixing operation, during which it may appear to separate ; nevertheless, with continued agitation a smooth stable cream, it is stated, will result.

CHAPTER 10

"SKIN FOODS"—LUBRICATING AND SKIN CONDITIONING CREAMS

THE designation "skin food", which is commonly applied to emollient creams of this type is, in the author's opinion, a misnomer. Even though it should be shown that the *cells* of the skin can be *influenced* by the external application of certain substances, it by no means follows that such substances can be classed as *foods*.

It is a *sine qua non* that, as the living cells of the epidermis progress outwards from the germinal layer (possibly owing to diminished supplies of certain necessary nutrients and almost certainly *owing to loss of moisture* and changes in hydrogen ion concentration and pressure) they cornify, forming the dead protective outer layer of the skin. Were we able to feed *this layer* (the one we see) it would not be dead, whilst if by feeding we refer to the immediate adjacent layers, subtending inwards from the corneous layer; then again, were we able to *affect* these *cells* by supplying necessary *nutrients* for their existence, they might no longer cornify to form the vital corneous layer essential for human life.

At the same time, the application of certain cosmetic creams may affect the *external appearance and condition* of the skin in a *desirable manner*. As discussed in Chapter 1, The Hydration of the Skin, there is no doubt but that the water content of the outer skin layers is defined within fairly narrow limits. If this is too high we get the appearance of a macerated skin with subsequent infection; if too dry owing to drying winds, central heating or other means of space heating, we get the characteristic appearance of "dry skin" in which painful cracks and fissures develop and may become infected.

The addition of cosmetic creams containing a suitable fatty material can *delay* the rate of water loss from the skin. In addition, by incorporating a suitable humectant (*see* Chapter 44) it is possible to retain an aqueous film consisting of moisture plus humectant in contact with the skin.

Such preparations can supply a valuable check to *premature* ageing of the skin in that they keep the outer corneous layer of the skin soft and supple, and prevent, or at least minimise, chapping and windburn, both of which are considered to produce an appearance of ageing in the skin; in delaying this, they do therefore delay the onset of wrinkles although they do not prevent the ultimate wrinkling of the skin.

The creams containing sex-hormones come into rather a different category, though even in the case of these preparations the author would not classify them actually as skin *foods*. In general the use of such preparations on senile skin has been observed to lead to an increased avidity of the areas for taking up fluids and to a greater succulence (again pointing to the importance of an adequate water and saline balance in the skin); their effect is seen also in the stimulation of proliferative activity, in other words they seem to stimulate the production of the new cells rather than to feed them or alter their normal metabolic process of cornification. It is, however, agreed that "hormone creams" present a problem in classification in that they appear to lie in the "no man's land" between true "skin foods" and lubricating and skin conditioning creams.

A large number of materials have been suggested for incorporation in lubricating creams. In general they may be classified into the following groups:

(i) Emollient fatty substances, of which lanolin is a leading example.
(ii) Vitamin preparations.
(iii) Hormonal preparations.
(iv) Other miscellaneous "additives", for example "biodynes" (from yeast extracts, etc.), lecithin, protein hydrolysates.

Lanolin

As stated in Chapter 4, all the evidence available at present suggests that lanolin, of all the various cosmetic materials available, is the one most closely akin to sebum, the natural skin lubricant. Indeed, this is not surprising, since it is the natural skin lubricant of the skin and wool of the sheep which has been suitably cleansed and purified. Modern research into the structure of the amino acids and X-ray diffraction patterns of the molecular structure of the keratins of skin, hair and feathers (*Brit. J. Derm.*, 1950, **62**, 1–15 [1]) has indicated that Nature is sparing in her use of fundamental materials and that she tends to build apparently dissimilar structures and compounds from a few fundamental and comparatively simple "bricks". Over very many years, lanolin has proved very efficacious in the treatment of chapped skin surfaces and in the prevention of industrial dermatitis. It has been shown that the addition of saponified oils to mineral lubricating oils has consistently led to a reduction in the

[1] *See* Molecular Structure of Skin and Hair, etc., "The Skin," Chapter I.

number of experimental tumours produced in animals and *no oil has been found so far which surpasses lanolin in this respect.* It is also remarkable for the manner in which it preserves the skin smooth and soft. (*See* Report of the Manchester Committee on Cancer, 1923-34; and also C. C. Twort and J. M. Twort, "The Utility of Lanolin as a Protective Measure against Mineral Oil and Tar Dermatitis and Cancer", *J. Hyg., Camb.*, 4 March 1935, **352**, No. 1.)

Simpson and Cramer (*Cancer Res.*, 1945, **5**, 1-4) have also drawn attention to the fact that lanolin has some action in preventing skin cancer following the application of chemical carcinogens. It is pointed out that *it is known that methycholanthrene suffers a considerable reduction in its capacity to produce cancer when it is dissolved in lanolin.*

Whilst in our present state of knowledge, too much should not be read into the above facts, the evidence available suggests that lanolin is a desirable ingredient of cosmetic and toilet preparations. It should be noticed that the emphasis is on lanolin *per se* and that no evidence is available to show that lanolin-derivatives possess the same properties as lanolin. As Malmstrom (*J. Soc. cosmet. Chem.*, June 1949, **1**, 4, 244) has pointed out: ". . . contrary to popular belief the benefits derived from lanolin are not centred about the properties of the individual fatty acids or alcohols present. . . . This mixture which we call lanolin, is essentially a chemical combination of fatty acids and alcohol in ester form. No evidence has been published to show that any chemical individual contained in the mixture is entirely or partly responsible for the properties of lanolin. . . . ."

I suggest that the value of lanolin as a skin lubricant may be due to the fact that it can hold moisture, either in the form of a water-in-oil emulsion or possibly as bimolecular leaflets. At the same time the barrier formed by lanolin is, in my experience, not impervious like that of petroleum jelly and other oils. Thus it may be able to *regulate* the water loss from the skin, and if in fact such water is held in bimolecular leaflets, a complex-lanolin-electrolyte balance may be the key to such regulating mechanism. In this event, lanolin *per se* would be expected to have virtues not necessarily shared by any of its single constituents. [*See* 'Sebum,' Chapter 20, also Bimolecular Leaflets, Chapter 41].

Lanolin, when used in comparatively low amounts in cosmetic preparations, has, however, an odour which it is difficult to disguise completely by means of sophisticated perfumes. Moreover, creams containing appreciable quantities of lanolin tend to be somewhat sticky in use. For this reason there has been a tendency towards the use of lanolin extracts, although we have no evidence that such extracts possess the desirable properties of lanolin *per se*. These extracts are available in varying degrees of purification as set out below :

Wool Wax Alcohols (Alcoholia Lanae) are prepared by the saponification of lanolin and the separation of a fraction containing cholesterol and other alcohols. Wool Wax Alcohols of the British Pharmacopoeia are described as a golden brown solid, somewhat brittle when cold but becoming plastic when warm, containing not less than 28 per cent. cholesterol. "*Hartolan*" *wax*[1] is a proprietary name for a similar preparation having slightly different chemical values.

Wool alcohols as described above contain a predominance of alcohols other than sterols in the mixture. Further purification of wool alcohols has resulted in the production of mixtures which are predominantly cholesterol, probably with other sterols and sterol-like substances. Two of these are available on the British market under the designation "Kathro" cholesterol and "Dastar" cholesterol. It has been suggested that such products, containing upwards of 50 per cent. cholesterol, should be termed "Wool Wax Steroids" or "Wool Steroids" to distinguish them from "Wool Wax Alcohols" sometimes called "Wool Wax Sterols".

"*Dastar*" *Cholesterol.*[1] An off-white to cream-coloured powder containing approximately 50 per cent. cholesterol, 5 per cent. agnosterol and lanosterol and some 45 per cent. of optically inactive alcohols.

"*Kathro*" *Cholesterol.*[1] A white amorphous powder containing 70 per cent. to 72 per cent. cholesterol, 2½ per cent. agnosterol and lanosterol, together with about 25 per cent. to 30 per cent. of optically inactive aliphatic alcohols.

Pure 100 per cent. cholesterol is obtainable in crystalline form, but it is much more expensive and its emulsive properties are inferior to those of the cruder extracts.

In addition to the above forms of lanolin concentrates, a number of so-called "absorption bases" are available. These in general consist of an intimate mixture of one or more of the lanolin derivatives mentioned above, dissolved in petroleum jelly, or a mixture of petroleum jelly with other emollient and fatty substances. These may be used in place of lanolin and at a lower concentration than would be necessary with lanolin, in the formulation of water-in-oil emulsions.

Well known examples of such "absorption bases" are, "Cremba" and "Isocreem" bases (Croda Ltd.), "Abracols" (SHO, ISL, VCH, VPX, VPY and VPZ, etc.), "Protegins" and "Iso-Lan" (Goldschmidt Chemical Corporation); "Falba" (Pfaltz and Bauer), etc.

[1] Proprietary designation, "Croda," Ltd.

More recently a new range of water-soluble derivatives of lanolin has become available; these have been prepared by reacting lanolin and polyoxyethylene sorbitol. Produced by the Atlas Powder Company, Wilmington, U.S.A., these derivatives differ in their hydrophilic balance and are available under a series of numerals ranging from lanolin *per se* insoluble in water, through G-1405; G-1401; G-1425; G-1431, etc., which are *dispersible* in water, to G-1441; G-1451; G-1475 and G-1471 which are soluble in water. Absorption bases of a new type may be prepared by the use of these derivatives; for example, the following formulation was quoted by Griffin, Carter and Behrens (*Drug Cosmet. Ind.*, Sept. 1948):

	per cent.
Arlacel C. (sorbitan sesquioleate)	6·0
G-1425 (polyoxyalkylene sorbitol-lanolin)	4·0
Ceresin wax	15·0
Mineral oil	45·0
Petrolatum	20·0
Lanolin	10·0

Procedure

Warm sufficiently to melt all ingredients and mix.

The range of water-soluble products manufactured in the United Kingdom is at present more limited. Polychols I.D. and I.M. (Croda Ltd.) are water-soluble polyoxyethylene condensation products of Wool Wax Alcohols and are non-ionic surface-active agents, consisting of mixed polyoxyethylene glycol ethers of cholesterol, lanosterol and straight chain alcohols.

Raisin Seed Oil. This oil appears to possess many qualities which make it of interest to the cosmetic manufacturer. It is an almost colourless, odourless oil, and appears to be entirely non-irritant. The experiments of Hume *et al.* (*Biochem. J.*, **32,** 2162) show that this oil appears to be an excellent source of vitamin F. The potency of a fraction of the unsaturated fatty acids from linseed oil was compared with a similar fraction from raisin-seed oil, and the latter was found slightly more potent, both as regards promotion of weight increase in rats, and in the healing of the skin lesions characteristic of a vitamin F deficiency. (*See* Unsaturated Fatty Acids in Chapter 4.)

Cod-liver Oil. This appears to be of value in dry skin. Steel (*Lancet*, 1935, pp. 229, 290) has found it very useful for promoting granulation and in the healing of wounds. A. J. Cameron (*Brit. Med. J.*, 1936, **2,** 785), Sandor (*Lancet*, 1934, pp. 231, 738) and Von Drigalski (*Z. Vitaminforsch.*, 1934, pp. 231, 737) ascribe its healing action to its content of vitamin A.

Dawson (*Lancet*, 1936, pp. 231, 737), however, does not agree with this conjecture. Bond (*Brit. Med. J.*, 1928, **1**, 338), after experimenting with irradiated ergosterol as a dressing for wounds, concluded that vitamin D was the active constituent.

M. Proto (*Ann. ital. Chir.*, **15**, 31), experimenting with vitamins A, C and D on the healing of wounds in rabbits, found that the process of healing was not modified at all by vitamin C, no matter how administered. Vitamins A and D by mouth slightly promoted healing, but when applied directly to the wounds healing was greatly favoured, and vitamin A was especially effective.

Hayashi (*J. orient. Med.*, Dairen, South Manchuria) believes that in the accelerated healing the lipoids are chiefly responsible.

The fact remains that, whatever the exact explanation, cod-liver oil is an excellent constituent of healing ointments for chafed hands and wounds. Perfuming of such a preparation is admittedly difficult, probably an oil-soluble rose perfume is as good as anything.

Turtle Oil. Turtle oil, as supplied by the leading manufacturers, is claimed to be pure turtle oil obtained from the giant sea turtle (*Chelonian Athacae*, specie *Spharigida*). Such turtles, it is said, are from 250-700 years old, the smallest caught usually having attained a weight of 300 lb. Their long life is attributed to the fact that they possess three hearts and can live as long as any one continues to beat.

It is said that turtle oil is readily absorbed by the skin and is also claimed to exert powerful astringent action. The author has found no confirmatory evidence for these claims. The raw oil, as expressed, has a very fishy odour and it is often supplied in a deodorised condition. The suitability of such oil, as compared to the raw product, requires further investigation, since such treatment may impair any therapeutic properties which it may possess.

Information regarding its composition and vitamin content requires further confirmation. The Imperial Institute has examined samples prepared experimentally, and found that while the specific gravity and saponification values did not differ greatly, the oil of the green turtle (*Chelonia mydas*) possessed a relatively low iodine value, while that of the *Dermochelys coriacea* possessed a high acid value. Lee (*Analyst*, 1935, **60**, 650-653) examined West African turtle oil and found no significant amounts of vitamin A, or of ergosterol or other pro-vitamin D, and absence of vitamin E. Tsujimoto (*J. Soc. chem. Ind., Japan.*, 1937, **40**, 185-6B) has examined green turtle oil from *Chelonia japonica*, Thunberg. Very little evidence was found for vitamin A, and the analytical figures agreed with those found by Lee for West African turtle oil.

Avocado Pear Oil. The oil of the avocado pear (Persa Gratissima), a native of tropical America, has been claimed to contain vitamins A, B and D, phytosterol and lecithin. Bacharach and Lester-Smith, however (*Analyst*, Nov. 1938, p. 811), examined a sample of commercial oil and found that only a very transient colour of low intensity was obtained with the unsaponifiable fraction of the oil, freed from sterols, indicating a negligible proportion of physiologically active carotenoids (pro-vitamin A). Biological tests for vitamin E indicated that the proportion present was not more than one-tenth of that in a good sample of wheat germ oil, whilst vitamin D was found to be present only in very small amount.

It is claimed that " avocado pear " oil has very penetrating properties and gives a finer emulsion and that in consequence of the above, its use is conducive to creams of a type less greasy than with other oils. My investigations into skin penetration (*see* Chapter 4) did not confirm this claim.

Vitamins in Cosmetics

The external application of vitamins is dealt with in Chapter 4; the internal administration of vitamins in relation to skin health in Chapter 3.

Hormones in Cosmetics

These are discussed in some detail in Chapter 4.

Lecithins in Cosmetics

Lecithin is not the designation of a single chemical entity but is a generic name for a group of phosphatides of the following structure:

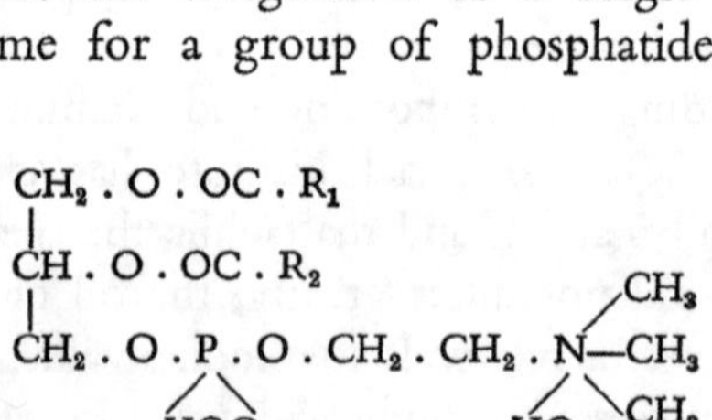

where OC . R_1 and OC . R_2 denote fatty radicles which may be palmitic, stearic, oleic, linoleic, linolenic or arachidonic. They are thus diglycerides in which the third $-CH_2OH$ group is linked to the choline ester of phosphoric acid.

Lecithins are an essential constituent of all animal and vegetable cells. Soya beans which contain about 1·6 per cent. lecithin, and egg yolk which contains 7 to 10 per cent. ovolecithin are commercial sources of this substance.

Lecithin is a constituent of human skin, being present to the extent of approximately 0·4 per cent. (Reward and Schwieger, *Biochem. Z.*, 1933, **258,** 180.) It is claimed that a mixture of lecithin and cholesterol stimulates glandular secretion, and such a mixture is often termed an artificial hormone, but this nomenclature is *erroneous. It is not a hormone,* nor does it produce any effects of true hormones.

The ratio of lecithin to cholesterol in such mixtures ranges in general, from 1 : 2 to 2 : 1. Creams containing lecithin must be carefully preserved, and also have the disadvantage of yielding coloured products.

Lecithin appears to assist dispersion of emulsified products and is claimed to exert an " emollient effect " but little clinical evidence is available to support such claims.

PROTEINS AND PROTEIN HYDROLYSATES

There is evidence that small amounts of protein may, under suitable conditions, penetrate the skin and also circulate in the blood. (Walzer *et al., Arch. Derm. Syph., Chicago.* 1940, **41,** 692 ; 1944, **49,** 427.) Recently, deNavarre (*Amer. Perfum.*, 1949, p. 205) has drawn attention to the introduction of a new material containing cystine and methionine in a hydrolysate, presumably derived from hair. Pointing out that Wiesenfeld had recently reported the value of an ointment containing a protein hydrolysate in the treatment of anterior poliomyelitis, in that, on massaging this ointment over a portion of the limbs in twelve children, there had been an increase in the circumference of the thigh so treated and an improvement in the muscular tone and colour, deNavarre suggested that such protein hydrolysates might be considered for inclusion in cosmetic preparations pointing out that milk had often been recommended for use, in the past, in toilet preparations.

In criticising this suggestion I would say that the possible introduction of *proteins into the blood stream always involves a risk of allergic shock.* For this reason I am not in favour of using proteins or hydrolysed proteins externally as a means of treating the skin " cosmetically ".

FORMULATION

In general no special difficulties in formulation are encountered and the basic formulae may be selected from cold cream formulae, from foundation cream formulae and from " all-purpose " creams. For this reason only a few illustrations are given in this chapter :

	per cent.
Lanolin	3·0
White oil	3·0
Petroleum jelly	3·0
Lanette wax SX	15·0
Sorbitol syrup	3·0
Glycerin	3·0
Water	70·0
Preservative	*q.s.*
Perfume	*q.s.*

	per cent.
Glyceryl monostearate (self-emulsifying)	14·0
Lanolin	2·0
Cetyl alcohol	2·0
Mineral oil	8·0
Spermaceti	5·0
Almond oil	8·0
Glycerin	5·0
Water	56·0
Preservative	*q.s.*
Antioxidant	*q.s.*
Perfume	*q.s.*

	per cent.
"Polawax" (Croda Ltd.)	18·0
Lanolin	2·0
Isopropyl myristate	4·0
White oil	4·0
Glycerin	7·0
Water	65·0
Preservative	*q.s.*
Perfume	*q.s.*

The following formulation (Courtesy Alginate Industries Ltd.) illustrates the use of sodium alginate, with olive oil, liquid paraffin and a relatively high proportion of lanolin in a "dry skin cream":

	Parts
Manucol SS/LH	2·0
Nipagin M (preservative)	0·1
Olive oil	10·0
Liquid paraffin	20·0
Lanolin	10·0
Beeswax	3·0
Glyceryl monostearate	5·0
Perfume	0·2
Water to	100·0

Procedure

Dry mix the SS/LH and Nipagin and disperse in olive oil. Add water and stir until dissolved, then stir in lanolin. Weigh the beeswax, glyceryl monostearate and liquid paraffin into a beaker, heat to 70° C., add mix to solution, homogenise slowly, stir until cool and then perfume.

The following water-in-oil cream is prepared with absorption base, "Protegin" X:

	per cent.
"Protegin" X (Goldschmidt)[1]	26·0
Tegin (glyceryl monostearate) [Goldschmidt]	1·0
Spermaceti	5·0
Lanolin	5·0
Cetyl alcohol	2·0
Vegetable oil	8·0
Glycerin	3·0
Mineral oil	5·0
Tegosept P (Goldschmidt)	0·15
Water	44·85

("Emulsifiers"—Goldschmidt Chemical Corporation.)

The following two creams, one oil-in-water, the other water-in-oil, are both based upon non-ionic emulsifiers and may be modified to give a lubricating cream of whichever phase is desired [from Griffin, Carter and Behrens, "Hydrophilic Lanolin Derivatives", *Drug Cosmet. Ind.*, Sept 1948].

OIL-IN-WATER ALL-PURPOSE CREAM

		per cent.
(A)	Stearic acid XXX	15·0
	Beeswax (white)	2·0
	Lanolin (anhydrous)	1·0
	Mineral oil (65/75)	23·0
	G-1425 (polyoxyalkylene sorbitol-lanolin)	5·0
	G-1441 (polyoxyalkylene sorbitol-lanolin)	1·0
(B)	Arlex (commercial sorbitol solution)	10·0
	Water	43·0
	Preservative	*q.s.*
(C)	Perfume	*q.s.*

Procedure

Bring (A) to 70° C. Bring (B) to 72° C. Add (B) to (A) slowly and under continuous agitation. Perfume at 45° C., and pour just before set point.

[1] Other absorption bases may be tried.

EMOLLIENT WATER-IN-OIL CREAM (COLD CREAM TYPE)

		per cent.
(A)	Petrolatum	35·0
	Mineral oil 65/75	15·0
	Paraffin wax	5·0
	Ceresin wax	5·0
	Lanolin	1·0
	Arlacel 83 (sorbitan sesquioleate)	2·0
	G-1425 (polyoxyalkylene sorbitol-lanolin)	4·0
(B)	Water	30·8
	Arlex (commercial sorbitol solution)	2·0
	Magnesium sulphate	0·2
	Preservative	*q.s.*
(C)	Perfume	*q.s.*

Procedure

Warm the oil phase (A) and water phase (B) separately to 70°-75° C. Add the water phase (B) gradually to the oil phase (A) while stirring. Add perfume at 55°-60° C. Homogenise at 55° to 60° C. filling directly into jars.

For other formulations which may be adopted for use as a lubricating cream or so-called " skin-food " *see* Chapters 5, 6 and 9. For required dosages of sex hormones in a hormone cream *see* Chapter 4.

CHAPTER II

FACE POWDERS, COMPACT POWDERS AND CAKE MAKE-UP

THE function of a face powder is to impart a smooth velvet-like finish to the skin by masking any shine due to the secretions of the sebaceous and sweat glands. To obtain this effect the powder must not be too transparent to mask the shine neither must it be sufficiently opaque to give a " clown-like " appearance. In addition, it must possess reasonable lasting properties in order to avoid the necessity of frequent re-powdering, i.e. it must be adherent to the skin and reasonably resistant to the mixed secretions of the skin. Finally, through intimate contact of its perfume-laden particles over a warm and relatively large area it should disseminate a pleasing odour, the psychological value of which is often under-estimated.

No single substance possesses all the desired properties : covering power, slip, absorbency, adhesiveness and bloom, hence a modern face powder is a blend of several constituents each one chosen for some specific quality. The materials most commonly used, grouped according to their function are (where a material has more than one property it is listed twice) :

(*a*) *Covering Power :* to cover skin defects, e.g. enlarged pores and skin shine.
Titanium dioxide, zinc oxide, kaolin, magnesium oxide.

(*b*) *Slip :* to ameliorate spreading and to give the characteristic smooth feeling.
Talc, metallic soaps, such as zinc stearate, and to a lesser extent, starch.

(*c*) *Absorbency :* to absorb sebaceous (oily) secretions and perspiration and thus reduce shine.
Precipitated chalk, magnesium carbonate, starch, kaolin.

(*d*) *Adherence :* to improve clinging to the face.
Metallic soaps, such as the magnesium and zinc salts of various fatty acids. Alternatively/or additionally, the incorporation of small quantities of oil or fatty material with the powder base.

(*e*) *Bloom :* to give the smooth velvet-like appearance of a peach to the skin.
Chalk, starch.

There should be a valid reason for the inclusion of every constituent in a face powder.

Colloidal Kaolin

Halpern, Powers and Bradney (*Proc. Sci. Sect. T.G.A.*, Dec 1950, p. 4) point out that : " Kaolin is not a primary mineral but is a generic term applied to several hydrated aluminium silicates. Not all aluminium silicates, however, may be called kaolin. On the basis of X-ray and physical studies Ross and Kerr [U.S. Geol. Surv. Prof. Paper, No. 165E ; 151 (1934)], established that three different groups of clay are classified as kaolin. These clays (kaolinite, nacrite and dickite) have essentially the same formula ($Al_2O_3 . 2SiO_2 . 2H_2O$). . . . It is generally regarded that the best sources for the pharmaceutical kaolins are England and the United States."

These writers point out that the method of manufacture of the kaolin is an important factor in determining the properties of the resultant product ; ordinary china clay is obtained by elutriation and on microscopic examination mica, quartz and felspar are readily discernible. Pharmaceutical grades of kaolin are obtained by a peptising process in which the clay is suspended in water containing a suitable electrolyte (e.g. sodium pyrophosphate) which confers an electrical charge upon the clay and keeps the finer particles in suspension. Removal of the suspension of fine particles, followed by removal of the electric charge (by addition of another electrolyte or by means of an electric field), yields the finest forms of kaolin.

Colloidal kaolin is an excellent material upon which to base a powder. It possesses good covering power, excellent grease-resisting properties and absorbs perspiration. Used alone, however, it lacks " slip " and is apt to appear a little harsh.

Precipitated Chalk

This is also an excellent medium although some manufacturers appear to be prejudiced against it. Today it is possible to obtain special grades of exceptional fineness, accurately balanced to prevent harshness, possessing good absorption and grease-resisting properties, in varying densities according to the purpose required. Precipitated chalk is also obtainable treated in a special manner, in which—it is claimed—its absorptive power for oils and grease is not affected, and which does not dry the skin. This material is claimed to be particularly adhesive. Both of the above chalks are guaranteed to conform to the U.S.P. specification for lead, arsenic, etc.

Up to 70 per cent. of chalk may be used in the formulation of such powders, providing this is one of the special brands prepared for this purpose. The majority of chalks, however, lack slip and are therefore modified by the inclusion of other constituents.

Talc

Talc is a hydrated magnesium silicate obtained from Italy, France, Japan, Norway, and Egypt, the quality varying with its country of origin. Only the Italian and French varieties used to be considered suitable for a high quality face powder ; more recently other supplies have become available. Japanese talc is not so good although it is sometimes used in cheap powders. The main function of talc in such powders *is to impart the quality of easy spreading and application*, i.e. *slip*. It possesses, however, a low covering power and hence it is usual to add ingredients to modify this defect. Up to 70 per cent. or more may be used in a high class face powder.

Rice Starch

In the face powders of the leading American brands rice starch is seldom used, although it is very popular in Europe. The objections to starch raised by McDonough ("Truth About Cosmetics", *Drug Cosmet. Ind.*, 1937, p. 110) are that it readily forms a sticky paste when wet, clogging the pores, and that it is an ideal nutrient, when moist, for bacteria. In addition it coats the hair shaft and so accentuates the downy hair, otherwise unnoticeable, on a woman's face.

However, it is only fair to mention that, *due to the coating of the hair shaft, starch helps to give the peach-like bloom which is considered to be attractive and desirable by many people.*

Decomposition can be reduced in many cases by the addition of perfume ; mention of clogged pores refers not to pores but to the openings of the hair follicles. (Pore openings are invisible by ordinary inspection.) There is no proof that starch can cause clogging of such openings. (*See* Cosmetic Facts and Fallacies.)

Zinc Oxide

Grady (*J. Soc. cosmet. Chem.*, July 1947, p. 17) has published an investigation into the characteristics of zinc oxide when used in face powder. The measurement of the covering power of a pigment has been a controversial subject for a long time, since, by varying the test condition one can obtain widely different values.

Grady calculated the covering power of several face powder ingredients from the refractive indices of the pigments and of the various media in which they might be used for cosmetics. Fresnel's law (R. W. Wood, *Physical Optics*, 1934, pp. 411, 512) states that "the reflectivity of an absorbing medium is proportional to the square of the difference in refractive index between the two components divided by the square of their sum" and is written

$$R = \frac{(n_2 - n_1)^2 + k^2}{(n_2 + n_1)^2 + k^2}.$$

Because the absorption coefficient K is very small in the case of a white pigment, Grady ignored the second term in numerator and denominator in calculating the data shown in Table I below. In each medium the covering power of zinc oxide has, arbitrarily, been designated as 100. (Actually the value decreases progressively from 100 to 37 to 21 as zinc oxide is placed in air, water and petrolatum respectively.)

Whilst the refractive index used in these calculations measures the ability of the substance to bend light and gather it to itself, the light must also be reflected back and this is done at the crystal surfaces. The greater the surface present, the more light will be reflected back, hence any discussion of covering power would be incomplete without reference to the influence of particle size. In general, greater covering power per pound results as the degree of subdivision is increased, but there are limiting factors as Grady illustrates in the following figure which is a calibration curve used for the routine checking of the particle size in plant operations, using the turbidimetric method described by Stutz and Pfund (*Industr. Engng. Chem.*, 1927, **19**, 1, 51).

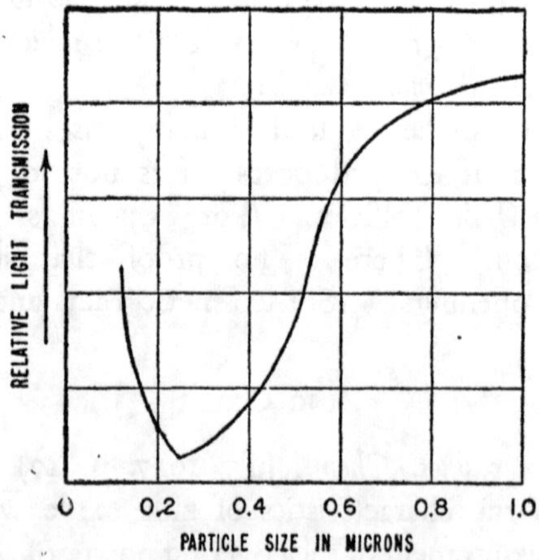

FIG. 14—Calibration curve relating particle size with relative light transmission.

It will be noted that a sharp maximum occurs in the neighbourhood of 0·25 micron; this is the particle size for optimum opacity of zinc oxide in water. Grady points out that the sharp decrease in opacity below 0·25 microns is due to the fact that the particles have become so small in respect to the wavelength of light that scattering becomes more dominant than normal reflection.

TABLE 1—CALCULATED COVERING POWER OF PIGMENTS

Pigment	*Refractive Index*	*Relative covering power*		
		In air ($n = 1{\cdot}00$)	*In water* ($n = 1{\cdot}33$)	*In petrolatum* ($n = 1{\cdot}475$)
TiO_2 . .	2·52	166	232	292
Zinc oxide	2·008	100	100	100
Chalk . .	1·658	55	29	15
Talc . .	1·589	46	19	6

A second desired function of a face powder is to eliminate skin shininess due to excessive oiliness in certain facial areas. The prime requirement of a material for this purpose is a high absorptive capacity. Zinc oxide of the desired particle size for optimum covering power will retain less oil perhaps than other materials specially prepared for this purpose but its oil absorption capacity is in the range of other face powder constituents. As face powder absorbs moisture and oil from the skin, its covering power decreases. Under these conditions the high-refractive index pigments, as shown in Table 2, lose less opacity proportionately than the materials of low-refractive index. Here again the desirability of such materials in a face powder is evident.

TABLE 2—RELATIVE COVERING POWER RETAINED AFTER WETTING DRY PIGMENT

Pigment	*With water per cent.*	*With petrolatum per cent.*
TiO_2 . . .	51	37
Zinc oxide . .	37	21
Chalk . . .	20	5
Talc . . .	15	3

Finally, Grady has drawn attention (*J. Soc. cosmet. Chem.*, July 1947) to the sun-screening action of zinc oxide and states that zinc oxide cuts off the ultra-violet more sharply than any other white pigment used in face powders and that zinc oxide, and to a lesser degree, titanium dioxide, should be quite useful in preventing severe sunburn. [It is interesting to note that in the experiments carried out on behalf of the U.S. Army Air Force in December 1942 on protective skin coatings for the prevention of sunburn (Luckiesh Taylor, Cole and Sollman, *J. Amer. med. Assoc.*, 1946, 130, 1), zinc oxide was found to be of definite value in preventing sunburn whilst titanium dioxide was not found to be a very dependable protective judged on a specimen containing 20 per cent. of this substance in petroleum jelly.—AUTHOR].

TABLE 3—ULTRA-VIOLET TRANSMISSION CHARACTERISTICS OF PIGMENTS

Pigment	*Per cent. transmitted of wavelengths*					
	4358	4047	3655	3342	3131	3023
Zinc oxide	46	40	0	0	0	0
TiO_2 . .	35	32	18	6	½	0
China clay	63	61	59	57	55	54
Chalk .	87	86	84	82	80	79
Talc . .	90	90	90	89	88	87

(*After* GRADY).

TITANIUM DIOXIDE

As shown in the above tables, titanium dioxide has considerably greater covering power *per se* than zinc oxide, about 1·6 times that of the latter in air and about 2·9 times the latter in petroleum jelly. On a moist greasy skin, its covering power relative to zinc oxide is probably of the order of 2·5 times. Titanium dioxide is not astringent but is physiologically inert and may be found, in any rare cases of allergy to zinc compounds or in cases of dry skin, preferable to zinc oxide. Its sun-screening properties are, however, inferior to zinc oxide.

MAGNESIUM CARBONATE

Magnesium carbonate confers fluffiness on the powder, assists in preventing it " balling " and is highly absorbent. It is a satisfactory substance with which to incorporate and mature the perfume. Five per cent. is ample for this purpose.

Zinc and Magnesium Stearates

Three to 10 per cent. imparts improved adherency to the powder and renders the ultimate product soft and fluffy. A number of patented proprietary products are also available for this purpose, these are in general zinc or magnesium salts of straight chain aliphatic acids having an odd number of carbon atoms. (*See* Patented Powder Bases.)

Powdered Silica

A very fine grade of pure silica has been introduced for cosmetic purposes. It is claimed that the use of this substance obviates the need for zinc and magnesium stearates. The addition of 10 per cent. to an ordinary powder mix exerts a marked effect in increasing its fluffiness. Up to 20 per cent. may be used in a face powder or 30 per cent. or more in talcum and baby powders. *While there is no clinical evidence to prove or disprove its value I should hesitate to recommend it until we know more of the causes of silicosis.*

Powdered Silk

A raw material for face powders (and other cosmetic preparations) which, apart from any unique or desirable properties it *might* have, will provide opportunities for the advertising agencies to produce rapturous copy writing, is powdered silk.

Like many other inventions which have gained acceptance in the U.S.A. and in other overseas countries, it was originally a British product. Some ten years ago a British patent (482,269) described a process for its preparation. Since then there have been two other patents, both British (555,044 and 519,544) dealing respectively with a technique for pulverising silk for producing silk powder. This cosmetic material has been discussed in *Schimmel Briefs* (No. 161, Aug. 1948) in which it is pointed out that raw silk consists of a protein fibre (fibroin) covered with a coating of gummy material called serocin. This coating is composed mainly of albuminoid substances with small amounts of fatty acids, resin and colouring matter. The silk is therefore first degummed by the conventional processes used in the textile industry, then treated with acid or alkali in order partially to hydrolyse the protein molecules. At an appropriate stage it is washed and dried and finally reduced to an impalpable powder by grinding.

It is claimed (*Parfumerie Moderne*, 1947, No. 4, 29) that the physical characteristics of silk powder make it well suited to serve as an ingredient of face powders, that it spreads easily and adheres tenaciously to the skin producing a velvety matt finish, and that it possesses a very high absorbent power in that it will absorb as much as three times its volume of water and still retain the appearance of a powder. The addition of large amounts of such materials as kaolin or chalk is not advised as it is claimed they tend to make the final product too dense and compact.

Patented Powder Bases

Various proprietary preparations have been marketed from time to time, having as their object the improvement of the adhesiveness of the face powder ; for example, British Patent 433,142 describes the use of the zinc or magnesium salts of fatty acids containing an uneven number of carbon atoms, i.e. undecylic acid, such a base being employed in a proportion of 5–10 per cent. in the finished powder. Many manufacturers prefer to correct any lack of adhesiveness in their product either by increasing the amount of zinc or magnesium stearates incorporated or by including in the powder mixture a couple of per cent. of petroleum jelly, mineral oil or cetyl alcohol. Vegetable oils are not used to any extent because of their fatty odour and their susceptibility to rancidity.

Water Absorbent Properties of Face Powders

The water absorbent properties of face powders or face powder constituents may be determined by the method of Hewitt (*Perfum. essent. Oil Rec.*, Feb. 1943), in which a known weight of the powder is shaken with excess water and filtered under a standard pressure through a Büchner funnel until no more water emerges. The wet powder is then transferred to a weighed, stoppered weighing bottle, and the increase in weight determined. Methods involving the addition of water from a burette, until the powder becomes semi-fluid, are open to the objection that different observers do not obtain concordant results and the end point is not easily determined.

Grease Absorbent Properties

It should be remembered that water absorption is by no means the main characteristic required in a powder, it must also be absorbent for grease. If a person's face is inclined to dryness a more greasy foundation is usually employed. A powder which is not *grease* absorbent will show a shiny nose or face which will necessitate re-powdering. Constituents of higher opacity such as zinc and titanium oxides tend to mask greasiness, while starch, chalks and kaolin absorb only a certain amount of grease.

Opacity or Covering Power of a Powder

Various published articles have sought to correlate the weight of various face powder constituents with their covering properties or opacities. However, it is not the *weight* with which the cosmetician is concerned, but the volume, inasmuch as a woman dips her puff into a powder and takes out a volume which depends partially on the adherent properties of the powder, on the size and type of the puff employed and the depth and pressure with which the puff is applied to the face powder container.

Comparison of the different covering properties, or opacities of different face powder constituents is not easy for the very simple reason that when the size of a certain powder is reduced the particles scatter more light and hence the opacity of that substance is increased.

To get a very rough idea of the average relative grade of opacity which prevails in cosmetic materials, I have determined the opacity of chalk, kaolin, magnesium stearate, rice starch, talc, titanium dioxide, zinc oxide, and zinc stearate by applying these materials by means of a swansdown face powder puff to similar areas of black velvet paper. The whiteness or opacity produced on the smooth black adherent surface was (*a*) estimated visually, (*b*) recorded photoelectrically. For the materials employed, the only particle size specification was that they should all pass completely through a 200 mesh sieve. The order of opacity obtained was as follows, the constituents being arranged in order of ascending opacities :

Talc,
Rice starch,
Magnesium stearate,
Chalk (light, precipitated),
Zinc stearate,
Kaolin,
Zinc oxide,
Titanium dioxide.

When titanium dioxide was used alone, its adherence to the puff was found to be poor, while, as would be expected, the zinc and magnesium stearates showed excellent adhesion to the puff. From what has already been said it will be apparent that to get a true comparison between the relative covering properties of the various face powder constituents it would be necessary to separate similar size particle fractions of each constituent and subject them to exact tests. However, the conditions of such a test, although scientifically more exact, would be so different from the conditions ruling in face powder formulation as to have little actual practical value. The opacities of various finished face powder formulae may be tested approximately by the above method. For a discussion of the relative covering properties of zinc and titanium oxides in relation to other face powder constituents, *as determined by calculation*, reference should be made to the paragraph (in this Chapter) headed Zinc Oxide. It should always be remembered that *the criterion of a face powder in respect of its water absorption, grease absorption, and covering properties or opacity is judged by the interval elapsing between powdering and repowdering the face; and that a woman judges this by the evidence of shine, which is a complex phenomenon not related to any one scientific test and often dependent upon a woman's skin, type of foundation cream used, and occupation.* These facts should be adequately considered by consumer trials, properly carried out and statistically evaluated. Such consumer trials must be carried out scientifically, as ill-conceived trials can be made to prove anything and often prove nothing.

Formulae

Multifarious variations in formulae could be listed, many of which, under laboratory conditions, show slight differences in respect to opacity, slip, absorbency, water and grease resistance, etc., but it is my experience that many of these variations cannot be detected by the average woman under normal conditions of use. The following formulae exemplify various types of face powder, the variations in which are sufficient to be detectable:

	per cent.
Talc	80·0
Zinc oxide	5·0
Zinc stearate	5·0
Rice starch	10·0
Perfume	*q.s.*
Colour	*q.s.*

This powder is a very transparent one, i.e. it is a "light" powder, and is favoured by persons who wish to impart some colour and bloom to the face without appearing to be "made up". The starch may be replaced if desired with precipitated chalk.

	per cent.
Talc	30·0
Zinc oxide	24·0
Zinc stearate	6·0
Precipitated chalk	40·0
Perfume	*q.s.*
Colour	*q.s.*

This powder has high opacity and gives a very definite opaque matt finish which tends to hide minor skin defects. It is more popular with certain people who like to have a definite powdered appearance without being in any way " clown-like ".

In between these two types of powders there are a number of popular variations such as the following :

	per cent.
Talc	65·0
Precipitated chalk	10·0
Zinc oxide	20·0
Zinc stearate	5·0
Perfume	*q.s.*
Colour	*q.s.*

	per cent.
Talc	60·0
Kaolin	20·0
Zinc oxide	15·0
Zinc stearate	5·0
Perfume	*q.s.*
Colour	*q.s.*

As previously stated both starch and precipitated chalk tend to impart bloom and the following powder is one of medium weight, i.e. medium opacity or coverage and bloom :

	per cent.
Talc	50·0
Rice starch	15·0
Precipitated chalk	15·0
Zinc oxide	15·0
Zinc stearate	5·0

If it is desired to obtain maximum coverage and still maintain a high talc content, this may be achieved by replacing the zinc oxide in any of these formulae by about one-quarter of its weight of titanium dioxide. deNavarre (*The Chemistry and Manufacture of Cosmetics*, New York : D. Van Nostrand Inc., 1941, p. 334) has drawn attention to the fact that in France, pure electrolytic zinc metal is burnt and the fumes collected to produce a pure zinc oxide. In America zinc-bearing ore is burned and the fumes collected. Such samples should be carefully examined in respect of " live " whiteness and contamination.

The following formula is prepared from precipitated chalk and a high proportion of zinc stearate is incorporated. To provide some grease resistance, kaolin and titanium dioxide are employed.

	per cent.
Waterproof chalk base	50·0
Zinc or magnesium stearate	10·0
Kaolin	20·0
Titanium dioxide	6·0
Talc	14·0
Perfume	*q.s.*
Colour	*q.s.*

Ralph Auch in 1934 (*Amer. Perfum.*, Sept. 1934), gave the following example of a face powder which had been made up and submitted to a testing panel of 150 housewives in about forty American States who, in their replies, were asked to include an answer to the question " How does this powder compare with your favourite brand of face powder ? " Seventy-eight observers reported " equal to or better than their favourite powder " ; 53 thought it " inferior ". Asked whether the powder was " too light ", " too heavy " or " satisfactory " in respect of texture, 103 out of the 150 housewives considered it " satisfactory " :

	per cent.
Talc	75·0
Zinc oxide	20·0
Zinc stearate	5·0
Perfume	*q.s.*
Colour	*q.s.*

S. P. Jannaway (*Alchemist*, Jan.-Feb. 1948) states that the following formula, gives a good medium powder, characterised by excellent slip, absorbency, adequate coverage, good velvety feel and adherence—and an indefinable improvement in mattness, etc., which is attributed to the rice starch :

	per cent.
Zinc oxide	16·0
Talc	37·0
Zinc stearate	5·0
Precipitated chalk (light)	18·0
Rice starch	8·0
Kaolin (best cosmetic grade)	16·0

Winter (*Alchemist*, May 1947, p. 188) has described a special kind of " fatty powder " which he states is much favoured by persons afflicted with a rough or dry skin :

	parts
Vaseline	50
White beeswax	40
Petroleum jelly	40
Stearin	20
Glyceryl monostearate	75

The procedure recommended is to melt the above fatty materials together and add, whilst stirring constantly,

Water (hot) . . . . 500 *parts*

Continue to stir until the emulsion has formed, then add

Talc . . . . 1000 *parts*

Knead, allow to dry, rub to powder, pass through a sieve and perfume.

Choice of Perfume

The odour of the face powder must be fragrant and pleasant and a preference is shown today for either a flowery fragrance or that of one of the newer synthetic bouquets. For the formulation of suitable products a monograph on perfumery should be consulted. Unless the manufacturer has had wide experience of perfume manufacture, and can afford to spend plenty of time both for experiment and subsequent *maturing*, it is far better to purchase the perfume from one of the firms specialising in such products.

One particular point should be noted : in most cases the odour of the same perfume is somewhat different when used in a powder base than when used in a cream, and some adjustment of its constituents may be necessary.

"Colouring" of Face Powder

The colours used consist of :

Pigments. Ochres, umbers, etc., are inexpensive but lack strength and vitality. They may be brightened, however, by the use of lakes or spirit-soluble dyes. The latter are preferable to water-soluble dyes since they dry more uniformly and quickly.

Lakes. May be prepared by the precipitation of harmless aniline colours on aluminium lakes. These lakes are strong and brilliant.

Water-soluble Colours. May streak out in warm or wet weather.

Synthetic Ochres and Iron Oxides. Form the latest class of colouring matters and consist of practically pure oxides or hydroxides of iron. They possess about four to five times the strength of the natural ochres and are free from grit. In order to minimise error in the case of strong colours, they may be diluted with one of the constituents before use.

Because of different proprietary names and numbers for various colouring matters, local regulations—as for example the use only of colouring matters certified by the F.D.A. in the United States—and different opinions amongst firms themselves as to what particular combination of colours gives their "particular" rachel, peach, tango, etc., no attempt has been made to list the multifarious colouring matters available. Instead, it is suggested that coal tar lakes, etc., be studied by consulting the U.S. Colour regulations [or by reference to R. G. Harry, *Cosmetic Materials*, 1948, London: Leonard Hill Ltd., Appendix II, wherein ninety pages are devoted to listing the properties of these colouring matters]. From a description of their solubilities, etc., it will be possible to rule out a number of these dyes; of the remainder belonging to the "colour classification desired", a number will be found to be obtainable of similar composition in the United Kingdom but without, in every case, the guarantee of various metallic and other impurity limits. A number of dye manufacturers will be found very helpful in respect of the above dyestuffs and certainly, so far as the smaller cosmetic companies are concerned, they will do well to seek the collaboration of such firms who will readily advise on suitable colouring matters, oxides, and earths and give advice concerning proportions for various colour matches which may be required.

The choice of milady's colour is usually a matter of taste. Formerly, it was considered that *naturelle* was suitable for blondes and *rachel* for brunettes. It is now considered, however, that *naturelle* suits very few complexions, and *rachel* is decidedly the most popular. Peach is useful also—particularly for blondes. In order that *naturelle* shall suit one's complexion this must not be milky white, but actually decidedly bluish. Florid complexions may be toned down by means of pale bluish-green powders.

As well as the actual complexion itself, varying colours of hair and dress all affect the apparent tint, which probably accounts for the multitude of colours in demand. (*See also* Application of Cosmetics.)

Manufacture

Mixing of the ingredients in face powders is usually carried out in a horizontal mixer with a screw agitator. If lakes are used they may be mixed with a small quantity of one of the constituents, chalk, zinc oxide or talc, and the colour concentrate so formed mixed with the main bulk. In the case of water or alcohol soluble dyes these are best sprayed on to the mix or alternatively on to one of the constituents which possesses good absorbency such as chalk, kaolin or magnesium carbonate, this being then dried and mixed into the main bulk. Machines are available which mix, sift and spray the perfume automatically.

The writer is opposed to the use of water- or oil-soluble colours in a face powder since they lead to streaking, darkening and staining of the skin when applied over ordinary make up. Chilson (*Modern Cosmetics*, 1st edn., p. 68) has drawn attention to the pebble mill method of mixing which obviates the making of a colour base. All the ingredients, including the colour and perfume, are milled together in a pebble mill for six hours, discharged and then sifted. He states that such a mill delivers an excellent product and is widely employed in preference to mixers. This method, however, is too slow to be recommended for large scale production. More recently micro-pulverisers are being increasingly employed in the United States. Only a rough pre-mixing is required, and the material which is obtained from the micro-pulveriser is finely ground and uniformly mixed. This method is fast and economical. Various other pulverisers such as disintegrators, hammer mills, attrition mills, etc., may also be used.

Pin-disc mills give good results, especially in respect of colour dispersion, providing the material is first given a rough pre-mix. Such mills are often supplied in conjunction with a turbine sifter.

The *Air Spun Process* employed by Messrs. Coty Inc. is described briefly by deNavarre (*The Chemistry and Manufacture of Cosmetics*, New York: D. Van Nostrand Co. Inc., 1941, p. 361) as follows:

". . . Purified and cold air, under great pressure (100 lb. per sq. in.), is permitted to rush in a continuous stream into a closed drum-shaped chamber. This chamber or mill is called a microniser because it reduces particles to micron size. (A micron is 1/1000 of a millimetre or 1/25,000 of an inch.) The speed of the air stream, the manner in which it is directed and the shape of the chamber itself, causes air to revolve about this chamber at a rate somewhat in excess of a thousand miles per hour. In this super cyclone all the ingredients are hurled against each other until they reduce themselves to the desired size and fluffiness. When this is attained such particles are emitted through a central exit while the heavier particles are forced to remain. It is claimed that the particle size was selected after numerous experiments had shown it to be the best for the appearance, effect and adhesiveness of a face powder.

Apart from this process various physical methods exist for preparing powders of a desired particle size range. These depend upon elutriation by means of air or water. Control of such separated fractions may be carried out by microscopic examination of the fractions, but this method involves the visual or photomicrographic inspection of a very large number of fields in the microscope and is tedious. Various sedimentation tests, some based upon passage of a beam of light through the sedimentation column into a photoelectric cell, have also been suggested. One of the simplest methods for the cosmetician is that based upon the principles of Stokes' Law described by Hinkley (*Industr. Engng. Chem.*, 15 Jan. 1942, p. 10). [*See also* Hibbot (*Perfum. essent. Oil Rec.*, Aug. 1947, p. 268), Hinkel, Nachod and Tainter (*Proc. Sci. Sect. T.G.A.*, Dec. 1948).] A useful variation is the method of Andreason in which volumes of the suspension, after definite times of settling (calculated from Stokes' Law), are pipetted into a tared dish, evaporated to dryness and weighed. Various air permeability methods are also widely used. *In cases of doubt the author infinitely prefers microscopic inspection, using a projection instrument in a darkened room.*

In some cases, particularly where the powder is prepared especially for use on a dry skin, a little oil is included in the formula. Up to 2 per cent. mineral oil is best, as vegetable oils may undergo oxidation with unfavourable result on the perfume.

Packaging is usually carried out by vacuum automatic filling devices, which minimise dusting.

In choosing powder boxes, care should be taken to see that these are prepared with an odourless glue, otherwise on storage the fragrance of the powder will be ruined.

Compact Powders; Cake Make-Up

Cake make-up as such is not new. Years ago compacts of face powder and of rouge were available in cake form. Such cakes differed from the present type of cake make-up chiefly in that they contained less fatty materials and were compressed using either gums, or soap as a binding agent. Macias-Sarria (*Amer. Perfum.*, Nov. 1944, p. 43) tells of the women of the Dutch East Indies " making their own cake face powder by soaking shelled rice for a day or two, exposing it to the sun to swell the grains, after which it is milled with water in their own stone mills. From this paste they make their cake by hand and when the cake has dried out they use a piece of wet cloth to rub the surface and smear the rice powder on their faces to produce the smooth-looking finish typical of oriental women."

In place of rice, read *a somewhat opaque face powder containing a fair amount of opacifying ingredients* such as zinc oxide or titanium dioxide, *treated as some face powders are with a little oil*, and instead of merely forming a cake by drying in the sun, read *compacting to form a suitable cake*, and, in essentials, we have a cake make-up. The well-known Max Factor patent claims (*a*) that the cake after application dries to form a substantially *water-repellent* powder film, and (*b*) the cake contains a wetting agent to enable the oil-treated powder to be readily picked up upon, and dispersed by a wet sponge.

Generally speaking, cake make-up may be described (Hilfer, *Drug Cosmet. Ind.*, March 1945) as a highly pigmented powder incorporated into a dehydrated cream. The addition of water by means of a moist applicator allows the formation of a film of cream which has the powder incorporated in it. After application of the film to the face, the water evaporates leaving a film of powder and dried cream.

It must be emphasised at this stage that (*a*) the term "Pancake" Make-up is protected by Max Factor; (*b*) U.S. Patents 2,034,679 and 2,101,843, together with British Patent 501,732 lay down a method of manufacture and a range of composition protected under letters patent. In suggesting any composition for a cake make-up, I am discussing the question purely from the scientific and technical aspect and *not* from the legal aspect. It may be that some manufacturer can claim and prove a prior right to his method of manufacture but in all cases I would most strongly advise any manufacturer seeking to produce a cake make-up to study the patents which have been issued in this connection, the method and formula by which he intends to produce it and the legal implications which *may* be entailed.

In British Patent 501,732 taken out by Messrs. Max Factor a number of claims are made among which the salient ones are as follows:

No. 4. *Appertaining to formulae.*

This covers the range,

oils and fats, 0·8 *per cent. to* 24 *per cent.*
water soluble dispersing agent, 1 *per cent. to* 13 *per cent.*
fillers, 35 *per cent. to* 80 *per cent.*
pigments and colours, 12 *per cent. to* 50 *per cent. by weight.*

the particles of fillers and pigments of said cosmetic being substantially *water repellent.*

No. 5. A make-up cosmetic as set forth in claim 4, wherein the water-soluble dispersing agents are selected from the group consisting of ethanolamine soaps and glycerin, glycol and glycol derivatives.

No. 6. A make-up cosmetic preparation as set forth in Nos. 4 and 5 above, in which the particles of fillers, colours and pigments are coated with oils and fats to be substantially water repellent, the make-up having the property of becoming suspended in water when a cake of it is rubbed with a moistened pad.

The method of manufacture covered by the patent, involves treating the powder, comprising of the *fillers,* such as talc, chalk, etc., and *pigments*, e.g. zinc, titanium and/or ferric oxides, etc., with an oil-in-water emulsion and a water-soluble dispersing agent (using 0·75 to 1·25 parts of the powder to 1 part of emulsion) drying the resulting mixture, pulverising the dry product and compressing to form a solid cake. For those who think this affords a means to get around the patent I would remind them that the mere addition of water to make a more dilute emulsion and thus circumvent the relationship of powder to emulsion would not, in my opinion, be valid inasmuch as in the course of the drying operation the preparation would at some stage pass through the phase covered in the Factor patent.

Other methods of *manufacture* undoubtedly exist, but the *formula* covered by the patent is extremely wide.

The Atlas Powder Co. (*Drug and Cosmetic Emulsions*, 1946, p. 29) quote the following formula for a cake make-up adding that it is merely indicative and that adjustment to personal taste will be required. It will be noted that the emulsifiers used in this preparation are non-ionic. Whether this circumvents the patent is a matter for legal advice in the country concerned.

PIGMENT BLEND

	per cent.
Talc	60·0
Kaolin	20·0
Zinc oxide	10·0
Titanium dioxide	5·0
Calcium carbonate, light	5·0
Iron oxide colours	*q.s.*

COMPLETED FORMULA

	per cent.
Pigment blend	81·4
Arlex (sorbitol)	4·1
Propylene glycol	2·4
Arlacel C (sorbitan sesquioleate)	9·7
Mineral oil or lanolin	2·4
Perfume	*q.s.*
Preservative	*q.s.*

The method of manufacture recommended is to mix the Arlex (sorbitol) with the propylene glycol and preservative and spray this mixture into the powder while it is being mixed in a dough mixer. Mix the Arlacel C and mineral oil. If lanolin is used, melt the lanolin with the Arlacel C. Add the perfume and spray on to the powdered mass which is agitated in the dough mixer. Transfer to a Fitzpatrick tablet granulator or an equivalent machine. After granulation, the mass is ready for preforming and compression.

Experiments are necessary to determine the optimum pressure; usually 100 to 125 lb. per sq. in. is adequate.

APPLICATION OF CAKE MAKE-UP. Macias-Sarria (*Amer. Perfum.*, Dec. 1944, p. 48) quotes Maurice Seiderman (make-up artist of R.K.O.) as recommending the application of cake make-up in the following manner: "To apply cake make-up correctly, wet and squeeze out a sponge and rub it lightly over the face. Smooth the cake make-up on the face and before it dries blend in the rouge. Carefully squeeze all water out of the sponge and rub it lightly over the face until the make-up is dry." Macias-Sarria adds that people who do not like a heavy make-up, should blot off the excess of water with a dry towel or facial tissue.

It is claimed that cake make-up is satisfactory in the case of the younger woman; in the case of persons in the later thirties, and even younger persons who suffer from dry skin, it is found to be rather drying. To cater to this market, to coincide with the general trend towards more greasy make-up as exemplified by many foundation creams, and possibly also with a view to cashing in on the flat type of pack in which cake make-up is packed, a greasy type of pack containing pigments of high covering power in a waxy base has been marketed.

Such products appear to be poured instead of being compressed in the usual manner. Wetting agents may be incorporated so that these products may be removed with a damp sponge. Formulation may be made along the lines discussed in Chapter 9.

Compact Powders

On account of their convenience, compact powders have enjoyed wide popularity. There are three common methods of preparation, viz.:

(1) The damp compression method.
(2) The dry compression process.
(3) The moulding process.

DAMP COMPRESSION METHOD. In the damp process, the powder, intimately mixed with a suitable binding agent, is milled to the requisite plasticity, compressed into suitable containers and dried for the requisite period in a current of warm air. In the dry process the mass is subjected to compression without being wetted to any appreciable extent. This process, although difficult to achieve satisfactorily in the first case, is probably the best to use for manufacturing compacts on a large scale, for when once the mix and suitable conditions have been determined, it can be rigidly adhered to.

The two methods already described are in use for the production of the best class products. In the moulding process the powder is mixed with plaster of Paris, wetted and then cast into moulds and dried.

The manufacture of a successful compact requires a considerable amount of experimental work, together with some mechanical ability. The smaller manufacturer will be well advised to purchase his supplies from firms specialising in the production of these products.

The following suggestions for a suitable binding agent, together with typical formulae, are given by G. S. Collingridge in an article dealing with "Compact Powder and Rouge" (*Mfg. Perfum.*, April 1937, **2**, 6), to which reference for more detailed particulars may be made.

BINDING AGENT

	per cent.
Gum tragacanth mucilage	10·0
Quince seed mucilage	7·0
Colophony tincture (10 per cent.)	1·0
Distilled water	82·0

A typical formula for a compact powder is:

	per cent.
Talc, Italian	40·0
Zinc oxide	20·0
Zinc stearate	8·0
Rice starch	10·0
Magnesium carbonate	10·0
Kaolin, extra fine	12·0

DRY COMPRESSION PROCESS. Winter (*Handb. der gesamten Parfum. Kosmet.*, 2nd edn., 1932, pp. 615-620) recommends an ammonia-stearin-starch compound containing white petrolatum, ammonia, starch and stearin for the manufacture of compact powder and rouge. The preparation of this compound is as follows:

. . . 100 g. of stearin and 20 g. of white petrolatum are melted together and 50 cc. of 97 per cent. ammonium hydroxyde solution is added and thoroughly stirred in while hot. Finally 250 g. of rice or maize starch is added to the warm mixture with vigorous stirring. The introduction of the starch presents difficulties and requires practice. During the addition thick lumps form in the starch powder, but, with vigorous stirring and pressing, these break down and mix with the starch. The crumbly mass is then rubbed up in a mortar and passed through a 70-80 mesh sieve. The mixture must be well cooled before being sifted.

Of the crumbled and sieved ammonia-stearin-starch compound 13-15 per cent. is added to the powder base. Together with the colouring matter the mixture is subjected to pressure. It is stated that such pressing should not be carried out suddenly but by gradually increasing the pressure. The writer is in full agreement with this view. Unless a little time is given for the air to escape gradually, it becomes entrapped in the compact with disastrous results.

It would appear that compacts can be prepared from almost any good face powder providing a suitable binding agent is employed and a suitable compact press utilised.

The maximum permissible proportion of starch in a compact is controversial. It is stated (*Perfum. essent. Oil Rec.*, Jan. 1930) that the starch content should be low, otherwise there is a tendency to hardness and non-removal of the powder when the puff is applied. A formula is quoted (*Perfum. essent. Oil Rec.*, Sept. 1932, p. 362) which includes 2·5 per cent. rice starch. Winter (*Handb. der gesamten Parfum. Kosmet.*, 2nd edn., 1932, pp. 615–620), however, considers that starch acts as a good binding agent and recommends a base containing about 13 per cent. starch; another article (*Perfum. essent. Oil Rec.*, July 1932) states that up to 20 per cent. starch is helpful in binding a compact.

Winter suggests the following powder base mixture:

	per cent.
Talc	26·7
Kaolin	56·7
Zinc oxide	3·3
Rice starch	13·3

to which may be added 13–15 per cent. of stearin-starch and the required colouring matters. Water is added to produce a dough-like paste which is dried, ground and passed through a 120 mesh sieve and the mass compressed into a suitable metal case or godet.

Today it is more usual to employ a soap such as sodium stearate or one of the amino stearates together with a few per cent. of fatty matter. The following formula will serve as an example:

	per cent.
Kaolin	20·0
Zinc oxide	15·0
Precipitated chalk	20·0
Talc	32·0
Starch (rice)	5·0
Sodium stearate	3·0
Oil or other fatty matter	2·0
Colours	3·0

The colours are ground with the powder constituents; the oil emulsified in the starch and water by means of the soap and the powder moistened with the oil-in-water emulsion (formed by the fatty matter, soap and water) to the consistency of a thick dough, dried, ground to pass a 60 mesh sieve, placed in suitable metal trays and compressed. The perfume may be incorporated into the powder during the grinding process with the colours, or added to the oil-in-water emulsion used to moisten the mass. In either case drying of the moistened mass should be carried out at a temperature which does not produce volatilisation of the perfume.

	per cent.
Kaolin	20·0
Zinc oxide	15·0
Precipitated chalk	25·0
Talc	32·0
Compact binder (e.g. soap)	8·0
Perfume	*q.s.*
Colour	*q.s.*

The method of manufacture is the same as that given for the previous formula.

Talcum Powders

These are widely used on account of the smooth and cooling feel which they impart, and to absorb perspiration in certain parts of the body where maceration would otherwise occur. They are also a popular application after bathing. Such powers, correctly formulated, exert a cooling effect, heat being lost continuously from their many-edged particles.

It is essential that good quality talc, free from gritty and alkaline matters be used in talcum powders. In order to confer upon the powder " mild antiseptic " virtues, it is usual to " borate " them by the addition of a small percentage of boric acid and it is possible that, apart from such action, the addition of the boric acid may act favourably *per se* in virtue of the fact that it *is* mildly *acidic*. (*See* pH of the skin in Chapter 1.) To improve the absorbency of such powders a proportion of starch is sometimes added, and metallic stearates have been suggested to improve the adherence of the powder to the body.

Within reason, such additions are legitimate *providing* the resultant talcum powder is *mainly talc*. I consider that the powder should contain a *minimum of* 50 *per cent. talc* and that 70 per cent. or upwards would be preferable.

The sale of powders containing very little, if any, talc, under the term " talcum powder ", is unjustifiable and steps have already been taken in this country to protect the consumer against such practices. On 23 June 1943, a London wholesale firm was fined £20 for selling chalk under the label of talcum powder. Defendants submitted that "talcum" was a trade name for a dusting powder and that what they sold was not talc but "talcum". The Magistrate decided, however, that the label was misleading (*Chem. and Drugg.*, 3 July 1943, p. 18). In a subsequent case in which a firm was prosecuted for selling as talcum powder a preparation containing 51·1 per cent. talc, 27·4 per cent. calcium carbonate and 18·3 per cent. magnesium carbonate, the case was dismissed (*Soap Perfum. Cosm.*, Feb. 1945, p. 118).

It would appear that, as one would expect, the term "talcum", whilst not synonymous with powdered talc, is taken as indicating that the dusting powder contains a very substantial proportion of talc.

The following are some typical formulae for preparations of this type :

	per cent.
Boric acid	6·0
Starch	10·0
Talc	84·0

	per cent.
Boric acid	5·0
Zinc oxide	5·0
Starch	10·0
Talc	80·0

	per cent.
Talc	70·0
Magnesium stearate	5·0
Starch	10·0
Colloidal kaolin	15·0

	per cent.
Boric acid	5·0
Talc	95·0

The use of boric acid as an antiseptic has a wide history of clinical usage behind it ; however, with the development of new antiseptics of proven efficacy there seems no reason why these should not either supplant or, if compatible with, supplement the usual boric acid.

Because of the particular conditions under which talcum powders are used, conditions of heat, moisture and friction against the skin occasioned by the movement of the external clothing, it is particularly important that all ingredients of such powders, antiseptics, perfume, etc., be dermatologically innocuous.

The manufacture of such powders follows the conventional lines, usually they are blended, mechanically sifted and remixed ; perfume being sprayed into the powder automatically between the sifting and remixing process.

Liquid Powders

So-called "liquid powders" are sometimes used as a basis for ordinary powder or to replace such powder, for evening wear, dances, etc.

In the past, solutions of phenazone have been used to "whiten the neck and shoulders for dances, etc."; a 20 per cent. solution of phenazone in water, tinted faintly pink with a trace of water-soluble dye, also forms, so Redgrove states (*Mfg. Chem.*, Sept. 1935, p. 287) a highly effective agent for whitening the hands. As pointed out by the writer (R. G. Harry, *Cosmetic Materials*, London: Leonard Hill Ltd., 1948, p. 237) the use of phenazone in toilet preparations is not justifiable. By suitable blending of chalks, zinc oxide, titanium, talc, etc., any desired degree of opacity may be achieved.

The following are more modern formulae which will serve as a basis for experiment:

	per cent.
Zinc oxide	3·0
Chalk (precipitated)	15·0
Kaolin	2·0
Colouring matter	*q.s.*
Glycerin	15·0
Water	65·0
Preservative	*q.s.*
Perfume	*q.s.*

	per cent.
Zinc oxide	10·0
Titanium dioxide	10·0
Talc	10·0
Colouring matter	*q.s.*
Gum tragacanth (0·5 per cent. solution)	25·0
Glycerin	15·0
Water	30·0
Preservative	*q.s.*
Perfume	*q.s.*

Procedure

The perfume may be previously incorporated in the powder base, the different constituents of which should be blended with the "insoluble" colouring matters and milled. Inert pigments and/or iron oxides may be used for colouring. The powder must be intimately ground with the pigments and should be sufficiently heavy to sink and not leave portions floating in the bottle which would be unsightly. Either a powder of suitable density should be chosen, or the lighter impurities should be water-floated off. The powder is then "wetted" with the glycerin and mixed into the aqueous phase.

CHAPTER 12

MAKE-UP PREPARATIONS

LIPSTICK

LIPSTICK is used to impart an attractive colour and appearance to the lips, accentuating their good points and disguising any bad ones. Narrow *bad tempered* lips are widened, and broad sensual lips made to appear narrower by its use. In fact, if applied intelligently it is capable of entirely altering the apparent facial characteristics.

Since lips are considered to be more alluring when they possess a slightly moist appearance, this is always achieved by the use of a greasy base which also exerts an emollient action.

There is no doubt that the wide use of lipstick among women has led to decrease in cracked and chapped lips, the crevices of which were always liable to bacterial infection. In addition, as in the case of many other cosmetics, it exerts a psychological effect difficult to assess, and induces a feeling of mental comfort.

CHARACTERISTICS OF A MODERN LIPSTICK

(*a*) It must colour the lips smoothly and attractively.

(*b*) It must be non-toxic and dermatologically innocuous.

(*c*) The colour must be reasonably permanent on the lips, but must be capable of being readily removed when desired.

(*d*) It must not possess a nauseous taste.

(*e*) It must be sufficiently hard to be massed into stick form, soft enough to melt instantly in contact with the lips, and yet must possess sufficient body not to *ooze* in the handbag under any conditions that might ordinarily be encountered.

(*f*) It must not sweat, crumble or cake.

(*g*) It must not develop a *bloom* on storage.

MATERIALS USED IN MANUFACTURE OF LIPSTICK

The desired consistency of a lipstick is achieved by the judicious blending of oils, fats and waxes, those in main use being beeswax, ceresin, paraffin wax, spermaceti, lanolin, and lanolin absorption bases, petroleum jelly, liquid paraffin, castor oil, cocoa butter, lard, cetyl alcohol, stearyl alcohol, hydrogenated vegetable oils, etc.

BEESWAX. Beeswax is a useful component in lipsticks, imparting firmness to the composition, it also appears to assist in blending castor oil with mineral oils and waxes. Providing the amount employed is not too high, sticks containing beeswax possess good gloss and contract readily, allowing their removal from the mould. However, I have not found the use of this substance as indispensable as a perusal of the literature would suggest and, providing the other ingredients in the base are suitably chosen and balanced, good lipsticks can be prepared *without* the use of beeswax.

CARNAUBA WAX. Carnauba wax is very effective in conferring firmness upon the stick; this effect appears to be thixotropic in that in a suitably balanced formula, such a stick, though firm, will spread very readily on the lips. Up to 20 per cent. carnauba wax may be employed depending upon the formula employed.

HYDROGENATED CASTOR OIL. (Hardened Castor Oil) up to 15-20 per cent. may be employed with advantage in certain formulations.

OZOKERITE. This wax, in amounts up to as high as 20-30 per cent., can be employed in lipstick formulations with satisfactory results.

CERESIN WAX. Mixture of ceresin wax with carnauba and or ozokerite waxes are sometimes used instead of beeswax. With a suitable balance of oils and soft melting jellies, and fatty alcohols and esters, thixotropic formulations may be prepared.

In the majority of cases, blends of two or more of the above waxes are employed.

The CORHYDROLS (L. Givaudan) are a range of hydrogenated vegetable oils not prone to rancidity which have extremely useful applications in lipstick, in rouge, and other make-up preparations discussed in this chapter.

PETROLEUM JELLY AND LIQUID PARAFFIN are used as lubricants, and tend to make the stick spread more smoothly and with less *tackiness.* The former should be of the *short fibre* type, and the latter possess a reasonably high viscosity. In general the amount of petroleum jelly should not exceed 10 per cent., and that of liquid paraffin should not be greater than 25 per cent. since otherwise the *adhesion* of the lipstick may be impaired. Moreover, they interfere with the solution of bromo acid, which is not readily soluble in hydrocarbons, and if a fairly high proportion of castor oil is included as a solvent, this will not form a satisfactory mixture with large proportions of hydrocarbons, unless a suitable " coupling agent " is employed. This is often used as a solvent for the dyestuff, particularly when bromo acid is employed.

Castor oil was employed very largely as a solvent for bromo acid in the days when other solvents were not available. Today, with the availability of many other bromo acid solvents, it is of less importance though still employed in many formulations. In my experience, quite small amounts of castor oil can be tasted in the finished stick by persons having a very sensitive palate.

CETYL ALCOHOL is often incorporated for its unctuous effect, its emollient action and the fact that it is considered to assist in the dispersion of the dyestuff. Only a small percentage, not greater than 4–5 per cent., should be used. Recently technically pure stearyl alcohol has been introduced as a substitute for cetyl alcohol, it being claimed to be effective in smaller proportions. It may be used for the same purpose.

LANOLIN AND LANOLIN ABSORPTION BASES. These possess emollient properties and by acting as a binding agent for other constituents tend to minimise sweating and cracking of the stick, giving it a certain degree of plasticity. Up to about 10 per cent. may be employed.

COCOA BUTTER is used because of its desirable characteristic of combining hardness with low melting-point and excellent emollient properties. Unfortunately such sticks on storage may exhibit a " bloom " similar to that found on chocolate. In view of the similarity of this problem to that of the chocolate manufacturer, the experiments of Clayton, Back, Johnson and Morse (*J. Soc. Chem. Ind., London*, 1936, **56**, 196T) should be of interest. These investigators found that oxidised cocoa butter possessed a marked capacity to inhibit fat bloom in chocolate and recommended the use of up to 1 per cent. for this purpose. Substitutes for cocoa butter are also available and appear to give satisfactory results.

By selective hydrogenisation of cottonseed oil, followed by fractional crystallisation from solvents, Kraemer, Smith and Bailey (*Oil and Soap*, 1944, 20, **11**, 235) have produced a hard butter which had similar properties to cocoa butter. It differed from it in composition due to the presence of iso-oleic acid and also showed minor physical differences, having a slightly longer plastic range, supercooling less and contracting less on solidifying whilst not showing such marked polymorphism. A yield of 28 per cent. was obtained from the cottonseed oil, the residue being used as a hardening agent in shortening products.

BROMO ACID SOLVENTS. As previously mentioned, castor oil was in general use in lipstick formulation as a dispersing agent for the halogenated fluoresceins. Unfortunately its solubility for such materials is very low, only about 1 per cent. Investigations were therefore undertaken to find a suitable, non-toxic and non-irritant solvent. In 1941, Fiore patented the use of tetrahydrofurfuryl alcohol (U.S. Patent 2,266,540) for this purpose. Subsequently Gottfried patented the use of the *esters* of tetrahydrofurfuryl alcohol (such as the acetate, stearate ricinoleate, etc.) for this purpose (U.S. Patent 2,506,921). By arrangement with Messrs. Croda Ltd. these esters have been marketed in the United Kingdom under the designation of "Eosols". The striking solubility of bromo acid in these solvents is well exemplified by the fact that the solubility of bromo acid in propylene glycol mono ether is less than 2 per cent. whereas its solubility in Eosol solvent is 28 per cent.

"*Eosol*" esters have been found to be stable against oxidation and polymerisation. With the exception of the acetate, which is miscible in all proportions, these esters are largely insoluble in water but can be mixed with alcohol, ether and chloroform. The product is miscible with most oils, fats and waxes used in cosmetic formulations and can be employed with the usual lakes, toners, oil-soluble dyestuffs and many inert pigments, etc.

Lipstick trials on over 200 women (50 of whom were either allergic to eosin or suffered in an acute state from herpes bucalis or herpetic stomatitis) were carried out for a period of sixty days without complaint, state the manufacturers. Skin tests were conducted, again with very satisfactory results. In fact it is stated that ". . . the solvents are reported to reduce risk of eosin dermatitis attributed to the action of undissolved eosin on the lips. . . ." (From the "Eosols"-Croda Ltd.). Physical advantages in formulation claimed from the use of "Eosol" are (1) superior staining power, (2) greater plasticity in the stick without causing crumbling, (3) convenience, since a stock solution of the halogenated fluorescein in "Eosol" esters can be stored indefinitely without having to employ continual agitation in subsequent manufacture.

Butyl stearate has been used to some extent as a bromo acid solvent. It is, however, considerably inferior in this respect to the "Eosols" mentioned above. Moreover, my experience has been that the use of this material leads to "sweating" of the stick, due to separation of this component from the rest of the mixture.

As will be seen from the table given below (*Soap Perfum. Cosmet.*, 1944, p. 924) some of the polyethylene glycols, the higher members of which are known as the carbowaxes, have quite a remarkable solvent power for bromo acid; however, they are still considerably inferior in this respect to the "Eosols".

Morel (*Soap Perfum. Cosmet.*, Aug. 1950) has suggested the use of diethyl sebacate as a good all-round solvent for lakes in bromo acid lipstick. Morel states that it is also said to be a good coupling agent for mineral and vegetable oils, including castor oil.

The use of Loramine wax O.M. 101 as a bromo acid (and Eosin salt) solvent in lipsticks is discussed later in this chapter.

WETTING AGENTS. Prior to the introduction of such solvents for Acid Eosin, the use of wetting agents had been advocated to assist dispersion of the insoluble dyestuff and also improve, possibly, the permanence of the stain upon the lips. The use of powerful synthetic wetting agents for this purpose is no longer necessary and the author is not in favour of their use.

	Eosin in solution at 20° C. per cent. approx.
Polyethylene glycol "4,000"	12·0
Polyethylene glycol "1,500"	10·0
Polyethylene glycol "400"	10·0
Hexa-ethylene glycol	9·0
Phenyl ethyl alcohol	8·0
Diacetone alcohol	6·5
Benzyl alcohol	6·0
Tetraethylene glycol	5·7
Hydroxycitronella	4·5
Citral	4·5
Triethylene glycol	4·0
Acetone	3·5–4·0
Diphenyl ketone	3·5–4·0
Diethylene glycol	2·5
Terpineol	1·9
Ethylene ricinoleate	1·9
Cyclohexanol	1·6
Ethyl ricinoleate acetate	1·4
Oleyl alcohol	1·0
Ethylene glycol	1·0
Lauryl alcohol	0·75
Myristyl alcohol	0·57
Stearyl alcohol	0·5
Glycol oleate acetate	0·4
Cocoa butter	0·35
Lauric acid	0·3
Myristic acid	0·3
Cetyl acetate	0·3
Ethyl oleate	0·3
Castor oil	0·2–1·7
Ethyl stearate	0·2
Glycol oleate	0·1

(Reproduced by permission of *Soap, Perfumery and Cosmetics* from their December 1944 issue, p. 924.)

The following are illustrative of some modern formulations:

	per cent.
Hardened castor oil	10·0
Cetyl alcohol	2·0
Beeswax	20·0
Ozokerite	6·0
Lanolin	10·0
"Eosol" (Stearate or oleate)	22·0
Liquid paraffin	20·0
Colours and bromo acid	10·0
Flavour	*q.s.*

	per cent.
Carnauba wax	16·0
Ozokerite	16·0
Lanolin	24·0
Liquid paraffin	24·0
Eosin solvent	10·0
Bromo acid and modifying lakes	7·5
Titanium dioxide	1·0
Flavour	1·5

	per cent.
Beeswax	10·0
Ozokerite	24·0
Carnauba wax	8·0
Paraffin wax	8·0
Lanolin	10·0
Liquid paraffin	22·0
Eosin solvent	8·0
Bromo acid	2·5
Modifying lakes	5·0
Titanium dioxide	1·0
Flavour	1·5

The following formulation is from the "Eosol" pamphlet (Croda Ltd.):

	Parts
Beeswax	40·0
"Eosol" stearate	15·0
Castor oil	15·0
Cocoa butter	20·0
Anhydrous lanolin	5·0
Bromo acid	2·0
p-Hydroxy benzoic acid	0·1
Carmine lake (inert pigment)	*q.s.*
Flavour	*q.s.*

Loramine wax O.M. 101 (Dutton & Reinisch Ltd.) is claimed to dissolve amounts of bromo acid as effectively as the tetrahydrofurfuryl esters and to have, so the makers claim, the following additional advantages:

(i) Loramine wax O.M. 101 is virtually without action on plastics in common use, and lipsticks containing them may be kept in plastic cases or in cases incorporating some plastic components;

(ii) this wax is claimed to be a solvent for eosin *salts* and the *salts* of other dyes whereas, it is stated "... these materials are substantially insoluble in all previously known lipstick components, even the tetrahydrofurfuryl esters, and could only be incorporated in lipsticks by some form of mechanical dispersion either direct or by precipitation from alcohol. O.M. 101 is able to dissolve these salts, and sticks may be prepared free from any gritty eosin particles. ..."

Loramine wax O.M. 101 should be regarded as a basic raw material and blended with the oils, fats and waxes normally employed. The dye is best dissolved first in the wax by agitation at 60°–65° C. and the other ingredients are then added. It is claimed that a solution of dye in O.M. 101 keeps practically indefinitely and may be prepared in the form of a "stock solution" which is then cast into slabs and stored away until required when the slabs are merely re-melted.

The following example is from *Loramine Wax O.M. 101* (Dutton and Reinisch):

	parts
Loramine O.M. 101	20·0
Lanolin	10·0
Cocoa butter	5·5
Refined beeswax	4·0
Ozokerite	18·0
Carnauba wax	4·2
Oleyl alcohol	7·0
Mineral oil (high viscosity)	29·3
Perfume	2·0 or *q.s.*
Insoluble lake	10·0 or *q.s.*
Bromo acid (or eosin salt)	2·0

The following lipstick formulation illustrates the use of butyl stearate in the base containing two proprietary dispersing agents:

	per cent.
Castor oil	15·0
Butyl stearate	5·0
Abracol I.S.L. (A.B.R.)	7·0

	per cent.
Emulsene 1212 (A.B.R.)	2·0
White beeswax	20·0
Spermaceti	10·0
Petroleum jelly	12·0
Hydrogenated palm kernel oil	15·0
Acid eosin	1·0
Titanium dioxide	1·0
Lakes	12·0

(From Technical Information Sheet No. 172, "Butyl Stearate for use in Cosmetics", A. Boake Roberts Ltd.)

An interesting variation on the above, in which diethyl sebacate is used as a bromo acid (i.e. acid eosin) solvent, and which employs isopropyl myristate is:

	parts
isoPropyl myristate	10·0
Diethyl sebacate	10·0
Beeswax	36·0
Mineral oil (heavy)	6·0
Hardened palm kernel oil	23·0
Lanolin	4·0
Emulsene 1212 (A.B.R.)	2·0
Acid eosin	1·0–2·0
Lake colours	12·0–14·0
Titanium dioxide	2·0
Antisept (A.B.R.)	0·15

(From Technical Information Sheet No. 144, "The Use of IsoPropyl Myristate in Cosmetics", A. Boake Roberts Ltd.)

Emul P7 (Polak and Schwarz) is a proprietary stearic acid ester, which it is claimed possesses the property of assisting the dispersion of the pigments in a lipstick. The following formulation (Polak and Schwarz, *Emulsifying Agents*), illustrates its use:

	parts
Emul P7	10·0
Beeswax (white)	17·0
Oleyl alcohol	9·0
Butyl stearate	4·0
Cetyl alcohol	4·0
Castor oil (finest)	40·0
Acid eosin	1·0
Lakes, pigments, etc.	14·0
Perfume	1·0

An example of a lipstick based upon a non-self-emulsifying grade of glyceryl monostearate (Tegin 515) is:

	per cent.
Tegin 515	42·0
Castor oil	36·0
Bromo acid	5·0
Mineral oil	6·0
White petroleum jelly	4·0
Carnauba wax	4·0
Lanolin	3·0

(From *Emulsifiers*, Goldschmidt Chemical Corp., New York.)

Finally, for manufacturers who merely wish to add colour and flavour to a proprietary base, the following formulation is illustrative :

	parts
Lipstick base P.50 (Polak and Schwartz)	84·0
Coloured lakes	14·0
Titanium dioxide	1·0
Acid eosin	0·5 to 1·0
Flavour	1·0 to 1·5

Lipstick is prepared from the uncoloured, unflavoured base, by dissolving the acid eosin in the melted base and stirring in the coloured lakes and titanium dioxide. The mass is then roller-milled several times (to ensure even dispersion of colours, etc.), reheated to 75° C., the flavour added and the resulting mixture run into moulds.

Manufacture of Lipsticks

The method of manufacture will depend to some extent upon the formulation and the plant available. The pigments, eosin and lakes may either be (*a*) milled separately with one of the oily ingredients of the base or (*b*) processed with the whole of the lipstick base. With the advent of the newer acid eosin solvents (such as the " Eosols ", Loramine Wax O.M. 101, diethyl sebacate, etc., mentioned above) it is possible to make up, separately, a solution of the acid eosin ; and where these solvents are employed, this course has much to commend it. In general, the process is as follows :

The dyestuffs are dissolved in the requisite amount of the solvent, and this mixed with any other liquid constituents. The fats and waxes are melted separately, keeping the temperature only a few degrees above the melting-point of the highest constituent to prevent overheating. After mixing, the mixture is milled several times. For all these operations a heated mill should be used. The milling is necessary since a mere mixing of the constituents is not sufficient to give a smooth and satisfactory product.

After milling, the temperature of the mass should be raised (just a few degrees above the melting-point of the stick) and transferred to a water-jacketed, air-evacuated tank and sufficient vacuum applied to remove the air that has been occluded in the process of milling and mixing. The mass should be kept rotating whilst under vacuum. When the air has been removed, the vacuum is shut off and the mass stirred and perfume added. The finished lipstick mass may then either be gently stirred until it solidifies, and " blocks " of this base gently remelted as and when required, or in firms operating on a larger scale, the mass may be run directly into moulds for casting.

Kempson-Jones (*Mfg. Chem.*, Aug. 1948, p. 341) has pointed out that moulds may be of the vertical split or automatic ejection type; and that for split moulds a cooling cabinet is required. A preheating device is stated to be useful in that the moulds can then be raised to a temperature of about 40° C. before filling with the lipstick mass, thus avoiding " flow marks " which would otherwise be visible on the moulded stick. With the water-jacketed automatic ejection mould a cooling cabinet is unnecessary. The jacket is filled with warm water, prior to pouring the lipstick mass, then the cold water is introduced and kept running to chill the lipstick mass.

It is stated (*Mfg. Chem.*) that with all types of automatic ejection moulds (whether air- or water-cooled), it is impossible to produce a good " bullet-shaped " stick because a small ring or ridge is left near the tip of the stick caused by the thickness of the metal edge of the ejection plunger. It is considered that such moulds are best for the wedge-shaped stick. After moulding, the sticks should be stored for about a week, prior to filling into the lipstick holders, after which they are flamed by passing rapidly through a small flame and capped.

Compact Rouge

Compact rouges may be prepared along the lines discussed for compact face powders (which see). Many modern high class products, however, employ the dry compression method as apart from the damp compression or moulding process. A modern binding agent consists of an oil-in-water emulsion containing a soap or other emulsifying agent. The ammonia-stearin-starch compound prepared from white petrolatum, ammonia, starch and stearin which is crumbled, sieved and incorporated into the rouge mass can also produce a useful compact.

In general, the vast majority of cosmetic textbooks steer clear of rouge formulation, much to the exasperation of the would-be enquirer. Rouge production is not as easy as producing, e.g. a cosmetic cream, but the difficulties are by no means insuperable. The following formulae are quoted as reasonable basic formulae upon which the experimenter can work to produce, by varying the constituents and pressures of compacting, a rouge compact to his liking. In view of different colour regulations existing between the different countries and the variations which exist between batches of the same colour when supplied by different manufacturers, the formulae are confined essentially to the base.

As rouges are highly coloured, a base of high opacity is not desirable otherwise an artificial effect is produced. The following formula, which is of the transparent type, will serve as a basis for experiments :

	per cent.
Talc	80·0
Zinc oxide	5·0
Zinc stearate	5·0
Rice starch	10·0
Perfume	*q.s.*
Colour	*q.s.*

The proportions of colouring matter may vary from 1½ per cent. in the case of the lighter shades to some 6 per cent. with the deeper shades. As binding agent 13-15 per cent. of starch-stearin mixture, as suggested by Winter (*Handb. der gesamten Parfum. Kosmet.*, 2nd edn., 1932, pp. 615-620), may be employed or alternatively a soap-oil mixture of about 3 per cent. sodium stearate or amino stearate and 2 per cent. oil or other fatty matter may be used. (*See* Compact Powder.)

In the case of the starch-stearin mixture this is prepared and added to the base which is moistened with sufficient water to form a very heavy dough-like mixture, dried at low temperature to avoid loss of perfume which may be included in the preliminary powder mixture, rubbed through a 90 mesh sieve and compressed. In the case of soap-oil mixtures it is more usual to emulsify the oil by means of the soap, in sufficient water, so that when mixed with the powder base it forms a heavy dough-like mix. This is dried again at low temperatures, rubbed through a 60 mesh sieve and compressed.

In compressing rouges, the powder is usually filled into a metal container called a godet and subjected to a *slowly increasing* pressure.

Preparation of Starch-Stearin (Winter, *Handb. der gesamten Parfum. Kosmet.*, 2nd edn., pp. 615-620) : 100 g. stearin and 20 g. white petrolatum are melted together and 50 cc. of 97 per cent. ammonium hydroxide solution added and thoroughly stirred in while hot. Finally 250 g. of rice or maize starch is added to the warm mixture with vigorous stirring. The introduction of the starch presents difficulties and requires practicc. During the addition thick lumps form in the starch powder but with vigorous stirring and pressing these break down and mix with the starch. The crumbly mass is then rubbed up in a mortar and passed through a 70 to 80 mesh sieve. The mixture must be well cooled before being sifted.

Cream Rouge

Although cream rouges are more difficult to apply than the dry type, it is claimed that their use gives better results, in that there is no obvious line of demarcation when correctly applied. This gives a more natural effect.

An effective cream rouge may be prepared along the lines of the following formula:

	per cent.
Petroleum jelly	70·0
Kaolin	30·0
Colours	*q.s.*
Perfume	*q.s.*

The method of manufacture is by grinding the colours with the powder constituent and then milling this into the warmed fatty base or alternatively by mixing all the ingredients and milling in a warmed ointment mill.

An emulsified form of cream rouge of the cold cream type may be prepared by the interaction of beeswax with an aqueous solution of borax:

	per cent.
Lanolin	5·0
Cocoa butter	5·0
Beeswax	14·0
Liquid paraffin	30·0
Cetyl alcohol	1·0
Water	44·2
Borax	0·8
Colour	*q.s.*

Disperse the finely powdered colour base with the melted fats, add the hot aqueous solution of borax at about 170° F. (both fats and water being at the same temperature to prevent crystallisation), mix well and finally mill.

Cream rouge of the vanishing cream type may be prepared as follows:

	per cent.
Stearic acid	15·00
Water	76·32
Potassium hydroxide	0·50
Sodium hydroxide	0·18
Glycerin	8·00
Colour	*q.s.*
Preservative	*q.s.*

If water or other soluble dyes are used in the above, they may be dissolved either in a portion of the water, or in the glycerin, and added to the main bulk of cream after saponification in the normal manner. (*See* Vanishing Creams.)

If desired one of the newer emulsifying agents may be used, e.g. diglycol stearate, glyceryl monostearate, etc.

	per cent.
Diglycol stearate	20·0
Water	70·0
Glycerin	10·0
Water-soluble colour	*q.s.* (from 0·6–1·0)
Preservative	*q.s.*

The difficulty in all cases where a water-soluble colour is introduced is to prevent evaporation, which leads to a darkening of the cream surface, due to concentration of the colour.

When such colours are used, it is necessary to incorporate sufficient hygroscopic constituents, e.g. glycerin, the glycols, etc. ; *d*-sorbitol would appear to offer interesting characteristics for this purpose, since it possesses a much narrower humectant range than glycerin, i.e. it absorbs less moisture in a moist atmosphere, but holds it better in a dry one. A further improvement might be the packing of such products in a well-capped tube.

In general, however, most of the colours employed in cream rouge are insoluble lakes, although sometimes oil colours are used. In the vanishing cream type, however, these lakes may be supplemented if desired by fluorescein dyestuffs, when, as stated above, it is necessary to incorporate a non-volatile solvent.

The following formulae for cream rouge are selected from the technical literature :

	per cent.
White beeswax	5·0
Stearic acid	7·0
Cetyl alcohol	3·5
Petroleum jelly (short fibre)	77·0
Mineral oil	7·5
Colours	*q.s.*

(This formula is from *Modern Cosmetics*, Thomssen).

An example of a cream rouge utilising the superior staining properties of the " Eosols " is :

	parts
Cetyl alcohol	3·0
Cocoa butter	3·0
White beeswax	3·0

	parts
Spermaceti	5·0
Lake colour	3·0
Acid eosin	2·0
Petroleum jelly	50·0
Absorption base (viscous)	20·0
"Eosol" acetate	10·0
Perfume	*q.s.*
Preservative	*q.s.*

(From E. S. Lower, *Mfg. Chem.*, 1947, **18**, 503.)

The following cream rouge is of the water-in-oil type, the emulsifier being Arlacel C (sorbitan sesquioleate). It is stated (*Drug and Cosmetic Emulsions*, Atlas Powder Co., Wilmington) that this formula provides a product which is soft and creamy, and which possesses tremendous spreading properties. Because it is of the water-in-oil type it has less tendency to dry out than *emulsified creams* of the *oil-in-water* type.

		per cent.
A	Arlacel C	2·0
	Lanolin (anhydrous)	2·0
	Mineral oil 65/75	16·0
	Petrolatum	30·0
	Preservative	*q.s.*
B	Brilliant red C-10-013 (Ansbacher)	10·0
	Arlex	5·0
	Water	35·0
	Perfume	*q.s.*

General Method of Manufacture

Where the base is entirely a fatty one, the colours are ground with the powder constituents (if any), and then mixed into the melted fatty base. In the case of oil-in-water creams of the vanishing cream type, or of the cold cream, or water-in-oil type, details of methods of manufacture of the base can be obtained by turning up the appropriate chapter heading. In the case of the above, water-in-oil cream rouge based on Arlacel C, the recommended method of manufacture is as follows: Heat (B) to 95° C. Melt (A) and bring to 90° C. Add (B) to (A) with agitation. When the emulsion has formed, slow down agitation and continue to stir to 45° C. Perfume and package at 45° C.

Liquid Rouge

This appears to have come into partial favour again, and such preparations are claimed to yield extraordinarily good results when skilfully applied. The difficulty occasioned in their application has been overcome by fitting a small wick in the neck of the container, the rouge being readily transferred by capillary attraction to the lip.

The essential requirements of such a preparation are that it should have sufficient viscosity to allow of ready and even application and that it dries reasonably rapidly.

Aqueous preparations are prepared by dissolving the requisite amount of a suitable water-soluble dye, adding a gum or synthetic derivative to increase the viscosity of the solution, and including a small proportion of a suitable wetting agent to allow of its easy spreading. A little glycerin may be included if desired.

	per cent.
Methyl cellulose	2·0
Wetting agent [1]	0·1–0·2
Water	to 100·0
Water-soluble red	*q.s.*
Preservative	*q.s.*

Alternatively, 0·4 g. gum tragacanth may replace the methyl cellulose in the above.

	per cent.
Sodium alginate	0·45
Calcium citrate	0·13
Wetting agent [1]	0·1–0·2
Water	to 100·0
Water-soluble red	*q.s.*
Preservative	*q.s.*

In this case the sodium alginate, dye and wetting agent are dissolved in about two-thirds of the water, the calcium citrate slurried in the other third portion and added to the alginate solution, as soon as thickening occurs on standing. By varying the proportion of the alginate and calcium citrate the viscosity may be altered at will. (A discussion of sodium alginate will be found under Hair Fixatives.)

In order to speed up the time taken in drying, 10–20 per cent. alcohol or more may be added to gum mucilages, but high concentrations must not be used with alginate products otherwise precipitation may occur.

The newest preparations of this type consist of a suitable alcohol-soluble dye dissolved in an alcoholic solution of ethyl cellulose or alcohol-soluble resin, a plasticiser being added to obtain the requisite flexible film. No wetting agent is of course necessary and by the use of suitable dyes, more permanent preparations are obtainable than with aqueous mixtures. Since evaporation of spirit will lead to increase in the viscosity of the product, it is particularly important that containers

[1] The term *wetting agent* in the above formulae does not indicate unqualified approval of all wetting agents, and any such substance should first be subjected to careful dermatological tests before use.

should be fitted with a well-fitted *wick* built into, or screwed into, the neck of the container, the whole being enclosed in a screw dust-cap. By this means, ready and even application is obtained with the minimum of care and with the least possible chance of covering the applicant's hands with sticky red varnish. The resultant lip rouge film is readily removed with a little alcohol, to which may be added if desired a small proportion of a relatively high boiling solvent to prevent too rapid evaporation of the *rouge remover*. It is important that all solvents used should be innocuous.

	per cent.
5 per cent. tincture of styrax	38·0
Alcohol (95 per cent.)	60·0
Castor oil	2·0
Spirit-soluble red	*q.s.*

The above solutions are prepared by simple mixture. Proportions of film-forming material, plasticiser and dye may be altered to suit individual requirements. The use of alcoholic preparations on the lips is likely to lead to "smarting" on application and dryness in some instances. Persons who suffer in this way should discontinue the use of these preparations and apply 40 per cent. solutions of aqueous glycerin occasionally and use an emollient lip *salve*.

The manufacture of liquid lipsticks of certain composition is covered by U.S. Patent 2,230,063 from which the following illustrative examples are quoted:

	per cent.
Ethyl cellulose	3·1
Ethyl alcohol	68·4
Petroleum ether	20·0
Hydrogenated methyl abietate	7·5
Rhodamine	1·0

	per cent.
Ethyl cellulose	3·06
Bleached wax-free shellac	4·94
Ethyl alcohol	65·00
Petroleum ether	14·66
Hydrogenated methyl abietate	12·00
Fuchsine	0·30
Saccharin	0·04

	per cent.
Ethyl cellulose	3·5
Ethyl alcohol	90·7
Castor oil	5·0
Tetra-bromo eosine	0·8

	parts
Ethyl cellulose	3·0
Bleached, wax-free shellac	2·5
Methyl abietate	7·5
Petroleum ether	11·0
Ethyl alcohol	77·0
Oil-red O	1·0

According to the patent quoted, accessory agents such as perfumes, preservatives, anti-oxidants, etc., may be added. The preparations are preferably clear and transparent and are of a viscosity ranging between 3 and 5 hundred centipoises, while best results are obtained in a range between 20 and 50 centipoises.

Mascara (Eyelash Cosmetic)

> . . . *Egyptian women soon discovered that smearing the eyelids with unguent and stibium* (i.e. *powdered antimony*) *not only eased the pain in the eyes and rested them but also added to the natural beauty of their faces. The whiteness of the whites of the eyes was emphasised by the darkened eyelids and the large dark pupils appeared like black pools in their midst, the whole effect being very striking. . . .*
>
> [*Dwellers of the Nile*, Sir Wallis Budge.]

The function of mascara is to increase the charm of the features by darkening and increasing the (apparent) length of the eyelashes, and it is claimed that by its intelligent use the brightness and expressiveness of the eyes is enhanced.

Mascara is marketed in cake, cream and liquid form, all of which must possess the following characteristics :

(*a*) It must be capable of even application.

(*b*) It must dry rapidly and should possess reasonable permanence.

(*c*) It must not cause the eyelashes to stick together.

(*d*) It must be non-toxic and non-irritant.

The colours usually employed are dark brown and black, the former being achieved either by the use of lakes, or sienna and umber, and the latter by carbon black. Oil blue (soluble) is also employed for this purpose.

Under the United States Food, Drug and Cosmetic Act, the use of coal tar colours in preparations to be applied in the area of the eyes is forbidden, even when those colours have been certified for use in cosmetics. *The area of the eyes is defined as " the area bounded by the supra-orbital ridge and the infra-orbital ridge, including the eyebrow, the skin below the eyebrow, the eyelids, the eyelashes, the conjunctival sac of the eye, the eyeball and the soft areolar tissue that lies within the perimeter of the infra-orbital ridge.*"

Thus defined, the "prohibited area" extends from the top of the eye socket to the top of the cheekbone.

Carbon black, bone black and oil black are permissible if they are pure colours. Pure vegetable colours are usable, including chlorophyll, except for the grade containing copper. Mineral and earth colours may be used, but suppliers are required (in the United States) to guarantee their product's freedom from certain impurities and that their arsenic content does not exceed 2 parts per million. Salts of cobalt may be used only if they are insoluble salts and will not react with other ingredients of the preparation to form soluble cobalt compounds. Finely powdered metals, such as silver and aluminium, have been widely employed in eye shadow and may be used if they consist entirely of the pure metal. *If they contain an appreciable content of copper they are considered to be harmful.*

CAKE MASCARA (BLOCK MASCARA). Earlier types of mascara were based on a mixture of soap and carbon black massed with sufficient water to produce a stiff paste which was dried at the requisite temperature, and then stamped out.

These could be readily applied, were fairly permanent, but since they were composed of a water-soluble base, tears and even heavy rain were capable of producing black streaks and smudges. Moreover, a trace of soap base in the eye produced extreme irritation. More recently attempts have been made to revive such preparations, using the soaps of the newer amino emulsifying agents, e.g. triethanolamine stearate whose reaction is less alkaline.

Jewel (*J. Ass. Off. Agric. Chemists,* 15 Nov. 1945, **28,** 74) states that fundamentally these products usually consist of a soap (generally triethanolamine stearate) modified in consistency with oils, waxes and colour. The colours used are bone black, ultra-marine blue, etc., and the pigments used are often iron oxides with titanium. The addition of organic dyes is prohibited in the U.S.A. The following formula is quoted as making a fairly satisfactory product very similar to a large majority of the mascara sold at present in the U.S.A.:

	parts
Stearic acid	27·0
Triethanolamine	12·0
Beeswax	30·0
Carnauba wax	50·0
Colour (bone black)	25·0

LIQUID MASCARA. These may be prepared by suspending the pigment in a mucilage, e.g.:

	per cent.
Gum tragacanth	0·2
Alcohol	8·0
Water	83·8
Lampblack	8·0
Preservative	*q.s.*

These, however, still suffer the drawbacks of water solubility and stickiness. More modern preparations are prepared by the use of an alcoholic solution of a resin in which carbon black is suspended. A little castor oil is often included in the formulae. These dry rapidly, producing a semi-permanent, waterproof colour, but are irritant if dropped actually in the eye, e.g.:

	per cent.
Rosin (10 per cent. alcohol solution)	3·0
Castor oil	3·0
Ethyl alcohol	84·0
Lampblack	10·0

Other resins, or ethyl cellulose, may replace rosin if desired.

Industrial methylated spirit is best avoided in such preparations as it tends to irritate.

CREAM MASCARA may be prepared by milling the pigment into a vanishing cream base, or by the use of a suitable oil-soluble dye, but in such cases it is often necessary to include a suitable wetting agent to lower the surface tension, otherwise the colour will not adhere to the brush.

In manufacturing mascara, the melted ingredients are mixed, milled, and ultimately passed through a warmed plodder the plate of which has a gate of the desired dimensions. The mascara strip is then cut to the desired lengths.

GREASY TYPES, which are more resistant, may be made by incorporating the pigment or dyestuff, about 10 per cent., with a greasy base, this being warmed slightly and applied with a fine brush.

	per cent.
Beeswax	4·0
Spermaceti	4·0
Cetyl alcohol	2·0
Cocoa butter	6·0
Petroleum jelly	64·0
Oil-soluble blue	20·0
Preservative	*q.s.*

	per cent.
Cocoa butter (odourless)	5·0
Petroleum jelly	50·0
Paraffin wax (uncrystallisable)	5·0
Lampblack	40·0

Melt and mix.

The following examples of mascara are from the technical literature:

Cake Mascara

	per cent.
Triethanolamine stearate	40·0
Paraffin	30·0
Beeswax	12·0
Lanolin	5·0
Lampblack	13·0

	per cent.
Glyceryl monostearate	60·0
Paraffin	15·0
Carnauba wax	7·0
Lanolin	8·0
Lampblack	10·0

Procedure

Melt and mix the ingredients, then cast, or extrude to the proper form.

(From "Readers' Questions", *Drug cosmet. Ind.*, Oct. 1942, **51**, 469.)

	parts
Cocoa butter	5·0
White petroleum jelly	55·0
Paraffin wax (m.p. 110°–118° F.)	5·0
Lampblack	45·0

(From *Perfum. essent. oil. Rec.*, Feb. 1949, p. 53.)

CREAM MASCARA. In the opinion of K. N. Richardson (*Soap Perfum. Cosm.*, 1945, **18**, 286) a reliable cream mascara which does not dry up in the tube and which stays on the eyelashes very well can be made up according to the following formula:

	parts
Mucilage of quince seeds	350·0
Sugar syrup	350·0
Gum arabic	75·0
Ivory black (or umber)	225·0

Procedure

The gum, and the ivory black (or umber, etc.), are ground up with the syrup (3 parts sugar to 2 parts water), then the mucilage containing a preservative (e.g. methyl *p*-hydrobenzoate) is added.

Eyebrow Pencils

These are used to modify the outline of the eyebrows after plucking. They consist of a suitable colouring material dispersed in the wax base of the lipstick type, in which, if desired, the proportion of beeswax or other high melting constituent may be increased to make a somewhat firmer pencil. Such sticks must, however, be capable of ready and uniform application and should not be brittle.

	per cent.
Hydrogenated castor oil	46·0
Hydrogenated cottonseed oil	12·0
Cocoa butter (odourless)	8·0
Castor oil	8·0
Lanolin absorption base	17·0
Lampblack (best)	9·0

If a brown stick is required, the lampblack may be replaced by umbers, burnt siennas, etc.

Eyebrow pencils are also prepared in the usual pencil style, in which form they are even more readily applied than in the stick type.

Eye Shadow

Eye shadow is marketed in a variety of shades, and is used, particularly for evening wear under electric lights, to produce an attractive background for the eyes, e.g.:

	per cent.
Cocoa butter (odourless)	2·0
Beeswax	3·0
Spermaceti	5·0
Lanolin	5·0
Petroleum jelly	55·0
Zinc oxide	30·0
Cosmetic lake	*q.s.*
Preservative	*q.s.*

	per cent.
Petroleum jelly	75·0
Cocoa butter (odourless)	8·0
Lanolin	7·0
Cetyl alcohol	3·0
Paraffin wax (uncrystallisable)	7·0
Cosmetic lake	*q.s.*
Preservative	*q.s.*

The colours in use are blue, bronze, silver, green and brown, which are milled into the base until a smooth product is obtained. To obtain scintillating effects a small proportion of powdered metal is sometimes added, i.e. gold leaf, bronze powder, powdered aluminium, etc.

CHAPTER 13

SUNBURN AND SUN-TAN PREPARATIONS

Effect of Light Exposure—Principal Events involved in Sunburn—Sunlight and Cancer—Erythemal and Tanning Effectiveness of U.V. Energy—Types of Sunburn and Sun-tan Preparations—Sun-screens, Transmission Spectra of some Sunscreens—Evaluation of the Efficacy of Sunscreens—The " Sunscreen Index ".

NO one will deny that the *moderate* exposure of the human organism to sunlight is beneficial, but if carried to excess, detrimental results accrue, varying from the preliminary stages of general irritability and depression (with or without an increase in bodily temperature) to inflammatory conditions of the skin, which may become septic.

It seems evident that excessive exposure of the human body to sunlight may not only precipitate a predisposition to cancer but can in itself produce malignant growth.

The effect of exposure to the sun's rays is first, the development of an erythema, and later, the formation of a tan, which the present civilised world appears to have adopted as a criterion of physical health.

According to Keller (*Strahlentherapie*, 1924, **16**, 537) one of the main effects of exposure to such rays is the degeneration of the *prickle-cell* layer of the skin (*see* Histology of the Skin), possibly by denaturation of its protein constituents. Histamine-like substances, which produce dilation of the blood vessels and consequent erythema, are released by all injured cells and are responsible for the boiled lobster like appearance resulting shortly after sun-bathing. In addition, melanin, the natural pigment of negro skin and present also to a lesser extent in the white races, passes upwards and outwards from the basal cell layer, where it normally resides, by the migration of pigment granules towards the stratum corneum, while a fresh supply of this pigment is slowly formed *in situ* in the basal cell layer. This migration of melanin produces some degree of protection as does also the human sweat secreted by the sweat ducts, *but the main protection is afforded by a thickening of the corneous layer itself, which then exerts considerable screening power.*

The following summary of the effect of light upon the skin is from an excellent survey of this subject by Klarmann (*Amer. Perfum.*, July-Aug., 1949). Blum (*Physiol. Rev.*, 1945, **25**, 483) has postulated a basic scheme of the several events involved in sunburn and its sequelae, in which he

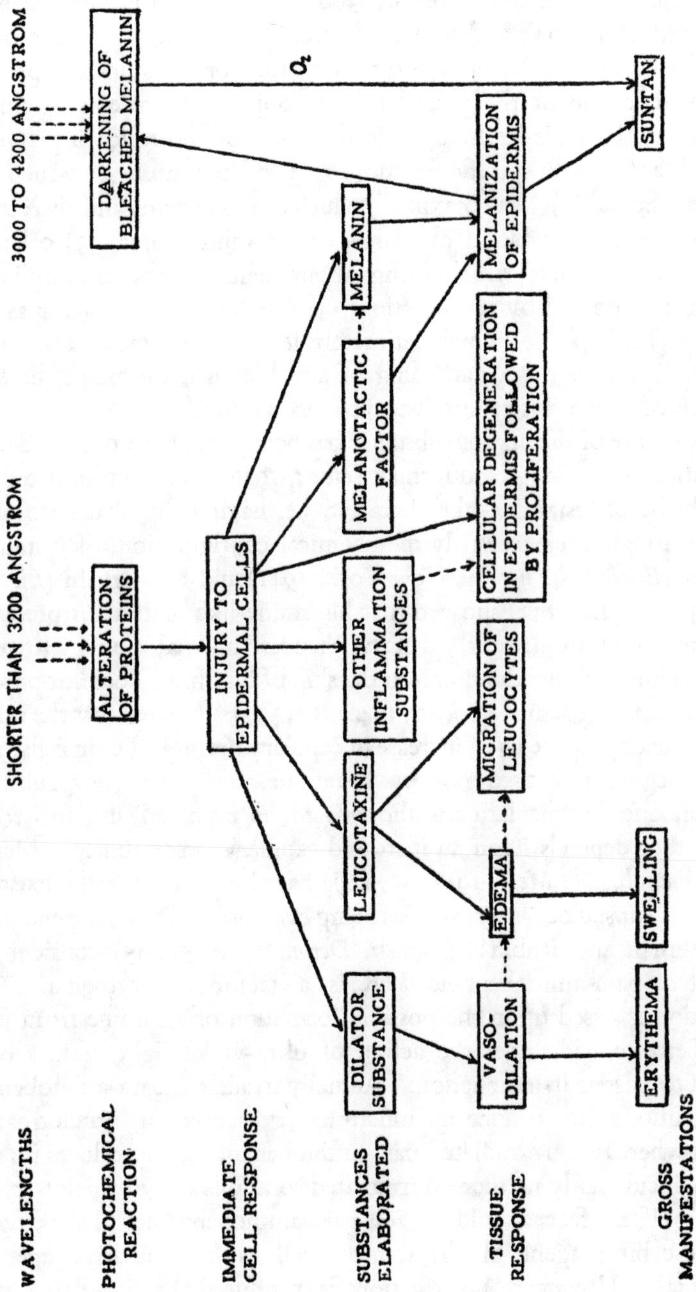

FIG. 15.—Summary of the effect of light on the skin.

[By courtesy of *The American Perfumer*

distinguishes between the effects caused by radiation of wavelength shorter than 3200 Å and those of 3000 to 4200 Å, the former being considered erythemal, and the latter directly melanogenic. The injury to the epidermal cells by the shorter wave radiation is assumed to produce first an alteration of the photolabile unconjugated proteins or nucleic acids, or both; this leads to the elaboration of the following five individual factors with specific functions: (1) dilator substance which produces erythema, (2) "leucotaxine", which causes oedema and also attracts leucocytes from the blood capillaries to the injured area, (3) other inflammation products which bring about cellular degeneration in the epidermis, followed by proliferation, (4) the melanotactic factor as well as (5) melanin *per se*, which ultimately leads to sun-tan. The longer wave radiation causes a darkening of any bleached melanin; here the presence of oxygen is required to produce tanning.

The nature of the dilator substance has been the subject of considerable speculation. Lewis and Zotterman (*Heart*, 1926, **13**, 203) postulated that it might be of histamine-like character, i.e. having the pharmacological action, though not necessarily the chemical configuration, of histamine. Ellinger (*Radiation Therapy*, New York, 1941) and Kawaguchi (*Biochem. Z.*, 1930, pp. 221, 232) showed that histamine-like material *is* present in irradiated skin in greater quantity than in normal skin. However, the experimental introduction into the skin of histamine does not produce pigmentation. Menkin (*Science*, 1944, **100**, 337) suggested that the migration of leucocytes due to an increase in capillary permeability in inflammatory processes is caused not by histamine, but by a new substance "leucotaxine": the latter is thought to be involved also in oedema which, too, depends upon an increased capillary permeability. Menkin (*Arch. Pathol. Lab. Med.*, 1943, **36**, 269) has also postulated the existence of another substance "necrosin" as being responsible for cell degeneration.

Rothman and Rubin (*J. invest. Derm.*, 1942, **5**, 445) consider that irradiated para-aminobenzoic acid is a factor in erythema. Their suggestion is based upon the possible formation of an imine from para-aminobenzoic acid under the action of ultra-violet light, imines being known to possess irritant action. Actually irradiated para-aminobenzoic acid solutions do produce an inflammatory action on intradermal injection whereas non-irradiated para-aminobenzoic acid produces no such effect; incidentally neither do irradiated solutions of tyrosine or tryptophane. These facts would suggest para-aminobenzoic acid as being the light-absorbing agent in the skin as well as the causative agent in erythema. However, no reaction is produced by irradiated para-aminobenzoic acid in the absence of oxygen, whereas oxygen deprivation during exposure to ultra-violet radiation does not inhibit subsequent development of erythema. Moreover, injection of irradiated para-aminobenzoic acid does not produce pigmentation.

If the release of a histaminic substance into the tissue were responsible for the symptoms observed in solar erythema then it could reasonably be postulated that the prior introduction of an antihistaminic would inhibit such phenomena. Kurtin, Bierman, and Yontef (*J. invest. Derm.*, 1947, **9**, 161) investigated the effect of the prior iontophoretic introduction into the skin of pyribenzamine in respect of its response to ultra-violet radiation. As a result of their investigation they attributed an anti-histaminic quality to pyribenzamine in respect of its capacity to prevent solar erythema. However, their conclusions were criticised by Baer, Kline and Rubin (*J. invest. Derm.*, 1948, **11**, 405) who showed that the protective action of pyribenzamine was due to its absorption of the active ultra-violet rays producing erythema, rather than to its antihistaminic action. This criticism is further supported by the fact that benadryl, which is also a powerful antihistaminic, displays but minor effect in checking ultra-violet erythema ; the explanation again lying in the fact that benadryl shows only a moderately high absorption for wavelengths of about 2537 Å. Similar conclusions were reached independently by Friedlaender *et al.* (*J. invest. Derm.*, 1948, **11**, 397).

Sunlight and Cancer

Evidence has converged from a number of sources to indicate that the ultra-violet radiations in sunlight are a major factor in the production of cutaneous cancer (H. F. Blum, *J. nat. Cancer Inst.*, 1940, **1**, 397), and further, that the wavelength of a maximum efficacy for carcinogenesis lies, also, between 2900 and 3000 Å (J. S. Mitchell, *Proc. roy. Soc.*, 1938–39, Ser. B, vol. CXXVI). Piers (*Brit. J. Derm.*, 1948, **60**, 10, 319) states " . . . it has been found that the wavelength limits are the same for carcinogenic and erythema-producing ultra-violet rays, and that therefore . . . a higher incidence of skin cancer would be expected to prevail in regions favoured with sunlight rich in the shorter ultra-violet rays. . . ."

The hypothesis that sterols in the skin are changed by such radiations into carcinogenic compounds receives no support from recent experiments. Bergmann *et al.* (*Amer. J. Cancer*, 1940, **38**, 81) have been unable to produce carcinogenic substances by exposure of various sterols to ultra-violet radiation *in vitro*. Evidence from wavelength studies (H. F. Blum and S. W. Lippincott, *J. nat. Cancer Inst.*, 1942, **3**, 211) indicates that the cells are directly affected by the radiation and that the corneum which must contain a large proportion of the sterols of the skin does not participate in carcinogenic action.

The evidence that " excessive " sunlight is an important factor in the production of skin cancer is impressive.

Roffo (" Para el Estudio y Tratamiento del Cancer ", *Bol. Inst. Med. exp. Cancer, B. Aires*, 1933-36) has shown that malignant growths occur mainly in those regions of the body which receive the greatest amount of light. In experiments in which he exposed 600 rats to sunlight, 365 died within the first few days and 70 per cent. of the remainder developed tumours. Ellinger (*Fundam. radiol.*, 1938, **4**, 181) has shown that tumour cells from Ehrlich's mouse carcinoma, implanted in mice, were definitely followed by development on irradiation of only two or three times the normal erythema threshold and of short duration. Professor Passey, making his report at the annual meeting of the Yorkshire Council of the British Empire Cancer Campaign (16 May 1938), stated that seamen who were exposed to intense sunlight over a number of years developed cancer of the skin more often than others.

It has been found in Australia that people of British descent are liable to develop skin cancer five to ten times more frequently than in Britain. Piers (*Brit. J. Derm.*, 1948, **60**, 10, 319), E. H. Molesworth (*Introduction to Dermatology*, London: Churchill Ltd., 1937) states that cancers of the skin in Australia exceed in number those of all other organs and that 99 per cent. of these are due to chronic sunburn. An extensive statistical survey carried out under the direction of Dorn on behalf of the U.S. Public Health Service (Elliott and Welton, *Arch. Derm. Syph., Chicago*, 1944, **53**, 307) in certain regions of the U.S.A. showed that the incidence of cutaneous cancer among the white population increased rapidly from north to south.

Piers (*Brit. J. Derm.*, 1948) has drawn attention to the fact that sunlight appears to be the paramount factor in the causation of cutaneous cancer in Kenya and considers that the outlook is rather gloomy for two reasons, (*a*) that old age is not yet of major importance in the colony but that with the general ageing of the population the cancer rate will rise, and (*b*) that *the town dweller following the command of fashion exposes himself voluntarily with a truly alarming recklessness.* In this country the danger is very much less, nevertheless we *occasionally* get summers during which *excessive* exposure to the sun could lay the seeds of future trouble.

Milder degrees of sunburn may produce various forms of solar dermatitis, and it is probable that eczema, rosacea, pruritis and lupus erythematous are at least exacerbated. Other types of dermatitis are produced by photo-sensitisation resulting from the application of certain dyestuffs and chemicals plus the effect of the sunrays. Examples of this are Berlock dermatitis resulting from the application of bergamot oil or

Cologne spirit to the skin followed by exposure to sunlight. Eosin and certain derivatives may produce similar effects, and this should be remembered in the formulation of lipsticks and nail lacquers. It is possible that some of the lesions reported from use of the latter may be due to the introduction of a trace of a photo-sensitising dyestuff into the skin or lip plus the effect of sunlight, especially by trauma from the nails.

In assessing the danger from exposure to sunshine it should be remembered that the percentage of the shorter wave-lengths present in the incident light will depend upon the time of the day, season of the year, and the presence or absence of moisture and dust particles. It is well known that the maximum intensity of sunshine occurs between 10 a.m. and 2 p.m. (G.M.T.), and that reflection from the water or sky is very active in the production of a sunburn. The fact that appreciable burn may result on a dull and hazy day near the sea coast or up in the mountains owing to the fact that *water vapour substantially does not absorb the shorter wave-lengths* is not realised. On the other hand, *smoke* (as in an industrial town) *possesses a high absorptive power for the shorter light rays and greatly decreases the amount of ultra-violet* which can reach the inhabitants.

It is true of course that *moderate* exposure of the human organism to sunshine results psychologically and physiologically in a general sense of fitness, peace of mind, and general well-being which it is difficult to estimate. *At the same time it should be remembered that tanning is not by any means a sign of health, but is actually part of the procedure by which nature is trying to minimise, to the best of her ability, the damaging effects which would otherwise be produced by exposure to light.* Tanning should therefore be produced very gradually. If the first exposure is excessive, a blistering is produced. The outer keratinous coat (which the body was thickening to absorb the light) will be thrown off, and not only will an open wound result with all the subsequent dangers of infection but also the protection against sunlight will be absent and exposure to sunlight will then exacerbate the condition.

The advent of the automobile, bringing with it increased opportunities for frequent week-end picnics by the sea, and the increase in sun-bathing have made the production of preventive and soothing applications not a matter of luxury but one of necessity.

Erythemal and Tanning Effectiveness of Ultra-violet Energy

Several investigators have studied the efficiency of ultra-violet energy in producing erythema and an erythemal effectiveness curve has been tentatively established by combining all the data available. However, little quantitative data concerning the spectral region between 3200 Å and 3600 Å and its effect was available until Luckiesh and Taylor (*Gen. Elec. Rev.*, 1939, **42**, 274) extended their previous studies from which they established a spectral tanning curve and also extended the spectral erythemal curve in the long wave region. Since it was found difficult to obtain monochromatic radiation of sufficient intensity to produce tanning—if its tanning effect is low—Luckiesh and Taylor used filters with varying degrees of transparency to radiant energy of various wavelengths. Seven such filters were chosen and a mercury arc operating between incandescent tungsten electrodes in clear quartz and Corex D bulbs used; a water cell was introduced to remove most of the heat from the beam.

It was found that the action on the exposed areas was dependent upon the wavelength of the energy to which they had been exposed. In those cases where the total effect was predominantly due to energy in the spectral region 2950 Å to 3150 Å there was no immediate visible effect, but after a few hours a definite erythema set in. In a few days the inflammation subsided and a tan formed. In the case of exposures through filters transmitting only those wavelengths longer than about 3300 Å, the areas appeared somewhat brownish or tanned immediately after exposure followed later by some erythema together with the tan. There was obviously definite latent tanning effect in the former case which might or might not be present in the latter case. Erythemal and tanning results were appraised by examination of the subjects immediately after exposure, on the next day, and at weekly intervals thereafter. It had been expected to find a progressively decreasing rate of tan with variations in the filters, for *it has been commonly assumed that tan is principally due to wavelengths longer than those which cause pronounced erythema. Luckiesh and Taylor found no appreciable difference in the rate of fading of the erythema and tan produced with the various filters. These observations lead these investigators to believe that for wavelengths longer than* 2950 Å *the spectral erythemal effectiveness curve cannot be separated from the tanning effectiveness curve, at least for such tanning effects as may be apparent within* 12 *hours, when the erythema has approximately reached its maximum.* The dotted curve in the figure shows the relative effectiveness of radiant energy of different wavelengths in the production of erythema as adopted by the International Commission on Illumination (I.C.I.) (*Trans. Illum. Engrg. Soc.*, July 1935, **30**, 568) and the solid curve gives the tanning effectiveness values determined by Luckiesh and Taylor. As the energy at 2804 Å and 2894 Å was very low in their tests they assumed the relative tanning effectiveness to be the same as the erythemal effectiveness for these two wavelengths. Consequently no significance, the authors state, should be attached to this portion of the curve. In the wavelength region longer than 2967 Å the tanning curve derived by Luckiesh and Taylor departs appreciably from the I.C.I. erythemal curve, and these workers believe this departure to be caused principally by inaccuracies in the longwave end of the present I.C.I. erythemal-effectiveness curve. They have suggested its revision.

RELATIVE EFFECTIVENESS OF ULTRA-VIOLET ENERGY OF DIFFERENT WAVELENGTHS IN PRODUCING ERYTHEMA AND TAN

Wavelength (Å)	*Erythemal Effectiveness (I.C.I.)*	*Tanning Effectiveness (Luckiesh and Taylor)*
2967	1·00	1·00
3022	0·55	0·50
3130	0·03	0·02
3342	0·000	0·004
3663	0·000	0·0012

From examination of tanned skin under ultra-violet light, Luckiesh and Taylor conclude that there may be a simultaneous production of erythema and tan, but that the presence of the tan may be obscured by a strong erythema. This is especially true in the case of sunlight with a great deal of energy in the region which Luckiesh and Taylor have found to produce direct tan. As a consequence these investigators consider it probable that the erythemal effectiveness curve heretofore tentatively accepted, is in actuality a combined erythemal and tanning curve for wavelengths longer than about 3000 Å.

As the energy must be absorbed to produce erythema or tan, they are related in some way to the depth of penetration of the energy. Erythema due to wavelengths in the spectral region 2500 Å to 2700 Å is quite superficial and disappears in a few days with little or no resultant tan. Consequently it was considered safe to assume that this short wave energy did not reach a depth sufficient to affect appreciably the tanning pigment or process. It appeared that the longer wavelengths, especially 3342 Å and 3663 Å, produced a direct or immediate tan, or its equivalent with less inflammation than that produced by the shorter wavelengths.

Luckiesh and Taylor have also studied the effect of sub-erythemal exposures to the sun lamp in the production of tan. None of the areas receiving an intermittent exposure showed any signs of erythema or tan while several of those which received a single exposure, which was actually 40 per cent. less than the total time received intermittently, did develop erythema and tan. *These results appeared to indicate that if tanning is desired the exposures should be long enough to produce some erythema. If it is desired to tan without appreciable erythema, it seems to be necessary to screen off the energy of wavelengths shorter than* 3300 Å. *This appears to be the action of the sun-tan lotions now on the market. Some are highly absorptive in the region shorter than* 3300 Å. *Quite long exposures to sunlight are necessary when using these lotions to result in tanning, but this is the condition usually desired by the user.*

Erythema and tanning following exposure of the skin to sunlight or to an artificial source of ultra-violet energy, give visible evidence that the subject has received at least a minimum exposure to erythemally effective ultra-violet energy. Thus everyone is his own " ultra-violet meter " ; the exposure required to produce a minimum perceptible erythema (MPE) varies over a considerable range with individuals. In discussing ultra-violet energy Luckiesh and Taylor (*J. opt. Soc. Amer.*, 1931, vol. 21) adopted as a unit of energy the E-viton. This is equivalent to 10 microwatts of energy at 2967 Å, where the relative erythemal effectiveness is a maximum. To produce a minimum perceptible erythema on an average untanned skin requires an exposure of approximately 40 E-viton minutes per sq. cm. of skin. Thus a minimum perceptible erythema is produced by any one of the following exposures :

1 E-viton per sq. cm., acting for 40 minutes.
10 E-vitons per sq. cm., acting for 4 minutes.
40 E-vitons per sq. cm., acting for 1 minute.

The intensity of erythemal ultra-violet energy in E-vitons per sq. cm. on a horizontal plane is shown in figures 16 and 17 for three specific days in 1936 and the hourly variations.

It is a very interesting fact that for about eight months of the year a clear sky contributes more than half of the erythemal ultra-violet energy in daylight at all times of the day incident on a horizontal plane. *In the midsummer months there are only a few hours in the middle of the day when the erythemally-weighted ultra-violet energy from the sun on a horizontal plane exceeds that from the sky.* These facts may appear surprising to those who believe that exposure to direct sunlight is necessary in order to receive the effects of ultra-violet energy.

Types of Sunburn and Sun-tan Preparations

Cosmetic sunburn and sun-tan preparations may be classified into three groups, namely :

(i) Those designed to allow tanning with the minimum of *sunburn* ; these preparations are termed " Sun-screens " and represent the most important group of preparations marketed by the cosmetic manufacturer.

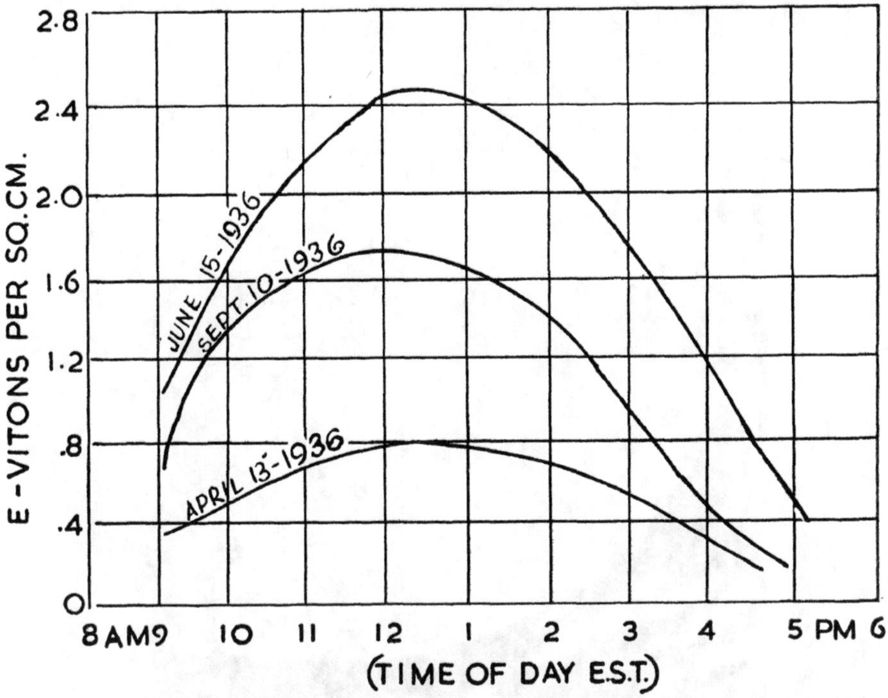

[*By courtesy of the American Perfumer.*

FIG. 16.—Erythemally-weighted or anti-rachitic ultra-violet energy incident on a horizontal plane on three clear days in April, June and September. An exposure of approximately 40 E-viton minutes per sq. cm. produces a barely perceptible erythema on average untanned skin.

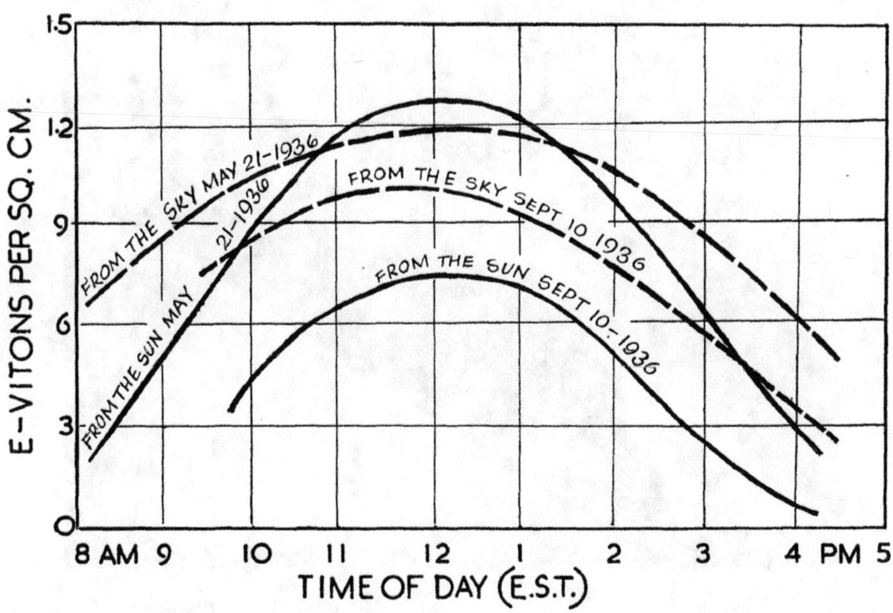

[*By courtesy of the American Perfumer.*

FIG. 17.—Erythemally-weighted or anti-rachitic ultra-violet energy incident on a horizontal plane from the sun and from the entire sky on two clear days in May and September.

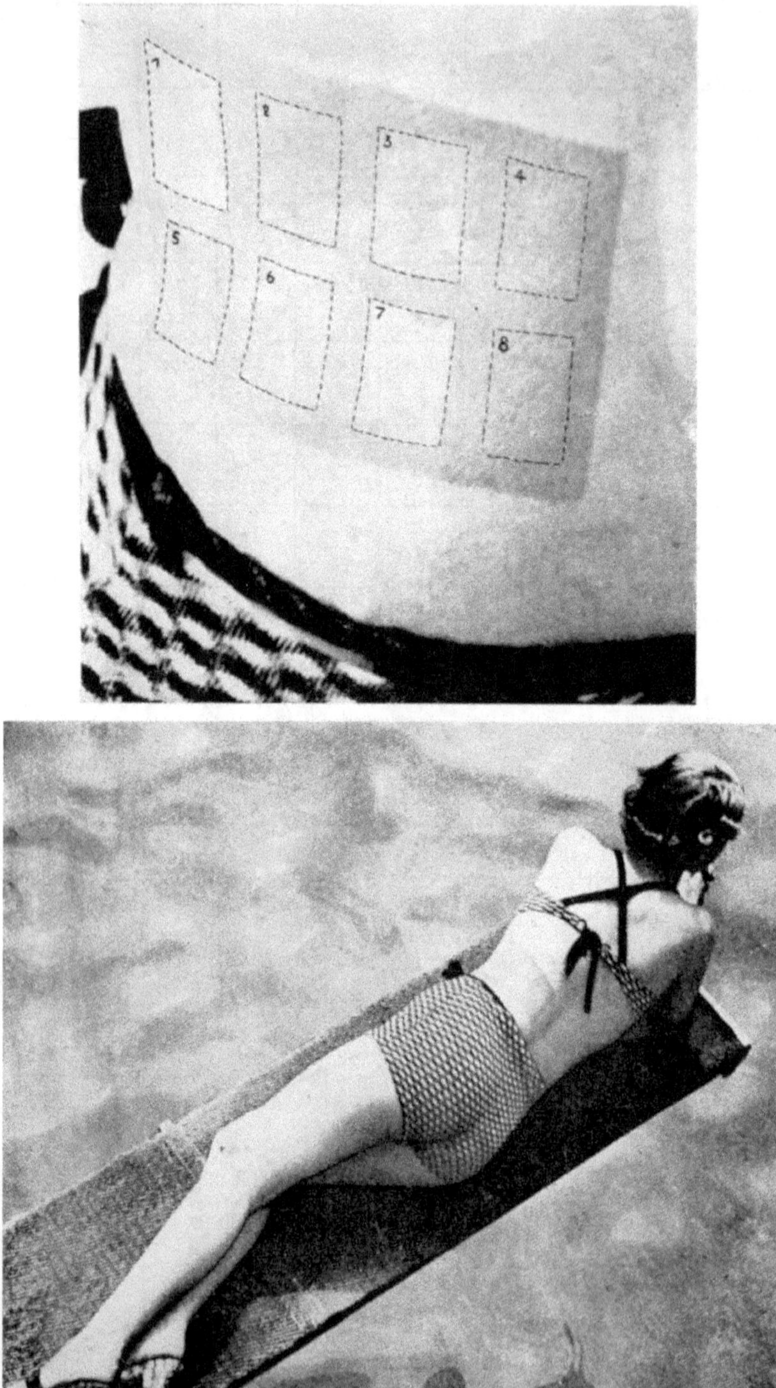

[By courtesy of Firmenich and Co.

FIG. 18.—The practical evaluation of various sunscreens may be checked by the practical tests along the " very pleasant lines " portrayed above. The (chemical) technique is self-explanatory.

(ii) Simulative preparations designed for those who wish to feign a brown skin in the minimum of time and with the least possible pain or trouble. These are essentially preparations which stain the skin brown.

(iii) Palliatives, designed to alleviate the pain and irritation resulting from excessive exposure to sunlight. This latter class of preparation must represent quite an appreciable market. Many such preparations are " pharmaceuticals " which are purchased from the local chemist and druggist.

COMPARATIVE ABSORPTIONS OF THE ANTIVIRAYS
FILM THICKNESS .0012 mm

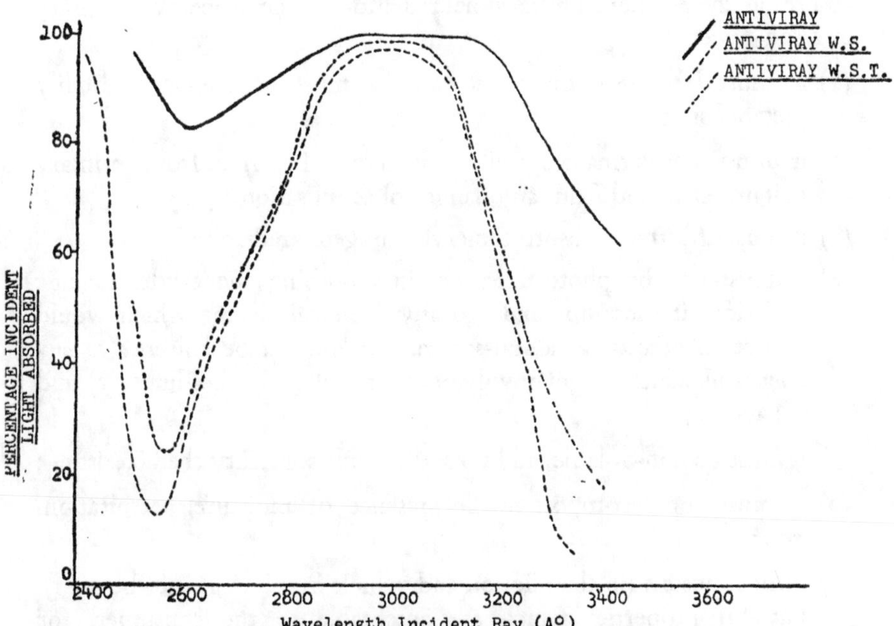

NOTE:
Calculated from extinction values, using the relation:

$$Ecd = \log_{10} \frac{\text{Intensity of incident light}}{\text{Intensity of transmitted light}}$$

Where c = Percentage concentration of the Antiviray solution
d = Thickness of the film (c.m.)
E = Extinction coefficient

Fig. 19.

Sun-screens

Sun-screens should either scatter the incident light effectively, or they should absorb the erythemal portion of the sun's radiant energy. Opaque powdered materials when applied to the skin either in the dry state or when incorporated into suitable vehicles will serve to scatter the ultraviolet light falling upon them. As discussed under Face Powders, etc.,

Chapter 11, zinc oxide is the most effective of such powders and is superior to titanium dioxide in this respect. Other powders which may be employed for this purpose with, however, very much less efficiency, are kaolin, calcium carbonate, magnesium oxide, talc, etc. Obviously the particle size of the powder employed is a factor of considerable importance in such preparations.

Although powders of this type rank but low down in the sales of anti-sunburn preparations, when applied as a second line of defence over a suitable sun-screening foundation, their light-scattering possibilities should not be ignored.

The most important class of sun-screens are those which operate by absorbing the erythemal ultra-violet radiation. The properties necessary in a sun-screen are:

(1) it must be non-toxic *per se*, and it must not influence bodily metabolism;

(2) it must be dermatologically innocuous, i.e. free from primary irritant effect and from any danger of sensitisation;

(3) it must effectively absorb the erythemogenic radiation;

(4) it must not be photolabile, i.e. in absorbing the erythemogenic radiation, it must not undergo any chemical change which would reduce its efficacy as a sun-screen, nor must it be *converted to any compound* which might involve any hazard under headings (1) and (2) above;

(5) it must be non-volatile, and possess suitable solubility characteristics;

(6) it must not decompose in the presence of moisture, perspiration, etc.;

(7) it must possess (in the dilution and vehicle in which it is to be used), physical properties which are acceptable to the consumer, for example, it must not be malodorous;

(8) it should not be absorbed through the skin.

Criteria (1) and (2) above are so obviously necessary in all cosmetic and toilet preparations that it might be considered unnecessary to include them in the above list of requirements. However, *sun-screens*, as Draize (*Arch. Derm. Syph., Chicago*, 1951, vol. 64) has pointed out, *are unique as cosmetics in that their manner of use may involve multiple and extensive daily applications to large areas of the body surface and—in addition—they may be applied to skin already damaged by sun or wind burn.* Further, they may be used on persons of all age groups and in varying conditions of health.

Draize states that "... pharmacological and toxicologic tests should establish an 8-fold margin of safety and that this involves acute and sub-acute dermal toxicities and potential sensitisation studies. . . ."

Potential sun-screen compounds are found amongst chemical compounds possessing widely different physical and chemical characteristics which make it extremely difficult to classify them into chemical families. The 1939-45 War led to systematic investigation of a number of materials of cosmetic interest (soldiers fighting in tropical countries and—even more—airmen shot down over tropical islands with little or no suitable protective kit, required sun protective creams, insect bite preparations and so on). Intensified research on these problems led to the introduction of many scores of new organic materials which in turn had to be screened for efficacy and toxicity.

Klarmann (*Amer. Perfum.*, July-Aug. 1949) has given a comprehensive listing of some of the more commonly used sun-screen compounds and classified them as follows:

". . . Para-aminobenzoic acid and its derivatives (ethyl, isobutyl, glyceryl esters; para-dimethylaminobenzoic acid).

Anthranilates (i.e. ortho-aminobenzoates; methyl, menthyl, phenyl, benzyl, phenylethyl, linalyl, terpenyl and cyclohexenyl esters).

Salicylates (amyl, phenyl, benzyl, menthyl, glyceryl and dipropyleneglycol esters).

Cinnamic acid derivatives (menthyl and benzyl esters; alpha-phenyl cinnamonitrile; butyl cinnamoyl pyruvate).

Dihydroxycinnamic acid derivatives (umbelliferone, methyl-umbelliferone, methylaceto-umbelliferone).

Trihydroxycinnamic acid derivatives (esculetin, methylesculetin, daphnetin, and the glucosides esculin and daphnin).

Hydrocarbons (diphenylbutadiene, stilbene).

Dibenzalacetone and benzalacetophenone.

Naphthosulphonates (sodium salts of 2-naphthol-3,6-disulphonic and of 2-naphthol-6,8-disulphonic acids).

Dihydroxy-naphthoic acid and its salts.

Ortho- and para-hydroxybiphenyldisulphonates.

Coumarin derivatives (7-hydroxy, 7-methyl, 3-phenyl).

Diazoles (2-acetyl-3-bromoindazole, phenyl benzoxazole, methyl naphthoxazole, various aryl benzothiazoles).

Quinine salts (bisulphate, sulphate, chloride, oleate and tannate).

Quinoline derivatives (8-hydroxyquinoline salts, 2-phenylquinoline).

Uric and violuric acids.

Tannic acid and its derivatives (e.g. hexaethylether).

Hydroquinone. . . ."

He points out that isomerism plays an important role in determining absorptive capacity and illustrates this fact with obscuration (absorption) curves for ortho-, meta-, and para-aminobenzoic acids ; the superiority of the para-isomer over the ortho- and meta-isomers is quite apparent. By

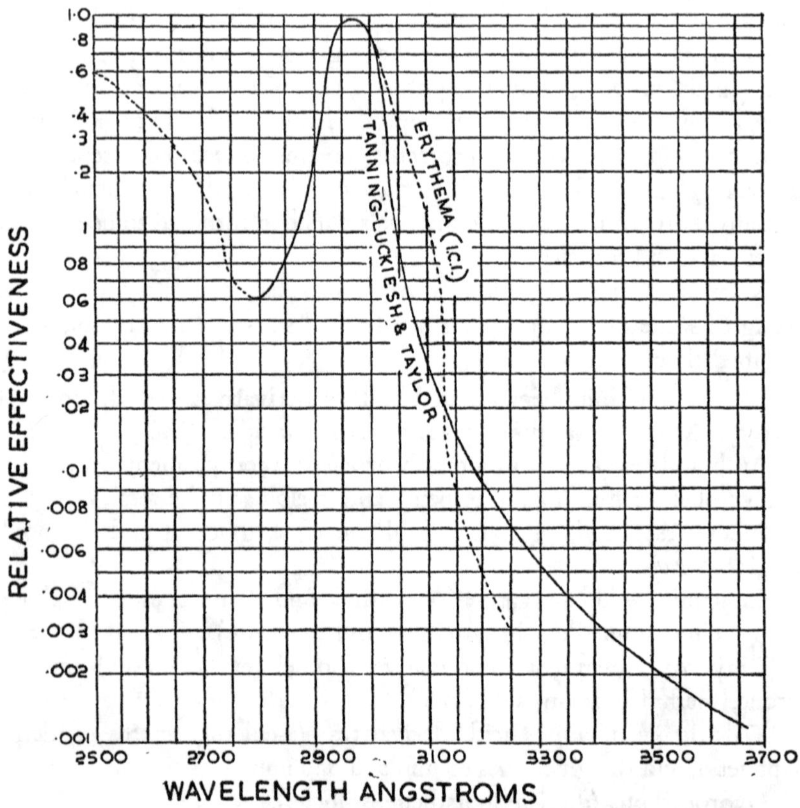

[*By courtesy of The American Perfumer*

FIG. 20.—Relative spectral effectiveness of radiant energy in the production of erythema (as adopted by the International Commission on Illumination) and tan (Luckiesh and Taylor).

way of contrast orthohydroxybenzoic (salicylic acid) has a high absorption value for erythemal radiation whilst parahydroxybenzoic acid has practically none.

Experiments on protective skin coatings for the prevention of sunburn have been carried out on behalf of the U.S. Army Air Forces. (*See* Luckiesh, Taylor, Cole and Sollmann, *J. Amer. med. Ass.*, 1946, **130,** 1.) In applying the results obtained to the cosmetic industry it must be remembered that the requirements of such a preparation for army use were exceedingly stringent and involved compliance with conditions which, *in toto*, are not likely to be generally encountered in the case of toilet preparations. Nevertheless, they give valuable indications of those substances which are of very definite value. Men marooned on life rafts or in the desert might be subject to very severe solar exposure without shelter and to either very high or very low temperature conditions, as well as to spray and waves. It was essential therefore that

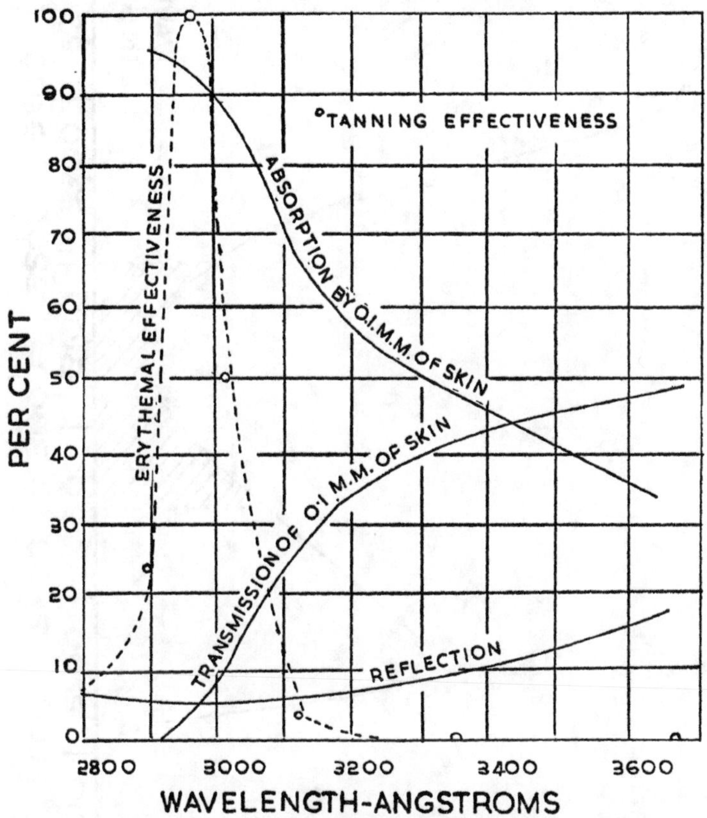

[*By courtesy of The American Perfumer*

FIG. 21.—Relative spectral erythemal effectiveness of radiant energy and the absorption (after Hasselbach) reflection and transmission (Luckiesh and Taylor) and transmission by 0·1 mm. of skin.

the substances chosen should give effective protection, should be stable at freezing and at tropical temperatures, should be free from rancidity, non-irritant, non-toxic and should be waterproof.

The screening agents tested included titanium dioxide, zinc oxide, phenyl salicylate, yellow petroleum jelly, amber petroleum jelly, zinc oxide ointment, lotions containing menthyl salicylate, a proprietary sun-preparation, dark red veterinary petroleum jelly, and several other

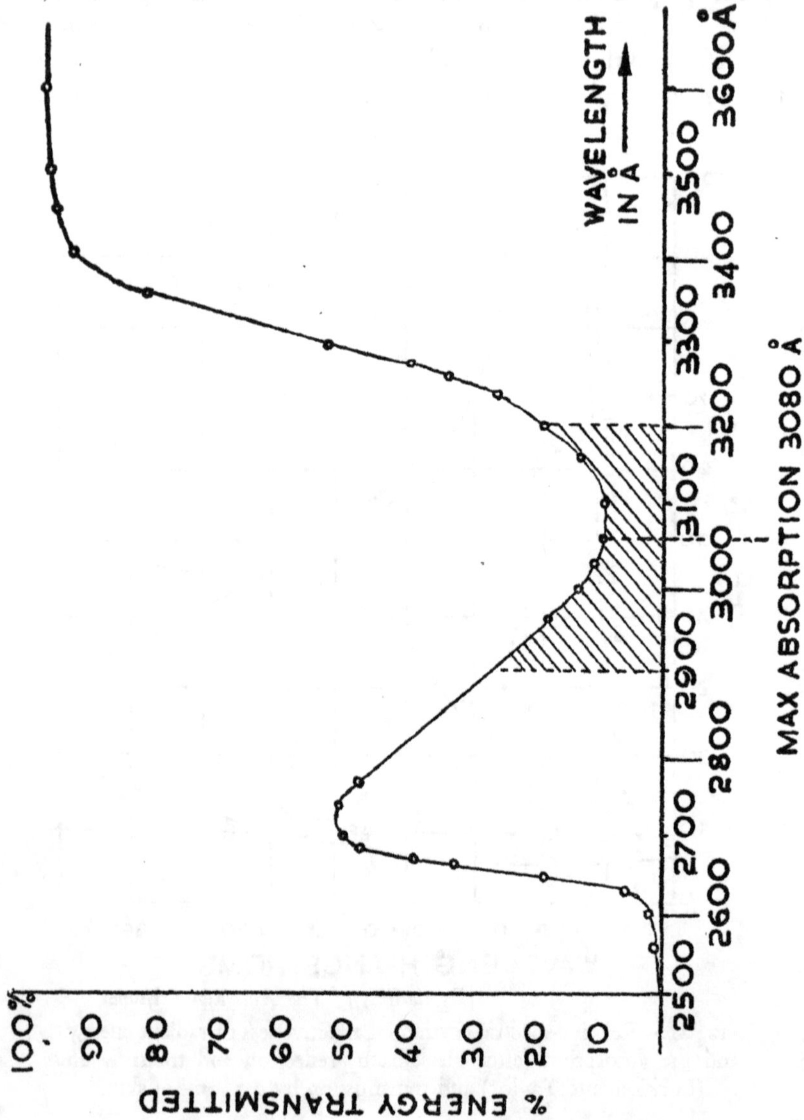

[*By courtesy of Givaudan & Cie.*

FIG. 22.—Transmission curve of ultra-violet rays through a bed of 0·02 mm. anti-solar preparation containing 5 per cent. of Parsol L.G.

grades of petroleum jelly. Various types of bases used included water-in-oil emulsions of lanolin and petroleum jelly, vanishing cream base, petroleum jelly base.

The specimens containing (*a*) titanium dioxide and vanishing cream, (*b*) phenyl salicylate in zinc oxide ointment, (*c*) proprietary sun-tan cream, (*d*) D. & R. sun-lotion containing menthyl salicylate, were found to be readily removed from the skin by slopping water over them, whereas the other products adhered tenaciously. Freezing experiments showed that it was advisable to avoid water in the compound. As a result of these investigations it was found that a dark red petroleum veterinary jelly (Standard Oil Co., New Jersey) was quite opaque to erythemal energy and served *on its own* to give complete protection to the skin in an exposure equivalent to 20 hours of the strongest sunlight measured during a four-year period in Cleveland. This compound was found to be non-irritant and to adhere tenaciously to the skin. Phenyl-salicylate (salol) was also found to be an excellent sun-screen when 10 per cent. was incorporated in a suitable base, such as petroleum jelly, particularly in a jelly having erythemal screening properties of its own. Experiments showed phenyl salicylate to be non-toxic. Zinc oxide was found of definite value also in preventing sunburn, but not in conjunction with phenyl salicylate with which results were not so good when zinc oxide was added. Titanium dioxide was not found to be a very dependable protective judged on a specimen containing 20 per cent. in yellow petroleum jelly. Menthyl salicylate and a mixture of Butesin, Metaphen and oleic acid ester amide diethylamine in cold cream were not found particularly good. Yellow petroleum jelly was found to possess dependable screening properties against ultra-violet energy at wavelengh 2967Å and 3022Å, far more than that possessed by white petroleum jelly.

A number of proprietary products have been based upon menthyl salicylate. Unlike some salicylates, the menthyl ester of salicylic acid is non-irritant, odourless and at concentrations of about 10 per cent. —initially—acts as a satisfactory sun-screen. However, as pointed out by deNavarre (*Chemistry and Manufacture of Cosmetics*, 1941, New York: Van Nostrand), menthyl salicylate undergoes chemical change on exposure to light with the result that its screening properties are "considerably diminished". Menthyl anthranilate is marketed under a proprietary designation by Givaudan-Delwanna Co. (U.S.A.) after carrying out a number of investigations into the screening properties of various salicylates (*The Givaudanian*, Dec. 1938). It is claimed that about 4 per cent. gives maximum effectiveness. The use of this material in cosmetic preparations is covered by U.S. Patent; licences under the patent are available.

The spectrophotometric transmission curve for menthyl anthranilate is given below:

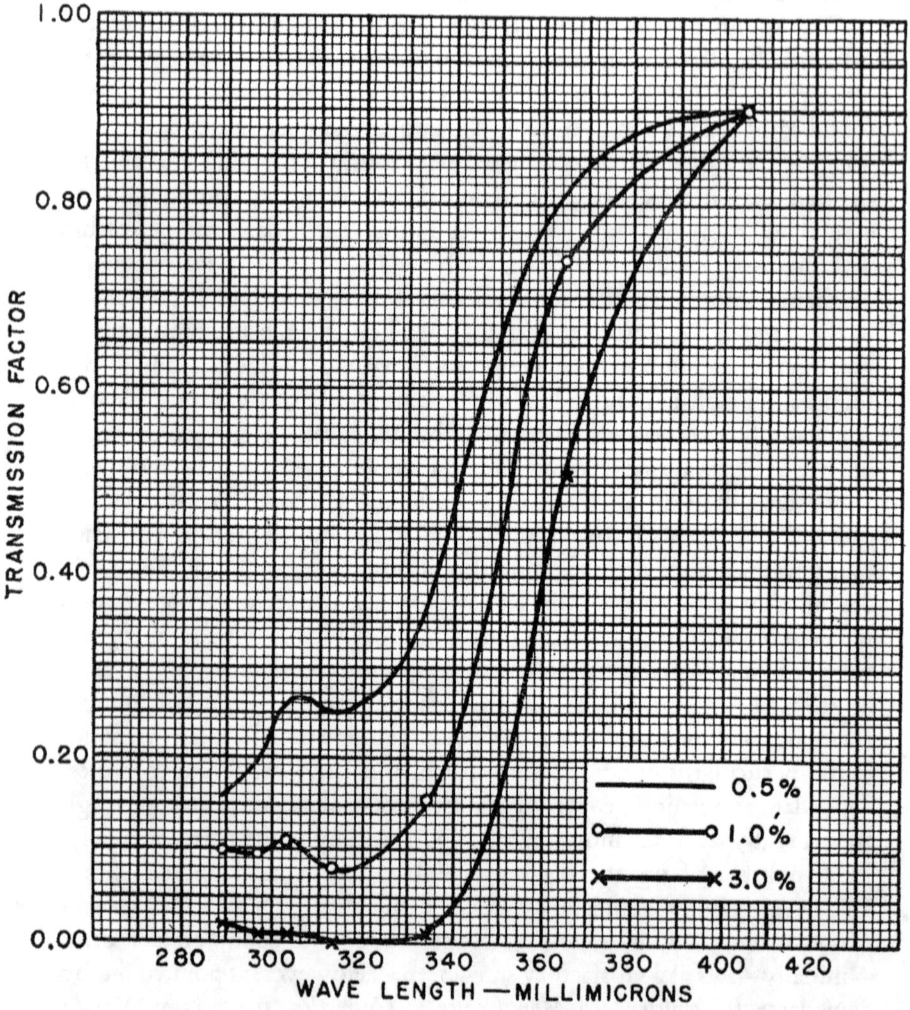

[*By courtesy of Givaudan-Delwanna.*

FIG. 23.—The spectrophotometric transmission curve for menthyl anthranilate. From Givaudan *Sunscreening Agents.*

A number of proprietary preparations are also available. It is not possible within the scope of this book to list all of these. One of these screens, with which the author has had excellent results, is "Solprotex", manufactured by Firmenich & Co. (Geneva). It is claimed by Firmenich that ". . . a team of research workers in collaboration with Professor Ruzicka, Nobel Prize Winner in 1939, tackled the problem of investigating sun-screen compositions . . . a suitable sun-screen would be the reverse of the curve of sensivity of the human skin to erythema. Such a product has been achieved in Solprotex. . . ." In a report on the physical, pharmacological and dermatological properties of Solprotex [L. W. Hazleton, J. Groopman and E. P. Morrish, *Proc. Sci. Sect. T.G.A.*, May 1950] it is stated that this material was an outstanding sun-screen preparation, upon which scientific tests had been conducted for the past fifteen years.

The spectrophotometric transmission curve of Solprotex together with a comparison of the sensitivity of the skin to erythema (after Hauser and Vahle)—with the absorption properties of this material—are reproduced on p. 250.

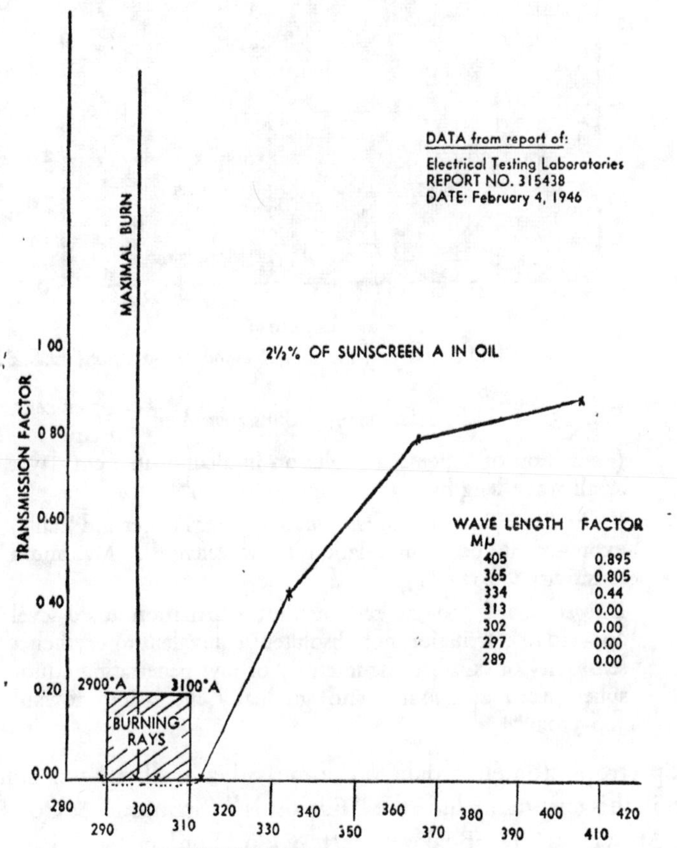

[*By courtesy of the Toilet Goods Association, U.S.A.*

FIG. 24.—Sunscreen A — "Solprotex". (From Hazleton, Groopman and Morrish, *loc. cit.*)

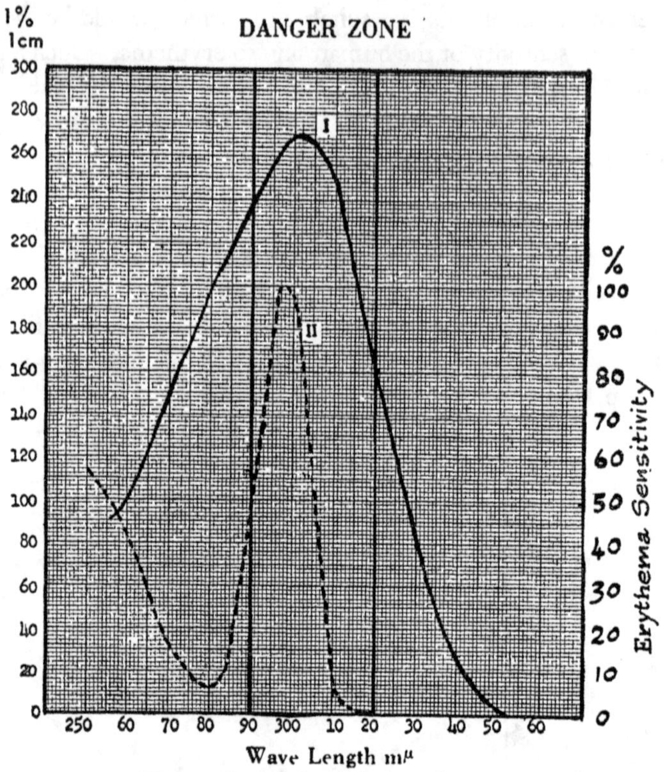

[*By courtesy of the Toilet Goods Association, U.S.A.*

FIG. 25.—I. *U.V. Absorption of Sunscreen A in E* $\frac{1 \text{ per cent.}}{1 \text{ cm.}}$ (extinction of 1 per cent. solution in alcohol in 1 cm. layer at all wave lengths in the range 250-350 m^{μ}).

II. *Erythema Sensitivity of Human Skin* (after Hauser and Vahle) expressed in per cent relation to wavelength. Maximum sensitivity: 297 m^{μ}.

Danger Zone; 290-320 m^{μ}, maximum irritation at sea level 295-310 m^{μ}. Irritation not absolutely equivalent to erythema sensitivity of skin because intensity of rays penetrating atmosphere zero at 290 m^{μ} and gradually increasing toward 300-310 m^{μ}.

Spectrophotometric data on some other well known sun-screens given in this chapter include the "Filtrosols" (Schimmel & Co., U.S.A.), the "Antivirays" (A. Boake Roberts & Co., England).; "Parsol L. G." (Givaudan & Cie.); "Iso-butyl-kelo-form" (Fries Bros.), etc.

Giese, Christensen and Jeppson (*J. Amer. pharm. Ass.*, Sci. edn., Jan. 1950) have prepared a list of a number of the sun-screens mentioned in the literature and have determined their extinction coefficients at

2970 Å, together with listing some of their physical properties. These are reproduced below:

Compound	*State*	*Solvent*	*Molecular weight*	*Extinction coefficient*	*Concentration per cent.*
Ethyl *p*-dimethyl aminobenzoate	Solid	Alcohol	194·13	27,000 27,300	1×10^{-4}
Ethyl *p*-aminobenzoate	„	„	165·19	21,750 21,450	2×10^{-4}
*Iso*butyl *p*-aminobenzoate	„	„	193·13	23,200 22,800	2×10^{-4}
Menthyl anthranilate	Liquid	„	275·374	941 956	5×10^{-4}
Homomenthyl salicylate	„	„	390·38	6,720 6,720	$2{\cdot}5 \times 10^{-4}$
Phenyl salicylate	Solid	„	214·08	3,850 3,900	5×10^{-4}
Menthyl salicylate	Liquid	„	276·19	4,540 4,600	5×10^{-4}
Amyl salicylate	„	„	208·12	4,150 3,970	5×10^{-4}
*Iso*amyl salicylate	„	„	208·12	348 381	5×10^{-4}
Benzyl salicylate	„	„	228·13	4,060 4,200	1×10^{-4}
Cinnamic acid	Solid	„	148·06	705 693	1×10^{-3}
Benzyl cinnamate	„	„	238·11	1,908 1,979	1×10^{-4}
Homomenthyl cinnamate	Liquid	„	300·32	505 530	5×10^{-4}
β-menthyl umbelliferone	Solid	„	176·066	8,510 8,560	5×10^{-4}
2-Naphthol-6-sulphonic acid	„	Water	304·28	3,310 3,240	5×10^{-3}
2-Naphthol-8-sulphonic acid	„	„	304·28	2,010 1,830	1×10^{-3}
3-Hydroxy-2-naphthoic acid	„	Alcohol	188·17	3,470 3,330	5×10^{-4}
Acetanilide	„	„	135·08	162	1×10^{-1}
Violuric acid	„	„	157·05	4,800 4,700	1×10^{-3}
Benzylacetophenone	„	„	208·196	24,200 23,900	1×10^{-4}
Quinine sulphate	„	„	548·39	3,500 3,500	4×10^{-4}

Pernich and Gallagher (*J. Soc. cosmet. Chem.*, Dec. 1950, p. 92) have reported transmission spectra data on a number of examples from the various "families" of sun-screens,[1] namely, two-*p*-aminobenzoates, several salicylates, pyrones such as cinnamates, umbelliferones, coumarins, naphthoic acid, benzylacetophenone, tannic acid, violuric acid and quinine sulphate.

These investigators found that ". . . on the basis of the transmission spectra compared on per cent. content of sun-screen, the following compounds head the list as efficient sunscreens : ethyl-*p*-dimethyl-amino-benzoate, isobutyl-p-aminobenzoate, coumarin, 8-methoxycoumarin, 5.7-dihydroxy-4-methylcoumarin, 6-aminocoumarin, umbelliferone, benzyl-b-methyl-umbelliferone, and benzylacetophenone, whilst the poorest are dicoumarol, 2-naphthol-8-sulphonic acid, 2-naphthol-6-sulphonic acid, 3-hydroxy-2-naphtholic and violuric acid. The other compounds fall in between."

The transmission spectra for the most efficient of these compounds are reproduced below :

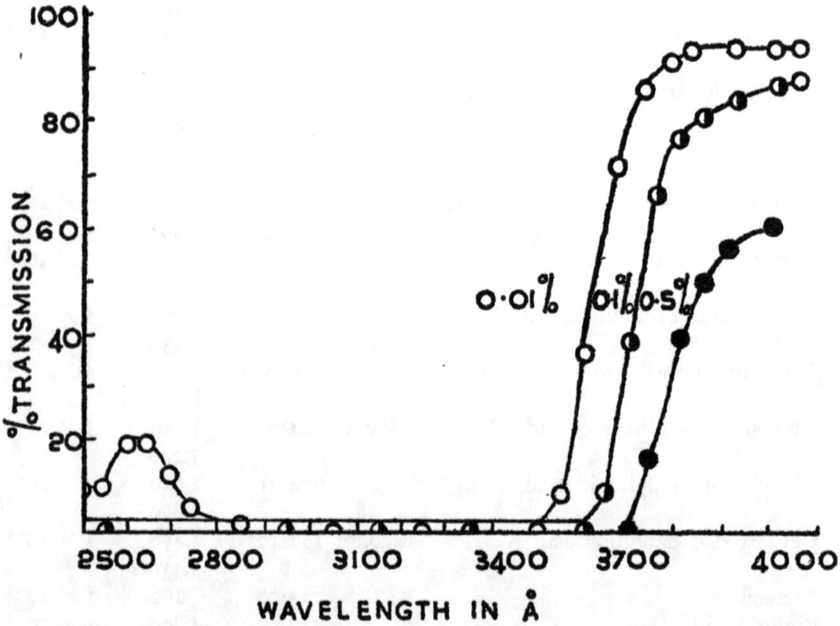

[*By courtesy of Pernich and Gallagher, J. Soc. cosmet. Chem., Dec.* 1950.

FIG. 26.—Transmission spectra of 0·5 cm. layers of umbelliferone (in alcohol).

[1] All the sun-screens used in this study were made available by the co-operation of the American cosmetic authority, Maison deNavarre, as were the various samples of oils also tested.

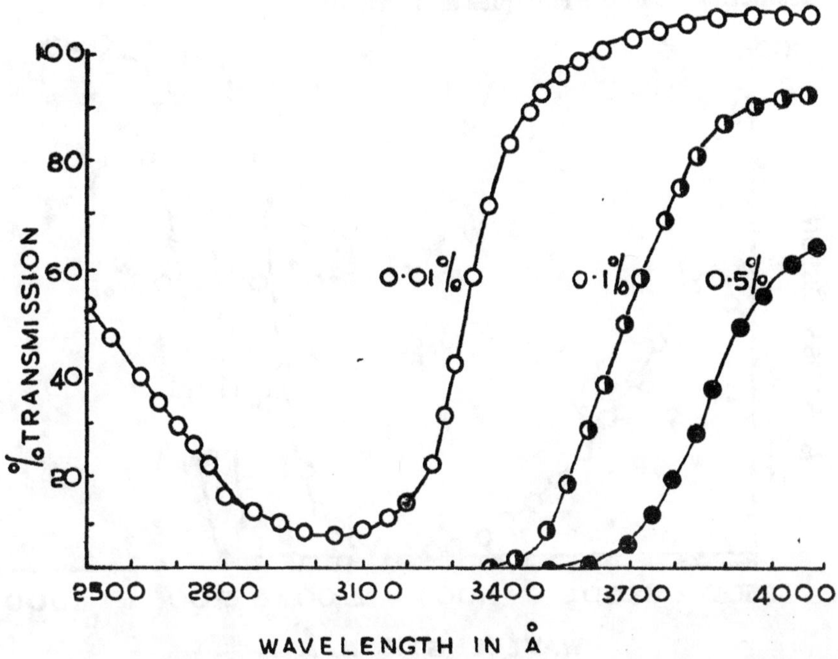

[*By courtesy of Pernich and Gallagher, J. Soc. cosmet. Chem.*, Dec. 1950.

FIG. 27.—Transmission spectra of 0·5 cm. layers of benzyl-acetophenone (in alcohol).

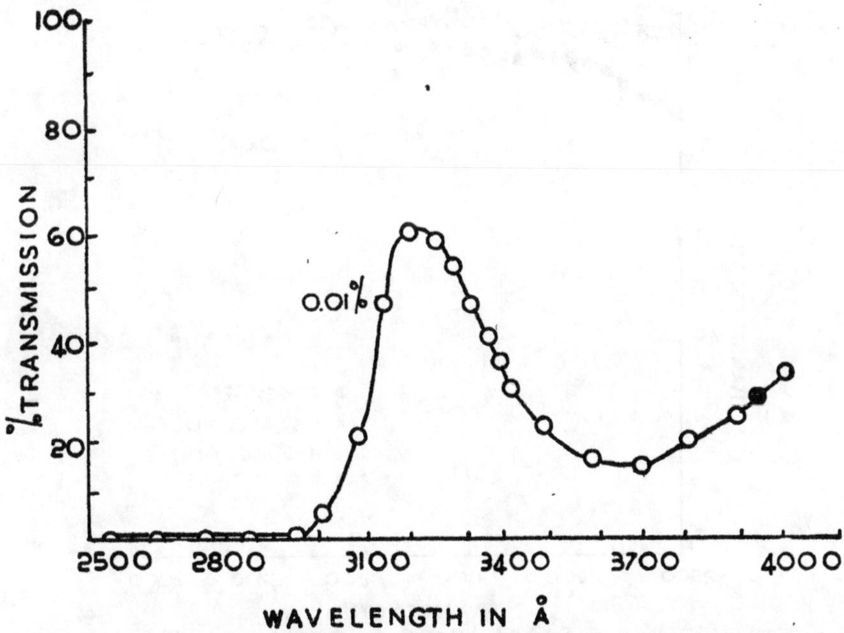

[*By courtesy of Pernich and Gallagher, J. Soc. cosmet. Chem.*, Dec. 1950,

FIG. 28.—Transmission spectrum of 0·01 per cent. 6-amino-coumarin in alcohol. The higher concentrations (0·1 and 0·5 per cent.) showed no transmission over the entire range.

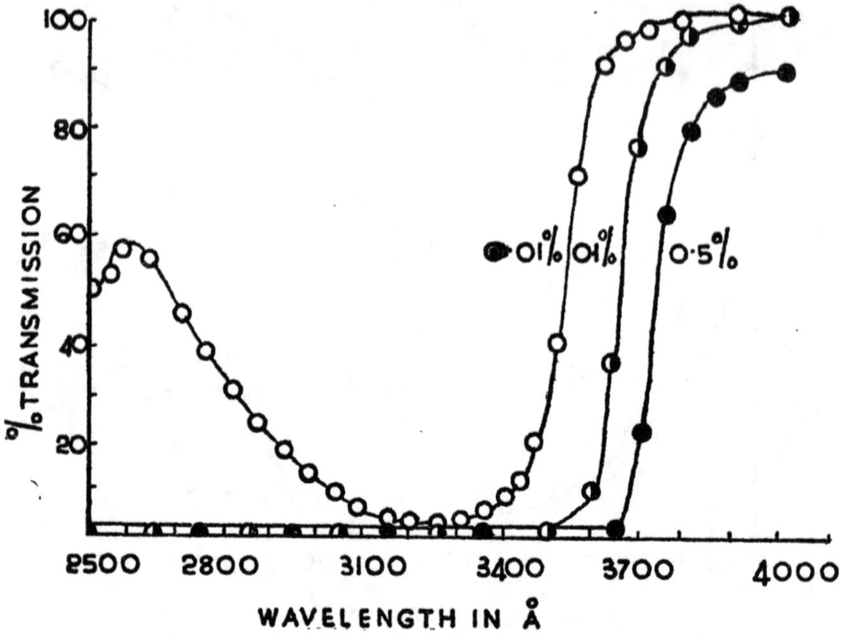

[*By courtesy of Pernich and Gallagher, J. Soc. cosmet. Chem., Dec.* 1950.

FIG. 29.—Transmission spectra of 0·5 cm. layers of benzyl-B-methyl umbelliferone (in alcohol).

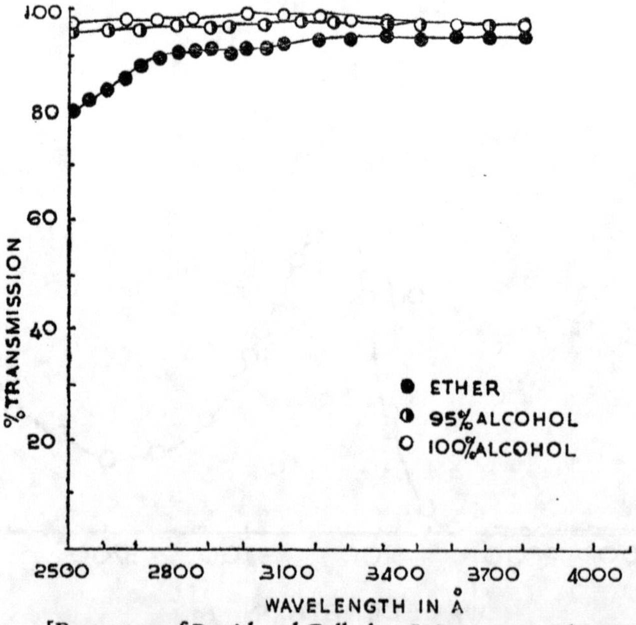

[*By courtesy of Pernich and Gallagher, J. Soc. cosmet. Chem., Dec.* 1950.

FIG. 30.—Transmission spectra of 0·5 cm. layers of absolute and 95 per cent. alcohol and of ether (control).

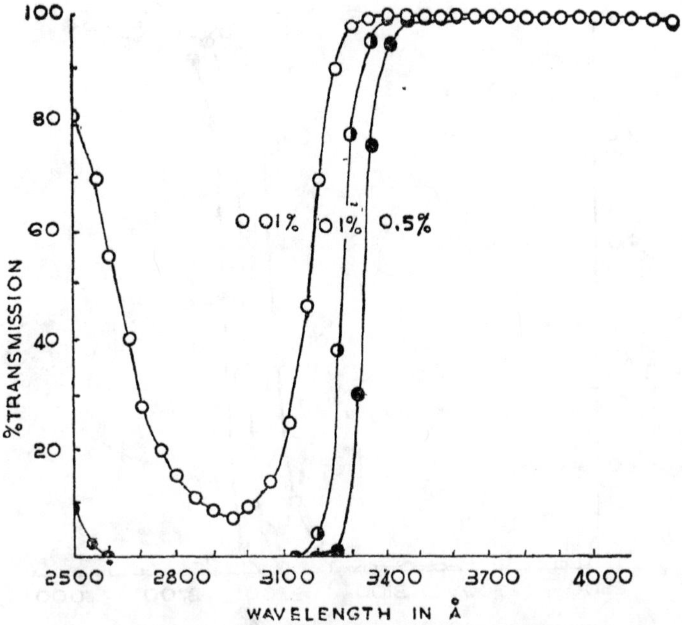

[*By courtesy of Pernich and Gallagher, J. Soc. cosmet. Chem., Dec.* 1950.

FIG. 31.—Transmission spectra of 0·5 cm. layers of isobutyl-*p*-aminobenzoate (in alcohol).

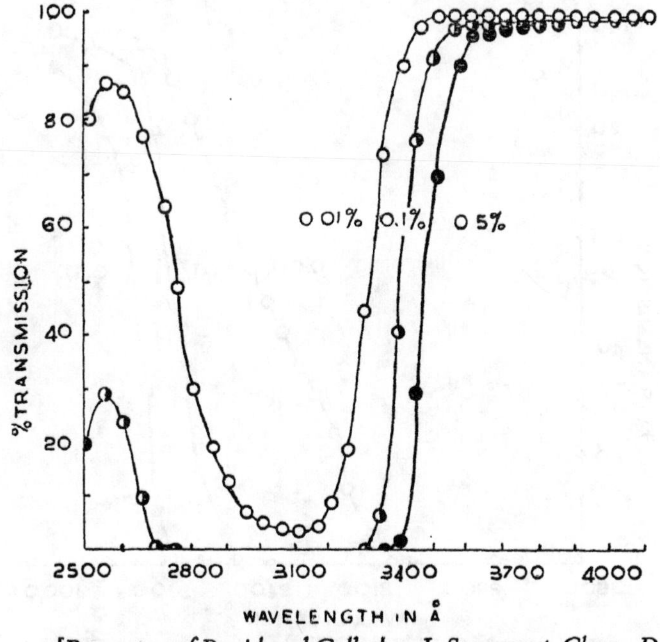

[*By courtesy of Pernich and Gallagher, J. Soc. cosmet. Chem., Dec.* 1950.

FIG. 32.—Transmission spectra of 0·5 cm. layers of different concentrations of ethyl-*p*-dimethyl-amino-benzoate (in alcohol).

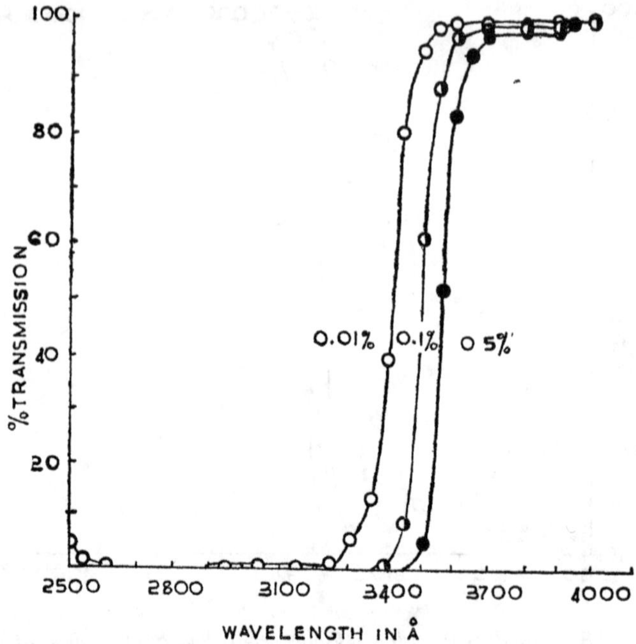

[*By courtesy of Pernich and Gallagher, J. Soc. cosmet. Chem., Dec.* 1950.

FIG. 33.—Transmission spectra of 0·5 cm. layers of coumarin (in alcohol).

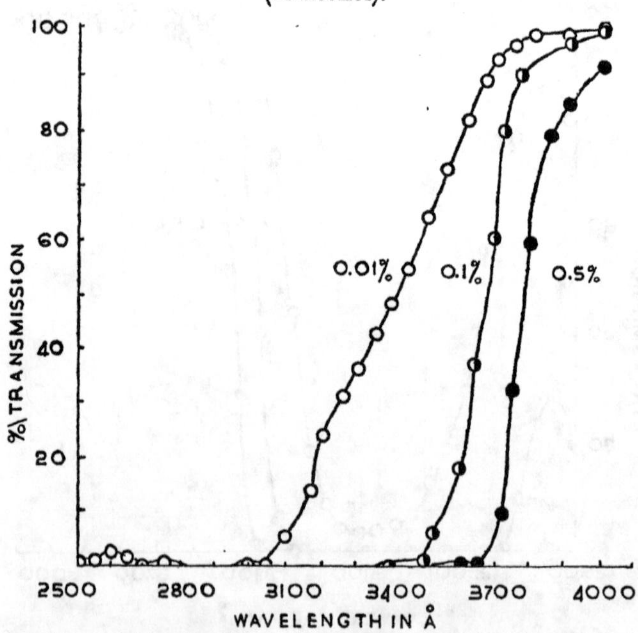

[*By courtesy of Pernich and Gallagher, J. Soc. cosmet. Chem., Dec.* 1950.

FIG. 34.—Transmission spectra of 0·5 cm. layers of 8-methoxy-coumarin (in alcohol).

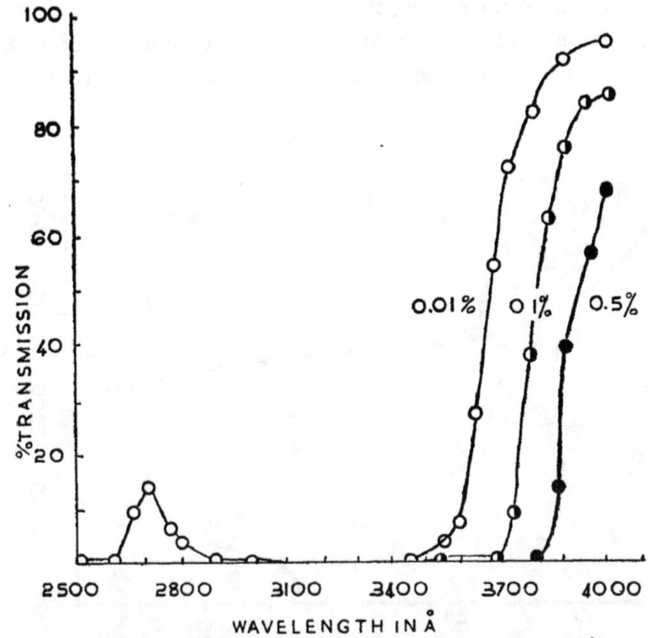

[*By courtesy of Pernich and Gallagher, J. Soc. cosmet. Chem. Dec.* 1950.

FIG. 35.—Transmission spectra of 0·5 cm. layers of 5, 7-dihydroxy-4-methylcoumarin (in alcohol).

EVALUATION OF THE EFFICACY OF SUN-SCREENS. Different authors have suggested different methods of determining the efficacy of a sun-screen.

In general these methods involve a preliminary sorting-out of materials by means of spectrophotometric tests, a further " weeding out" of such materials on the grounds of toxicity, sensitising properties, physical attributes, etc. The ultimate test can only be made by means of carefully controlled user tests.

The following description by Klarmann (*Amer. Perfum.*, July-Aug. 1949) is of Stambovsky's method (*New Jersey J. Pharmacy*, Aug. 1947): " . . . this method provides for the use of radiation generated by a quartz mercury lamp and filtered with Corex D glass ; the latter is practically impervious to radiation of 2800 Å but it transmits 50 per cent. of energy of 2950 Å and 72 per cent. of 3000 Å.

" The calibration is carried out first by determining the time required to produce the minimum perceptible erythema at a given distance from untreated, untanned skin. A 500 watt lamp will produce such erythema usually in one minute at a distance of 12 inches from the skin. To this end the anterior portion of the forearm is used (which is rarely exposed to the sun and therefore retains its sensitiveness to erythemal radiation).

Starting 1 in. below the elbow, three ½ in. sectors are outlined with strips of adhesive tape. The sectors are numbered consecutively 1, 2 and 3. With a sheet of opaque paper, sectors 2 and 3 are covered while sector 1

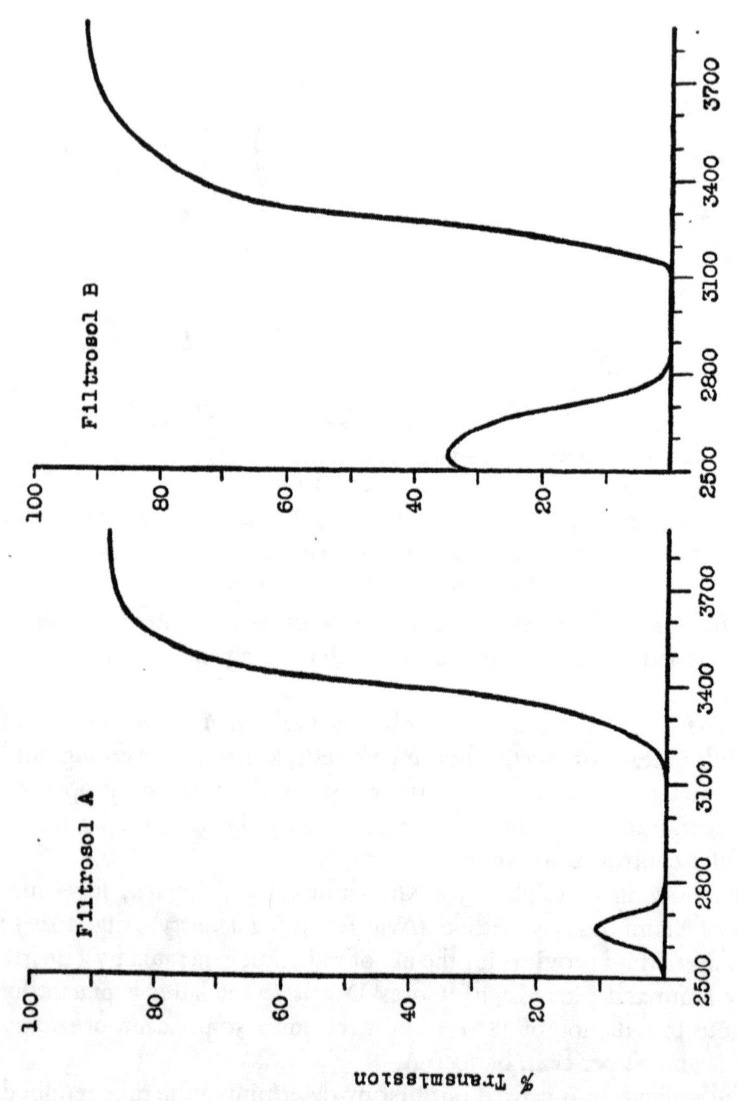

FIG. 36.—Transmission spectra of Filtrosols A and B. [*By courtesy of Schimmel & Co., U.S.A.*

is irradiated for 1 minute. Then sector 2 is exposed and finally sector 3; thus sector 1 receives a total exposure of 3 minutes, sector 2 one of 2 minutes and sector 3 one of 1 minute. Readings are taken after about 10 hours at which time the test of the particular sun-screen is started.

"The preparation under investigation is applied to the other forearm in the same manner as would be used in practice. Again strips of adhesive tape are attached; but this time five sectors are exposed. Using opaque

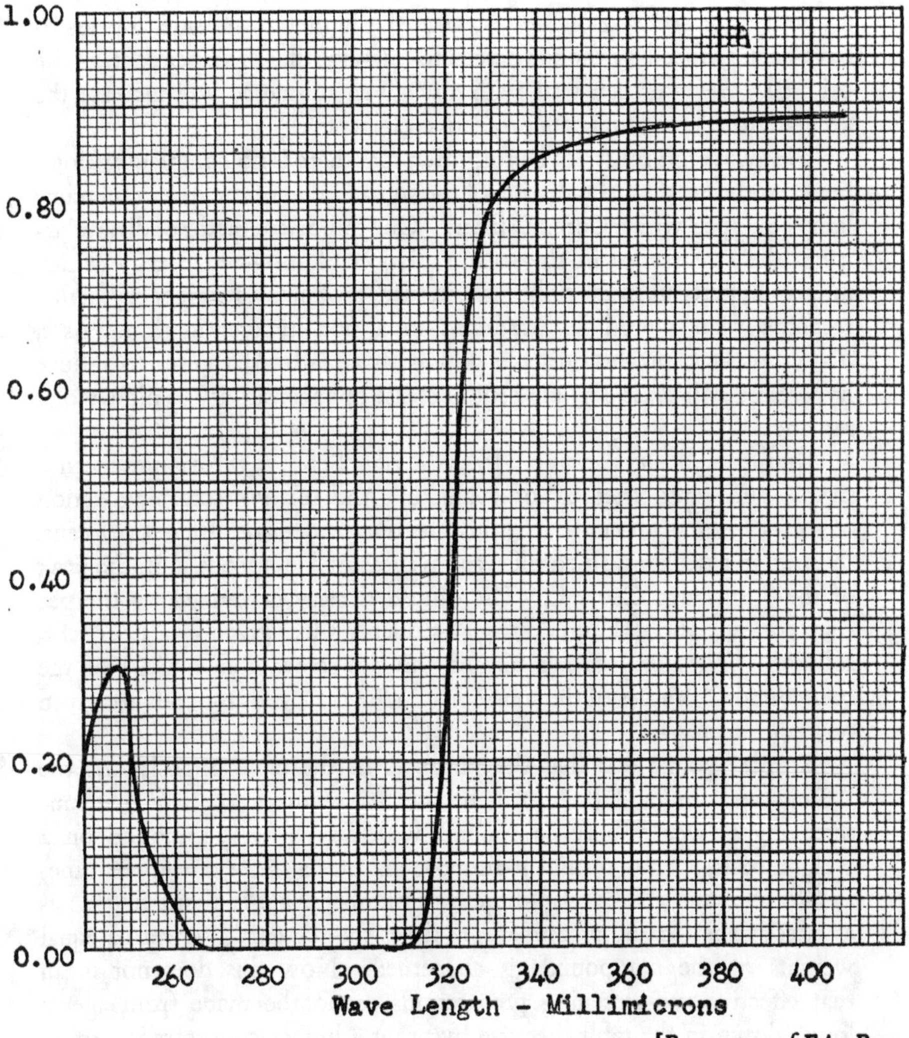

[*By courtesy of Fries Bros.*

FIG. 37.—U.V. transmission of iso-butyl kelo-form sample (0·5 gm. per cent.).

paper to cover the other sectors, sector 1 is irradiated first for 2 minutes, then the paper is moved so as to expose sectors 1 and 2, and radiation is continued for 2 minutes, etc. In this fashion at the end of the irradiation period, sector 1 will have been exposed for 10 minutes, sector 2 for 8 minutes, sector 3 for 6 minutes, sector 4 for 4 minutes, and sector 5 for

2 minutes. If after 10 hours sector 2 shows a perceptible erythema while sector 3 shows no response, then the effect produced in sector 2 will be comparable to that in sector 1 of the control irradiation. Since the latter required an exposure time of 1 minute on the control arm against that of 8 minutes for sector 2 of the test arm, the light transmission appears to have been reduced by the sun-screen to one-eighth, i.e. 12 per cent. of the original. Several such tests with any given substance will increase the accuracy of determining its protective efficiency.

" However, it must not be forgotten that there is no complete analogy between the erythemal radiation of the sun and that of the quartz mercury lamp equipped with a Corex D filter. One important factor of dissimilarity is the occurrence in the solar radiation of infra-red energy which induces hyperemia in the skin; this, in turn, produces a stronger erythemic response than would be produced in a non-hyperemic skin. As a matter of fact, pre-heating the skin with an infra-red lamp to induce hyperemia will cause a 33 per cent. increase in its sensitivity to ultra-violet radiation."

Kumler (*J. Amer. pharm. Ass., Sci. edn.*, Sept. 1952) has proposed a simple and rapid method of evaluating the relative screening action of sun-screen compounds. In this, the optical density of a 0·1 per cent. solution in a 0·1 mm. fused silica cell is measured at 3080 Å unit, the peak of the " Sunburn Curve ". The optical density is divided by the per cent. concentration, thus reducing all values to those given by a 1 per cent. solution. These values are termed the sun-screen index (S.I.) of the compounds. Values of the sun-screen index for 45 compounds are given on opposite page.

Kumler points out that the numbers in the table opposite for the " Sun-screen Index " (S.I.), can be used to compare the effective sun-screening power of any compound with any other compound on a weight basis. Thus propyl *p*-amino-benzoate is 9·0/3·0 = three times as effective, and the ethyl *p*-dimethylaminobenzoate is about five times as effective as 3-carboxycoumarin as far as the screening power of equal weights of the compounds is concerned. Now this does not mean that effective sun-screening preparations cannot be made from agents lower down in the table, because by using a higher concentration of an agent low in the list the same screening can be achieved as with a low concentration of some other agent above it. Thus a 3 per cent. solution of 3-carboxycoumarin would have as much protective action as a 1 per cent. solution of propyl *p*-aminobenzoate, considering only the relative absorbing characteristics of the compounds themselves.

Sometimes other factors enter into the effectiveness of the ultimate preparations, such as the thickness of the film that is formed on the skin

Compound	Sunscreen Index (S.I.) Optical Density at 3,080 Å Conc. 1 per cent.
Ethyl *p*-dimethylaminobenzoate	14·8
Ethyl *p*-aminobenzoate	9·6
Isobutyl *p*-aminobenzoate	9·2
Propyl *p*-aminobenzoate	9·0
n-Butyl *p*-aminobenzoate	8·0
β-Methyl umbelliferone	7·7
p-Aminobenzoic acid	7·4
Dehydracetic acid	7·0
3-Carbethoxycoumarin	6·6
Benzilidine camphor	6·6
Heliotropine	6·5
Umbelliferone acetic acid	6·0
Salicylic acid	4·3
Sodium *p*-aminosalicylate	4·3
Methyl salicylate	4·0
Salicylamide	3·9
Methylenedisalicylic acid	3·0
3-Carboxycoumarin	3·0
Thiosalicylic acid	2·7
Brightener W/450	2·7
p-Hydroxyanthranilic acid	2·6
Sodium salicylate	2·4
Digaloyltrioleate	2·3
α-Reslorcylic acid	2·2
Salicylaldehyde	2·2
p-Aminosalicylic acid	1·9
Dipropyleneglycol salicylate	1·9
Pyribenzamine	1·8
Pyrianisamine maleate	1·7
Sodium gentisate	1·7
Fluorescent white	1·6
Ethnolamide of gentisic acid	1·5
Ethal gallate	1·4
Sodyum sulphadiazine	1·2
Ethiyl vanillate	1·1
Sodium sulphapyridine	0·95
Lauryl gallate	0·85
Totaquine	0·80
Barbituric acid	0·19
Chlorophyll	0·15
Amberlite IR-4-B	0·15
Salicyl alcohol	0·05
Anisic acid	0·01
Uvitex RBS	0·01
Uvitex RS	0·005

when the preparation is applied, the decomposition of the compound in the presence of light, etc. If this film is twice as thick in one case as in another, the protective action of the one preparation would be double that of the other, although the two preparations might contain equal amounts of the same sun-screen compound. Factors of this type are not taken into account by the figures in the table. This and perhaps some other factors can be evaluated only by actual tests on human subjects. However, one is frequently concerned not with these other factors but only with the relative effectiveness of various compounds on a weight basis in absorbing the rays that cause sunburn, and on that basis, the values of the sun-screen index given in the table have significance.

The " Sun-screen Index " (S.I.) of the compound can be used to calculate the per cent. of the compound that should be incorporated to screen out a certain percentage of the sun-burn-producing rays under any given set of conditions. For example, U.S. armed forces have set up specifications that a preparation shall not transmit more than 1 per cent. of the rays in the sunburn region through a film 0·001 inch thick. One can calculate what per cent. of any one of the above compounds would have to be incorporated in a preparation to give this amount of screening. The figures in the table are for a cell 0·1 mm. or $0{\cdot}1/10 \times 2{\cdot}5 = 0{\cdot}004$ inch thick. A transmission of 1 per cent. corresponds to an optical density of 2. Therefore if x is the per cent. of the compound that would have to be incorporated for 1 per cent. transmission under these conditions, then

$$x = \frac{2 \times 4}{\text{S.I.}} = \frac{8}{\text{S.I.}}.$$

Thus for *n*-butyl *p*-aminobenzoate, x would be equal to $8 = (8/8) = 1$ per cent. and for methyl salicylate it would have a value of $x = (8/4) = 2$ per cent. This signifies that a 1 per cent. solution of the former and a 2 per cent. solution of the latter when present in a film 0·001 inch thick would transmit 1 per cent. of the rays in the sunburn region. Since the specifications call for a transmission of less than 1 per cent. the actual concentration used would have to be higher. Allowing for a safety factor of 100 per cent., the concentration for *n*-butyl-*p*-aminobenzoate should be 2 per cent. and for methyl salicylate 4 per cent.

The choice of base for a sunburn preparation is controversial. Where aesthetic considerations are dominant, the oily or greasy base may well be criticised on the grounds that such a preparation picks up sand and grit and is messy in use (some people even state they " frizzle " under the fats). Such persons will choose a non-greasy cream or lotion. On the other hand, the experiments carried out on behalf of the U.S. Army Air Forces, reported earlier in this chapter, show that the fatty base *per se*, may play an important part in skin protection ; moreover, such preparations are not washed off in swimming, so that those who prefer a lasting " screen " may choose a screen of the greasy, or of the water-in-oil type.

The following are some examples of bases of various types. It should be remembered that the *concentration of active sun-screen* necessary (and desirable), *will vary with the particular screen* chosen for test (as a result of studying the above data on various screens) so that it is not possible to give detailed examples except in specific instances. Moreover, it will be found that very many of the creams and lotions listed in other chapters in this book (*see* Chapters 5, 6, 9, 10, 39, etc.) may be used with suitable modification, in the formulation of such products.

Sun-tan oil

	per cent.
Sesame oil	25·0
Mineral oil	50·0
Isopropyl myristate	25·0
Sun-screen	*q.s.*
Perfume	*q.s.*
Antioxidant	*q.s.*
Colour	*q.s.*

	per cent.
Sesame oil	40·0
Olive oil	10·0
Solprotex	2·5
Mineral oil	47·5
Antioxidant	*q.s.*
Perfume	*q.s.*
Colour	*q.s.*

Procedure

By simple solution (in each of the above instances).

Cream type

	per cent.
(*a*) Stearic acid	15·00
(*b*) Potassium hydroxide	0·50
(*c*) Sodium hydroxide	0·18
(*d*) Cetyl alcohol	0·50
(*e*) Lanolin	2·00
(*f*) Glycerin	5·00
(*g*) Water	76·82
(*h*) Sun-screen	*q.s.*
(*i*) Preservative	*q.s.*
(*j*) Perfume	*q.s.*

Procedure

(1) Heat (*a*), (*d*) and (*e*) at 75° C. until homogeneous.

(2) Heat (*b*), (*c*), (*f*), (*g*) and (*i*) until homogeneous. Adjust temperature to 75° C.

Add (2) to (1) with gentle but continuous stirring. Stir down to 45° C. Incorporate perfume. Stand 24-48 hours. Mill or homogenise.

[Note: Sun-screen compound will be dissolved in the oil, or the aqueous phase (according to its solubility), and included in the cream. If the screen is not stable at elevated temperature, or not stable to alkali, etc., it may be dissolved in a separate portion of one of the constituents; in some cases, for example, Solprotex 3, it may be simply stirred into the finished cream. Such cream must not contact iron but should be stored in opal jars or in aluminium.]

The following creams are based on non-ionic emulsifiers:

	per cent.
(*a*) Polawax (Croda)	14·0
(*b*) Lanolin	2·0
(*c*) Petroleum jelly	2·0
(*d*) Mineral oil	1·0
(*e*) Glycerin	7·0
(*f*) Sun-screen [1]	*q.s.*
(*g*) Water	74·0
(*h*) Preservative	*q.s.*
(*i*) Perfume	*q.s.*

Procedure

(1) Heat (*a*), (*b*), (*c*) and (*d*) to 75° C.

(2) Heat (*e*), (*g*) and (*h*) to 75° C.
(If stable, dissolve (*f*) in the appropriate phase (1) or (2).)

Add (2) to (1). Stir down to 45° C., perfume and continue stirring to 25°-30° C.

	per cent.
(*a*) Hysterene T.70 (70 per cent. stearic acid)	15·0
(*b*) Isopropyl palmitate	1·0
(*c*) Arlacel 60	2·0
(*d*) Tween 60	1·5
(*e*) Arlex (Atlas commercial sorbitol soln.)	2·5
(*f*) Water	78·0
(*g*) Sun-screen	*q.s.*
(*h*) Preservative	*q.s.*
(*i*) Perfume	*q.s.*

Procedure

(1) Heat together (*a*), (*b*), (*c*) and (*d*) until dissolved.

(2) Heat together (*e*), (*f*), (*g*) (if water-soluble and stable at this temperature) and (*h*) and raise temperature of this solution to 95° C.

Add (1) at 90° C. to (2) at 95° C. with thorough agitation. Perfume at 50° C. Stir occasionally, stand 24 hours and pack.

[This formula is identical with a formula given in *Drug Cosmet. Ind.*, Feb. 1950 (Advert. Sect.), but with sun-screen included.]

[1] If the amount of sun-screen chosen is large, the water content of this cream should be reduced to compensate for it.

More greasy creams of this type may be made along the following lines :

	per cent.
Glyceryl monostearate (self-emulsifying)	16·0
Cetyl alcohol	1·0
Mineral oil	10·0
Sesame oil	10·0
Glycerin	7·0
Water	56·0
Sun-screen	*q.s.*
Antioxidant	*q.s.*
Preservative	*q.s.*
Perfume	*q.s.*

or along the lines discussed for cold creams, all-purpose creams, foundation creams and " make-up " preparations. (*See* Index.) For the formulation of liquid creams and milks refer to the appropriate chapters. Manufacturing procedure will be found under these preparations.

Amongst " type formulae " quoted by Klarmann (*Amer. Perfum.*, July-Aug. 1949) for sunburn preparations are the following :

Sun-tan Cream (liquid)	per cent.
Diethyleneglycol monostearate	2·0
Stearic acid	1·5
Cetyl alcohol	0·5
Menthyl anthranilate	5·0
Triethanolamine	1·0
Water	90·0
Perfume	*q.s.*

Sunshade ointment	per cent.
Calamine	15·0
Petrolatum, yellow	37·5
Lanolin	12·5
Water	35·0
Perfume, colour	*q.s.*

Quartermaster Corps sunburn cream	per cent.
Glycerylmonostearate	13·00
Lanolin	4·70
Propylene glycol	4·70
Titanium dioxide	2·50
Sodium lauryl sulphate	0·05
Isobutyl-*p*-aminobenzoate	2·00
Isopropyl myristate-palmitate	20·00
Water	53·05
Colour	*q.s.*

Sun cream (N.F. VIII)	*per cent.*
Phenyl salicylate	5·00
Ethyl aminobenzoate	2·00
Titanium dioxide	1·00
Neocalamine	1·00
Yellow ferric oxide	0·10
Coumarin	0·10
White wax	2·00
Triethanolamine	0·50
Stearyl alcohol	8·00
Stearic acid	2·00
Glycerin	10·00
Water	68·30
Perfume	*q.s.*

The following two examples are from Schimmels Briefs, No. 205 April 1952:

Sun-tan lotion	*per cent.*
Methyl cellulose	0·5
Glycerin	2·0
Alcohol	10·0
Water	80·5
Filtrosol B	7·0
Perfume	*q.s.*

Sun-tan cream	*per cent.*
Stearic acid	6·00
Cetyl alcohol	0·50
Filtrosol A	5·00
Preservative	*q.s.*
Veegum [1]	2·28
Water	85·42
Borax	0·50
Potassium hydroxide	0·30
Perfume	*q.s.*

Preparations Simulating Skin-tan

These may be formulated in either oils, creams, lotions or powders, and consist of a solution of a suitable dye in oil or water, or alternatively of a powdered pigment. Water-soluble dyes, however, will streak on exposure to rain or moisture, and oil-soluble dyes are used instead. A vegetable product may be obtained by extracting cudbear and henna with warm deodorised olive oil (8 and 2 per cent., respectively), the ratio of the vegetable dyestuffs being altered as desired.

[1] R. T. Vanderbilt Co.

A more modern procedure is the use of suitable oil-soluble dyestuffs for this purpose. Heavily pigmented face powders, or modifications of the " cosmetic stocking ", may also be used. In conjunction with suitable shades of make-up excellent effects may be obtained.

PALLIATIVE PREPARATIONS

Preparations for the relief of sunburn may be formulated on the basis of calamine lotion, or other zinc preparations, or upon tannic acid.

In connection with this, manufacturers should note that sun " burns " are quite capable of producing exactly the same injury as steam burns, and the consequent risk of infection by bacteria and of absorption of the damaged proteins is still present. For this reason such preparations should be antiseptic.

Calamine lotion type	*per cent.*
Colloidal calamine	20·0
Glycerin	5·0
Water	75·0
Antiseptic	*q.s.*

Nadkarni and Zopf (*J. Amer. pharm. Ass., Sci. edn.*, 1948, **9**, 212) have suggested the following improved calamine lotion :

Zinc oxide	8·0 g.
Prepared calamine	8·0 g.
Polyethylene glycol 400	8·0 cc.
Polyethylene glycol 400 monostearate	3·0 g.
Lime water	60·0 cc.
Water *q.s. ad*	to 100·0 cc.

Triethanolamine milks are also soothing :

	per cent.
Triethanolamine stearate	4·80
Liquid paraffin	10·00
Water	85·20
Antiseptic	*q.s.*

If desired 10 per cent. colloidal calamine may be added to this mixture, which is prepared by heating the stearate and oil to 70° C. and adding to the water at the same temperature or preferably by preparing the triethanolamine stearate *in situ*. The choice of a suitable antiseptic is a matter of individual preference, many of the new chlorinated compounds (*see* Antiseptics) are good germicides and are non-irritant and innocuous in ordinary concentrations. For badly burnt areas the inclusion of a local anaesthetic or analgesic is indicated, but in view of the dangers of absorption this should be chosen with care. The treatment of a serious burn should be carried out under medical supervision. Tannic acid may be used on minor burns when no lesion is present, but modern medical opinion is against its routine use for burns.

	per cent.
Tannic acid	2·0
Glycerin	5·0
Water	92·5
Phenol	0·5

In general greasy preparations should not be used in the treatment of sun burn. They only retain the heat of the burn and prevent the use of an antiseptic capable of mixing with the secretions and preventing bacterial infection.

All such preparations should be either aqueous solutions or oil-in-water emulsions which are capable of exerting both a protective and cooling effect.

CHAPTER 14

ACNE PREPARATIONS

ACNE vulgaris, often termed simple " acne ", is an inflammatory disease of the skin involving the sebaceous glandular system, occurring generally in adolescence and post-adolescence. It is characterised essentially by the appearance of comedones (blackheads) which may be accompanied by papules and occur usually on the face, although the neck, back and shoulders may be involved. Unfortunately, acne is still regarded by the general public as a somewhat trivial complaint which will cure itself in time. Actually, when neglected, serious and permanent scarring of the skin may result. Treatment of acne should be carried out by a dermatologist. The frequency of its occurrence in adolescence and the reluctance of the sufferers to seek medical aid, however, make it desirable to record briefly some facts about this complaint and details of simple palliative measures, since the treatment of spots at adolescence is still regarded by the layman as within the province of the " beauty specialist ", or, even worse, as within his or her own capabilities.

As Williams (*Practitioner*, May 1948, p. 367) has pointed out, " . . . certain factors concerning the relationship between the sex hormones and the skin are well known. Acne vulgaris commonly, almost physiologically arises at the time of puberty and persists for varying periods, up to perhaps the age of 30. It is more common in males than in females. . . . Whatever may be its cause or causes, and the literature is vast and contradictory, and at whatever time of life it occurs, the essential fact is that androgens predispose to acne and oestrogens inhibit it." It is pointed out that the severity of the condition depends upon individual susceptibility, on tissue susceptibility and on secondary factors such as dirt and infection and that it is against these secondary factors that treatment must first be directed.

The determining cause of acne is seborrhoea, but such excessive secretion of sebum, providing its exit is not mechanically obstructed is not necessarily associated with acne. Certain contributing factors are recognised, including of course, age and sex, septic foci in the body, dyspepsia, constipation, irregularities of menstruation, etc. ; but these factors are in no way causal and few *cures* would be achieved by simple correction of them.

Blackheads, i.e. comedones, may be described as consisting of "concentrically arranged layers of horn cells, enclosing considerable numbers of *corynebacterium acnes* and a variable quantity of sebum". The minute *acarus desmodex follicularium* may sometimes be present (B. C. Tate, *Practitioner*, March 1950). The blackening of the comedone is probably due to oxidation and possibly also the presence of surface dirt.

Formerly it was thought that the causative agent was the acne bacillus and that this organism on entering an open follicle set up irritation causing proliferation of the horny layer of the skin. It was also thought that a secondary infection by *staphlococcus epidermidis albus* led to papule formation and the characteristic pustular stage. It is now considered that the formation of a comedone is a physiological effect and that the mechanical obstruction caused may account for the subsequent suppuration. At the same time scratching, shaving, rubbing the face harshly with a towel, or any other form of trauma, may result in bacterial infection of the pustule.

The relation between the rate of sebum excretion and diameter of the hair follicle is probably very variable in different persons, the former being governed by glandular conditions while the latter is an anatomical feature. Variations in this relationship would account for the fact that not everyone suffers from acne during puberty. In connection with glandular activity it is interesting to note that according to Hamilton (*J. invest. Derm.*, 1942, **5**, 473; *J. Clin. Endocrin.*, 1941, p. 570; *Amer. J. Anat.*, 1942, **71**, 451) eunuchoid and castrate men do not develop seborrhoea or acne, but that administration of male hormone in the majority of such cases led to the development of seborrhoea and comedones. Rony and Zakow (*Arch. Derm Syph., Chicago*, 1943, **48**, 601) have shown that androgen has a stimulating action on the sebaceous glands of boys in the prepubertal stage increasing decidedly their number and size.

Studies, F. W. Lynch (*J. Amer. med. Ass.*, 1939, **113**, 1792), suggest that the incidence and severity of the cases in males is greater than in females. The existence of a probable endocrine dysfunction in acne has been assumed for years.

Tate has pointed out (*Practitioner*, March 1950), that it can be shown experimentally that administration of *androgens causes proliferation and increased* activity of the sebaceous glands, whereas *oestrogens produce the reverse changes and further, that the administration of oestrogens in sufficient quantity will cure acne in both sexes.* Williams (*Practitioner*, May 1948) has drawn attention to the fact that (i) it is advisable not to use such hormones at all in women under the age of 20 and (ii) the risk of permanent sterility in males, following administration of oestrogen, is so grave that *it is doubtful whether the use of oestrogens in males is ever justifiable.* (In this connection it must be noted that the dosage to *produce comparable effects* in men with the oestrogens must often be as high as five times that required for women.)

Discussing the mode of action of androgens, Tate refers to changes which have been shown to occur in the composition of human hair fat at puberty (*see* Hair, Chapter 20) and suggests that the sebaceous secretion, in cases of acne, may itself contain factors which are conducive to keratinization of the mouths of the hair follicles.

As might be expected, there is no evidence that acne is related in any way to intelligence. Lipman Cohen (*Brit. J. Derm.*, Dec. 1947), after investigating cases of acne in the army among men who had been graded intellectually by means of the progressive matrices devised by Penrose and Raven [Progressive Matrices, Sets, A, B, C, D, and E, London, Lewis, *Lancet*, 1942, 1, 115] found no difference between the intelligence of men with acne and the general population from which they were drawn. (It is, of course, well known that "nervy" individuals, by the very act of rubbing or scratching their skin, increase the irritation and the chances of infection.)

It would appear that the rational *cosmetic* treatment of acne must be limited to means designed to reduce the oiliness of the skin by local applications and to remove, as aseptically as possible, the comedones from the face. The avoidance of foods known to increase oiliness may be helpful, as also the avoidance of a high carbohydrate intake. (For more active steps to be taken, the proper procedure is to consult one's medical practitioner.) [Acneform eruptions may be produced by the ingestion of iodides and bromides in persons possessing an idiosyncrasy to them. Shelmire (*J. Amer. med. Ass.*, 9 June 1928, **90**, 1869) quotes six personal cases of acne due to ordinary iodised table salt.]

"Squeezing" should never be attempted until a proper comedone extractor has been obtained and after its use, a little local antiseptic should be applied. The use of the finger-nail to remove a blackhead may well result in a septic infection. The comedone extractor itself should be placed in dilute antiseptic before use.

Degreasing of the skin may be achieved by the use of plenty of soap and water or by a detergent, or cleansing lotion. Comedones may be removed by first treating the skin with hot towels for some 5 minutes; a little resorcinol ointment (or other suitable skin ointment) is then applied and after the ointment has been in contact for about 2–3 minutes, a comedone extractor is applied and a spot of antiseptic subsequently dabbed on.

SULPHUR OINTMENTS AND LOTIONS

Sulphur, on account of its antiseptic, keratolytic and keratoplastic properties, is widely used in the formulation of lotions and ointments for the treatment of acne. A favourite preparation, Lotio Potassae Sulphur Sulphuratae (B.P.C.), is often termed Lotio Alba. This contains zinc sulphide *freshly* precipitated by the chemical interaction of sulphurated potash and zinc sulphate, together with hydrogen sulphide gas:

	per cent.
Sulphurated potash[1]	2·29
Zinc sulphate	2·29
Distilled water	to 100·0

The solution must not be corked for about half an hour after mixing to allow the excess of gas, which the solution cannot dissolve, to escape. It is upon the presence of this gas that the efficacy of the solution depends. As dispensed by a pharmacist the solution is fresh and effective, but in the interval between its preparation by a manufacturing chemist and its subsequent retail disposal the solution may become valueless. Gustafson (*Amer. Perfum.*, Sept. 1938, p. 31) has studied the *p*H values of freshly prepared lotio alba as compared with solutions which had been aged and showed that the freshly prepared solution had a *p*H of 6·9 and contained a fair amount of hydrogen sulphide gas, the *p*H remaining constant despite various moderate dilutions with distilled water. Old solutions, however, had a *p*H of 4·8, and the acidity of the lotion was further increased on the addition of distilled water. He has suggested that the determination of the hydrogen-ion concentration might be used to test the effectivity of commercial preparations.

In view of these facts it is best for the lotion to be put up into two separate containers to be mixed before use, the one containing the required proportion of sulphurated potash and the second the zinc sulphate.

Sulphur may be employed in simple suspension, e.g.:

	per cent.
Precipitated sulphur	10·0
Glycerin	10·0
Spirit of camphor	10·0
Distilled water	70·0

	per cent.
Precipitated sulphur	15·0
Tinc. quillaia	15·0
Glycerin	5·0
Distilled water	65·0

[1] See British Pharmaceutical Codex, 1934.

Wrong ("The Treatment of Acne with Sulphur Lotion", *Brit. J. Derm.*, Dec. 1950, p. 491) has investigated the efficacy of a special sulphur lotion proposed by MacKee (MacKee, Sulzberger, Hermann and Baer, *J. invest. Derm.*, 1945, **6**, 43, and MacKee, Wachtel, Korf and Herrmann, *J. invest. Derm.*, 1945, **6**, 309) and reported that of 125 unselected university students treated with the special lotion, 57 of these students were "followed" over a period of three months. In 75 per cent. of these 57 patients there was a moderate or excellent improvement at the end of three months or longer; the term "cure" was not thought to be applicable to any of them. No severe reaction suggestive of a true sensitivity occurred in any of the patients, although a reaction occurred within the first two weeks in some patients but disappeared within a few days (this was considered a desirable effect). Wrong concluded that although this lotion was far from being a "cure-all", it was probably one of the best sulphur lotions available today; its composition was as follows:

	parts by weight
Sulphur	7·5
Sodium mixed alkyl benzene sulphonates	110·0
Antipyrin	154·0
Triethanolamine	100·0
Propylene glycol	560·0
Water	168·6

Fanburg (*J. med. Soc. N.J.*, 1950, **47**, 19) states that he has found the following cosmetic base, which *incorporates resorcin* and sulphur, an excellent aid in the topical treatment of acne. This preparation, it is stated, has exceptional covering properties and the medications act over a long period of time. Applied during the daytime to the skin it is said to act as a great boost to the morale of the acne vulgaris patient since the lesions can be almost completely hidden. The product consists of the ingredients blended to produce a flesh-coloured cake, which is put up in the form of a compact. (It is understood that the preparation is available commercially in the United States):

	per cent.
Isopropyl stearate	32·0
Lecithin	1·0
Lanolin	3·0
Cetyl alcohol	2·0
Titanium dioxide	42·0
Kaolin	6·0
Ceresin	4·0
Resorcin	2·9
Sulphur	8·0

Various methods of wetting and suspending sulphur, calamine and other powders are available, for example, wetting of the material with "Veegum", magnesium aluminium silicate (R. T. Vanderbilt, U.S.A.), or with one of the detergent or surface active agents discussed in this book. (*See* Chapter 22, Hair Shampoos, and Chapter 41, Emulsions and Dispersions.) Gelatinous hydrated aluminium oxide (Unemul) may also be used for this purpose (*Mfg. Perfum.*, 1940, **11**, 103). It is inert, can be used for edible products and is unaffected by electrolytes. The addition of about one-fifth of its weight to sulphur or other water-repellent substances enables them to be readily wetted and suspended in a mixture of the oxide and water, and finally homogenised to yield a lotion which does not sediment so readily as the pharmacopoeial preparations. Sulphur and calamine may also be incorporated into cetyl/stearyl alcohols, 10 per cent. sulphated. Miller (symposium; *J. invest. Derm.*, 1940, **3**, 143) has successfully employed a zinc oxide ointment containing 10 per cent. kaolin and 10 per cent. precipitated sulphur.

Resorcin in low concentration possesses astringent and keratoplastic properties, but in proportions of 10 per cent. and upwards is caustic. In paste form it is used, clinically, to produce desquamation in acne. It is dangerous in large concentrations if applied over a fairly large area, and a fatality has occurred in the use of paste containing 25–30 per cent. resorcin over a large surface. (*Extra Pharmacopoeia*, vol. 1, 1936, 21st edn.) More recently it has been discovered that its prolonged use may produce Myxoedema due to a specific anti-thyroid action of this substance (G. M. Bull & R. Fraser, *Lancet*, 1950, 851; O. J. G. Hobson (*Proc. R. Soc. Med.*, 1951, **44**, 164). In my opinion there is no longer justification for its use in a cosmetic preparation.

Detergent Preparations

In Germany the use of medicated detergents is considered a better treatment than the use of medicated ointments, and the following formula has appeared in the German literature:

	per cent.
Triethanolamine lauryl sulphate, liquid	80·0
Salicylic acid	2·5
Sulphur (precipitated)	0·5
Alcohol	5·0
Lavender oil	0·5
Rose water	6·5
Glycerin	5·0

Sodium lauryl sulphate is widely used in the cosmetic industry, and the triethanolamine salt combines excellent detergent properties with a very mild *pH*. The use of tar, sulphur and salicylic acid is on the lines of a well-known medicated soap. With the development of antiseptic and germicidal substances which are active in soap, as for example " G.11 " (Givaudan) and " Actamer " (Monsanto Chemicals Ltd.), the dermatologist has available antiseptics which can be applied automatically by the patient in the course of washing, probably without even realising that he, or she, is so doing. Other substances such as D.C.M.X. (dichlormeta xylenol), are, at the time of writing, under investigation. The importance of such developments should not be minimised. If pleasant-smelling, effective, germicidal soaps are available to or used by acne patients the reduction of total bacterial flora on the skin will reduce the risk of septic infection. Combined with sulphur or other suitable treatment, to reduce oiliness of the skin, these substances are likely to prove a useful addition to the dermatologist's armament.

For a more detailed discussion of such substances, *see* Chapter 42, Antiseptics and Preservatives, and Chapter 27, Toilet Soaps.

Schwartz and Blank (*J. Amer. med. Ass.*, 1944, **125**, 30), found a mixture containing 25 per cent. sulphated oil, 25 per cent. mineral oil and 50 per cent. water very satisfactory as a cleansing agent for patients with acne vulgaris. It was suggested that the face be massaged with the mixture for a few moments followed by a thorough rinsing with warm water, three times a day; the number of applications being reduced as the skin became less greasy. These investigators found that in the juvenile type of acne vulgaris, such a method of cleansing was sufficiently drying and that lotions were unnecessary, although borated alcohol (prepared by mixing equal parts of saturated aqueous boric acid and alcohol) might be used. The patients were shown how to remove comedones in the correct manner and a diet which eliminated chocolate was recommended.

CHAPTER 15

THE APPLICATION OF COSMETICS

(A Simplified Technique for Beauty)

THE term *make-up* applied to cosmetic preparations is psychologically unsound.[1] To obtain the maximum results from the use of such preparations they must be regarded as *beauty adjuvants* designed with the object of:

(1) Enhancing the general appearance by minimising facial defects and unobtrusively directing attention towards any individual *qualities.*

(2) Preventing *premature* ageing and wrinkling of the skin due to *external* causes by keeping the skin soft, supple and clean and protecting it from wind-burn, excessive sunlight, etc.

To attain the former object the shades of the various cosmetics, when used in daylight, must approximate the natural colouring of the purchaser, minor variations, in good taste, being permissible to add sparkle or piquancy.

Electric lighting (unless corrected by a blue filter) gives light of a yellowish cast which alters the apparent colour of the complexion and cosmetic; consequently for evening wear more latitude is permissible, and a cosmetic containing more pink or a little mauve (according to the complexion) may be used.

From the dermatological aspect the choice of any particular type of cosmetic preparation should depend on the condition of the customer's skin.

A perusal of the varying advice offered in different beauty columns, textbooks, and instructions issued by different cosmetic manufacturers is apt to prove confusing. In this brief chapter, the technique for beauty has been stripped of all but essentials and reduced to a bare minimum.

THE CONDITION OF THE SKIN IN RELATION TO TYPE OF COSMETIC EMPLOYED

The fortunate possessor of a normal skin should cleanse it by means of a good toilet soap and water, rinsing well with plenty of the latter. As a

[1] I have used the title *make-up preparations* in Chapter 12 solely because it is commonly used in the trade, and also for lack of a substitute word which would be acceptable.

powder base vanishing cream is usually satisfactory ; one of the modern pigmented foundation make-up preparations may be used if desired. The opinion has often been expressed that the use of powder on top of a cream will lead to clogging the pores ; this is not true. Scientific investigations by the writer ("The Removal of Powders from the Skin Surface", *Brit. J. Derm.*, March 1941, **53**, 79), in which the removal of luminous powders was studied under ultra-violet light showed that powders are somewhat more readily removed from the skin (by ordinary washing with soap and water) when applied on top of vanishing cream (or other oil-in-water emulsion) than when applied directly to the skin.

The choice of cream or compact rouge is immaterial and merely a question of taste. In winter a little cold cream may be applied to counteract any tendency to dryness of the skin, or wind-burn.

Apart from the above, the possessor of such a skin may experiment with the whole gamut of skin preparations and may derive considerable psychological pleasure in so doing, without detriment, except to her pocket.

The possessor of a *dry* skin is in a different position. Such skin is often supersensitive because it lacks the normal amount of protective sebum and moisture (Chapter 4). In such cases of skin hypersensitivity a complexion milk is occasionally preferred for cleansing purposes. These preparations contain upwards of 10 per cent. emulsified oil and possess valuable cleansing properties combined with very mild reaction, alternatively a cleansing cream may be used.

Vanishing cream sometimes proves too drying for use as a powder base for dry skin, and in this event a non-greasy cold cream, or an all-purpose cream may be employed. Cream rouge should be used in preference to powder rouge.

Liquid powder preparations and astringent lotions should be avoided.

In the case of *greasy* skin the reverse procedure should be adopted. For example, cleansing creams and milks containing oil should be avoided, though cleansing lotions containing borax, sodium bicarbonate (or certain soapless detergents) may be employed with advantage until the greasiness has been sufficiently reduced. A greasy skin will itself act as a powder base and a greasy cream is better avoided. If a powder base is required, a liquid powder containing zinc or titanium salts may be used. Mild astringent lotions containing glycerin, alcohol and witch hazel can be used if desired.

Hot face packs provide another method for reducing excessive oiliness.

FACE MASSAGE. Friction increases the supply of blood to the skin, and skilful massage assists in keeping the skin supple.

Ageing of the skin is accompanied by a diminution in elasticity, and merely applying creams to the face and then vigorously rubbing without following any preconceived plan may lead to the production of skin folds (i.e. wrinkles) the very opposite of the result desired.

Charts designed to show the paths which should be followed in facial massage have been prepared by various cosmetic manufacturers. The chart given opposite is reproduced by courtesy of the Icilma Co. Ltd.

As stated (Chapter 1, Ageing of Skin)—so far as we know at present—no externally applied preparations appear to *feed* the skin. *The regular use of a face cream can prevent the premature (not ultimate) ageing of skin due to external causes and thus delay the appearance of lines produced by loss of elasticity or diminution in subcutaneous fat which the beauty columnists term wrinkles.* They cannot, however, prevent the natural ageing of skin due to metabolic processes nor wrinkling caused by ill-health, psychogenic factors or certain diseases.

Wrinkles must be differentiated from the lines produced by the emotions, e.g. constant scowling or sneering. The best cure for these is to cultivate a placid disposition.

Cosmetic Technique

The usual technique for beauty treatment employed after cleansing the face is firstly the application of a vanishing cream or other powder base (in the case of a very greasy skin this is not necessary), then the application of powder, followed by rouge and lipstick. If the technique is more formal, mascara, eyebrow pencil (and sometimes eye shadow) may also be used.

VANISHING CREAM.[1] This is generally purchased on its perfume, consistency, texture, vanishing, and powder-adhesive qualities according to the personal preference of the user. To apply it correctly a portion should be dabbed on the forehead, tip of the nose and chin and on each cheek. It is then spread so as to produce a smooth, even film, using as little as possible of the cream.

FACE POWDER. To obtain the most flattering effect, the powder should be applied generously to the face by means of cotton-wool, or a clean puff, and *the excess brushed off by means of a soft brush.* Alternatively, the powder may be applied and spread with a powder-puff. This is more usual, but the cosmetic effect is usually inferior to that obtained by

[1] *Foundation Cream*: Recent tendency is to place more emphasis on the use of a cream as a *foundation* for powder, rather than on its ability—in itself—to remove shine and " vanish " rapidly. Such creams termed *Foundation Creams* are usually characterised by an increased content of fatty matter or glycerin and contain powder. They are often flesh in colour.

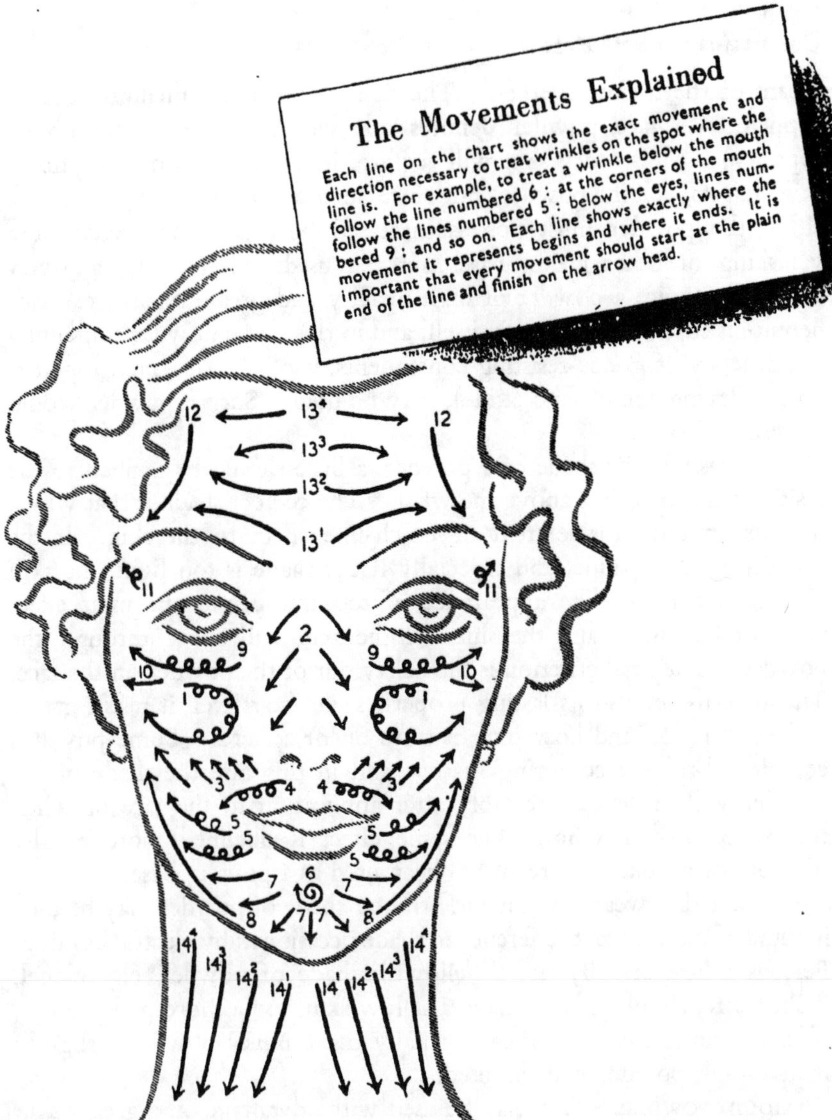

CHART (*copyright*).

Area	No.	Movement	Pressure
Cheeks	1.	Two or three fingers .	*Light.*
Nose	2.	Two fingers	*Medium.*
Cheeks	3.	Two fingers	*Medium.*
Upper Lip	4.	Two fingers	*Light.*
Chin	5.	Two fingers	*Light.*
Chin	6.	One finger .	*Light.*
Chin	7.	Two fingers	*Rather heavy.*
Chin	8.	Four fingers	*Heavy.*
Eyes	9.	Two fingers	*Very light.*
Cheeks	10.	Three fingers	*Medium.*
Forehead	11.	Two fingers	*Light.*
Forehead	12.	Four fingers	*Heavy.*
Forehead	13.	Four fingers	*Medium.*
Neck	14.	Thumb and two fingers .	*Rather heavy.*
Neck	15.	Pass four fingers round the back of the neck, from front to back, finishing downwards towards the spine . .	*Rather heavy.*

Fig. 38.—Massage diagram.

means of the former method. The designation light, medium, heavy, applied to a face powder denotes not weight but covering power (opacity). Thus a dry skin will require, in the absence of exceptional skin defects, a light powder, but since such a skin is lacking in grease either the powder must possess increased powers of adherence or a vanishing or other cream base must be used. Conversely, a greasy skin will require a powder of high opacity and grease resistance. Adherence is supplied by the skin itself, and in this case a powder containing a sufficiency of grease-resisting constituents, kaolin, chalk, etc., together with a drying agent (zinc oxide), may be used. Such a powder would be termed heavy.

To examine the shade of a powder, a little should be applied to the inside of the arm, just above the wrist. The correct shade is that which imparts an unobtrusive matt or peach-like effect to the skin. If the powder is too opaque, and especially if the shade is too light, the skin will have a clown-like appearance, if too transparent the matt effect will not be visible and the shine of the skin will show through the powder. The final criterion is the behaviour of the powder on the face. This determines also its lasting properties, i.e. how well it resists grease and perspiration and how long it stays on or adheres. Some powders contain oil-soluble colouring matters and in this case the shade of the powder will deepen appreciably after application to the face or when the person becomes hot. The same effect is obtained more rapidly if a cold or all-purpose cream has been used as a powder base.

For evening wear a somewhat brighter shade of powder may be used in view of the apparent difference in shade occasioned by electric lighting. Persons who normally use a yellowish shade of powder, e.g. rachel, flesh, ochre, should, if they have a sallow skin, use a more pinky shade. If their skin is clear and they normally use a pinky powder a slightly mauve-pink powder may be used.

LIQUID POWDER. This may be used with advantage on a greasy skin since zinc and titanium salts possess a drying action. The suspension of powder should be shaken well before use, poured into a shallow glass or china container and applied by means of cotton-wool. After the face has dried, ordinary face powder and rouge may be applied in the usual way.

ROUGE. Cream rouge, properly applied, has a more natural appearance and possesses better lasting properties than compact rouge and is particularly recommended where it is desired to use rouge on a dry skin as it is, in effect, a coloured cold cream.

The use of cream or compact rouge is optional in the case of normal skin but the latter is recommended in the case of a greasy skin.

Whichever type of rouge is employed, the Helena Rubenstein convention for rouge may be studied with advantage. This recommends the following method for application :

TYPE OF FACE	POSITION OF ROUGE
Oval	Apply rouge in a triangle from temple towards the nose downwards from a point parallel to the tip of the nose and thence to the ear.
Round	Apply high on cheek bones, just beneath the eyes and close to the nose to give length to the face.
Broad	Carry rouge downwards in a slightly elongated line.
Long	Apply lower than usual and spread over a comparatively large area.
	If the nose is a trifle long a touch of rouge beneath the tip makes it appear shorter.
For evening wear	Place rouge nearer the eyes to intensify their sparkle and touch the tips of ears and chin with rouge to make face look piquant.

The correct shade of rouge is that which most nearly matches the colour of the consumer's cheeks when flushed either through blushing or exertion.

Rouge should be applied in such a manner that it diffuses unobtrusively into the surrounding skin. It should never possess a hard outline.

LIPSTICK. Lipstick is used to impart an attractive colour and appearance to the lips. Narrow, *bad tempered* lips are widened and broad sensual lips made to appear narrower by its use. Applied intelligently it is capable of altering the apparent facial characteristics.

In applying lipstick it is best to accentuate the arches of the lips (Cupid's Bow) and to spread it in such a manner that it is unobtrusively faded out at the corners. The correct colour of the lipstick is that which most nearly matches the inner mucous membrane of the lip. Slight variations in colour may be used according to taste, but orange shades confer a somewhat bizarre effect. Even in sunburn the lips retain their normal colour.

MASCARA. The function of mascara is to increase the charm of the features by darkening and increasing the apparent length of the eyelashes, and it is claimed that by its intelligent use the brightness and expressiveness of the eyes is enhanced.

Mascara is best applied to the upper eyelashes only. For black or dark brown eyelashes, black mascara is satisfactory. Blue mascara applied to blue or grey eyes increases the apparent blueness of the eye.

Blondes and red heads sometimes use green mascara in an endeavour to obtain exotic effects.

EYE-SHADOW. Eye-shadow is used to confer apparent depth to the eyes and to make them appear more luminous. It is not generally used in daylight but is sometimes employed with evening wear.

EYEBROW PENCILS. These are used to modify the outline of the eyebrows after plucking. A more natural effect is obtained by applying the eyebrow pencil in a series of parallel lines at about 30° than by one hard line (i.e. ///// instead of ——).

For medium and blonde hair a dark brown pencil is best, for red heads a reddish brown pencil may be used.

THE SUN-TANNED SKIN. The technique for a sun-tanned complexion differs but slightly from the foregoing instructions. The powder and rouge may be matched as previously mentioned, though in this case the matching should be carried out on the sunburned skin. To modify the whiteness of ordinary vanishing cream it may be mixed with sunbronze or peach powder—just before use [1] or a sun-tan powder cream may be applied. Brown eye-shadow may be used in conjunction with the shade of mascara and eyebrow pencil normally employed.

Orange lipsticks are sometimes employed with a sun-tanned complexion. Although they may be striking they are *not* natural, as the natural colour of the lips is not affected by the sun.

Minimising Defects

SKIN DEFECTS. Minor skin defects and blemishes can be minimised by the use of a flesh-coloured powder cream of high covering power (i.e. opacity).

SPECTACLES. Persons who have to wear glasses may apply a little mascara and eyebrow pencil (but *not* eye-shadow) to distract attention from the frame of the spectacles. In this case the eyebrows may be modified to follow the curve of the glasses providing these are not of a bizarre shape.

[1] Mixtures of cream and powder—prepared in this manner—are liable to mould growth and are best prepared in small quantities every two or three days. Proprietary preparations are, or should be, free from this defect.

CHAPTER 16

THE TOOTH AND PATHOLOGICAL DENTAL CONDITIONS

Histology of the Tooth—Fluorescence of Teeth—Tartar—Gingivitis—Pyorrhoea—Dental Caries—Factors Influencing Dental Caries—Fluorination of Water Supplies—Fluorides in Tooth-pastes—Mechanism of the Action of Fluoride on Enamel—The Use of "Therapeutic" Tooth-pastes and Tooth-powders, i.e. Ammoniated Dentifrices, Chlorophyll Tooth-paste, Penicillin in Dentifrices, Anti-Enzyme Dentifrices.

THE tooth is distinguished macroscopically by the *crown* (that portion of the tooth above the gum) and the *root* (the portion embedded in the gum), the constricted portion separating these being termed the *tooth neck*.

The chief substance, or tissue, composing the tooth is termed dentine (the so-called ivory), which surrounds the tooth pulp. The dentine matrix is perforated by a large number of tiny canals which radiate from the pulp cavity to the surface, termed *dentine tubules*. These contain processes from the odontoblasts, the cylindrical connective tissue cells which form the outer surface of the dental pulp adjacent to the dentine, lining the pulp cavity, by which the dentine obtains nourishment. Although dentine is extremely sensitive to trauma, as, for example, when the enamel protective surface is chipped, it has not been possible to demonstrate actual nerve fibres in it.

Dentine is protected in the crown of the tooth by a cap-like covering of enamel becoming thinner in the neck, and in the neck also by a thin layer of cement becoming thicker towards the root, which it encases with a bone-like protective covering, the *cresta petrosa*, often termed the cement.

Enamel consists of long, somewhat irregular hexagonal prisms, 3-6μ in length, consisting almost entirely of calcium salts, arranged vertically to the tooth surface, and covering the entire thickness of the enamel. Their exact course is extremely complicated as they show a distinct spiral bending, which in places amounts to a whorl. These prisms are the hardest tissue in the human body and contain practically no organic matter. Any interruption in the process of calcification of the enamel produces transverse markings which may be demonstrated after suitable acid treatment. These are distinct from the so-called parallel lines of Retzuis which exhibit a more or less brownish coloration and may always be recognised in ground tooth sections. These depend upon the deposition of the enamel in layers.

Sheldon, Bibby and Bales (" The Relationship between Microscopic Enamel Defects and Infantile Debilities ", *J. Dent. Res.*, **24**, 109) microscopically examined ground sections of ninety-five teeth from thirty-four patients with detailed medical histories to determine whether defects in the enamel structure were related to the occurrence of systemic ailments. In more than 70 per cent. of the cases there was a positive correlation between the time of formation of a band of definitely defective enamel and the existence of some systemic disability. Deficiencies of vitamins A, C and D and also of calcium and phosphorus were the commonest causes of defective enamel formation.

Fluorescence of Teeth

For many years it has been known that when human teeth are irradiated with ultra-violet light they fluoresce. Since, in general, fluorescence of a substance is sensitive to slight differences in structure it was thought that by the application of a suitable technique details of tooth structure, not evident by other means of examination, might be obtained.

Recently Dickson, Forziati, Lawson, Jr., and Schoonover (" Fluorescence of Teeth : A Means of Investigating their Structure ", *J. Amer. dent. Ass.*, Dec. 1952, **45**, 661) have developed such a technique, and photomicrographs of the fluorescence of tooth sections show details of structure not revealed by other means. These researches are proceeding. Meanwhile, two illustrations of such fluorescence photographs, by courtesy of these investigators are shown in Fig. 39. The first of these illustrates the strong fluorescence of dentin as compared with enamel and illustrates clearly that developmental lines in dentin are sharply outlined ; fluorescent tufts extending outward from the dentino-enamel junction are clearly visible. In the second illustration, an area of bright fluorescence near the outside surface of enamel, it is stated, may be an indication of *penetration of materials* into tooth.

Tartar

The term *tartar*, which it is believed was introduced by Paracelsus (1493-1541) (more correctly *salivary calculis*), is commonly used to denote incrustations formed on neglected teeth, which may range in colour from buff to black according to the presence and proportion of decomposed blood or chromogenic bacteria mixed with the concretion. The origin of *tartar* is due to its comparison, in those days, with the deposits formed in wine casks.

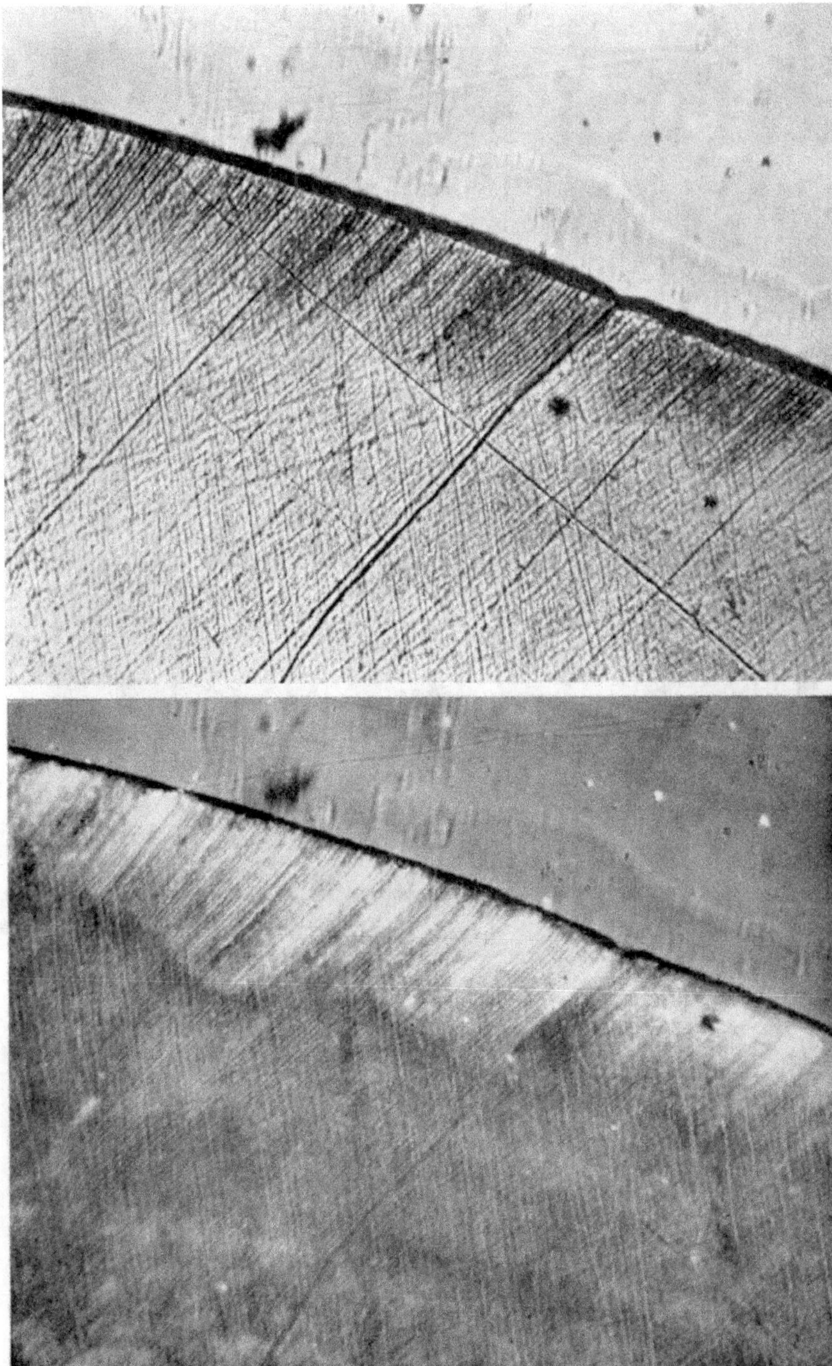

[*By courtesy of Dickson, Forziati, Lawson, Jr. and Schoonover.*

FIG. 39.—Comparison of visible light illumination, above, and fluorescence below, of enamel section. Area of bright fluorescence may be an indication of penetration of materials into the tooth. (Magnification—*c.* × 200.)

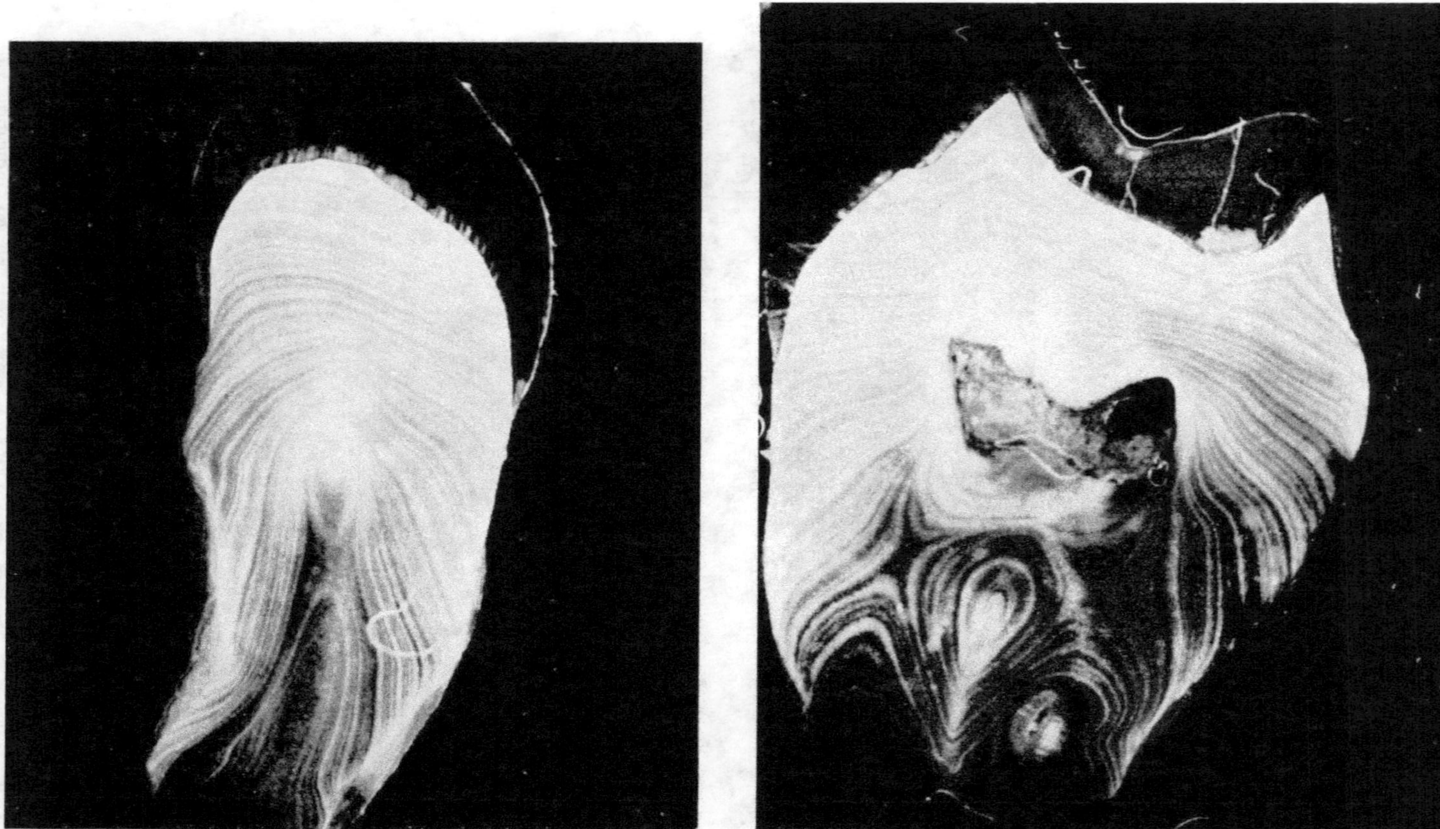

[By courtesy of Dickson, Forziati, Lawson, Jr. and Schoonover.

Fig. 40.—Fluoromicrographs of tooth sections. Note that dentin fluoresces much more intensely than enamel and that development lines in dentin are sharply outlined. It can also be seen that tufts extending outwards from dentino-enamel junction fluoresce brightly. (× 8.)

The relationship of lime salts to such incrustations was recognised as early as 1895, when H. Burchard (*Dent. Cosmos*) stated : " This much is accepted beyond cavil, that they are in large part composed of salts of calcium (almost entirely the phosphate and a small quantity of carbonate) combined with organic matter, the lime salts being held in suspension or solution in the saliva and for some insufficiently explained cause precipitated in favourable situations." Talbot (*Interstitial Gingivitis*, 1913) considered that tartar was due to excretion of the excess of calcium salts in the blood which remained soluble in the saliva until they reach the mouth cavity where precipitation occurred. G. V. Black (*Special Dental Pathology*, 1915) stated that he was of the opinion that the precipitation of calcium salts from the saliva so long held by himself and others was a myth, and that it would appear that salivary calculus (tartar) comes into the mouth as a finely divided calco-globulin, which collects in masses on hard substances, the colloidal elements become decomposed and a hard stony calculus forms. Kirk has suggested that the precipitation of salts by the escape of carbon dioxide from the saliva causes a combination of the colloidal mucin and such salts, which deposits on the teeth as tartar.

ROLE OF MICRO-ORGANISMS IN TARTAR FORMATION. Bullied (" An Experimental Study of Leptothris buccalis ", *Guy's Hosp. Rep.*, 1924, **74**, 444) pointed out the importance of leptotrichea in the formation of tartar. (*See also Brit. dent. J.*, 1925, **46**, 287.) Bibby (" Formation of Salivary Calculus ", *Dent. Cosmos*, 1935, **77**, 668) showed the importance of bacteria and incriminated leptotrichea rather than actinomyces.

Naeslund (" Studies of Tartar Formation ", *Acta path. microbiol. scand.*, 1926, **3**, 637) found numerous bacteria in tartar, chiefly leptothrix and actinomyces and demonstrated that loss of carbon dioxide and protein decomposition were of little importance under intraoral conditions in tartar formation. He suggested that the actinomyces may have a chemical influence through proteolysis and may also exert a physical effect in providing a tenacious framework for deposition of calcium salts.

The presence of alkaline phosphatase in the mouth has been demonstrated (Smith, " Factors Affecting the Deposition of Salivary Calculus ", *Aust. J. exp. Biol. med. Sci.*, 1930, **7**, 45 ; Adamson, " The role of Enzyme Action in the Formation of Dental Calculus ", *J. exp. biol. Med. Sci.*, 1929, **6**, 215 ; Glock, Murray and Pincus, " The Origin and Significance of Salivary Phosphatase ", *Biochem. J.*, 1938, **32**, 2096 ; Zander, " The Distribution of Phosphatase on Gingival Tissue ", *J. dent. Res.*, 1941, **20**, 347).

Citron (" The Role of Actinomyces Israeli in Salivary Calculus Formation ", *J. dent. Res.*, April 1945, **24**, 87) studied six strains of

Actinomyces israeli and found that they contained alkaline phosphatase. He suggested that these organisms may therefore cause precipitation of calcium phosphate from the saliva and initiate tartar formation.

INFLUENCE OF AN ENAMEL FILM OR PELLICLE ON TARTAR. King (National Institute of Medical Research) in a letter published in *Nature* (10 Nov. 1945, p. 572) on the enamel cuticle (Nasmyths membrane) in relation to tartar deposition in the ferret refers to a form of parodontal disease in the ferret caused by the formation of salivary calculus (*see also* J. D. King, *Brit. dent. J.*, 1944, **77**, 221, 245; J. D. King and E. R. Glover, *J. Path. Bact.*, 1945, **57**, 353) in which both tartar deposition and gingival disease were prevented by including in the diet short lengths of bone, this tartar-preventing action being ascribed largely to the mechanical friction set up by the bone.

While the precise cause of these calcareous accretions is still undetermined, King states that a series of recent observations has led him to believe that the enamel cuticle (Nasmyths membrane) plays an important part. Microscopical preparations of teeth and parodontal tissues clearly demonstrate the very firm adherence of the organic constituents of tartar to the enamel cuticle, even after decalcification and sectioning of the teeth, and the implication is that some association exists between the organic constituents of tartar and the enamel cuticle. Moreover, there is evidence to indicate that in ferrets given bone to gnaw, not only are they free from tartar and parodontal disease but also in time the enamel cuticle is largely removed by friction, and on subsequent withdrawal of bone from the diet the teeth still remain free from all but a trace of tartar in the most sheltered grooves distant from the gum margin.

King states that, finally, under certain conditions calcium-containing material is laid down *in vitro* on pieces of enamel cuticle on incubation in human saliva, and reports that further investigations are in progress.

Chase (*Anat. Rec.*, 1926, **33**, 357) found in 84 per cent. of human teeth, films whose insolubility in water and acid or alkali was as great as that of the enamel; similar films were found on the teeth of practically all domestic animals. These films withstood fairly vigorous brushing for some time, but could be removed, especially by the use of a toothpaste or a mild abrasive. Dobbs (*J. dent. Res.*, 1932, **12**, 581) found that mechanical cleansing of extracted teeth with pumice did not destroy the acid resistance of such surfaces but that tryptic digestion did so, and he concluded that organic protective membranes occurred on unworn enamel. Dobbs (*J. dent. Res.*, 1932, **12**, 853) produced similar surfaces *in vitro* and considered that mucus deposited on the teeth, particularly during sleep, became denatured and transformed into resistant plaques.

Manly (*J. dent. Res.*, 1943, **22**, 479) has shown that a structureless pigmented pellicle is formed on the teeth of persons who do not use dentifrices, and Valoton (*J. dent. Res.*, June-Aug. 1945, pp. 161-187) has confirmed the existence of such a pellicle and suggests that this protein is a denatured or otherwise altered mucin.

H. Mathis (*Z. Stomat.*, 1935, **33**, 1106), from optical crystallographic studies, stated that the crystalline constituent of tartar is hydroxylapatite, that little calcium carbonate is present and that the onion-like character of its deposition is brought about by variations in the flow of saliva during day and night.

H. Prinz (*Diseases of the Soft Structure of the Teeth and their Treatment*, H. Kimpton, London, 1937, p. 386) gives the following typical analysis of saliva and tartar respectively, with the proviso that as the composition of saliva changes, within limitations, continuously, it is natural to assume fluctuations in the composition of tartar.

Composition of saliva

	parts
Water	99·42
Epithelium and mucin	0·22
Ptyalin	0·13
Inorganic salts	0·22
Potassium sulphocyanide	0·10

Salivary Calculus (average of 5 samples)

	parts
Water	5·68
Water-soluble substances	5·24
Mucus and food debris	15·16
Magnesium phosphate	1·31
Calcium carbonate	9·14
Calcium phosphate	63·42

PREVENTION AND TREATMENT OF TARTAR. The presence or absence of tartar is accepted as a criterion of cleanliness of the teeth, and it is with preparations designed to reduce this to a minimum that the cosmetic and toilet technologist is intimately concerned.

Broadly speaking, apart from organic disease which may effect tartar formation, e.g. diabetes mellitus, tartar is produced by any condition which allows stagnation of the saliva, as for instance indentations of the teeth which allows the residence of stale food particles. Black has shown that when first deposited upon the teeth or dental plate, tartar may be readily removed with a tooth-brush and water within 5–12 hours of its deposition. After 24 hours it has begun to harden and is difficult to remove by means of a brush alone. In a week it cannot be brushed away at all, and continues to harden for one or two months, at the end of which time it is so hard that instruments are required to scrape it away. The hardness of tartar in its purest form is stated to be about 2·9 on Moh's mineralogic scale.

Gingivitis (Bleeding Gums)

This condition, though commonly seen in adults, is rare in young children. Bleeding of the gums is a characteristic of gingivitis ; it may be due to several causes, for example, the formation of tartar at the base of the tooth where it fits into the gingival collar ; inflammation results and the gums may then bleed when they are brushed or in severe cases even by simple pressure. When gingivitis is due to tartar formation, removal of the tartar by scraping should lead to disappearance of the gingivitis. On the other hand, gingivitis may be due to anatomical defects between the teeth which allows deposition of food and subsequent irritation. Though a diet adequate in vitamins B and C and in calcium and phosphorus is advisable, gingivitis is considered to be a condition of the mouth occasioned primarily by neglecting to brush the teeth regularly. An exception to this statement occurs in *hypertropic gingivitis* in which the gums become overgrown and surgical removal is necessary. This condition is, however, much rarer than what is ordinarily termed gingivitis.

Pyorrhoea Alveolaris

Neglect of gingivitis may result in the deeper tissues of the gum becoming involved. The gum tissue surrounding the tooth becomes loosened and pus collects in the pocket formed by this loosening of the attachment between tissue and tooth, resulting in what is called pyorrhoea. The majority of cases of pyorrhoea are of this type and can be cured by proper dental treatment. There is also a much rarer form of pyorrhoea which shows no preliminary symptom of gingivitis (no bleeding, no signs of infection, no tartar in the crevices, etc.), and apparently healthy teeth, then, all of a sudden, appear to separate from the gums. This form appears to be due to some nutritional deficiency.

Dental Caries

A conference held at the University of Michigan in 1947, to evaluate and correlate all available information on the aetiology and control of dental caries, unanimously adopted the following definition (Michigan Workshop Conference, *J. Amer. dent. Ass.*, 1948, **36,** 3) :

" . . . Dental caries is a disease of the calcified tissues of the teeth. It is caused by acids resulting from the action of micro-organisms on carbohydrates, is characterised by a decalcification [1] of the inorganic portion and is accompanied or followed by a disintegration of the organic substance of the tooth. The lesions of the disease predominantly occur in particular regions of the tooth and their type is determined by the morphologic nature of the tissue in which they appear. . . ."

Dental caries is ubiquitous and very few people are normally free from it. It is stated (*Dental Caries*, American Dental Association) that " . . . it may begin soon after the primary (first) teeth appear in the mouth, is common by the third year of life and may continue as long as the teeth are present. As high as 50 per cent. of 2-year old children have one or more carious teeth. The average person at the age of 16 years has seven teeth that have been attacked by caries, with an involvement of fourteen tooth surfaces.

Prior to the above adoption at the Michigan conference, there have been two schools of thought concerning the origin of dental caries : (i) nutritional, and (ii) microbiological, with the latter theory consistently gaining ground, though there is no doubt that an adequate diet is essential for the health of the whole body, including the teeth.

NUTRITIONAL. Experiments on rats have shown that a deficiency of phosphorus in the diet increases the *susceptibility* to, but does not produce, dental caries. A study of varying climatic conditions and the diet of the people inhabiting such regions does not lead to any definite conclusions. Shohl (*Mineral Metabolism*, A.C.S. Monograph, No. 82, New York, 1939) has pointed out that " the tropical sun of India does not prevent caries ; dental caries exists in Puerto Rico, but rickets are absent showing that there is no serious deficiency in Vitamin D. Caries occurs not only in Scotland, but also in Hawaii, the land of sunshine and fruit." Among Indian tribes caries seldom occurred—prior to the advent of the white man. Indian diet formerly consisted of *meat, Indian corn, nuts and berries.* Eskimos, *who live almost entirely on meat* are relatively immune, and so are

[1] It should be noted that whilst the bacterial theory of caries is generally accepted, that of " acid-decalcification " has many critics. As discussed under Ammoniated Dentifrice, Jenkins, Wright and Miller, point out that a number of workers believe that the initial attack on the tooth is of *proteolytic* origin. Pincus (1st International Congress of Biochemistry, Abstract 348/5, Section 5) has postulated a new theory. This authority believes that micro-organisms associated with the carious process elaborate enzymes, e.g. " sulphatase ", which can split off free sulphuric acid from the conjugated protein materials of enamel and dentin (i.e. that the acid is derived from the teeth themselves rather than from any external or dietary source, see " Anti-Enzyme Dentifrices).

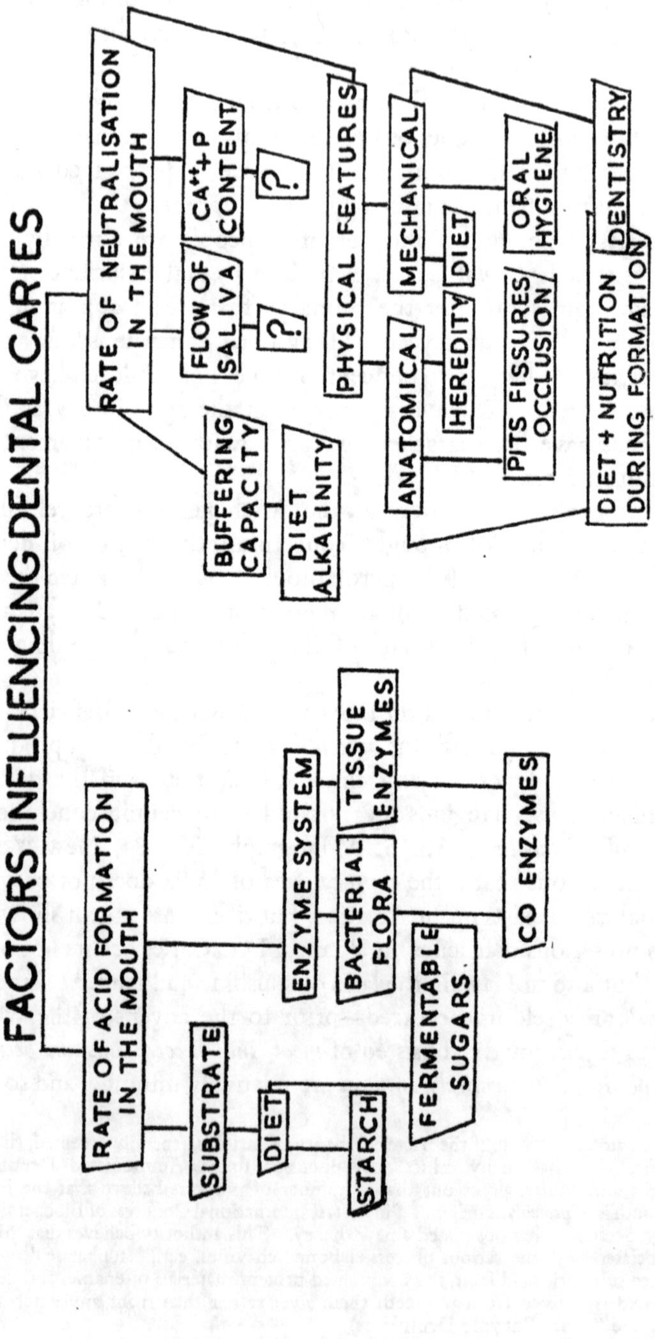

FIG. 41. [*By courtesy of the Toilet Goods Association, U.S.A.*

the Sikhs who live on milk products, green vegetables and wheat, and eat practically no meat.

MICROBIOLOGICAL. As far back as 1891, Miller (*Dent. Cosmos*, 1891, **33**, 689, 789, 913), considered that dissolution of teeth was the result of the chemical action of acids produced by bacterial fermentation of carbohydrate accumulation on the teeth and his contentions subsequently received the support of such eminent workers as Black, Goodby and Williams.

Fosdick (*Proc. Sci. Sect.* (U.S.) *T.G.A.*, May 1950, p. 13) has published a chart to indicate the mechanisms that take part and control the formation of acid in the mouth ; this is reproduced on page 290.

In the light of the above definition of dental caries, certain possible methods of control present themselves, viz :

(i) *Curtailment of purified carbohydrate intake.*

Dental caries can be controlled in a large number of cases by a curtailment in the intake of sugars, as for example, elimination or reduction, in sweets, jams, jellies, sweetened drinks, cakes.

Guttorm Toverud (*J. Amer. dent. Ass.*, Aug. 1946, **39**, 127) drew attention to the decrease in caries frequency in Norwegian children during World War II. During this period also, it was noted that in parts of Europe where the diet was restricted (and in prisoner of war camps in Germany and Japan there was a reduction in caries). *However, it is known that some children and adults can eat much larger amounts of refined sugars than others without showing evidence of dental decay.* Jay (*Amer. J. Orthodont.* (Sect. on Oral Surgery), **33**, 162, March 1947) points out that " . . . *as they grow older caries becomes inactive in many of these individuals despite the fact that they continue to maintain a very high level of carbohydrate consumption. There is no satisfactory explanation for this transition except that it is accompanied by a change in the bacterial flora of the mouth, characterised by a decline in the growth of the lactobacilli. . . .*"

[If one changes this last statement to read . . . " *is accompanied by a change in the* microbiological *flora of the mouth* " this statement would be in line with modern thought—Author!] The real answer to the problem is not then to curtail carbohydrate drastically, a scheme at best unlikely to achieve much success since few adults and fewer children would exchange their life for one free from dental fillings and " free from all the sweet things that make life pleasant ", but rather to find out the nature of the protective mechanism in the cases quoted above with a view to stimulating such natural protective factors. Moreover, Haggard and Greenberg

("Dent. Survey", through *Sci. News Lett., Wash.*, 1949, **56**, 376) point out out that trying to avoid tooth decay by avoiding sugar is impractical because almost all starch foods, produce sugars and the micro-organisms involved make no distinction as to the source of the sugar.

(ii) *The use of an enzyme inhibitor.*

Fosdick (*Proc. Sci. Sect. (U.S.) T.G.A.*, May 1950, p. 13) points out that "... the prevention of acid formation by means of enzyme inhibitors has been tried many times on a laboratory basis but only a few clinical investigations have been reported...." Theoretically this method offers some advantages. (See Anti-Enzyme Dentifrices.)

(iii) *The fluoridation of drinking water supplies.*

(iv) *The use of a "Therapeutic" tooth paste.*

(i) Has been briefly discussed above (ii) is discussed later in this chapter. The large scale experiments have rather been confined to (iii) and (iv) which hence will be discussed in greater detail.

FLUORIDATION OF DRINKING WATER SUPPLIES. Experimental investigations (*U.S. Public Health Reports*, 1939, **54**, 862; 1941, **56**, 761; R. F. Sognnaes, *J. dent. Res.*, 1941, **20**, 303; R. F. Sognnaes and Armstrong, *J. dent. Res.*, 1941, **20**, 315; M. C. Smith and H. V. Smith, *Amer. J. publ. Hlth.*, 1940, **30**, 1050 and many other publications) make it quite plain that the consumption of water or foods containing traces of fluorides—upwards of one part per million fluorine—greatly increases the resistance of teeth ot caries though it leads to mottling of the teeth in a number of cases, which, judged from an aesthetic point of view, might be considered undesirable. In the U.S.A. experiments are in progress in which small amounts of fluoride have been added to the community water supply to determine whether the addition of such fluorides in very small quantities, i.e. parts per million, will prevent the decay of teeth. It is too early at present to evaluate the outcome of these long term experiments. In order to allay any apprehension that might arise concerning such fluorination procedures a joint statement was released in 1951, by the Council on Pharmacy and Chemistry and the Council on Foods and Nutrition of the American Medical Association. This states (*J. Amer. dent. Ass.*, Dec. 1951, p. 733) that the Councils are "... *unaware of any evidence that fluoridation of community water supplies up to a concentration of 1 part per million would lead to structural changes in the bones or to an increase in the incidence of fractures. The only difficulty so far revealed is a possible increase in mottling of the tooth enamel ... After considering the evidence available at this time, the Councils believe* *that the use of drinking water containing up to one part per million of fluoride is safe. . . ."*

In Great Britain it has been recently stated that . . . " as fluoridation of water supplies was the only measure which so far gave any promise of preventing or reducing the incidence of bad teeth, the Ministry of Health announced on 13 December 1953, acceptance of the recommendations of the medical mission that had visited the U.S.A. There were many areas in Britain where there was already enough fluorine in the water supply and where no more would be added. There was no scientific basis for the allegation that fluorides in quantities of 1·0 to 1·5 parts in a million had any harmful effect. . . ". (" Medical Notes in Parliament ", *Brit. Med. J.* 6 February 1954, p. 340.)

FLUORIDES IN TOOTH-PASTE. It was suggested (Editorial, *Brit. med. J.*, 1st April 1944) that legislation should be introduced to render compulsory the inclusion of specified amounts of fluorine in every dentifrice sold. Presumably the fluorine would be added in the form of soluble fluoride, i.e. sodium or potassium fluorides. This proposal was criticised, and it was pointed out (*Chem. & Drugg.*, 22 April 1944) that at best, this would only prevent caries in those persons who used tooth-pastes while leaving many victims of caries untouched.

The author has been uncompromisingly against the addition of fluorides to dentifrices since the suggestion was first mooted. The distribution of a substance as toxic as sodium fluoride, quite apart from the pharmacological and therapeutic effects of such addition, would in itself require very careful manipulation to avoid local concentration of fluoride. In the case of some of the smaller manufacturers it would be difficult, if not impossible, to insure the adequate and effective distribution of fluoride in such minute amounts throughout the whole of production batches of tooth-paste. Moreover, although the amounts involved in drinking water are of the order of one part per million, the volume of water imbibed per day is so very much larger than the small amount of paste that comes into contact with the tooth, that to achieve the same results the concentration of sodium fluoride necessary would be more like 0·4 per cent., which would make the paste a very toxic and dangerous product. In the light of the above points, the addition of a soluble fluoride to a tooth-paste is, in my opinion, a very hazardous procedure which should be unhesitatingly condemned !

MECHANISM OF THE ACTION OF FLUORIDE ON ENAMEL. Using the polystyrene-silica surface replica technique in conjunction with an electron microscope, Chamberlain and Gerould (*The Dow Diamond*, March 1946) have compared the internal structures of normal and fluorosed teeth. In this technique the surface to be examined is polished and acid etched. A negative replica of the surface is made by moulding polystyrene against the etched surface. Evaporation of silica on this polystyrene moulding results in a positive film which is then used in the electron microscope. (*See* Fig. 43).

Contrary to popular opinion it was observed that fluorosed teeth (those containing more than the normal quantities of fluorine) were softer, rougher and often whiter than normal teeth, *yet they resisted decay.*

It was found that fluorine, entering the child's system during the years when teeth were forming, is laid down as calcium fluor-apatite, whereas the indications were that fluorine absorbed directly on to tooth enamel after it is formed is laid down as calcium fluoride. Examination of an impacted tooth never exposed to drinking water showed it to be fluorosed, bearing out the theory that fluorine entering the mouth from drinking water is absorbed through ingestion and not by direct absorption on the tooth enamel. Nevertheless, *there is evidence that absorption can occur from local application to the tooth surface per se* in a concentrated solution and that such topical application can aid in resisting decay. This method is, in fact, in widespread dental use and may be especially valuable for adults whose teeth are already calcified and consequently will reap no benefit from taking fluorine into their system.

In the light of their findings Chamberlain and Gerould have postulated the theory that as bacteria become concentrated in the protected regions of a fluorosed tooth, their acid attacks the tooth, producing a fluoride solution at the point of attack which " stews the bacteria in their own juice " as it were. Thus fluorosed teeth release a counter weapon at the precise point of attack to destroy or inhibit the bacteria.

The Use of " Therapeutic " Tooth Pastes

Dental Caries and " Ammoniated Dentifrices "

A study of caries-resistant persons, reported by R. G. Kesel (University of Illinois, *J. dent. Res.*, April 1948, **27**, 44)[1] revealed that persons resistant to caries developed ammonia in their saliva (upon incubation) at a more rapid rate than did the saliva of caries-susceptible subjects. It was found that the ammonia nitrogen had an inhibiting effect on Lactobacillus acidophilus and certain other acidogenic bacteria.

As a result of testing various ammonium salts for their efficacy in inactivating Lactobacilli, it was found that dibasic ammonium phosphate

[1] *See also* Kesel, Kirch, O'Donnell and Wach (*Oral Surg.*, April 1949, **2**, 459) ; Henschel and Lieber (*J. dent. Res.*, June 1949, **28**, 248) ; " Dental Caries, Symposium and Discussion " (*J. Soc. cosmet. Chem.*, Dec. 1950, pp. 57–88).

was the most practical for clinical use. It was also found that when urea was combined with the diammonium phosphate, the anti-bacterial action was increased and the degradation of glucose to lactic acid prevented. Clinical studies were then carried out as a result of which it was suggested that a concentration of 5 per cent. di-ammonium phosphate and 3 per cent. urea was a desirable and suitable mixture for this purpose. This combination used consistently in a dentifrice and as a mouth wash, produced marked reduction in oral Lactobacilli counts.

The use of such a tooth-paste has been patented and widely sold, particularly in the United States. Experiments on these lines are still in hand, but it would seem that some of the early claims were premature and the present position would appear to be that the evidence either for, or against, the efficacy of the ammoniated dentifrices is not *conclusive*.

Jenkins, Wright and Miller (*Nature*, 1950, **164**, 606) showed that the inhibition of lactate production by the Lactobacilli acidophilus was not the prerogative of the ammonium ion alone and that alkaline sodium salts gave rise to similar inhibition. It was concluded that, if the *p*H of the final mixture of salt and saliva exceeds 7·8, and the concentration and, therefore, buffering power of the salt is sufficient to maintain the *p*H above this figure, then inhibition occurs. In further tests they concluded that it was the urea which was the most powerful inhibitor of the Lactobacilli and that the part played by the ammonium phosphate was merely that of a buffer and an additional safeguard against the breakdown of urea. They further state, " We do not doubt that these mixtures would reduce acid production and maintain a high *p*H in the oral cavity at least for some time after use. We do not, however, believe that ammonium salts play the part which Kesel *et al.* stated. . . ." Finally, these investigators challenge the whole idea that reduction of acid-producing organisms in the saliva necessarily reduces tooth decay. They contend that this opinion is, at least, controversial, since a number of workers believe that the initial attack on the tooth is of proteolytic origin rather than an acid decalcification. They concede that large amounts of urea might interfere with proteolytic bacteria, but observe that further tests are necessary to clear up this point.

Davies and King (" The effectiveness of an Ammonium Ion Tooth-powder in the Control of Dental Caries ", *J. dent. Res.*, Oct. 1951) carried out an experiment designed to determine the effectiveness of a commercial ammonium ion dentifrice in controlling dental caries, when the actual brushing procedure was not under rigid supervision. According to these investigators the experimental ammoniated tooth-powder failed to reduce the annual increase in new caries when its effect was compared with that of a non-ammoniated powder used under identical conditions. (Some examples of Ammoniated Dentifrice formulations are given in Chapter 17.)

CHLOROPHYLL IN TOOTH-PASTES. Chlorophyll as found in nature is usually a mixture of three parts of a component Chlorophyll A ($C_{55}H_{72}O_5N_4Mg$) and one part of another component, Chlorophyll B ($C_{55}H_{70}O_6N_4Mg$).

The chloroplasts of vascular plants contain four pigments, namely chlorophyll A, chlorophyll B, carotin and xanthophyll, together with fatty, protein and mineral substances. Commercial chlorophyll is obtained by the extraction of suitable green vegetable matter with alcohol or acetone followed by a system of purification worked out by the manufacturer in question. The chlorophyll so obtained is in the form of a concentrated " plant extract " containing other substances closely related to chlorophyll and obtained in the process of extraction and purification during which some decomposition of the chlorophyll occurs. Extracts of the above nature, containing up to about 15 per cent. chlorophyll or its derivatives form the supply of oil-soluble chlorophyll used for various colouring purposes. When intended for use as soap colours they are usually treated with copper salts in order to obtain the maximum green coloration and light fastness.

By treating commercial chlorophyll with alkali, under appropriate conditions, one may obtain the salt of a dicarboxylic acid, viz. chlorophyllin. Apart from the loss of the phytyll and methyl residues, Mitchell (*J. Soc. cosmet. Chem.*, Nov. 1951, **3**, 183), this compound has the same structure as the original chlorophyll. The potassium and sodium salts of this acid are soluble in water and such salts constitute the active constituents of the so-called " water-soluble chlorophylls."

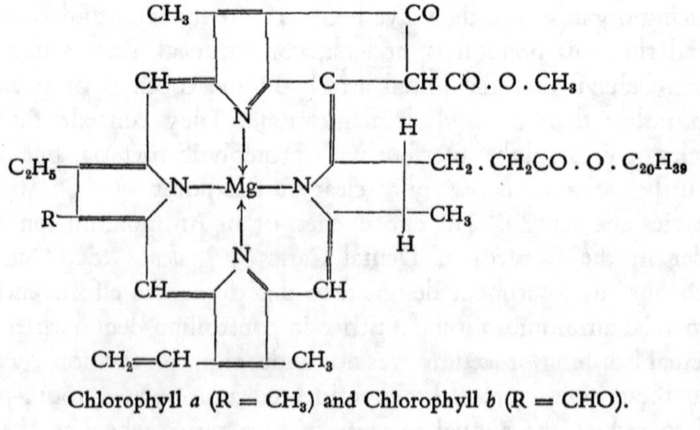

Chlorophyll *a* (R = CH_3) and Chlorophyll *b* (R = CHO).

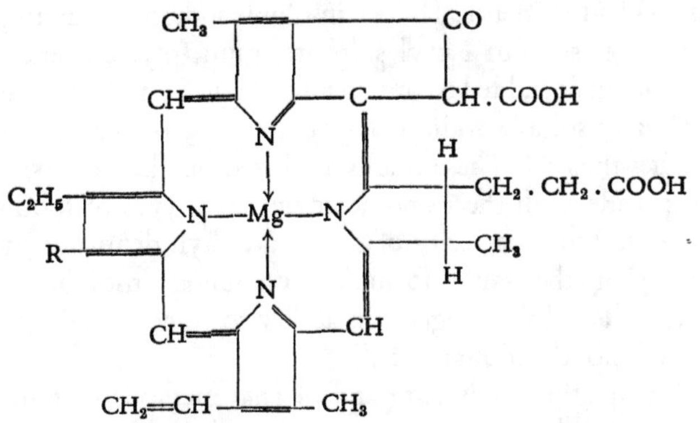

Chlorophyllin *a* (R = CH) and Chlorophyllin *b* (R = CHO).

CHLOROPHYLLINS IN TOOTH-PASTE. Gruskin (*Amer. J. Surg.*, 1940, **49**, 49) drew attention to the remarkable reduction in the odour of wounds to which " a substantially pure water-soluble chlorophyll was applied ". Bowers (*Amer. J. Surg.*, 1947, **73**, 37) reported that chlorophyll was first used at Winter General Hospital in a group of compound fracture cases, which were so malodorous as to deprive patients and attendants of appetite. The first observation made following the use of chlorophyll was that this odour immediately disappeared and was accompanied by an acceleration in wound healing. These observations are in accord with studies by Moss *et al.* (*J. Amer. med. Ass.*, 1949, **140**, 1136) under the auspices of the Therapeutic Trials Committee of the Council on Pharmacy and Chemistry of the American Medical Association. They too found that chlorophyll consistently acted as an effective deodorant when used on foul-smelling wounds.

Westcott (*N.Y. St. J. Med.*, 1950, **50**, 698), in an investigation of the value of water-soluble chlorophyll in the treatment of human secondary and nutritional anaemias, observed a very distinct decrease in urine odour. In particular the characteristic odour caused by the ingestion of vitamin B was largely suppressed. Westcott also carried out *in vitro* tests and showed that water-soluble chlorophyllin had a significant effect in reducing the odours of benzyl mercaptan, thioglycollic acid and trimethylamine.

A spate of papers dealing with chlorophyllins in all kinds of products subsequently appeared and chlorophyll " went to town " in almost every type of preparation, including tooth-pastes. In tooth-pastes it has been claimed to (i) eliminate mouth odours, (ii) reduce dental decay.

Barail (" A Study of the Deodorizing Properties of Chlorophyll in Dentifrices ", *J. Soc. cosmet. Chem.*, March 1952, **3**, 1) has reported the results of a large number of tests on 50 subjects (29 men and 21 women) in which two dentifrices were simultaneously tested on the same subjects.

These dentifrices had an identical base : insoluble sodium metaphosphate,[1] calcium phosphate, sodium lauryl sulphate, gum, glycerin and water. One of them contained, added to this identical basic formula, 0·1 per cent. of an active water-soluble sodium copper chlorophyllin. Barail concludes his studies thus : " These results are based on close to 1000 odour measurements made with the osmometer on both types of tooth-paste. They demonstrate the superiority of the chlorophyll dentifrice over the plain dentifrice of the same formula, containing insoluble sodium metaphosphate as a polishing agent, in ability to remove and retard the development of mouth odours. . . ."

Killian (" Evaluation of *in vitro* and *in vivo* methods of testing deodorants with particular reference to chlorophyll and its Derivatives ", *J. Soc. cosmet. Chem.*, March 1952, p. 30) found, in brief, that where chlorophyllins could contact the odour-producing substances they were able in many cases to deodorise them but that *direct contact* was necessary.

The case for chlorophyllin as a deodorant in tooth-pastes rests upon the above and similar tests. In the laboratory it can be shown quite definitely that aqueous solutions of chlorophyllins are capable of deodorising a number of malodorous substances. There is no adequate proof concerning the possibility that deodorisation of evil-smelling breath (arising from within the body) is produced by the use of chlorophyllin-containing tooth-pastes but it must be conceded that, providing the concentration of chlorophyll is adequate [it is usually about 0·10 per cent. concentration expressed as sodium (potassium, or potassium-sodium) copper chlorophyllin], and the solution can contact the surfaces of the substances, surfaces, plaques or cavities, producing the odour, some reduction in odour may occur. As far as the action of chlorophyllins in reducing the number of bacteria causing production of acids in the mouth is concerned, evidence at the present time appears to be inconclusive. In November 1951, the Council on Dental Therapeutics of the American Dental Association issued a preliminary report on a chlorophyll dentifrice (*J. Amer. dent. Ass.*, Nov. 1950, p. 43). This suggested that a conservative attitude be adopted regarding the efficacy of chlorophyll in dentifrices until further evidence is available.

PENICILLIN IN DENTIFRICES. The use of penicillin in dentifrices has been found by several investigators to lead to a reduction in the incidence of dental caries. Zander (*J. Amer. dent. Ass.*, May 1950, **40**, 5, 569) has reported the results of a two-year toothbrushing study in Walpole, Mass., in which 325 elementary school children participated. As a result of thorough dental examinations including full-mouth and bitewing

[1] *See* discussion on sodium metaphosphate and calcium phosphate in Chapter 17, paragraph dealing with action of dentifrices on the tooth structure.

roentgenograms of all the children before and after the study, Zander concluded that the use of a dentifrice containing penicillin reduced the incidence of dental caries significantly as against the use of a control dentifrice, without penicillin.

I have been consistently against the indiscriminate use of penicillin in cosmetic and toilet preparations and in 1948 (R. G. Harry, *Cosmetic Materials*, London: Leonard Hill Ltd., 1948, pp. 224-229) stressed the possible dangers arising from such use, under two headings:

(i) that penicillin-resistant strains of organisms might develop;
(ii) that penicillin may sensitise the patient.

I see no reason to alter my opinions.

The undesirable "bacteria-stimulating effect" of certain drugs and antibiotics was pointed out by Professor L. P. Garrod in his Kettle Memorial Lecture (*Brit. med. J.*, 3 Feb. 1951, p. 205); through *Chem. & Drugg.*, 10 March 1951, p. 307) who cited that there is clinical evidence that penicillin can stimulate the growth of bacteria, and increase the mortality in mice suffering from certain infections. Attention was drawn to the fact that penicillin might stimulate the growth of the tubercle bacillus which is highly resistant to penicillin and forms penicillinase. It was mentioned that certain workers have reported that the maximum enhancement of growth with many organisms was produced by about one-fifth of the amount of penicillin required to inhibit growth.

In May 1950, and again in October 1952 (*Drug Cosmet. Ind.*, Nov. 1952, p. 517), the Council on Dental Therapeutics of the American Dental Association issued a report on the current status of penicillin in dentifrices. The Council states the major problems as:

(i) the possibility of sensitising a significant portion of the population to penicillin;
(ii) the development of penicillin-resistant micro-organisms in those using the dentifrice.

Because of (*a*) the contradictory nature of the evidence from the therapeutic usefulness of penicillin dentifrices when employed with or without supervision and (*b*) the tendency for development of a higher percentage of micro-organisms resistant to 0·5 units or more, of penicillin per cubic cm., in the mouths of those using the penicillin dentifrice, the Council concludes that: "On the basis of available evidence, penicillin dentifrices should not be distributed at the present time except on a prescription basis. Qualified individuals or institutions should continue to conduct further investigations concerning the therapeutic usefulness and safety of antibiotic dentifrices. . . ."

ANTI-ENZYME DENTIFRICES. In August 1953, Fosdick and co-workers (*J. Dent. Res.*, August 1953, **32**, 4, 486) stated that the dental plaque was the source of most of the enzymes involved in the production of dental caries and that it served as a sponge to hold the sugars and acids in contact with the tooth surface. These workers endeavoured to find an enzyne-inhibitor which would attach itself to the dental plaque.

As a result of laboratory tests on 381 compounds, two compounds were found to be effective and fill all the desirable requirements of compatibility, flavour, colour and absence of toxicity. These substances were sodium *N*-lauroyl sarcosinate and sodium dehydroacetate. Subsequently Fosdick *et al.* published a clinical report (*Bull. Northw. Univ. med. Sch., Dent. Res.*, 1953, **54**, 3) which indicated that in a preliminary one-year test with *N*-lauroyl sarcosinate in a dentifrice, caries activity was reduced. However, Forscher and Hess [*J. Amer. dent. Ass.*, February 1954, **48**, 2, 201, "The Validity of Plaque *p*H Measurements as a Method of evaluating Therapeutic Agents"] have recently made a study of the *p*H of dental plaques using different instruments and types of subjects. These investigators found that:

(i) the actual *p*H measurement of a single plaque sample was reliable;

(ii) plaque samples from different regions of the mouth differed in *p*H;

(iii) a dentifrice containing 2 per cent. sodium N-lauroyl sarcosinate did not prevent acid formation in the dental plaque.

Forscher and Hess point out that whilst there is no doubt that the true *p*H of the plaque is the *p*H registered on the *p*H meter, the use of such readings on small samples, as a basis for conclusions concerning the whole mouth, or all the surface plaques in the mouth, may be questionable. Forscher and Hess found pronounced differences in the *p*H of plaque samples from different regions of the same mouth, and hence on the basis of their investigations question the validity of a screening test based on *p*H changes of plaque.

Summarising briefly the large amount of research on the therapeutic efficacy of dentifrices which has been carried out in recent years it appears to me that whilst such researches cannot fail to extend our general knowledge of the mouth, and of the mode of action of the decay processes and may well eventually lead to results of general benefit, *there is as yet no statistically significant and convincing scientific evidence that any of the dentifrices, available generally to the public, materially decrease the incidence and severity of dental caries by reason of the action of any specific active therapeutic ingredient in them.* This should *not*, however, be taken to mean that dentifrices have no prophylactic value; they undoubtedly have!

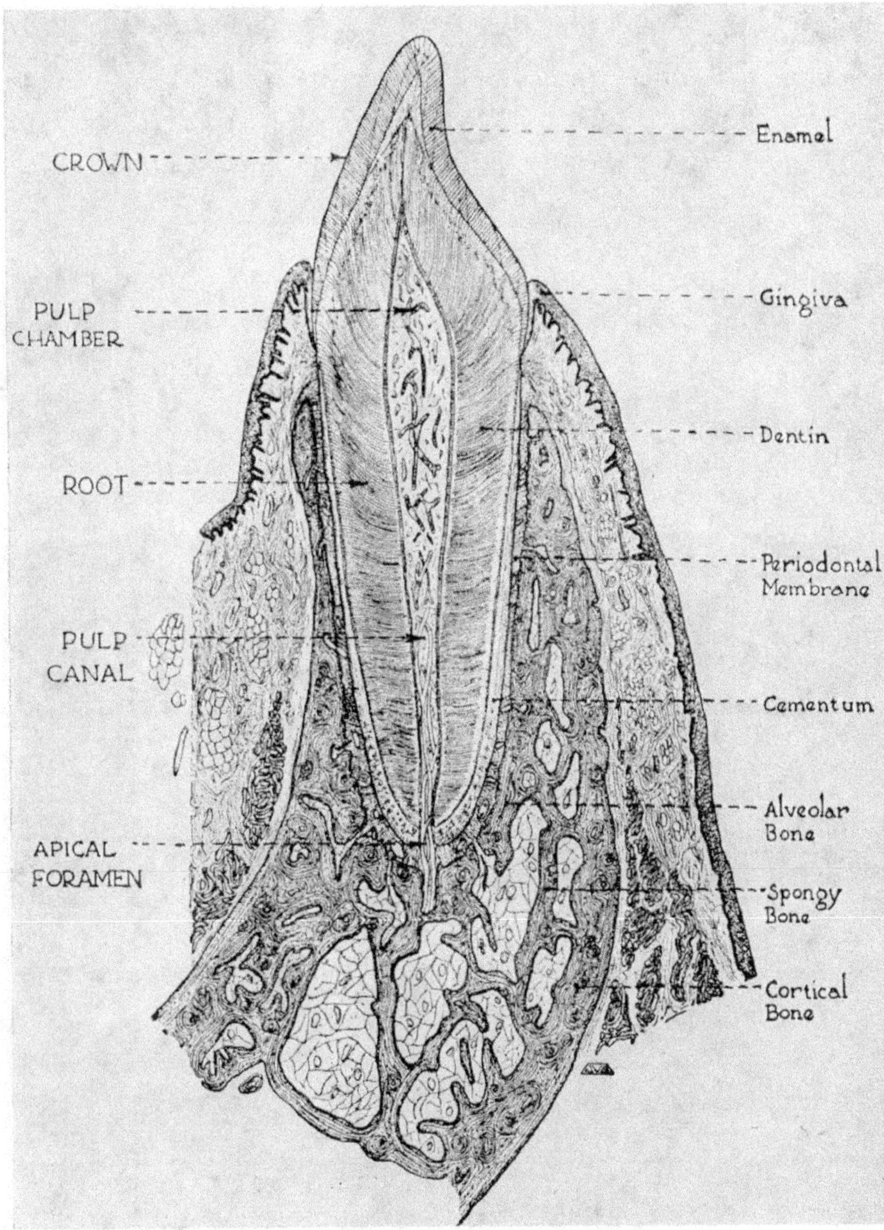

[*By courtesy of Lea and Febiger.*

FIG. 42.—Diagrammatic representation of the dental tissues (from Noyes, Schour and Noyes).

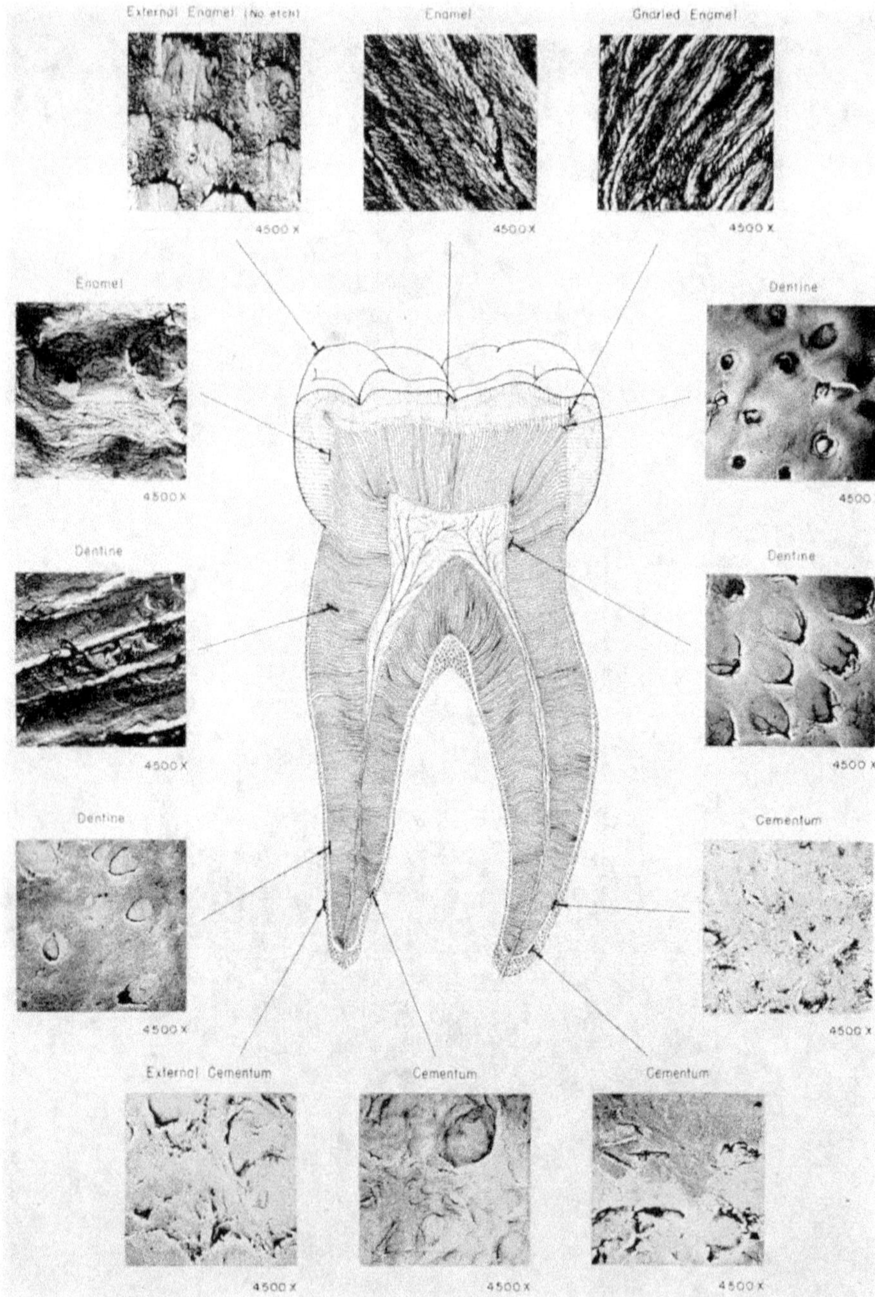

[*By courtesy of the Dow Chemical Co., Michigan.*

FIG. 43.—Cross-section of tooth enlarged. Tooth surfaces in above cases were polished, etched, reproduced by the replica technique and then photographed in the electron microscope.

Role of Dental Preparations

The role of dental preparations in the light of the above is thus obvious. Both as regards tartar formation and dental caries, they should assist the removal of food debris from the tooth surface and from open fissures which can be reached by the paste and brush. Their mild abrasive action and the wetting effects of incorporated soap or soapless detergent, assist in the prevention of tartar, if brushing is carried out regularly night and morning, and even in *its removal* if used within a day of its formation. They cannot, however, by themselves remove old-established tartar which has formed impermeable concretions over several weeks. This necessitates a preliminary removal of the incrustation by mechanical means. There is no doubt, however, that a tooth-brush plus a dentifrice is a far more efficient cleanser than a tooth-brush and water alone. The abrasive used in such preparations must be such that it will not damage the enamel. No essential difference exists between the cleansing power of a tooth-paste and of a tooth-powder, the latter in any case becomes a paste on wetting with water prior to application.

CHAPTER 17

TOOTH-PASTES AND TOOTH-POWDERS, DENTURE CLEANSERS

Abrasives—Detergents—Excipients—Sweeteners—The Abrasive and Lustre-Producing Properties of Dentifrices—Measurement of Lustre—Dentifrices and the Tooth Structure—Tooth-powder and Tooth-paste Formulations—Solid Dentifrice—U.S. Federal Specifications—Denture Cleansers.

> . . . . *No dentifrice, under ordinary conditions of use can or should sterilise the mouth. Not only is the period of contact too short, but dilution occurs by saliva and the water introduced in brushing; nor would sterilisation of the mouth—if achieved—be desirable. The health of the body, and its various tissues and organs—including the mouth—depends upon the maintenance of the normal microbiological and enzyme systems. The functions of a tooth-powder or tooth-paste, is to cleanse, polish and whiten the teeth without abrasion, impart a pleasant fresh taste to the mouth and disguise any disagreeable odour.—The Author.*

TOOTH-PASTES may be considered as tooth-powders suspended in a suitable excipient and binder. The exact differentiation between these two terms is not absolutely defined, as many substances are capable of acting in both capacities. In general, the term *excipient or vehicle* refers to the material imparting the necessary *fluidity* to the paste whilst the *binder* prevents separation. Tooth-pastes are manufactured in various colours: ordinary white paste, green (containing chlorophyllins), pink, and vivid red (to tint the gums).

The various components of tooth-powders and tooth-pastes and their effect on the tooth structure, where known, are described below prior to giving examples of dentifrice formulations.

ABRASIVES. Precipitated chalk is probably the most widely used abrasive in tooth paste formulations.[1] According to the conditions of precipitation and purification, precipitated chalks of different densities may be obtained. The crystalline structure is also influenced by the methods of precipitation, for instance, calcium carbonate precipitated from cold limewater by carbon dioxide has the calcite structure; from hot water, crystals of aragonite are produced. (Calcite, which is considered to be the stable form at ordinary temperatures and pressures, differs from aragonite in that its crystalline form is rhombohedral hexagonal whilst crystals of calcite are orthorhombic.) Some manufacturers prefer to

[1] In Great Britain but not in the U.S.A.

use a precipitated chalk which is essentially aragonite in structure. [The measurement of the proportion of calcite and aragonite in precipitated chalk has been described in the *Journal of the Society of the Chemical Industry*, London, 1937, p. 56, *Transactions*, pp. 283-287. Microscopical examination of the sample is valuable but requires great care. X-ray examination probably gives the most accurate representation of the ratio of aragonite to calcite but a rough test which is extremely useful is the Meigen Cobalt salt test (*See Ber. naturf. Ges. Freiburg. i. B.*, 1905, **15**, 38, 55 ; also *Mergen Centr. Min.*, 1901, p. 577).]

Chalk is cheap, and has been considered to clean well without scratching the enamel. Investigations by Phillips and VanHuysen (*Amer. Perfum.*, Jan. 1948, p. 33) reported in greater detail in this chapter under Dentifrices and the Tooth Structure, have, however, thrown some doubt about this supposition of " non-scratching " and further work on the abrasiveness of chalk on tooth enamel would appear to be eminently desirable. Alternatively to chalk, dicalcium and tricalcium phosphates, heavy magnesium carbonate, etc., have been used. Kaolin adheres tenaciously to the teeth when wetted and requires vigorous brushing to remove it. This is of advantage perhaps in some ways, but the difficulty of removing it rapidly makes the inclusion of some wetting agent necessary, additional to that normally used in a tooth-paste.

Various other materials, some of them patented, have been advocated for use in dentifrices. One of these is composed of a mixture consisting of insoluble metaphosphate and tricalcium phosphate (U.S. Patent 2,216,816, October 1940, assigned to Pepsodent Co.). The abrasive properties of " what appears to be a similar material ", in comparison with those of chalk are discussed by Phillips and VanHuysen.

Insoluble silicates having a hardness on Moh's scale of between 2 and 3 have been claimed to have a hardness sufficiently high for use in dentifrices but not high enough to be detrimental to teeth (U.S. Patent 2,059,396). Micas such as Muscovite, Paragonite, Lepidolite, Zinnwaldite, Biotite and Phlogopite were specifically suggested.

Aluminium hydroxide having a particle size substantially in the range 0·025–0·5 microns has also been suggested (U.S. Patent 2,550,207, 1951).

Of somewhat different type, the following materials have also been patented for use as an abrasive in dentifrices : a solid artificial resin in the form of a powder (U.S. Patent 2,211,369, Aug. 1940, assigned to Monsanto Chemical Co.) ; hemicellulose treated to form a " gelatin " which is warmed with solutions of carbohydrates and sulphonated fatty acids to give a clear transparent tooth-paste (Swiss Patent 524/50). Reference has also been made in the technical press to a new dentifrice based on powdered pulp left over from apple processing, the detoxicating

JOHN AND E. STURGE LIMITED

PRECIPITATED CALCIUM CARBONATE

Grade	Nature of P.C.C.	*Size analysis by weight. Percentage in each fraction of equivalent sphere diameter in microns*								*Weight median diameter in microns*	*Surface area by nitrogen adsorption* m^2/g	*Equivalent spherical diameter from ads. surface area in microns*
		+16	10–16	8–10	6–8	4–6	3–4	1½–3	< 1½			
Light "F"	Aragonitic	3·4	14·8	11·4	18·1	20·1	10·1	14·8	7·3	5·7	6·5	0·34
Aeromatt	Calcitic	1·4	2·4	1·7	14·1	43·3	25·1	10·0	2·0	4·5	4·4	0·50

Weight Median Diameter

The weight median diameter is defined as follows: If 50 per cent. by weight of a P.C.C. sample (as determined by size analysis) has a particle diameter greater than *d*, then *d* is known as the *weight median diameter* of the sample.

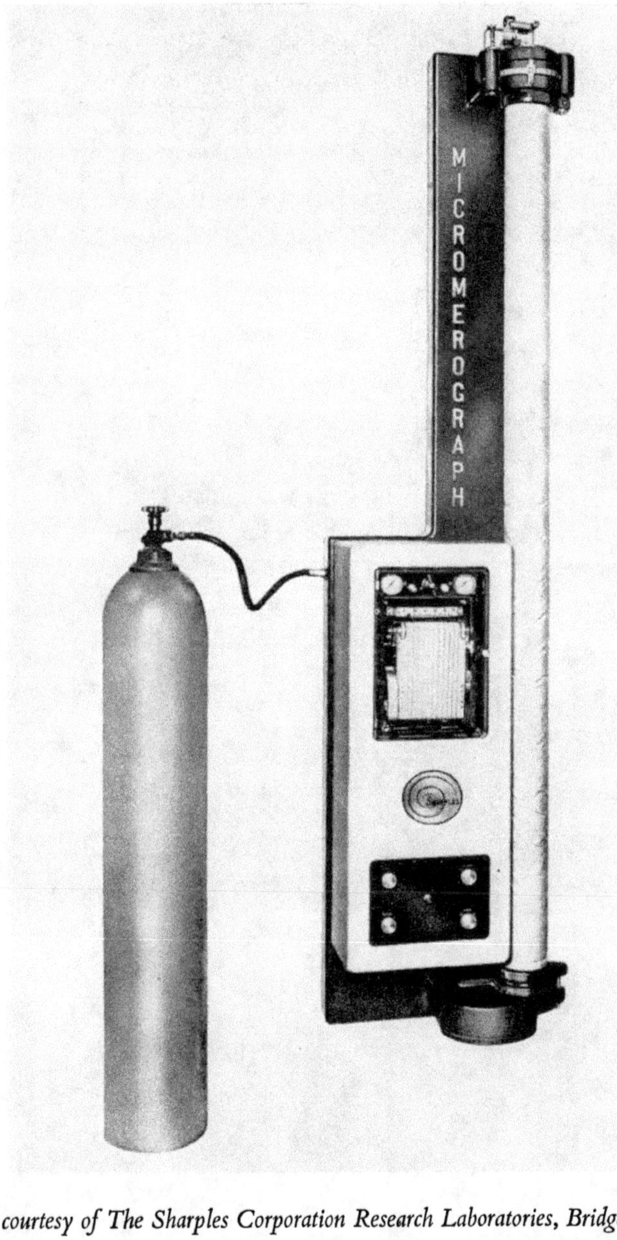

[*By courtesy of The Sharples Corporation Research Laboratories, Bridgeport, Penn.*

FIG. 44.—The Sharples Micromerograph. This is a new particle size distribution analyser which gives rapid, accurate and reproducible results on powders in the range of 1–100 microns. Designed for use in production control as well as research work, the instrument is comprised of a highly efficient deagglomeration device, a gaseous sedimentation tube, and an unusually rapid response servo-electronic recording balance of high sensitivity.

effect of which, it is claimed, promises a most effective and tasty guard against tooth decay. (Parke, Davis and Co. through *Drug Cosmet. Ind.*, Sept. 1951, p. 309).

Two new dentifrices based upon calcium lactate have been patented (U.S. Patents 2,554,464 and 2,554,465). These compositions are free from soap and detergent and, it is claimed, depend for their cleansing action upon the liquefaction of mucin, a viscous component of human saliva. The use of such dentifrices is based on the use of calcium lactate to serve as a substrate for an oxidising enzyme, lactic dehydrogenase.

DETERGENTS IN DENTIFRICES. Whilst soap was the detergent agent in the older dentifrices and *is still extensively used by a number of leading manufacturers*, there is increasing evidence of the use of synthetic detergent materials in tooth-pastes and several of the leading dentifrice manufacturers have gone over to a soapless formula. The fact that a number of these synthetic detergents have all " . . . *been components of widely used dentifrices for some years, without evidence of untoward effect would indicate them to be reasonably safe for use in dentifrices as long as the amount is not increased over what has been used to the present time.* . . ." [F. E. Walter and H. J. Carbson, *J. dent. Res.*, April 1949, **28**, 124].

The most widely used synthetic detergent in dentifrices would appear to be sodium lauryl sulphate (a mixture comprising essentially R . OSO_3Na, where R designates an alkyl group which is predominantly lauryl ($C_{12}H_{25}$)).

Other widely used materials are Nacconal LAL, the more recent name of which is Lanthanol LAL (Socium lauryl sulphoacetate).

$$Na\ O_3SCH_2COOR$$

where R again stands for the lauryl radicle ; and Sulphocolaurate which is a mixture stated to contain 91 per cent. by weight of the lauric acid ester of the potassium salt of sulphoacetic acid amide esterified with β-amino ethyl alcohol. The formula for this is given as

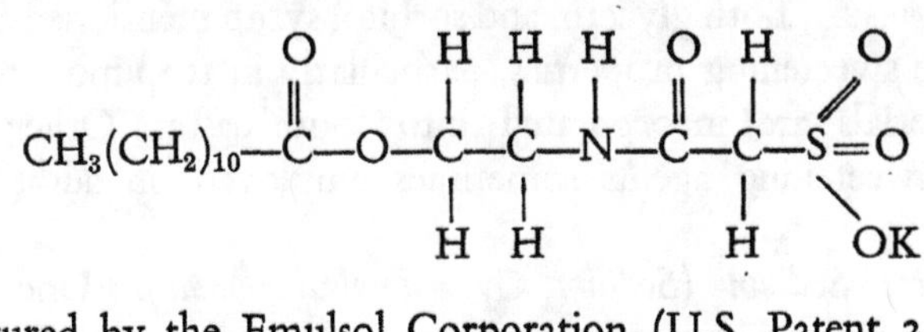

[Manufactured by the Emulsol Corporation (U.S. Patent 2,184,770).]

Dioctyl Sodium Sulphosuccinate (Aerosol OT), formula

$$C_8H_{17}—OOC—CH_2—CHSO_3Na—COO—C_8H_{17}$$

is also employed in dentifrices.

A factor which was of importance in leading to the adoption of synthetic detergents on a larger scale in the U.S.A. was that, by the use of such detergents in place of soap, many of the difficulties encountered in the formulation of ammoniated dentifrices were overcome. Apart from this, however, at least one leading United States dentifrice manufacturer has sponsored the use of sodium alkyl sulphate for many years.

EXCIPIENT AND HUMECTANT. Because tooth-paste is essentially a moderately firm dispersion of " solids in a liquid ", having certain necessary characteristics, viz. that the paste should not very readily dry out even if the cap of the tube is left off, the choice of the excipient is of great importance. Of necessity it must be non-toxic, non-corrosive, and have at least " a not-unpleasant " flavour. For a great many years glycerin has been the most popular excipient in tooth-pastes.

During wartime, it became necessary to endeavour to formulate paste without such addition, using instead certain sugar syrups and by-products. Some of these were moderately successful; nevertheless, the best indication of the value of glycerin in a tooth-paste was the immediate post-war scramble by manufacturers, in spite of the cost of glycerin—to get back to the use of this material.

Its nearest rival for use in tooth-pastes would appear to be sorbitol syrup, which tests have shown to have no irritating effect on the buccal membranes, which does not contribute to the formation of dental caries and which has been accepted for use in dentifrices by the Council on Dental Therapeutics of the American Dental Association (*J. Amer. dent. Ass.*, June 1940, p. 959) through *Drug and Cosmetic Emulsions* (Atlas Powder Co., Wilmington).

Propylene glycol has also been suggested for use in tooth-pastes but in my opinion glycerin and/or sorbitol syrup are more suitable, in general, for this particular purpose.

All of the above materials possess the very necessary property of " humectancy ". (*See* Chapter 44, Humectants.)

SWEETENERS. Both glycerin and sorbitol syrup mentioned above have appreciable sweetening properties, particularly in the amounts in which these materials are incorporated into tooth-paste. Other powerful synthetic sweetening agents sometimes employed, in addition to the above are:

Cyclamate Sodium (*Sodium Cyclohexylsulphamate*). Under normal conditions of use this material appears to be quite safe. Evidence indicates that it has a somewhat greater stability than saccharin when exposed to temperatures required for cooking. (*Accepted Dental Remedies*, 1952, p. 143.)

Cyclamate Calcium has very similar properties.

Saccharin (Gluside) in the form of its sodium salt (which is very soluble in water) is widely employed for sweetening dentifrices. Chemically this substance is 2,3-Dihydro-3-oxobenzisosulphonazole, i.e. ortho-sulphobenzimide.

OTHER ADDITIVES. *Cellulosic* derivatives such as sodium carboxy-methylcellulose, and methyl cellulose are sometimes used to assist in maintaining a satisfactory consistency.

Mineral oil may be included as a lubricant to assist in minimising any tendency for the cream to harden and to assist its extrusion from the tube.

Mucilage. Unless one of the cellulosic derivatives mentioned above is incorporated, it is usual to employ gum tragacanth as a peptising agent and protective colloid in tooth-pastes. According to the composition of the formulation, amounts employed may vary from about 0·1–1·0 per cent.

FLAVOURS. These, in the case of tooth-paste, are usually based either upon peppermint or upon spearmint oils ; modifiers included are usually selected from clove, wintergreen, eucalyptus, aniseed, rose, lavender, etc. Menthol is sometimes included in order to back up the peppermint effect and to exert a cooling flavour, but because of its burn and unpleasant after-taste it must be employed only with discretion. (In some instances it is possible to use a chemical method of stabilising the flavouring.) It has been pointed out (Schimmel Briefs, No. 201, Dec. 1951) that "... this chemical method of stabilisation can be applied only to volatile compounds which have in the molecule a reactive group such as hydroxyl or carbonyl. In general it is not applicable to the volatile esters but methyl salicylate (synthetic wintergreen) is an exception. This ester contains a free phenol group and reacts with alcoholic sodium hydroxide to form a non-volatile crystalline salt. The powdered sodium methyl salicylate may be used in tooth-powders to secure a long-lasting wintergreen flavour since the salt hydrolyses in the mouth, yielding free methyl salicylate...." (U.S. Patent 2,519,665.)

A new development is also the use of sorbitol as a matrix for dispersing flavouring or perfume oils (U.S. Patent 2,566,410).

"SPECIAL" ADDITIVES. To enhance the whitening effects of tooth-pastes and powders and to assist in the removal of stains, the following oxygen salts are sometimes incorporated : sodium perborate, magnesium peroxide, hydrogen peroxide-urea compounds, stabilised hydrogen peroxide compounds, etc.

Sodium Perborate. The Report of the Council on Dental Therapeutics of the American Dental Association, states that there is no carefully controlled evidence that sodium perborate is beneficial to the gums, bleaches the teeth, or prevents diseases of the gums ; it also states that, unless the powder and the alkali, resulting from its decomposition, be thoroughly removed, inflammation and necrosis of the oral membrane may result.

So far as the *peroxide compounds* are concerned, hydrogen peroxide-urea compounds—like the majority of peroxide compounds—possess only a limited stability. Hydrogen peroxide is sometimes added directly to a tooth-paste, but it is at least doubtful whether under such conditions the tooth-paste has any " peroxide " activity.

Ricinoleate and Sulphoricinoleate Derivatives. Various papers have appeared in the past to show that these compounds have detoxifying powers, for example (*Proc. Amer. Acad. Arts Sci.*, June 1932, through *Nature*, 18 Feb. 1933, p. 244 ; *J. Lab. clin. Med.*, Oct. 1932 ; *Dent. Cosmos*, 1930, **72,** 830). As pointed out (R. G. Harry, *Cosmetic Materials*, 1948, London: Leonard Hill Ltd., p. 305) " . . . considerable evidence has been accumulated to show that sodium ricinoleate has the property of detoxifying bacteria. In cases of gingivitis and infections of the gums and sockets the application of a *solution* of sodium ricinoleate has given excellent results. . . ." As to whether such advantages are conferred to the user of a *tooth-paste* containing such additions, can be ascertained only by careful clinical trial.

The Abrasive Action—and Lustre-Producing Properties—of Dentifrices

Because biological material in the form of extracted teeth, animal and human, is fairly readily available, researches on the relative effect of various dentifrice ingredients on teeth have been carried out by a number of investigators, research chemists, physicists and dentists. Moreover, since some observations can be made directly on human teeth without extraction, testing panels of human volunteers on quite a large scale are available for practical trials under actual usage conditions.

The properties of greatest interest to the dentifrice manufacturer are :

(i) the abrasive and/or chemical effect of the preparation being tested, upon the enamel and dentin of the tooth ;

(ii) the assessment of the relative polish, gloss, or lustre produced on the tooth by the dentifrice under test as compared with competitive products.

THE ABRASIVE ACTION OF DENTIFRICES. Before admission of a dentifrice to the Accepted Dental Remedies in the United States, the results of abrasion tests have to be furnished, together with samples of the product. Before discussing the abrasiveness of such products, it is worth while considering the prevalence of abrasion in teeth and also whether a completely non-abrasive dentifrice would be acceptable.

A number of papers have been published concerning the prevalence of abrasion in teeth ("Cervical Exposure and Abrasion in Human Teeth for Different Age Classes", P. C. Kitchin, *Science*, 18 July 1941, **94**, 65; "The Prevalence of Tooth Root Exposure and the Relation of the Extent of such Exposure to the Degree of Abrasion in different Age Classes", P. C. Kitchin, *J. dent. Res.*, Dec. 1941, p. 565; "Prevalence of Toothroot Exposure and Abrasion Among Dental Patients, J. C. Ervine and E. M. Bucher, *Dental Items of Interest*; "The Abrasion of Cementum and Dentin by Modern Dentifrices", R. S. Manley, *J. dent. Res.*, Dec. 1941, **6**, 583, etc.).

These investigations indicate that even moderately abrasive dentifrices result, over a long period of use, in some degree of abrasion and that the brush plays an insignificant part in such abrasion since Manley (*J. dent. Res.*) found that a dry brush abraded dentin only about 1 per cent. as much as the average of leading tooth-pastes and powders.

At the same time it should be realised that "a certain amount of abrasiveness" is necessary in order to keep the tooth surface clean. It has been pointed out (*Accepted Dental Remedies*, 10th edn., p. 86) that ". . . liquid dentifrices represent one extreme with respect to abrasiveness. It has been claimed that the lack of abrasiveness of these products is advantageous. In cases of gingival recession this may be plausible. On the other hand, the available evidence indicates that liquid dentifrices are not so effective as conventional tooth-pastes and powders under ordinary conditions of usage. Claims for superior cleansing properties are therefore unwarranted. . . ."

Manly ("A Structureless Recurrent Deposit on Teeth", *J. dent. Res.*, Dec. 1943, **6**, 479) has found that in the case of persons who use no abrasive in their oral hygiene, a thin structureless organic pellicle appeared in a number of cases. This deposit can readily be removed by one or two brushings with dentifrice abrasives and will recur whenever abrasive brushings are omitted for one or two weeks. Valloton (*J. dent. Res.*, June-Aug. 1945) confirmed Manly's observations.

Apart from those cases in which the gum line has receded, or where the dentin has become exposed (and these represent pathological conditions which require treatment by a dental practitioner), it is my opinion that it is not the presence or absence of abrasion *per se* that is important but rather the *degree* of any such abrasion in comparison with the efficacy of the product. I should imagine that in comparison with masticating hard sweets or gnawing bones such abrasion would be slight. Many manufacturers have assumed that the results of abrasion losses on metal plates, etc., can be related in some way to the amount of abrasion to be anticipated on teeth.

In *Accepted Dental Remedies* (American Dental Association, 10th edn., p. 86) it is stated, in relation to such tests, that *while data on these substances are listed it is not yet possible to draw definite conclusions concerning differences between the various products in regard to their action on tooth structures under actual conditions of use.*

Epstein ("Practical Significance of Abrasives in Dentifrices Council on Dental Therapeutics", *J. Amer. dent. Ass.*, 1 March 1944, p. 400) concludes (1) there is a definite relationship between particle size and the hardness of insoluble constituents, and the amount of abrasion caused by dentifrices. The larger or harder the particles, the deeper the abrasion. (2) Within reasonable limits the concentration of the dentifrice will not affect the amount of abrasion. (3) *No test material other than teeth is satisfactory for evaluating the amount of abrasion that can be caused by the use of a dentifrice on tooth structure. There is no correlation between tests on various metal plates and test teeth.*

Tainter (*Proc. Sci. Sect.* (U.S.) *T.G.A.*, 26 Jan. 1944, p. 27) as a result of tests carried out on metal plates of copper, silver, and antimony against a considerable number of tooth-powders whose abrasion had already been determined on teeth, showed that *there is no correlation between the results on metal and those on the teeth, and therefore the use of metal surfaces as test objects is useless since the information obtained thereby cannot be transferred in any useful way to the problem at issue.*

The use of glass slides as standard test objects was similarly investigated. Glass is much closer in hardness to the human tooth enamel than the metals normally employed such as copper, silver and antimony. It was found that if a fairly heavy pressure were applied and the abrasion was carried out with a moist material, there was a moderately good correlation between the degree of scratching of the glass and the demonstrated effects on teeth. However, a few tests were entirely aberrant and the test failed completely if an adequate degree of pressure were not applied since thereby enough force was not exerted, even with the most abrasive material, to cut through the glass surface. The major difficulty with the glass slide procedure seemed to be that the observed increases in scratching of the glass were small compared to those on the teeth.[1] As a result it would be very difficult with this technique to determine with the desired degree of accuracy how abrasive a given material might be on teeth.

[1] These results are of interest, since the U.S. Federal Specification FFF-D-191, Abrasion Tests F-1e(1) stipulates glass as a medium.

The main point of application of the glass slide procedure would seem to be to detect traces of highly abrasive materials, since these scratch the glass even though present in very minute amount. By this technique 0·016 per cent. flour of pumice or 0·0037 per cent. of 240 mesh silica in a standard calcium carbonate could be detected.

In experiments upon the abrasiveness of dentifrices on teeth, using a modification of the Pepsodent Abrasion Testing Machine, Tainter (*Proc. Sci. Sect.* (U.S.) *T.G.A.*, 26 Jan. 1944, pp. 24–28) records the following data:

CONCENTRATION OF THE SLURRY. Tests carried out with slurries of calcium carbonate U.S.P. having a mean particle size of 3·8 microns with practically all the particles less than 15 microns in diameter showed that the abrasion was only increased by 20 per cent. by a 700 per cent. increase in the concentration of the slurry which would indicate that *in brushing the teeth it makes little difference how much of the dentifrice is used, provided, of course, that enough is applied to have it always operating in the field of the tooth-brush.*

SENSITIVITY OF THE TEST. Data on this were obtained by mixing various amounts of a silica of 240 mesh fineness in the standard chalk. It was found that 0·16 per cent. increased the amount of abrasion from 100 per cent. to 158 per cent. while 5 per cent. silica increased it to 308 per cent. When the amount of added silica was reduced to 0·08 per cent. the added abrasive was found to be too low a concentration to be reliably detected by this method.

PARTICLE SIZE. The relationship between the particle size of a substance and its abrasiveness was investigated using various brands of calcium carbonate and dicalcium phosphate. *It was found that with calcium carbonate, doubling the size of the particles produced almost doubling of the abrasive power while in the case of dicalcium phosphate the inherent abrasive power was so much less that the diameter of the particles could be varied over a wide range without producing any substantially increased abrasiveness. These tests would indicate that control of particle size in calcium carbonate dentifrices is of greater importance than in the case of dicalcium phosphate dentifrices.*

Tainter found discrepancies of considerable magnitude in a number of powders sold to the industry with definite specifications as to their particle sizes. This may be due to the firms having used different methods of measuring their particle sizes or to stratification of the powders before use so that the samples were not representative of the material in general, or more likely, adequate control of particle size on the manufacturing scale was not maintained.

Smith (Research Laboratories, J. and E. Sturge Ltd., Birmingham, England, " Value of the Antimony Plate abrasion Apparatus in Testing

Dentifrices", *J. Amer. dent. Ass.*, Feb. 1939, p. 206) has drawn attention to the difficulty of obtaining reproducible biological surfaces such as teeth. Using an antimony plate surface with a revolving table type of apparatus, it has been shown that the abrasiveness of a series of precipitated chalks, so Smith states, followed the particle size whereas in comparing different powders, the hardness was a very important factor (Smith, *J. Soc. chem. Ind.*, 1936, p. 269). Smith agrees that unfortunately there is no correlation between such tests and actual tests upon teeth. However, various workers have concluded, as a result of brushing tests upon extracted teeth, that with the normal run of dentifrices now available, enamel is hardly damaged though there is a possibility of cutting into the softer tissues. Smith also draws attention to differences existing in particle size and aggregation of the various chalks used by different workers, so that it is difficult to apply the results of such experiments in a general way.

FLOW OF SURFACES. Discussing the flow of metal surfaces, Smith states that it is known that flow does occur in the polishing of surfaces and it is acceptable that in using finer powders a flow layer will tend to build up more readily as there will be less rapid removal of the top surface than with coarse powders, but it is pointed out that surface flow may also occur quite readily with any crystalline surface and that there is a possibility that flow occurs in the case of the polishing of enamel. Smith adds that to check this point an electron diffraction study would be of interest.

THE MEASUREMENT OF "LUSTRE" ("GLOSS", OR "POLISH") PRODUCED BY DENTIFRICES. The measurement of this quality is by no means such a simple and straightforward procedure as one might imagine, since the measurement is complicated by a number of factors which make assessment difficult and complex.

The "gloss" (which may be taken to be the same thing as "lustre") of a surface is its power to reflect light specularly (as distinct from a mirror surface).

Unfortunately, as R. S. Hunter ("Methods of Determining Gloss", U.S. National Bureau of Standards, Research Paper, RP. 958, Jan. 1937) has pointed out, it is impossible to measure specular reflectance and diffuse reflectance as separate entities in any but an approximate way. Hunter describes *six different kinds of gloss*, viz.:

(i) *Specular Gloss.* Identified by "shininess".

(ii) *Sheen.* Identified by surface shininess at grazing angles.

(iii) *Contrast gloss.* Identified by contrasts between specularly reflecting areas of surfaces and other ones.

(iv) *Absence-of-bloom gloss.* Identified by the absence of reflection haze or smear adjacent to reflected high lights.

(v) *Distinctness-of-reflected-image gloss.* Identified by the distinctness of images reflected in surfaces.

(vi) *Absence-of-surface-texture gloss.* Identified by the lack of surface texture and surface blemishes.

Fortunately these six types of gloss do not occur together. Sheen and contrast gloss usually occur in the case of surfaces of low gloss, specular gloss with a surface of somewhat greater gloss, whilst the other three types occur with surfaces of high gloss.

For reasons which will be apparent when we discuss the psychological aspect of lustre determination, it is extremely unlikely that any laboratory method will provide infallible results when compared with the opinion expressed by a number of observers judging merely on " sight " and " opinion ". *Complicated methods of measurements are therefore out of place unless it can be shown that they yield results which are concordant with expressed opinions.*

The simplest method of measuring, in the laboratory, the " lustre " of different teeth appears to be that in which the " specular plus diffuse reflection " is measured and then the diffuse reflection deducted.

In the " Goerz " method, this is accomplished by measuring the intensity of the light reflected at the angle of specular reflection and then turning the measuring apparatus so that it is then re-measured at right angles to this direction. The *ratio* of these intensities gives a gloss number, an arbitrary one as Harrison (V. G. W. Harrison, " Definition and Measurement of Gloss and Smoothness of Paper ", *Paper Mkr. Lond.*, 1945, Midsummer Special, Vol. CIX) has pointed out, but one which does bear a closer relationship to the *sensation* of gloss than do certain types of glossmeters.

It should be remembered that *opinions on the lustre of teeth are " built up " from observations of the tooth at many angles. If one is asked to express an opinion upon an extracted tooth, one picks it up, carries it to a good source of light and ROTATES it in the hand, and then, as a result of ALL of these observations at different angles of incident lighting (and acceptance angles by the eyes) one comes to a considered " opinion ". If an opinion is requested upon teeth in a person's mouth, then similarly, the person is asked to turn his head slowly whilst the teeth are similarly studied.*

As Harrison points out : " Hardly any attention has been given to the philosophic basis of the subject. . . . Gloss, texture and smoothness are not physical objects or quantities that can be measured in the same way as mass or length ; they are *sensations*, or more correctly, sense data ; they are neither material nor purely mental ; they are dependent upon our minds ; and their study involves, or should involve, a knowledge of the theory of sense perception, which is an important and difficult branch of philosophy. Without such knowledge one may easily go seriously astray. It is easy enough to devise instruments for measuring something that looks as if it should be related to the quality or property we are trying to assess ; but unless we have been very careful in the first instance in choosing that something, it is likely that we shall measure the wrong combination of physical qualities and end up with figures or meter readings that are either worthless or still worse, misleading. . . ."

In the paint and lacquer industry a test method has been worked out and described (American Society Testing Materials, D 523-44T, 1946), the basic principle of which is the illumination of the test specimen with a parallel beam of light and the measurement of the reflection of this beam at a predetermined angle. From consideration it appeared to M. L. Tainter and co-workers that this method could be modified for the measurement of directional reflectance. Considerable refinement of apparatus and technique was necessary to adapt this method to measurements of gloss on teeth because of the small size and curvature of the enamel surface. As a result of their experiments Tainter, Alford, Hinkel, Jr., Nachod and Priznar published, in 1947, their quantitative method for measuring polish produced by dentifrices (*Proc. Sci. Sect. T.G.A.*). For full details the original paper should be consulted ; the schematic set up of the apparatus is briefly as set out below.

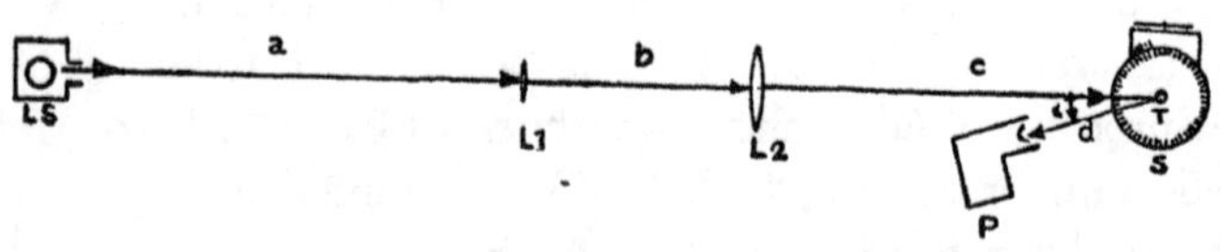

FIG. 45.

The angle of reflection adopted was 11°.

The above investigators claim that the method described affords a convenient means for evaluating the polishing power of dentifrices in terms of either absolute or relative figures and that it measures quantitatively the amount of " mirror polish " produced in values which can be calculated as ratios of an absolute standard for directional reflectance as defined by the American Society for Testing Materials.

In my opinion, the position so far as the measurement of gloss on teeth is concerned is simple. If dentifrice *A* produces more gloss than dentifrice *B*, then it is very helpful to have a *reproducible laboratory* method of *comparing A and B and recording such differences* and also of comparing dentifrice *A*, with say A_1, A_2 and any other changes in the formulation which may be made, *but the ultimate criterion of such gloss-producing properties is that the improvement in gloss must be readily discernible visually by a panel of independent, reasonably intelligent people. If such a panel can detect no difference (which is statistically significant), then I would say that the laboratory readings mean nothing.* Providing the test correlates with practical opinions, the position is different. Then laboratory methods can be standardised and are available whenever required. *The writer would stress this point because he has observed on many occasions the use of elaborate laboratory tests designed to show product A better than product B, and yet—when the product has been subjected to an ordinary user test, under the very conditions for which it was designed, the fallacy of the artificial test has been demonstrated.*

DENTIFRICES AND THE TOOTH SURFACE. R. W. Phillips and G. Van Huysen (*Amer. Perfum.*, Jan. 1948, p. 33) have investigated the action of dentifrice polishing agents on the tooth surface. In this study two methods were employed, (i) visual objective observation of lustre changes by comparison with a series of standards, and (ii) microscopic study of the tooth before and after brushing as it was considered that both methods were essential for correlating and interpreting the effects of abrasives. [These investigators point out that it should be kept in mind that polish or lustre is a surface phenomenon and is entirely independent of tooth colour. In other words, it is possible for a yellow tooth to possess as high a sheen or polish as a white tooth.]

After a standardised mechanical brushing procedure using a standard concentration of the dentifrice component as an aqueous slurry, the lustre of the teeth was compared with the lustre prior to such treatment (i.e. before and after each test). Each of the dentifrice abrasive components was tested for (i) its ability to raise the lustre on a dull surface, (ii) its tendency to dull the lustre on a highly polished surface. [Comparison of lustre was made against a control series of lustre standards composed of eight teeth which progressed proportionally in lustre from very low to extremely high lustre. Difficulties of lustre measurement and of retaining standards for comparison was thereby overcome.]

The abrasive components of dentifrices, selected for this study, were those used in varying proportions in commercial dentifrices. They were:

(1) Di-calcium phosphate.
(2) Tri-calcium phosphate.
(3) Calcium carbonate (extra heavy grade).
(4) Calcium carbonate (standard "drug" grade).
(5) Sodium meta-phosphate and tri-calcium phosphate.

Phillips and VanHuysen report as follows. "The ability of each abrasive to polish a dull tooth surface is summarised in the table below, which shows the average rise in our lustre divisions from the original 'low'.

Abrasive	*Lustre change*
$CaCO_3$ (extra heavy)	0
$CaCO_3$ (standard drug)	0
$Ca_3(PO_4)_2$	+ 1
$Ca_2H(PO_4)$	+ 1
Meta-phosphate plus calcium phosphate	+ 5

From this table it can be seen that the only agent which exhibited a definite polishing action is 'meta-phosphate + calcium phosphate', which produced a marked increase in lustre after brushing. The other agents, particularly the carbonates, do not appreciably polish a tooth which possesses a low degree of lustre.

"In order to detect any tendency towards dulling a polished tooth surface the abrasives were tested on teeth possessing a very high original lustre. The average results after the standardised time of brushing were as follows:

Abrasive	*Lustre change*
Meta-phosphate + calcium phosphate	0
$Ca_3(PO_4)_2$	— 0·7
$Ca_2H(PO_4)$	— 1·0
$CaCO_3$ (standard drug)	— 6·0
$CaCO_3$ (extra heavy)	— 6·3

"Thus, when starting with a high polish, all of the abrasives except meta-phosphate + calcium phosphate produced a dulling action, particularly the carbonates which lower the lustre almost the complete length of our lustre scale from a 'super-high' to a 'low'. . . ."

. . . Figs. 47 and 48 showing the abrasive action of calcium carbonate; number 52 showing the same tooth brushed with "meta-phosphate + calcium phosphate" agent and 49 showing a tooth brushed on one half with heavy chalk and on the other half with the "meta-phosphate + calcium phosphate", Fig. 50 shows the high polish produced by meta-phosphate + calcium phosphate.

Phillips and VanHuysen (*Amer. Perfum.*, Jan. 1948) summarise their study as follows:

"Many experimental data and substantiating photographs, with various alterations from this general method of approach, could be offered but very briefly the action of these agents can be summarised as follows:

(1) Calcium carbonate, both extra heavy and standard, produces a marked abrasion of the tooth surface. Because of this resulting rough

surface, these abrasives possess no polishing action and will actually cause extreme dulling of a naturally smooth, lustrous enamel surface.

(2) Di-calcium and tri-calcium phosphate are rather inert in regard to their polishing action. They raise the lustre very slightly on a dull surface and do not produce any marked dulling of a highly polished surface.

(3) The ' meta-phosphate + calcium phosphate ' agent is superior to all of those tested in terms of its ability to polish the enamel surface. It will raise the lustre on a dull tooth, sometimes as high as five lustre divisions. Microscopically it shows no abrasive action. [By abrasive action, we mean scratching of the surface, not cleansing action which can possibly be achieved without scratching. . . ."]

It is pointed out that before one could offer an opinion concerning the practical clinical significance of these observations, the effects of these agents *in dentifrices* has to be studied, as it is quite possible that when they are placed in commercial dentifrices, their behaviour is markedly altered due to reduced concentration and the influence of other ingredients. Some of these dentifrices contain mixtures of these agents and their action together might be different from when considered individually.

Phillips and VanHuysen add : " However, our research with the popular dentifrices, has led to the conclusion that in general the action of the dentifrices closely parallels that of its principal abrasive. For example, Fig. 49 shows the microscopical photograph of a tooth, the left half of which was brushed with a typical chalk dentifrice, while the right side was brushed for an equal period of time with a dentifrice containing meta-phosphate + calcium phosphate as its principal abrasive agent. The diagonal line of demarcation between the two is very pronounced with the calcium carbonate dentifrice having a scratched, abraded surface as compared to a smooth polished enamel produced by the other dentifrices (the dark vertical line is of course a crack in the enamel). . . ."

It is concluded " . . . It would appear that the smoother surface produced by meta-phosphate + calcium phosphate, or some similar acting agent, might be advantageous :

(1) Aesthetically because of the higher polish.

(2) A smoother surface might be less receptive to the retention of dental plaque and debris. It would seem probable that the rougher the surface, the easier foreign material would adhere. A smooth surface would thus aid in keeping the area clean.

(3) The apparent lesser abrasiveness of meta-phosphate + calcium phosphate might be advantageous in reducing the degree of abrasion and erosion. . . ."

't the above study is of importance to the cosmetician, … inferences drawn and work done, (ii) because the im- … this work will apply even more to tooth powders which …n simple mixtures ; which contain no excipient, such as glycerin …d which, since they are applied to the tooth surface in a concentrated form—represent conditions not far removed from those existing in the above experiments, and (iii) as illustrative of the type of work which needs doing in the cosmetic industry in all its many branches, i.e. practical scientific investigation on the various components which "custom has assured" a place in certain formulations, to see whether these really have unique properties or whether, in the light of newer knowledge, they cannot be supplanted with materials better suited to the end in view.

Typical Tooth-powder and Tooth-paste Formulations

The following are typical examples of basic formulae for tooth-powders and tooth-pastes. They can, of course, be "elaborated" as desired by the inclusion of various other materials in an endeavour to provide a suitable sales story. It should be noted that the use of such substances as chlorophyll, penicillin, ammoniated dentifrices, anti-enzyme dentifrices, etc., is discussed in the preceding chapter (Chapter 16).

Tooth-powders

	per cent.
Precipitated calcium carbonate	95·0
Dental soap	5·0
Flavouring	*q.s.*
Sweetener	*q.s.*

	per cent.
Dicalcium phosphate	97·0
Synthetic soapless detergent	3·0
Flavouring	*q.s.*
Sweetener	*q.s.*

The first is essentially a standard chalk-soap formulation ; soap level is given as 5 per cent. which appears to be adequate. Some persons may prefer a higher soap level. The second formulation is a soapless type in which the polishing agent is dicalcium phosphate. This substance is considered to be relatively free from the tendency to scratch teeth but its glycerin adsorptive properties are relatively low. It, however, is useful in a soap-free powder formulation as the above.

PRECIPITATED CHALK

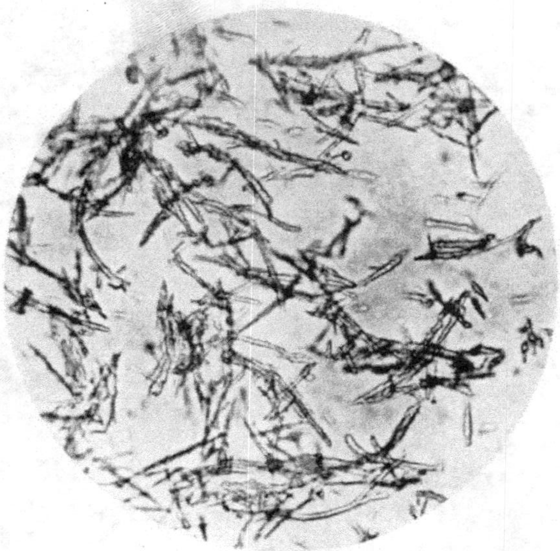

ARAGONITE.

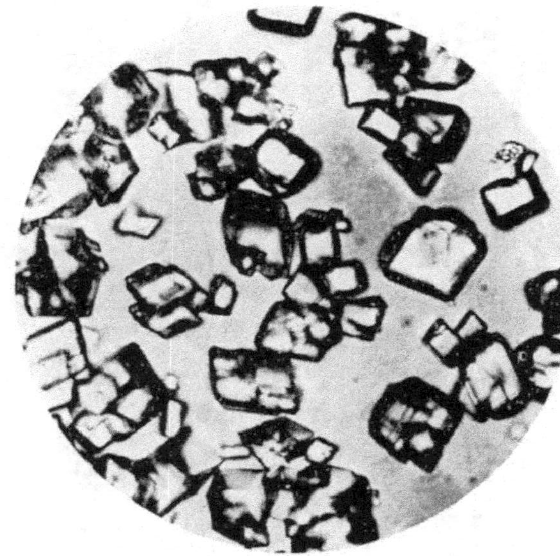

CALCITE.

[*By courtesy of Messrs. John & E. Sturge Ltd.*

FIG. 46.

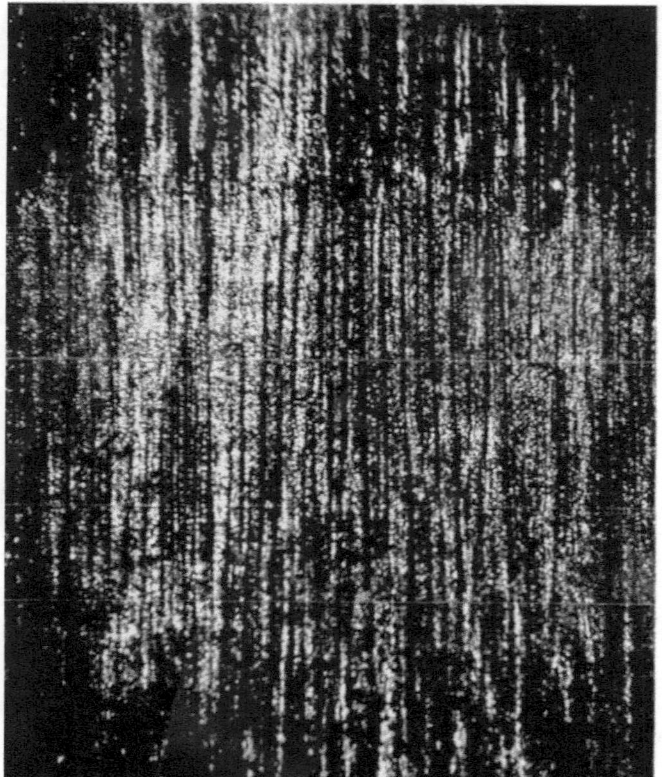

FIG. 47.—Photo-micrograph (120 ×) showing graphited tooth surface which was brushed with $CaCO_3$ (standard).

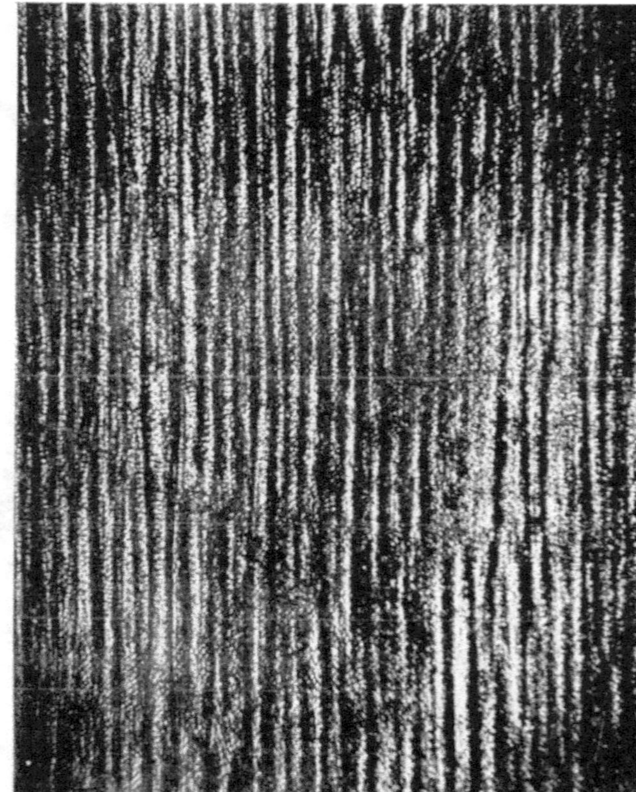

FIG. 48.—Tooth surface brushed with $CaCO_3$ (extra h

[*By courtesy of Phillips and Van Huysen, loc. cit.*

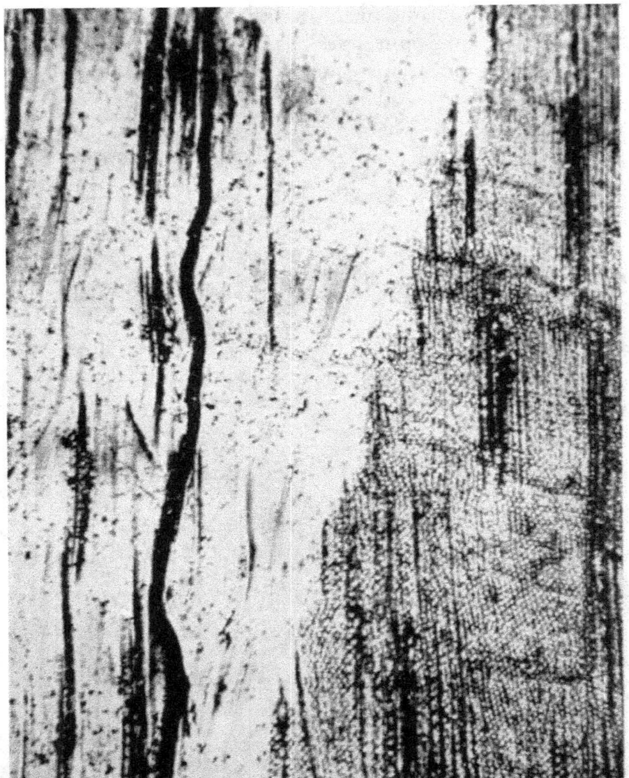

Fig. 49.—Left diagonal half of tooth brushed with chalk dentifrice while right side was brushed with dentifrice which contained metaphosphate plus calcium phosphate.

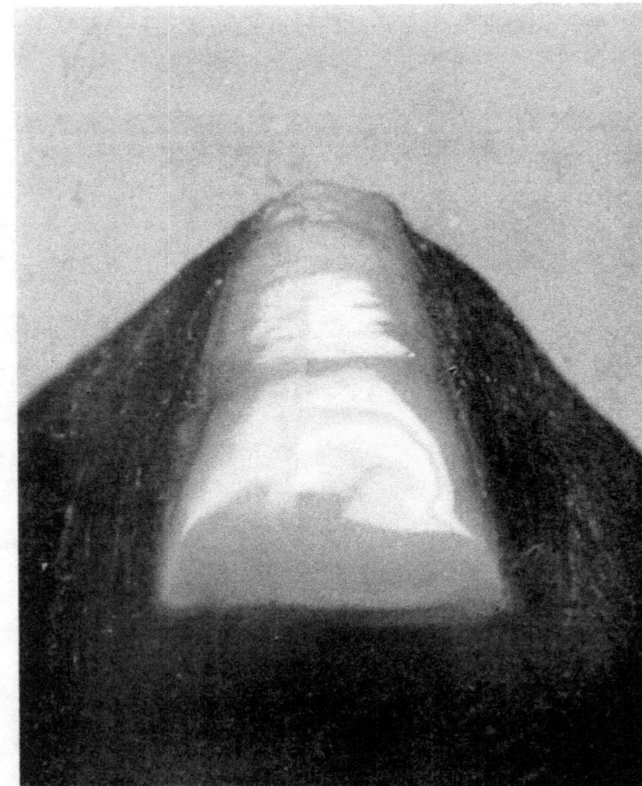

Fig. 50.—High polish on right produced by metaphosphate plus calcium phosphate.

[*By courtesy of Phillips and Van Huysen, loc. cit.*

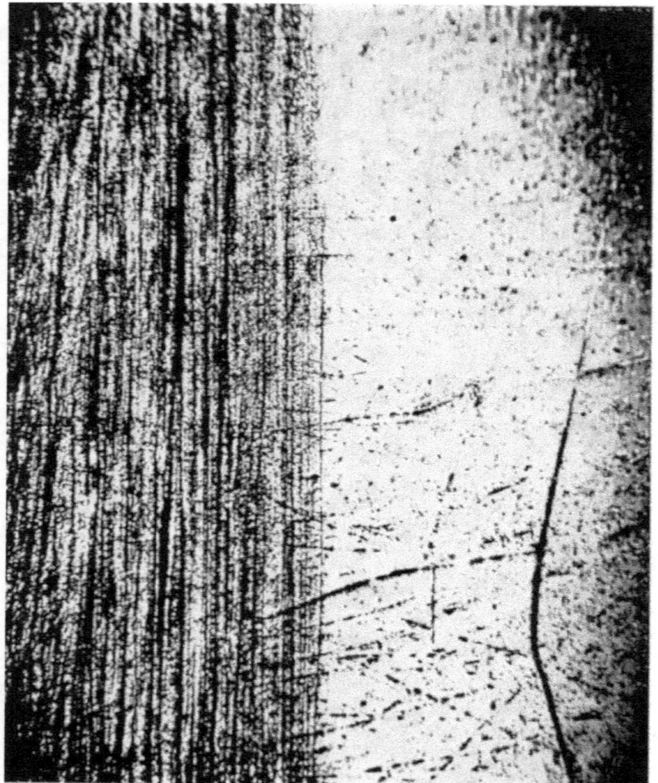

FIG. 51.—Microscopical appearance of tooth brushed with $CaCO_3$ (extra heavy) on left side and with metaphosphate plus calcium phosphate on right.

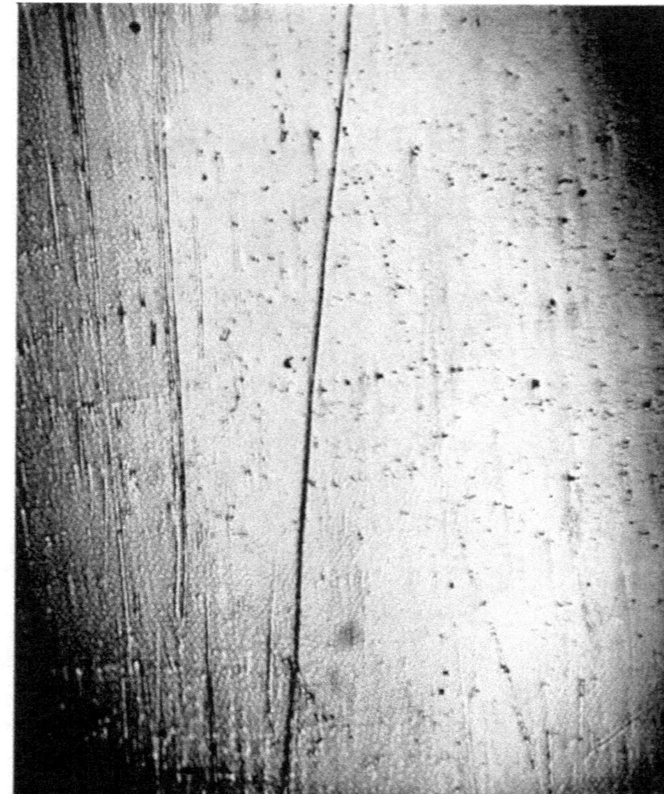

FIG. 52.—Same tooth as in Figs. 47 and 48 brushed with metaphosphate and calcium phosphate agent.

[*By courtesy of Phillips and Van Huysen, loc. cit.*

Oxygenated powder

	per cent.
Precipitated chalk	95·0
Synthetic detergent powder	3·0
Magnesium peroxide	2·0
Flavour	q.s.
Sweetener	q.s.

The proportion of detergent will depend upon the foaminess desired in the product and its solubility; similarly an increase may be made in the content of magnesium peroxide, the precipitated chalk content being adjusted to bring the total to 100 per cent.

The use of sodium perborate as an oxygenising agent has been suggested but the author is not in favour of it.

METHOD OF MANUFACTURE. The method of manufacture of the above powders is simple: the sweetener and flavour, together with a little alcohol if desired is rubbed up with some of the precipitated chalk, which is then incorporated with the main bulk with careful mixing.

SOLID DENTIFRICE. Solid dentifrice is a product in many ways more akin to a soap preparation than a tooth-powder. It consists essentially of a tooth-powder, suspended in a soap base. The proportion of soap may vary within fairly wide limits from about 12 per cent. up to 28 per cent. depending upon the glycerin content of the dentifrice, the method of manufacture and the hardness desired in the finished product. Because of the nature of the product it is advantageous to employ a rather higher level of flavour than is used in a tooth-paste. Such solid dentifrices are usually coloured. A formulation of this type is:

	per cent.
Dental soap	18·0
Abrasive materials (usually chalk)	79·0
Glycerin	3·0
Colour	q.s.
Flavour	q.s.
Sweetener	q.s.

In preparing such a product, the soap and abrasive material are milled with the glycerin, and *sufficient water to give a mass of suitable plasticity*, colour and flavour is included; the mass is plodded and the extruded bars or billets, cut and stamped in the manner of a soap tablet. (For discussion on plodding, stamping, etc., of soap, *see* Chapter 27.) Soapless solid dentifrices can also be prepared providing a suitable plasticising medium is employed.

The manufacture of solid dentifrice requires careful attention to detail, plant, etc., and is not recommended for the smaller manufacturer.

TOOTH-PASTES (DENTAL CREAMS). The properties desirable in such a product are pretty obvious, viz. the flavour should be clean and pleasant, the paste should adequately cleanse the teeth without damaging their structure, and it must of course be non-toxic. It should maintain its consistency over that temperature range likely to be encountered in practice, usually 5° to 42° C. will cover such conditions as are likely to be met in this country. Overseas specifications may need to be more severe. (*See* Federal Specification 1916.) From the manufacturers' point of view it should be made from inexpensive materials, in free supply, and should be non-corrosive to the tube container. To avoid aeration such creams should either be made under vacuum or alternately must be of such composition that, when made, the air may escape readily on standing, prior to setting up. The following are examples of straightforward tooth-paste formulae:

	per cent.
Glycerin	23·0
Gum tragacanth mucilage (5 per cent in water)	14·0
Precipitated chalk	50·0
Bentonite	3·0
Synthetic Detergent [1]	3·0
Water	7·0
Saccharin	*q.s.*
Flavour	*q.s.*
Preservative	*q.s.*

	parts
Magnesium silicate	18·0
Tricalcium phosphate	9·0
Precipitated chalk	24·0
Glycerin	32·0
Neutral dental soap	3·0
Gum tragacanth mucilage (2 per cent.)	14·0
Saccharin	*q.s.*
Flavour	*q.s.*
Preservative	*q.s.*

The glycerin content may be reduced if desired and the gum tragacanth content increased to about 1 per cent. pure gum.

The following formula may be taken as typifying a good soap-chalk dentifrice having no particular *frill*, or claims except that it is

[1] Chosen from the detergents already discussed, having regard to flavour and solubility.

a good dentifrice and assists the tooth-brush in cleansing the surfaces of the teeth :

	per cent.
Precipitated chalk	46·0
Neutral dental soap	4·0
Glycerin	20·0
Water	28·0
Gum tragacanth	1·0
Flavour	1·0
Saccharin	*q.s.*

The choice of the precipitated chalk is a matter of importance. If a *light* chalk is used and gently processed or milled, the mass will set hard in a few days, but by intensive mixing a smooth, soft paste is obtained which keeps its characteristics indefinitely. On the other hand, in dealing with heavier chalks of low absorptive power, prolonged processing does not prevent such setting, and hence light chalks should be used for dental creams and the product efficiently processed. In powders, heavier grades of such chalks are used.

The above formulae may be modified, if desired, by alteration in the grade of chalk used, or by varying the proportion of vehicle and powder, but in all cases adequate processing should be given, and this is best determined by withdrawing samples at different recorded intervals, and shelf-testing them, the sample found most satisfactory being then standardised. It is possible to obtain special grades of chalk of varying densities, which are accurately graded under a cipher.

MANUFACTURE. In the manufacture of such products, the gum tragacanth and soap (or soapless detergent) may be mixed " dry " and then wetted with the glycerin and water mixture ; alternatively, a stock of gum tragacanth mucilage may be prepared as required, the soap or synthetic detergent " wetted " with the glycerin and water and suspended in the tragacanth mucilage. The blended solids are then mixed in, preferably *in vacuo*, the flavour incorporated towards the end of the process and the tooth-paste either milled or homogenised.

The following basic suggestion for an antiseptic tooth-paste utilising quaternary ammonium compounds has been made (Rohm & Haas Co.),

	parts
Quaternary ammonium compound	0·25
Foaming agent	1·00
Methyl cellulose (4000 cps.)	0·70
Glycerin	8·00
Tricalcium phosphate	5·00
Calcium carbonate	43·00
Water	41·61
Flavour, etc. to	100·00

but *it is clearly pointed out that* it is by no means regarded as a finished formulation and that *no chemical, toxicological or sensitisation studies have been conducted on this product and hence no warranty is expressed or implied.* The quaternary ammonium compound in the suggestion is one of the Hyamines, the foaming agent, one of the Tritons.

It is pointed out (*Soap, N.Y.*, March, 1949, through *Amer. Perfum.*, 1948, **52**, 397) that using the wet filter paper method at 37° C. and staphylococcus aureus as a test organism, the killing time was found to be 2 minutes in a 1 : 8 dilution and 5 minutes in a 1 : 50. The pH of the paste was 8·8. One trouble with such a preparation is that claims for its antiseptic action have to be so whittled down that practically all sales appeal is taken out of the term " antiseptic ". It is of course impossible to sterilise the oral cavity although the bacterial count can be reduced. For this reason the F.D.A. frowns upon the use of " antiseptic " claims in a dentifrice.

Whilst the above attitude is quite correct there may be some merit in using an antiseptic paste in respect of its *self-sterilising action on the tooth-brush*, for example, under suitable conditions detergents are adsorbed upon hair fibres. Anyone who has ever seen the results of total bacterial counts upon ordinary tooth-brushes in use, might be inclined to view any method that will make the tooth-brush a more " healthy " tool with approval. Few people will bother to dip a tooth-brush in antiseptic regularly ; if they did, they would probably use the wrong type of antiseptic at an increased concentration for the wrong time and so damage the brush. Any tooth-paste that, without any risk of toxicity and without any unpleasant flavour helped to reduce the bacterial count of the brush (owing to an adsorbed film held in contact with the fibres whilst the brush is not in use) might be considered helpful to dental hygiene providing the tooth-paste was satisfactory also in respect of innocuousness and all other pertinent aspects.

" MANUCOL " (SODIUM ALGINATE) IN TOOTH-PASTE. Manucol (Grade SS/LL, Alginate Industries Ltd., London) may be used partially or wholly in replacement of gum tragacanth or other colloidal materials which are incorporated in tooth-paste to confer stability upon the paste. It is claimed that a cleaner tooth-brush, owing to diminished clogging of the bristles, and a smoother and more homogeneous paste is obtained. The amounts of Manucol to use must be determined by individual experiment depending upon the formulation involved, but they usually lie between 0·5 per cent. and 2 per cent.

One difficulty which may, in the author's opinion, be encountered in such pastes is a slow but progressive tendency to hardening due to the formation of calcium alginate. In chalk free dentifrices this may not occur and there is evidence than even in dentifrices containing chalk, by means of a proper balance of materials and possibly the use of some sequestrant, this tendency may be reduced.

AMMONIATED DENTIFRICES. Whilst it is possible to make additions to certain dental creams with but little change in formulation, as for example, the substitution of ricinoleate soaps for other soaps, the addition of chlorophyll, etc.; in the case of the ammonium ion, or ammoniated dentifrices special formulation is required in order to avoid loss of ammonia, etc. "Glycerin Facts" [Glycerine Producers Association, New York, December issue, with the co-operation of L. A. Kramer (Victor Chemical Works)], suggests the following as a starting point for the formulation of such dentifrices:

	per cent.
Tricalcium phosphate	26·67
Glycerin	45·40
Water	15·40
Flavouring (peppermint)	0·58
Gum tragacanth	0·96
Saccharin	0·10
Surface-active agent (Nacconal LAL)	2·89
Diammonium phosphate (powdered FF)	5·00
Urea (100 mesh)	3·00

Procedure

Allow the gum to expand in the water at room temperature for 30 minutes, add the glycerin and mix well. Slowly add the tricalcium phosphate to this solution and mix thoroughly. Mix in the remaining constituents in the following order: saccharin, flavouring, diammonium phosphate, urea and surface-active agent. After adding the surface-active agent, mix no longer than is necessary to obtain distribution.

The above reference draws attention to the fact that *all such products are sold under licence from the University of Illinois,* and that a formula of the above type should not be marketed without suitable patent arrangements.

According to the literature [Anon., "Accelerated Ageing Tests for Ammonia-Urea Tooth-pastes to be made by Licensees", Chicago, University of Illinois Foundation, 4 June, 1949, through M. A. Lesser, *Drug Cosmet. Ind.*, Feb. 1950, p. 146] the original formula suggested for ammoniated dentifrice powder was modified to:

	parts in g.
Dibasic ammonium phosphate	50·0
Carbamide (i.e. urea)	30·0
Bentonite	50·0
Chalk, precipitated	846·0
Soluble saccharin	2·0
Menthol	2·0

	parts in g.
Oil of peppermint	2·0
Oil of cinnamon	2·0
Oil of wintergreen	6·0
Sulpholaurate	10·0

Again, the patent position must be kept in mind.

One of the drawbacks of the ammoniated tooth-pastes in the author's opinion is their flavour. All of the ones so far tasted have been very considerably inferior in flavour to a plain peppermint "flavoured tooth-paste".

The following formula for a tooth-paste is based upon the use of "Veegum", a complex colloidal magnesium aluminium silicate gel. It is claimed that this material has exceptional protective colloidal characteristics and stabilises with high viscosity for low solids concentration. It is stated that the viscosity of pastes made with "Veegum" tends to remain constant upon ageing:

	per cent.
"Veegum" (R. T. Vanderbilt) Gel	26·42
Tragacanth gum powdered	1·00
Saccharin (soluble)	0·18
Sodium benzoate	1·00
Glycerin	19·80
Superlight chalk	43·85
Neutral white soap	5·00
Light mineral oil	0·20
Flavour	1·80
Calcium sulphate (dihydrate)	0·75

Procedure

Add the gum tragacanth, soluble saccharin and sodium benzoate to the glycerin. Mix well on a pony mixer and while mixing add the Veegum and one-half of the chalk. When homogeneous add the soap and the flavour oil dissolved in the mineral oil. Continue mixing on the pony mixer until uniform and then add the remainder of the chalk and finally the calcium sulphate dihydrate. Mix well and mill finely with an ointment roller, or colloid mill.

[*Note*: It is stated that the amount of calcium sulphate dihydrate is very critical. If the calcium sulphate content in the above formula is increased from 0·75 per cent. to 1 per cent., the resulting paste is much stiffer in consistency. This ingredient therefore provides a most satisfactory method of controlling the stiffness or viscosity of a paste of this type. In pastes containing no calcium sulphate, the viscosity is most easily controlled by adjusting the chalk to the proper value. From R. T. Vanderbilt, *Information about Veegum for Cosmetics* (revised edn.).]

PRESERVATIVES IN DENTIFRICES. Although it is usually assumed that the essential oils present as flavouring materials in tooth-pastes are sufficiently bactericidal to render the paste sterile, it is by no means certain that this is always the case. Theobald [Sf.Zg. 65-38-1029 through Schimmel Briefs, No. 110, May 1944] found that with the exception of a few so-called foaming tooth-pastes containing a high percentage of medicinal soaps, the pastes examined contained bacteria and he found it likely that oil pastes including those which have been proved sterile, originally contained ubiquitous cocci and spores (this is to be expected—author). Benzoic acid and various other additions are often made to tooth-paste with a view to " preserving " the tooth-paste. The amount and type of humectant, composition and level of the flavour, etc., all play an important part in the resistance of the paste to micro-organisms. (For a discussion on Antiseptics and Preservatives, *see* Chapter 42.)

U.S. Federal Specification : Dentifrice

1. CLASSIFICATION. 1.1 *Grade and types.* The dentifrice, covered by this specification, shall be of but one grade and the following types, as specified : Type I : Tooth-paste ; Type II : Tooth-powder.

2. APPLICABLE SPECIFICATIONS AND OTHER PUBLICATIONS. 2.1. The following Federal Specifications, of the issues in effect on date of invitation for bids, form a part of this specification : P-S-598—soap, liquid and paste ; (for) automobile, floor, and general cleaning ; P-S-616—soap, toilet ; floating, white ; P-S-621—soap, toilet ; milled.

2.2. *Other publications.* The following publications, of the issues in effect on date of invitation for bids, form a part of this specification : *Governmental :* Federal Food, Drug, and Cosmetic Act, and General Regulations for its Enforcement ; *Nongovernmental :* Pharmacopoeia of the United States.

2.3. Specifications and other publications applicable only to individual departments are listed in section 7.

3. REQUIREMENTS. 3.1. *Material.* The dentifrice shall be free from materials other than those specified and shall be uniform in composition.

3.2. *Type I and Type II.*

3.2.1. The dentifrice shall be free of lumps or particles which are palpable in the mouth as separate or discrete particles.

3.2.2. The dentifrice shall, when used in the normal manner, assist in the removal of the usual daily accumulation of debris and deposits from the exposed surfaces of the teeth without injury to the teeth, mucous membrane of the mouth, or body in general.

3.2.3. The dentifrice shall not irritate the mucous membrane of human subjects or produce unpleasant symptoms.

3.2.4. The flavour shall be distinct and pleasant or shall be as specified in the invitation for bids.

3.2.5. The colour shall be (*a*) white, (*b*) cream, (*c*) light tan, (*d*) pink, or as specified in the invitation for bids.

3.2.6. The dentifrice formula shall accompany the bid proposal (see 6.2.)

3.2.7. All deliveries shall conform in all respects to the provisions of the Federal Food, Drug, and Cosmetic Act of the issue in effect on date of invitation for bids. Particular attention is called to section 201 (i) and 601 of the June 25 1938 issue of the Act.

3.2.8. *Composition.* Dentifrice shall be made from combinations of two or more of the following ingredients and within the limits specified:

3.2.8.1. Forty per cent. or more (by weight) shall be from the following detergents: calcium carbonate, dicalcium phosphate, tricalcium phosphate, magnesium carbonate, magnesium hydroxide.

3.2.8.2. The following detergents, preservatives, and flavours are limited in their use (if used) as follows: soap (hard or soft) U.S. Patent, Federal Specifications P–S–598, P–S–616, P–S–621 (not over 20 per cent.); sodium benzoate (not over 2·5 per cent.); thymol (not over 0·2 per cent.).

3.2.8.3. Sugars and saccharin are permitted, except as limited by flavour or other tests.

3.2.8.4. Synthetic detergents considered safe for use by Public Health authorities, and one or more of the following detergents, plasticity and acidity regulators, in proper amount, shall be permitted:

1. Sodium bicarbonate
2. Sodium borate
3. Sodium carbonate
4. Sodium chloride
5. Boric acid
6. Acetic acid
7. Cream of tartar
8. Gelatine
9. Gum karaya
10. Gum tragacanth
11. Irish moss
12. Sodium alginate
13. Petroleum jelly
14. Mineral oil
15. Alcohol
16. Glycerine
17. Water
18. Starch
19. Sorbitol
20. Sorbitan monooleate
21. Sorbitan mololaurate
22. Propylene glycol

3.2.8.5. The use of flavours and colours, permitted by the U.S. Food and Drug Administration for use as food dyes and flavours, in proper amounts, shall be permitted.

3.2.9. Dentifrice shall not contain appreciable amounts of the commonly recognised poisonous elements such as arsenic and heavy metals.

3.2.10. The pH value for the dentifrice shall be greater than 4·9 and less than 10·1 when measured at 25° C.

3.2.11. The dentifrice shall not scratch glass when tested in accordance with 4.3.6.

3.3. *Type I.*

3.3.1. Ninety-five per cent. of the paste shall extrude from the tube in a continuous mass at a temperature of 10° C (50° F.) without the application of excessive force which would cause injury to the tube.

3.3.2. Paste extruded from the tube (orifice down) to a length of 10 mm. at a temperature of 20° C. (68° F.) shall remain attached to the tube for at least 15 seconds.

3.3.3. The paste shall not segregate, ferment, or deteriorate when cooled to a temperature of – 15° C. (5° F.) for 1 hour or when heated to a temperature of 45° C. (113° F.) for 72 hours.

3.4 *Type II.*

3.4.1. Type II shall be a free-flowing powder and without lumps.

4. SAMPLING, INSPECTION, AND TEST PROCEDURES. 4.1 *Sampling.* One or more containers of each type of dentifrice shall be taken from each delivery to determine compliance with the requirements of this specification :

4.2 *Inspection.*

4.2.1. *Consistency.* The dentifrice shall be inspected to determine whether it can be properly extruded in the case of Type I ; or whether it is free of lumps or particles and free-flowing in the case of Type II. (See 3.2.1, 3.3.1, 3.3.2, and 3.4.1.)

4.3. *Tests.*

4.3.1. *Irritability.* Apply undiluted dentifrice to the mucous membrane of the cheeks and gums for a period of 2 minutes. (See 3.2.3.)

4.3.2. *Flavour and colour.* Inspections for flavour and colour shall be made on the bid sample prior to awarding the contract. Material difference in flavour or colour of the dentifrice delivered on contract shall be sufficient cause for rejection. (See 3.2.4. and 3.2.5.)

4.3.3. *Purity.* The methods specified in the current Pharmacopoeia of the United States shall be used for the detection of poisons and impurities. (See 3.2.9.)

4.3.4. Requirements 3.2.7 through 3.2.9 may be regarded as in compliance when verified against 3.2.6. When doubt exists, special investigations and tests shall be made to cover the items in doubt. (Analytical and test methods outlined in standard texts shall be employed.)

4.3.5. *pH values.* The glass electrode and potentiometer shall be used for the determination of *p*H values. Dilute the tooth-paste with four parts of freshly distilled water to one part of paste by weight. Similarly, add four parts of water to one part of powder. (See 3.2.10.)

4.3.6. *Abrasion.* The dentifrice shall be placed on glass and rubbed with a metal instrument having a surface similar to the curved surface of a 5-cent coin. Add freshly distilled water to powder to give it a paste-like consistency before rubbing with the metal instrument. The glass shall be chemically clean and of the usual soda lime grade such as is used in non-corrosive microscope slides. The metal instrument shall be approximately the same hardness as the 5-cent coin. One hundred double strokes shall be made. A thrust of 16 oz. shall be applied during the test. A control test of the metal instrument and glass shall be made using a lubricant such as glycerine, petroleum jelly, or a known non-abrasive paste. Make this control test on the glass near the spot where the primary test was made. After both tests are completed, place the glass in hot nitric acid to remove particles of alloy adhering to the glass. View the glass in transmitted and reflected light without the use of a microscope. If the dentifrice test shows more scratching on the glass than does the control test, repeat the test to eliminate the possibility of accidental defective spots in the glass surface. If the repeat test shows excessive scratching by the dentifrice, the dentifrice shall be rejected. Ignore apparent polishing effects which may in some illuminations appear to be changes in surface, but which are not line scratches. (See 3.2.11.)

4.3.7. *Segregation and fermentation.* The paste under test shall be placed in glass test-tubes and stoppered. One or more shall be heated to a temperature of 45° C. (113° F.) for 72 hours after which examination shall be made for homogeneity and fermentation. The other tube, or tubes, shall be cooled to a temperature of – 15° C. (5° F.) for 1 hour and observed for homogeneity. (See 3.3.3.)

4.3.8. *Attack on container.* Heat one or more tubes of paste to a temperature of 45° C. (113° F.) for 72 hours. Extrude part of the paste and examine for contamination on the paste. Slit the tube, remove the paste and examine the surface of the tube and cap for corrosion, chemical attack, and other injury.

5. PREPARATION FOR DELIVERY. 51. *Packaging.*

5.1.1. Unless otherwise specified, each tube of paste shall contain not less than 2 oz. of paste and each package of powder shall contain not less than 1 oz. of powder.

5.1.2. Unless otherwise specified, each dentifrice container shall be packaged in a standard commercial carton according to best trade practice.

5.1.3. *Type I.* The container for the paste shall be a collapsible tube having a non-corrosive screw cap. The cap shall have a diameter at some point of 15 mm. or over. The container, including the cap, shall not.be attacked, chemically, by the paste. (See 4.3.8.) The area of the orifice through which the paste is to be extruded shall be greater than 13 sq. mm.

and less than 50 sq. mm. Orifices shall not have minor dimensions less than one-third the major dimension. Paint on the fold or crimp end of the tube shall not extend nearer than 3 mm. to the end of the tube when unfolded. Wax-lined tubes will not be accepted except upon specific agreement included in the bid request.

5.1.4. *Type II.* The powder packages shall be of glass, metal, or plastic, as specified, shall be non-leaking, of convenient shape and so constructed that the powder may be dispensed in normal amounts under control of the user and without danger of contaminating the powder in the package.

5.2. *Packing.* Unless otherwise specified, the product shall be packed in substantial commercial containers of the type, size, and kind commonly used for the purpose, so constructed as to permit acceptance by carrier for transportation at the lowest applicable rate, and to afford maximum protection from normal hazards of transportation.

5.3. *Marking.*

5.3.1. *Dentifrice containers.* Unless otherwise specified, each dentifrice container shall be lithographed to show the new weight, trade name of the contents, and the name or trade-mark of the contractor.

5.3.2. *Cartons.* Unless otherwise specified, individual cartons shall be marked with the type and trade name of the contents, the name or trade-marks of the contractor and manufacturer, and the net weight.

5.3.3. *Shipping containers.* Unless otherwise specified, shipping containers shall be marked with the name and type of the material as defined by the contract or order, the quantity of each type contained therein, the name of the contractor, the number of the contract or order, the name and address of the consignee, and the gross weight.

6. NOTES. 6.1. *Ordering data.* Purchasers should specify type, colour, and flavour required and should exercise any desired options offered herein. (See 1.1, 3.2.4, 3.2.5, 5.1.1, 5.1.2, 5.2, and 5.3.)

6.2. *Bid Samples.* Two-ounce samples are required with bid for the purpose of determining compliance with the requirements of this specification as to colour and flavour. (See 3.2.4 and 3.2.5.) The sample shall be from the formula required in 3.2.6.

6.3. Federal specifications do not include all the types, classes, sizes, etc., of the commodities indicated by the titles of the specifications, or which are commercially available, but are intended to cover the types, etc., which are suitable for Federal Government requirements.

6.4. *Transportation description.*

6.4.1. *Transportation description applicable to these items is:* Toilet preparation NOIBN: In barrels or boxes—carload weight 24,000 lb. subject to R34; truckload weight 24,000 lb.

7. DEPARTMENTAL REQUIREMENTS. 7.1. The following specifications and standards, of the issues in effect on date of invitation for bids, and special requirements, form a part of this specification for purchases made under this specification by the respective departments.

7.2. *Army, Navy and Air Force.*

7.2.1. *Applicable specifications and standards: Military Standards—* MIL–STD–105—Sampling Procedures and Tables for Inspection by Attributes; MIL–STD–129—Marking of Shipments.

Navy Department Specification—General Specifications for Inspection of Material.[1]

7.2.2. *Sampling.* Sampling shall be in accordance with Military Standard MIL–STD–105.

7.2.3. *Inspection.* Inspection will be made by the Government to determine compliance with this specification.

7.2.3.1. *Inspection procedures (Navy only).* General inspection procedures shall be in accordance with Navy Department General Specifications for Inspection of Material.

7.2.4. *Marking.* In addition to any special marking specified in the contract or order, shipments shall be marked in accordance with Military Standard MIL–STD–129.

(Reproduced by courtesy of the U.S. General Services Administration.)

DENTURE CLEANSERS

These cleansers are marketed either in powder or tablet form. Though such preparations may differ widely in detailed composition they comprise essentially:

(i) an oxydising agent;
(ii) an electrolyte;
(iii) an alkali.

The oxydising agent usually employed is either sodium perborate or sodium percarbonate. Sodium percarbonate is more soluble than sodium perborate in water but is not quite so stable though its stability for most purposes is adequate. As pointed out in the literature "Sodium Perborate and Sodium percarbonate", Laporte Chemicals Ltd., "... Sodium perborate is a white free-flowing powder which is available commercially in two forms, viz.:

(*a*) *Sodium Perborate Tetrahydrate* usually written as $NaBO_3 . 4H_2O$ although $NaBO_2 . H_2O_2 3H_2O$ is more correct. [Theoretical active oxygen 10·38 per cent., sold on basis of 10 per cent.]

[1] Applicable to Navy purchases only.

(*b*) *Sodium Perborate Monohydrate*, corresponding to $NaBO_3H_2O$ or more correctly $NaBO_2 . H_2O_2$. [Theoretical oxygen content of which is 16 per cent. but is usually sold on a basis of 15 per cent.]

Sodium percarbonate, like sodium perborate, is not a true persalt but is an addition compound corresponding to the formula

$$2Na_2CO_2 . 3H_2O_2. \ldots$$"

The purpose of a denture cleanser is to loosen the debris, which consists of saliva and food particles from the denture. This action results from (i) the evolution of bubbles of oxygen in the solution, (ii) solvent action of alkali on certain food residues, and (iii) flocculating effect of electrolytes such as sodium chloride on saliva and mucus. The combined effect of the above is to so loosen the debris (after a suitable period of soaking in water), that it is easily brushed away. In addition, owing to the evolution of oxygen and the *p*H of the solution, the plate is rendered very much cleaner bacteriologically. Tobacco and other stains which form on the plate in the case of certain smokers are very much more readily removed than by the use of a tooth-brush and tooth-paste alone.

The amounts of sodium perborate, or percarbonate, employed may vary from 20–50 per cent. Alternatively, hydrogen peroxide in solid form or one of the stabilised solid forms of chlorine-evolving preparations may be used. In such cases, care must be taken to ensure that the preparation does not bleach or otherwise alter the colour of the dental plate, which in most cases has been very carefully matched to suit the natural gum and tooth colours of the patient's natural gums and teeth.

The electrolyte employed in such preparations is almost invariably common salt (sodium chloride) which assists in the coagulation and removal of organic debris from the denture.

The alkali employed is anhydrous trisodium phosphate in amounts of from 10–30 per cent., or sometimes even higher. Sodium carbonate, sodium bicarbonate, sodium silicate (in tablets), disodium phosphate, etc., are sometimes included. Enzymes, catalyst accelerators, deodorants —such as chlorophyll, etc., may also be included. [Because of the *direct contact* of the chlorophyllin with the denture over quite a fair period of time, the deodorant action of such preparations would be expected to be greater than in tooth-paste, etc. (*See* Chapter 16 for discussion on chlorophyll in tooth conditions and preparations.)]

A few illustrative formulae of such preparations are set out below:

	per cent.
Sodium perborate	40·0
Sodium chloride	30·0
Trisodium phosphate	30·0

	per cent.
Flavour	q.s.
Colouring matter (if desired)	q.s.

A formula without trisodium phosphate is given by:

	per cent.
Sodium percarbonate	40·0
Sodium chloride	40·0
Sodium carbonate	20·0

Tablets can be prepared from simple mixtures such as:

	per cent.
Sodium percarbonate	88·0
Sodium chloride	10·0
Sodium silicate and/or other binders	2·0
Flavour	q.s.

or from a more conventional mixture on the lines of the first formula.

Where an effervescent preparation is desired some of the sodium carbonate, or other alkali, may be replaced by an organic acid such as tartaric acid.

The difficulties with which the manufacturer is faced are those of (i) obtaining fairly rapid solution, (ii) adequate clarity, (iii) avoidance of "caking" in the powder, (iv) adequate shelf life and stability. Moisture is one of the things which *must* be kept out of the finished product until it is used.

CHAPTER 18

MOUTHWASHES [1]

ANTISEPTIC mouthwashes have as yet but little sale in this country, although they are more popular abroad.

After having been *body odour conscious* and *cosmetic skin conscious*, I have no doubt that a little judicious advertisement could make us *mouth conscious*.

However, such products, if they are to hold any permanent position, must be

(1) reasonably antiseptic at the *dilution* and in the time normally used;

(2) refreshing in flavour, imparting a *clean* odour to the mouth;

(3) inexpensive;

(4) attractively packed and displayed.

Laboratory tests show that mouthwashes require the application of several minutes to insure sterility. This, however, is not a necessity since absolute sterility of the mouth, even if attained, could not persist many minutes, nor indeed would it be desirable.

Even in the absence of sterility, the *virulence* of the organisms present may be so impaired as to render them almost innocuous, even if their number is not reduced.

The ultimate effect is exerted as a result of a combination of three factors, (*a*) the mechanical effect of rinsing, (*b*) the effect of the antiseptic contained in the mouthwash, and (*c*) the effect of the essential oils used in flavouring. In connection with (*b*) and (*c*) there is possibility of synergistic action. This will be discussed later.

CHOICE OF ANTISEPTIC

The antiseptics usually employed in the preparation of such washes include phenol, thymol, salol, formalin, tannic acid, boric acid, the esters of hydroxybenzoic acid, chlorinated cresols, chlorinated thymols, etc.

[1] Because of possible differences in the quality, strength and specification of the active antiseptics used and of differences in the strength of any alcohol or alkali employed, it is essential that no mouthwash be marketed without adequate tests for toxicity and potential irritation. Except where innocuous, such solutions should be labelled with a suitable cautionary notice and distinctively packaged.

PHENOL

Phenol exerts an antiseptic action which varies not only with its concentration but also with the solvent used, the proportion of salts present, and the temperature. A 1 per cent. aqueous solution destroys the virulence of most putrefactive and septic bacteria but not resistant spores. An aqueous solution is often employed as an antiseptic mouthwash preferably as sodium or potassium phenate, e.g.:

	per cent.
Phenol	3·6
Sodium hydroxide solution (3·5 per cent. w/v)	9·6
Glycerin	12·0
Water	to 100·0

Dilute with 5–10 times its volume of water before use.

Caution: The above mouthwash is poisonous and should be coloured red.

p-CHLORMETACRESOL

The more recently introduced esters of *p*-hydroxybenzoic acid, although excellent for preventing certain mould growths, cannot be considered antiseptic, and no antiseptic mouthwash should be based solely upon a single one of these compounds (*see* R. G. Harry, *Mfg. Chem.*, Aug. 1936; also H. Davis, *Quart. J. Pharm.*, 1935, **8**, 361). Their place for such purposes is more satisfactorily taken by para-chlormetacresol. In the proportion of about 0·1 per cent., this latter substance forms an excellent aqueous mouthwash. Its solubility in water is, unfortunately, slight, viz. about 0·4 per cent. at 20° C., which would allow of a 1 : 4 dilution if it is to exert its maximum efficiency. It is, however, readily soluble in alcohol and could be marketed in this form, ready for dilution in water. Alternatively, the half sodium salt of para-chlormetacresol may be used for the same purpose. This is more soluble than the former, it being possible to prepare aqueous solutions of from 0·8–1 per cent. concentration, e.g.:

	per cent.
Para-chlormetacresol	0·2
Glycerin	20·0
Water	79·8

Add an equal volume of water before use.

(It is desirable to colour this solution red.)

TANNIC ACID

Tannic acid is strongly astringent but somewhat irritant. Like the salts of aluminium it coagulates albumin and proteins. A 2 per cent.

solution in alcohol has proved valuable in the treatment of spongy and receding gums. A useful mouthwash may be prepared using 2 per cent. aqueous tannic acid with glycerin and borax.

Alum (Potassium Aluminium Sulphate)

Alum is a valuable styptic for bleeding points, especially after tooth extraction. A 10 per cent. solution incorporating a little glycerin may be used, this being diluted with 8 parts of water before use. It is believed that *its use as a general mouthwash is undesirable, unless very quickly removed by rinsing, leading possibly to destruction of the teeth. It is not in itself antiseptic, and if for use with open wounds or raw gums, a suitable antiseptic should be included.*

Saponaceous Mouthwash

These are favoured by some on account of the clean taste in the mouth, e.g.:

	per cent.
Powdered soap (neutral)	2·0
Glycerin	15·0
Alcohol	20·0
Water	63·0
Flavour	*q.s.*

If a foaming wash is wanted the use of about 1 per cent. of sodium lauryl sulphate powder appears to be useful, in combination with other desired substances.

Liquor Formaldehyde (Formalin)

This is an aqueous solution containing between 37 per cent. and 41 per cent. w./v. of actual formaldehyde H . CHO, and is a powerful germicide. *It may be used up to 1 per cent. as a mouthwash, this being diluted 1 : 5 before use.* (*Note*: A 1 per cent. solution of formalin is indicated in the above, i.e. 1 per cent. of the pharmacopoeial solution containing 40 per cent. of formaldehyde.)

Myrrh

Myrrh, an oleo-gum-resin obtained from the stem of *Commiphora mohol* and other species, is a mild disinfectant and a local stimulant to the mucous membrane. The tincture may be employed as a wash for spongy and ulcerated gums, often in combination with borax, e.g.:

	per cent.
Tincture of myrrh	4·0
Eau de Cologne	65·0
Water	15·0
Borax	4·0
Syrup	12·0

Thymol (Isopropyl Metacresol)

This is a crystalline substance obtained from the volatile oils of *Thymus vulgaris*, *Monarda punctata* and *Carum copticum*. Thymol resembles phenol in its action, but is absorbed more slowly and is less irritant to wounds. Although its germicidal value is greater, it is only about one-quarter as toxic. Its insolubility limits its general application but in concentrations of 1 : 3000 it may be used as a mouthwash, in combination with boric acid or borax, e.g.:

	per cent.
Thymol	0·03
Alcohol	3·00
Borax	2·00
Sodium bicarbonate	1·00
Glycerin	10·00
Flavour	*q.s.*
Water	to 100·00

For a mild mouthwash dilute 1 teaspoonful with a wineglass of water. In cases of inflamed throat a dilution of up to 1 : 5 may be used.

Hydrogen Peroxide

This is an excellent *non-poisonous antiseptic*. It does not combine with albumins and may be used for cleansing ulcers and abscesses in the mouth, etc. A solution of 1 part hydrogen peroxide (10 vols.) diluted with 8 parts of water is useful as a mouthwash, or twice the strength may be used for cleansing septic cavities. In view of its ready deterioration, however, it does not usually enter the composition of proprietary mouthwashes. Sodium perborate may, however, be put up in powder form, and requires only solution in water to produce an oxygenated mouthwash, since it is soluble in water (about 1 : 40) with decomposition yielding an alkaline solution containing free hydrogen peroxide. In practice 17 g. of such a powder with 6 g. of citric acid will, on the addition of about 80 ml. water, make a solution of 10 vols. strength. This requires diluting 1 : 8. Tonsilitis has been treated with a gargle of sodium perborate 1·6 per cent.

In addition to the above, a number of simple mouthwashes are prepared with dilute alcohol containing aromatic essential oils, e.g. eucalyptol, menthol, peppermint, clove, wintergreen, anethol, etc.

Flavouring of Mouthwashes

This is carried out by the judicious addition of a blend of essential oils already mentioned. This flavouring is an essential point in the production of a popular mouthwash, and money spent on purchasing the best quality oils is usually found to be justified by the sales.

Precautions should be taken in the choice of flavours for an oxygenated product, since many essential oils are oxidised and their taste ruined. In many cases it is preferable for the smaller manufacturer to purchase flavours compounded for this particular purpose.

Ti-tree oil might also be used on account of its high antiseptic value, as the following table exemplifies, in which its value, as determined by A. R. Penfold, has been inserted among the Rideal-Walker coefficients for a number of other essential oils (S. Rideal, E. K. Rideal, A. Sciver and N. E. G. Richardson, *Perfum. essential Oil Rec.*, 1928, **19**, 285 ; 1930, p. 341).

Rideal-Walker Values

	per cent.
Thymol	20·0
Ti-tree oil [1]	13·0
Palmarosa oil	9·0
Eugenol	8·6
Clove oil	8·0
Cinnamon leaf oil	7·5
Geraniol	7·1
Bay oil	5·5
Coriander oil	5·4
Citral	5·2
Linalool	5·2
Citronellal	5·0
Spearmint	2·8
Lavender	1·6

The actual value of such essential oils against *mouth organisms* is difficult to assess, since the R-W value, although of undoubted value, is only a measure of their effectivity against one particular strain of organism, and varying bacteria show wide resistances to different antiseptics under varying conditions.

[1] Dr. W. G. Reynolds (*Mfg. Perfum.*, Jan. 1938, p. 3), who has examined various samples of this oil from various Australian sources, has not obtained a sample having a carbolic acid coefficient of more than 2 calculated on a 100 per cent. basis.

For this reason the use of a mouthwash containing a mixture of flavouring agents in combination with a suitable antiseptic offers the widest range of germicidal activity. It is obvious that the essential oils used in flavouring also possess a definite germicidal value, in particular thymol, eugenol and clove.

Abiotoxines

J. Risler (*C.R. Acad. Sci.*, 1936, **203,** 517) states that mixing two essential oils of different volatility lengthens their antiseptic value from a matter of days (when used separately) to about four years (when combined) and quotes as examples the preservation of Egyptian mummies. Risler terms such substances capable of prolonging the duration of the antiseptic value *abiotoxines* and suggests that when oils and aromatics are mixed, compound abiotoxines are produced which are more powerful than those present in the individual oils. In addition the author claims that mixing essential oils greatly enhances their immediate bactericidal effect.

These results, if confirmed, would be of the greatest value, and it is to be hoped that further researches in their direction will be undertaken.

Halitosis

H. Prinz (*Dent. Cosmos*, July 1930) has discussed the principal causes of halitosis, and concluded that an antiseptic mouthwash in conjunction with a dentifrice and correct prophylactic dental care will eliminate this complaint. A modern mouthwash for Halitosis might be based on the use of the chlorophyllins (*see* Chapter 16).

In conclusion, it is necessary to consider types of antiseptic washes for artificial teeth. These require special treatment, as if they are constantly brushed with a dentifrice, the fitting of the plate may be spoiled. Solutions of chlorinated soda have been recommended, but these have rather an unpleasant smell, and impart a taste to the plate. Moreover, some vulcanite dentures are discoloured by its use.

Antiseptic mouthwashes can readily be adapted for use with dentures and this fact can be mentioned on the container, since the use of a contaminated plate may give rise to serious trouble. *See also* Denture Cleansers (Chapter 17).

CHAPTER 19

EYE LOTIONS

"I have nothing to offer but blood . . . tears and sweat."
(*Sir Winston Churchill* 1940.)

In view of the sensitivity of the human eye to inappreciably small dust particles, hot or smoky atmosphere, chemical irritants, intense light and other forms of nervous strain, it is hardly surprising to find that eye lotions are among the oldest of our medicinal preparations.

The main considerations in their manufacture are that they should be non-irritant and soothing to the eye and that they should not affect, adversely, the natural biological protective agencies in the eye.

For some time it has been realised that the indiscriminate application of quite weak solutions of certain chemicals, in themselves innocuous, produced intense irritation in the eye and this has been explained on the grounds that to avoid irritation it is imperative that the lotion should have the same osmotic pressure, or tonicity, as the surrounding tissue and tears. Opponents of the theory that only the tonicity was really important have stressed the importance of the hydrogen concentration ion.

It now appears that both of these factors are important and that their importance is related in that the human eye can tolerate moderately wide variations in the *p*H value if the osmotic pressure is controlled within narrow limits and fairly wide variations in the osmotic pressure if the *p*H is controlled within fairly narrow limits.

The Tonicity of the Tears

There is no longer valid evidence to support the assumption that a 1·4 per cent. solution of sodium chloride is isotonic with the tears.

Hind and Goyan (*J. Amer. phar. Ass., Sci. edn.*, 1947, **36**, 33) point out that freezing-point determinations on a number of contact lens solutions judged to have optimum wearing qualities by the majority of a large number of patients, were found to have freezing-points of −0·54° C. which, these investigators point out, is the approximate freezing-point of physiological saline and contrary to the value of 1·4 per cent. sodium chloride solution generally advocated for isotonic ophthalmic solutions.

These results are in line with those of Krogh, Lund and Pedersen (*Acta physiol. scand.*, 1945, **10**, 88) who found that the osmotic concentration of lachrymal fluid was equivalent to 0·90 per cent. sodium chloride (freezing-point —0·52° C.).

More recently this value has been confirmed (Pedersen-Bjergaard and Smidt, *Acta derm.-venereol.* 1952, **2** (Suppl. 29), 261) by relative measurements of the conductivity and the vapour pressure of lachrymal fluid from 25 females and 25 males. This fluid was found in conductivity measurements to correspond to a 0·9 per cent. sodium chloride whereas in the vapour pressure determinations it corresponded to a 0·93 per cent. sodium chloride solution. The slight difference between these two results is ascribed to the content of sodium hydrocarbonate in the tears.

According to the work on contact lens solutions reported by Hind, the eye has been shown to have a wide range of tolerance to solutions of osmotic pressure. Freezing-point values of —0·331° C. to —1·244° C. (in terms of sodium chloride 0·50 per cent. to 2·0 per cent. concentration) may well be tolerated. (These observers point out, however, that the instillation of one or two *drops* of a medicating eye lotion has such a transitory osmotic effect on the eye tissue that, for practical purposes it need not be accurately adjusted as long as it is maintained within reasonable physiological limits.)

Natural Bactericidal Effect of Tears

Thompson (*Arch. Ophthal., N.Y.*, 1941, **25**, 491) points out that "... post-operative infections of the eye were relatively infrequent even in pre-Listerian days ..." and that organisms placed in the conjunctival sac rapidly disappeared therefrom.

Tears are described as mixtures of lachrymal and conjunctival secretions containing exfoliated epithelial cells, occasionally leucocytes and probably some Meibomian secretion normally only in minute quantities, according to Schirmer (*v. Graefes Arch. Ophthal.*, 1903, p. 67).

Thompson (*Arch. Ophthal.*, 1941), points out that Fleming (*Proc. roy. Soc.*, 1922, **93**, 306) showed that tears, among other biological secretions (such as nasal mucus, egg-white, etc.), had the remarkable property of dissolving certain saprophytic cocci rapidly and completely and obtained evidence that the agent, or agents was an enzyme to which Fleming gave the name of "lysozyme", or lytic enzyme.

Subsequent investigations by a team of investigators showed that this active lysis-producing agent in egg-white is a basic protein or polypeptide enzyme, stable to heat and filtration in an acid medium but insoluble and heat-labile in an alkaline medium.

This agent was inactivated by oxidising agents and by some heavy metals but not by boric acid or zinc sulphate.

James (*History of Ophthalmology to 1800*, 1933, London : Cambridge University Press) makes references to the use of the white of egg, as far back as the earliest Anglo-Saxon periods. Thompson (*Arch. Ophthal.*, 1941) refers to the use by Melnik and Natanson (*Bull. Inst. Metchnikoff* 1936, **3**, 133) of egg-white in cases of infection.

In the light of the above, it is evident that substances incorporated in eye lotions sold for *cosmetic* effect should contain no substances known to interfere with the natural biological protective agency of the human eye, but should be confined to soothing lotions of *p*H and tonicity as close as possible to that of a healthy eye.

The Hydrogen Ion Concentration of Tears

Hydrogen ion concentration *per se* has been briefly discussed in Chapter 6.

Horsford and Hicks (*Arch. Ophthal.* 1935, 13, 14) found the *p*H value of lachrymal fluid to be 7·35. Pedersen-Bjergaard and Smidt, using the glass electrode *p*H meter in the case of 50 normal individuals (25 male and 25 female) found an average *p*H of 7·4. These workers point out that it is difficult to establish the *p*H of lachrymal fluid with high accuracy because of the technical difficulties arising from the fact that the *p*H *in vitro* is evidently increasing with time, the rate of increase being dependent on the ease of escape of carbon dioxide.

From the aspect of cosmetic formulation, it is very fortunate that in sodium chloride and boric acid we have substances which may be used over a fairly wide range of concentration without giving rise to irritation, or to extremes in *p*H values, and that these substances (and zinc sulphate), do not appear—so far as is known—to interfere with the natural protective agency of the eye.

The Preparation of Isotonic Solutions

K. Pedersen-Bjergaard and co-workers have made a marked contribution to the study of isotonic solutions. In careful investigations these workers have made allowance for the " water fraction " which separates as ice before the solution itself freezes and have determined, as already mentioned, that the human lachrymal secretion is almost iso-osmotic with blood serum, i.e. equivalent to a 0·9 per cent. solution of sodium chloride. (Freezing-point $-0{\cdot}52°$ C.)

The usual question to be determined by the cosmetician then is how much sodium chloride has to be added to a hypotonic solution of a certain substance in order to obtain a solution iso-osmotic with a 0·9 per cent. sodium chloride ?

Pedersen-Bjergaard (*Schweiz. Apoth. Ztg.*, 1952, **90**, 650) points out that the iso-osmotic concentrations of a solution of several different substances can usually be found by adding together the freezing-point depressions of each single substance. This does not apply, however, where a reaction occurs. Thus when acids react with sodium carbonate solutions, carbon dioxide is evolved and the freezing-point depressions of the prepared solutions are smaller than the sums of the freezing-point depressions of the components. Also when boric acid is neutralised with sodium hydroxide, the solution of sodium borate thus formed gives a smaller freezing-point depression than the sum of the freezing-point depressions of boric acid and sodium hydroxide. In the latter case the effect is not due to volatile compounds but is ascribed to the transformation of orthoborate to tetraborate.

Pedersen-Bjergaard and his co-workers have made freezing-point determinations (and determinations of the relative vapour pressures) of aqueous solutions of a large number of substances used for the preparation of eye drops, etc. The fundamental basis of variation of concentration with freezing-point was investigated and the results corrected by a double system of logarithmic co-ordinates which allowed straight line relationships to be obtained. After the necessary equation had been calculated it was transferred to the arithmetical system with sufficient points to enable a more or less arched curve to be drawn accurately. By this means it has been possible to publish accurate graphs for a number of medicaments showing variations of depression of freezing-point with change of concentration (C. G. Lunde, E. Peulicke, Neilson and K. Pedersen-Bjergaard, " Contributions from the Danish Pharmacopoeia Commission ", Vol. 2—*The Preparations of Solutions Iso-osmotic with Blood, Tears and Tissue*, London: Heinemann Medical Books Ltd., 1947).

By the ingenious super-imposing of a reversed sodium chloride curve, it is possible to find rapidly the amount of sodium chloride which must be added to a hypo-osmotic solution of one of the substances to make it iso-osmotic. The concentration of the substance that is prescribed in the solution is sought out in the ordinate. Through the ordinate point of the concentration in question is drawn an imaginary line parallel to the abscissa, and through the point of intersection of this line and the curve of the substance in question is drawn an imaginary line parallel to the ordinate. The ordinate of the point where the latter line cuts the mirrored (i.e. reversed) sodium chloride curve gives the amount of sodium chloride that must be added to the solution to obtain a solution iso-osmotic with blood and tears.

The following is a typical example of such curves for, amongst other substances, boric acid, borax, sodium chloride and zinc sulphate together with the super-imposed "mirror" curve (i.e. reversed curve), sodium chloride.

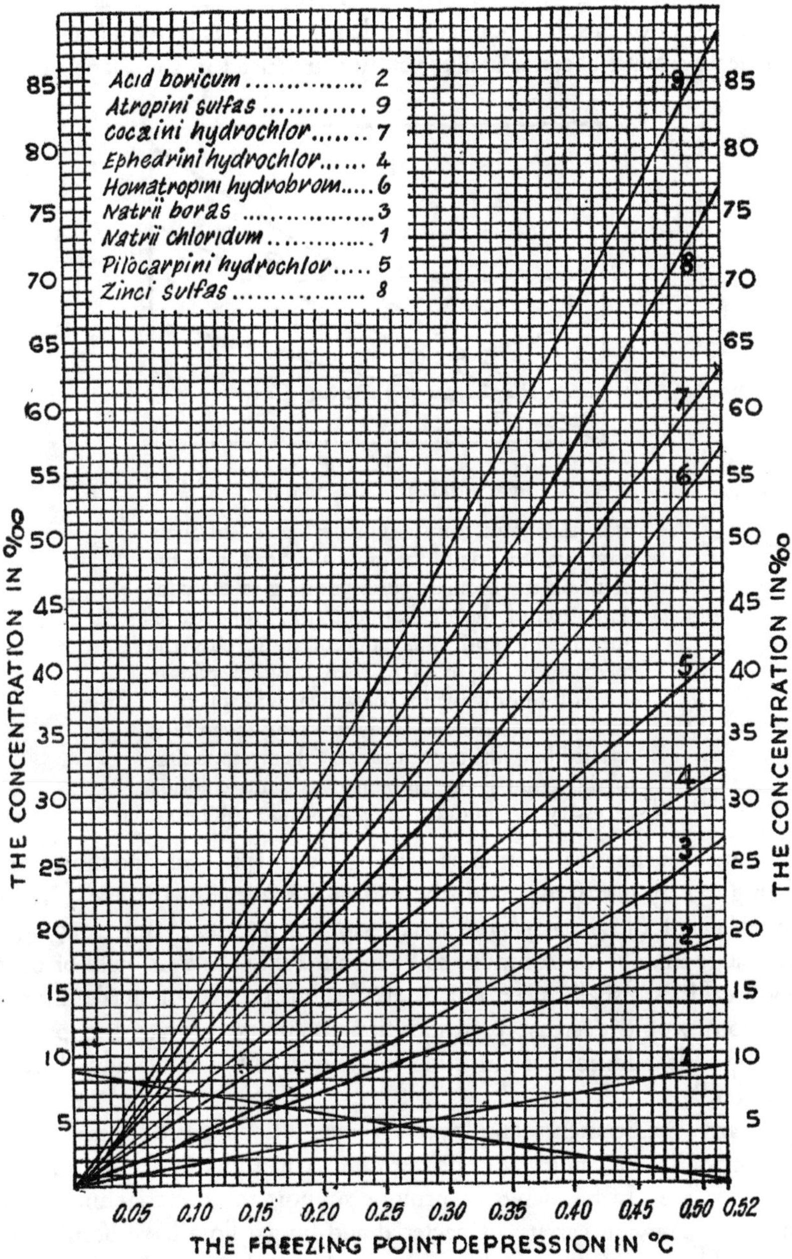

FIG. 53—Freezing point depression Curves (°C) with super-imposed "mirror" curve for sodium Chloride. [*By courtesy of Dr K. Pedersen-Bjergaard and Einar Munksgaard.*

The Preservation of Eye Lotions

There is some difference of opinion as to whether eye lotions *need be sterile*. Although the technical literature refers almost invariably to the necessity of this, it is pointed out that the eye has its own bactericides for dealing with bacteria inadvertently introduced in the shape of dust,

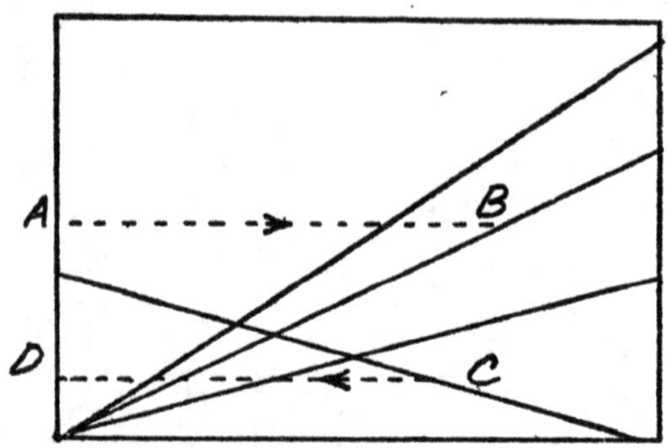

Practical use of graphs.

Fig. 54. shows from a practical point of view how easy it is to use the graphs. Start from the point on the ordinate corresponding to the concentration of the medicament (*a*); now travel horizontally until this concentration cuts the medicament curve (*b*); then travel vertically upwards or downwards (downwards in this case) until the "mirrored" sodium chloride curve is reached (*c*); the concentration (*d*) corresponding to this point is the amount of sodium chloride necessary to produce an iso-osmotic condition.

etc., and that the introduction of "strong" antiseptics may do more harm than good by interfering with the natural lysozyme of the eye. White and Vincent (*J. Amer. pharm. Ass., Pract. Pharm. edn.*, Aug. 1947, 3, **8**, 411) state that "... solutions to be instilled into the eyes, nose or other body cavities, usually need not be sterile, but the use of sterile diluting solutions would decrease predisposition to mould growth and prevent the possible addition of infecting organisms into an already diseased location."

Many medicaments employed in eye lotions possess little or no bacteriostatic or fungistatic power and consequently their aqueous solutions are always liable to provide support for bacterial and fungal growth. A wide variety of bacterial and fungal flora have been found in a viable condition, in such solutions as borax, boric acid, etc. Whilst it is relatively easy to sterilise eye drops and lotions, it is rarely possible to pack them commercially in such a manner as to prevent reinfection with air-borne micro-organisms in use.

Any antiseptic or preservative employed in such preparations should :

(i) be non-irritating to the eye ;

(ii) not interfere with the lysozyme of the eye ;

(iii) be stable in aqueous solution, even under heat-sterilisation conditions ;

(iv) be approximately neutral in reaction ;

(v) be compatible with any other medicaments added ;

(vi) be effective in inhibiting the growth of fungi and bacteria ;

(vii) possess suitable solubility characteristics at an effective concentration and over a widely varying temperature range.

The use of Methyl, Ethyl and Propyl esters of parahydroxybenzoic acid has been widely recommended in the preservation of eye lotions (" The National Formulary ", 1949 ; Simonelli and Marri, *Boll. Soc. ital Biol. sper.*, 1939, **14**, 289 ; Arrigoni and Tozer, *J. Amer. pharm. Ass., Pract. Pharm. edn.*, 1946, **7**, 292) though the value of the various esters for this purpose has been disputed by Spengler and Kessler (*Pharm. Acta Helvet.*, 1943, **18**, 660).

Although the official bodies still recommend " Nipagin-M " and " Nipasol-M " (i.e. methyl and propyl para-hydroxybenzoates) as suitable preservatives for eye drops in average concentrations of 0·04 per cent. Nipagin-M plus 0·02 per cent. Nipasol-M, Nipa Laboratories have for some time developed a special preparation called "Nipasept", which consists of a combination of the methyl-, ethyl- and propyl-para-hydroxybenzoates. It is understood (Dr. Boehm, personal communication) that Nipa Laboratories have found that each ester by itself is selective in its bacteriostatic and fungistatic action and that one alone does not cover the whole range of bacteria and fungi. By using the " Nipasept " combination, it is claimed that it is possible to produce a preparation which will function efficiently against all bacteria and fungi. The recommended concentration of "Nipasept " is 0·08 per cent. w./v. [This is best added in the form of a stock solution prepared by adding 0·8 g. to 1 l. of distilled water and boiling for a few moments to effect solution ; it is claimed that this solution will keep indefinitely.]

Chlorbutol (0·5 per cent.) and Chlorocresol (0·03 per cent.) have been suggested ; the former may well produce temporary smarting when dropped into the eye. Hind and Gayon (*J. Amer. pharm. Ass., Sci. edn.*, 1947) state that they have for several years used successfully alkyl dimethyl benzyl ammonium chloride (Zephiran-Winthrop Chemical Co.

or "Phemerol" Aqueous, Parke, Davis & Co.) in a concentration of 1 : 50,000 and found it perfectly satisfactory in preventing mould growth in ophthalmic solutions.

Having discussed briefly the background of eye lotions in relation to modern theories of tonicity and *p*H, including the role of lysozyme and preservation, it is possible to consider various cosmetic formulations.

From a therapeutic point of view, the following formulations are isotonic with the tears, non-irritant and should act as soothing lotions:

	per cent.
Sodium chloride	0·90
"Nipasept"	0·08
Distilled water	99·02

	per cent.
Boric acid	1·90
Distilled water	98·02
"Nipasept"	0·08

If a mildly alkaline solution is desired:

	per cent.
Sodium bicarbonate	1·40
Distilled water	98·52
"Nipasept"	0·08

However, from a sales point of view, they would appear to the layman to lack body (if the formulae were published on the bottle), and hence additional substances are often added to increase their complexity.

Such substances are often mild astringents, e.g. *Polygonum bistorta* (Linn.), commonly termed snakeweed or adderwort; and also *Erigeron Canadense* (Linn.), termed fleabane, coltstail or prideweed.

Other useful astringents are zinc sulphate, alum and various herbal distillates (e.g. *Liq. Hamamelidis*); this latter also exerts a cooling effect. Other soothing[1] preparations may include *aqua camphor* which has long enjoyed a reputation as a mild sedative for contusions and for tired eyes; and *aqua laurocerasi*. *Euphrasis officinalis*, commonly termed eyebright, has a reputation among herbalists in the formulations of lotions for the general treatment of eye disorders. The above extracts may be prepared as 1 : 1 solutions by steeping the drug in an equal volume of water and then pressing out the aqueous solution; such solutions, however, are inadvisable as they are likely to contain

[1] The eye is constantly kept bathed in fluid (the tears) by means of the eyelids which are sensitive to external stimuli, and if the eyeball tends to become too dry, blinking results and tears are shed. For this reason *local anaesthetics should not be indiscriminately incorporated into eye lotions for use by the public*, as by so doing the eyelid is no longer sensitive and serious damage may result to the eye while the tear supply is immobilised.

spores and other types of microbiological life. If aqueous extracts are desired, it is best to sterilise them after they have been prepared, or to use a distilled extract or alcoholic extract.

Zinc sulphate is often employed in the treatment of inflammation and conjunctivitis, in a concentration up to approximately 0·2 per cent.

As a vasoconstrictor and haemostatic, or in conjunctivitis, an addition of 1 part adrenaline in 4,000 parts of lotion may be made.

The following lotions are slightly more complex than those already mentioned :

	per cent.
Boric acid	1·90
Zinc sulphate	0·10
Distilled extract witch hazel	12·00
Preservative	*q.s.*
Distilled water	86·00

	per cent.
Sodium chloride	0·90
Tinct. euphrasis	1·00
Dist. extract witch hazel	10·00
" Nipasept "	0·08
Distilled water	88·02

	per cent.
Boric acid	1·90
Camphor water	5·00
Preservative	*q.s.*
Distilled water	93·10

One well-known proprietary product has the formula :

	per cent.
Liq. ext. Potentill erect.	0·50
Liq. ext. Polyg. bistort.	0·50
Liq. ext. Erig. Canad.	0·50
Liq. ext. Euphras. off.	0·50
Liq. ext. Hamam. virgin.	0·50
Boric acid	2·00
Sodium borate	0·50
Sodium salicylate	0·08
Zinc sulphate	0·10
Liq. Hamam. virgin.	25·00
Distilled water	69·82

This illustrates how herbals may be used to build up any formula which may be decided upon.

The tincture of euphrasia may be prepared by steeping the small cut fresh plant in an equal amount of 90 per cent. alcohol, macerated, pressed and filtered. This method may also be used for tinctures of other herbals. The possibility that the *net* result of a mixture of herbals in an eye lotion may be *greater than what we should expect from their sum*, owing to synergistic action, must be remembered in the criticism of proprietary preparations.

The method of manufacture is simplicity itself: the ingredients, together with preservative, being dissolved in the distilled water, any fluid or distilled herbal extracts added, the mixture transferred, preferably to containers, and then sterilised. Alternatively, the lotion may be sterilised and then transferred to sterile containers.

The former treatment is the more likely to achieve the desired result. In either event the lotion is sterilised either by autoclaving, by Tyndallization, i.e. heating for one hour at 80° C. on three successive days, or by filtration through a Berkefeld, Pasteur-Chamberland, or Seitz filter.

The reaction of the collyrium (eye lotion) is often affected adversely by alkali dissolved from the glass container. Dissolved silica also may ruin the product. For these reasons the use of ampoule-glass containers tested in accordance with the pharmacopoeia, is preferable. Such containers are especially suitable for the heat sterilisation of such products.

CHAPTER 20

THE HAIR

Histology of Hair—Hair Growth—Keratin—Mineral Constituents of Hair—Grey Hair—Diet and Hair Health—Effect of Cutting, Shaving and Singeing Hair—Sebum : the natural hair lubricant—The Endocrine Glands and Hair Growth—Pityriasis sicca (" dandruff")—Seborrhoea oleosa—M-type Baldness——Human Hair and Primate Patterning—Alopecia areata—Hair Tonics and Lotions.

ALTHOUGH fine, relatively unpigmented and inconspicuous hair covers almost the whole of the body, exceptions being the palms of the hands, soles of the feet, lips, etc., it is essentially that which covers the scalp with which we are concerned when speaking of " the hair ".

Whatever protective or other biological function hair may have played in the past, there is little doubt that its main function today is decorative. By changing its shape, its colour, and its style, women are enabled to alter, to a very considerable degree, the *apparent shape of the features.*

Before puberty the only hair that is well developed occurs on the scalp, the eyebrows and the eye-lashes ; such hair is coarse and usually fairly heavily pigmented. At puberty changes occur, leading to hair growth in the axillae and over the pubes in both sexes ; whilst in the male coarse hairs start to grow on the face, the " beard ".

Danforth (*Physiological Rev.*, 1939, **19**, 94) points out that after puberty the hairs of the body may conveniently be classified into three types:

(*a*) hair which is the same in both sexes, the growth of which is apparently uninfluenced by sex hormones (e.g. the eyebrows, eyelashes and the vellus—the fine velvety hair which grows over the body).

(*b*) hairs which are stimulated to coarse growth at puberty in both sexes, e.g. the pubic and axillary hairs ;

(*c*) hairs which are truly secondary sex characteristics, e.g. the male beard and male chest hairs.

Whilst many of the features of hair apply to all the above three types it is essentially the hair of the head which we shall consider.

In certain regions of the skin, the outer corneous layer (the so-called horny layer) is not immediately thrown off in the form of flakes but is first built up into a definite structure which we term " the hair ". (Compare Histology of the Nail.)

The hair is therefore a modified epidermal structure, the growth of which is limited. On attaining its normal span of life, it is replaced in a normal healthy head by a new hair. The close relationship existing between the hair and skin is seen when one studies the molecular relationship of these substances. (*See* Chapter 1.)

A hair consists of:

THE SHAFT. The shaft is the whole or that part extending outwards from the skin surface. This consists of an external layer of lubricated horny cells, i.e. the cuticle, surrounding a mass of flat epithelial cells containing pigment (the cortex). The centre of the cortex is traversed by a column of super-imposed cells (the medulla) in the form of a central canal, which, although nucleated near the papilla, lose their nuclei with increasing distance. Lanugo, i.e. downy hair, has no medulla.

THE ROOT. The whole of the buried portion is termed the root. This contains, at its lower end, a bulb (concave on its under surface), resting upon the papilla through which run the blood vessels which supply the hair with nourishment. Each hair is contained below the skin surface in an invagination of the skin termed a follicle. This consists of a narrow pocket formed partly by the dermis and partly by the epidermis, the outer sheath of which is continued down from the Malpighian layer, while the inner sheath is derived from the horny layer of the epidermis. (For an explanation of these terms *see* Histology of the Skin.) This follicle is continuous with the hair, and if the latter be forcibly detached, the former accompanies it and is then visible to the naked eye. The bottom of this pocket contains a finger-like projection, which consists of connective tissue from which the new hair develops and is termed the papilla.

The follicle does not run straight down into the skin, but is set at an angle so that that part of the hair above the surface has a "natural slope" to one side. Attached to the under side of each sloping hair follicle is a small non-striped muscle, the *Arrectores pili*, so called because it is this muscle which causes the hair "to stand on end" when contracted by fear, etc.

Many present-day dermatological works still express the view that contraction of the *Arrectores pili* muscle mechanically stimulates the excretion of sebum. This is denied, however, by MacLeod and Muende (H. K. Lewis, *Practical Handbook of the Pathology of the Skin*, London, 1940), who state that muscular contraction seems to have little or no action on the excretory process, and that it is now generally believed that such excretion is the result of the pressure produced by the continuous evolution of fat by the sebaceous cells. Other factors which affect the activity of the secretion are endocrinal and the influence of the autonomic nervous system.

The sebaceous glands are lobular structures situated in the dermis and are connected with hair follicles, except in the glans penis, prepuce, labia minora and the red border of the lips. They secrete a fatty substance termed *sebum* which the hair absorbs by capillary attraction, and which serves to give it lustre and pliability, and keeps the skin surface soft and supple. The condition of the endocrine glands exerts a great influence on the secretion. At puberty they become very active, but their activity usually decreases after middle age. (*See* Sebum ; also Acne Preparations.)

Hair Growth

Unlike animal hair, human hair does not undergo periodic loss but goes through a steady cycle of events, growth, fall and (in the case of a normal healthy head) replacement. At the end of its life span,

By courtesy of Edward Arnold Ltd.

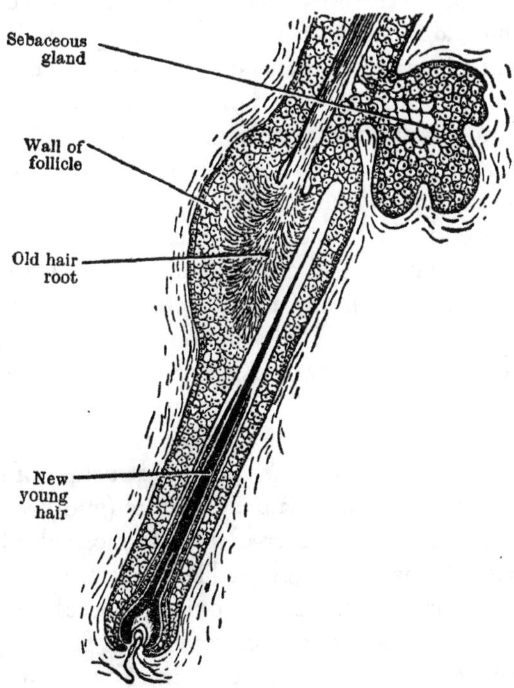

Fig. 55

Illustration of hair shedding, showing the freshly formed new hair below. (After Unna.)

the bulb of the hair loosens and separates from the papilla, it rises in the follicle and slowly moves to the surface, where it is shed. The new hair is believed to be formed by the process of mitosis (cell subdivision) from a growing point at the root of the hair around the papilla. Behrman (*loc. cit.*) gives the average " hair life " as 180 days, adding that in summer the hair displays a superior longevity, maintaining an average of 197 days before shedding.[1]

It has been estimated that a healthy adult head of hair contains an average of about 120,000 hairs, these varying according to the type of individual. In the case of a blonde the hair is finer, and the number estimated at 140,000, while black hair is thicker, and an average head of this colour would contain about 108,000.

Matsuura (*Arch. Derm. Syph., Wien*, 1902, **62**, 273) claimed that variation in the normal hair width was produced by illness but this has not been substantiated.

Hair is composed of keratin, a name derived from the Greek word " Keras " meaning horn. Hair, feathers, nails and horn have been known for a great many years to have certain features in common, for example, their insolubility in dilute acids and *dilute* alkalis, water and organic solvents and their resistance to digestion by pepsin, trypsin, etc.

It has been shown that the keratins can be divided into two groups which, although they had very similar physical properties, differed in their molecular ratios of basic amino acids, e.g. arginine, histidine and lysine. The group comprising horn and hair was termed " eukeratins " (acid hydrolysis showed a molecular ratio of histidine, lysine and arginine of approximately 1 : 4 : 12), the other group not showing this ratio was termed " pseudokeratins ".

Block (" Chemical Classification of the Keratins ", *J. Soc. cosmet. Chem.*, May 1951, **4**, 235) in the table which is reproduced on opposite page, gives the amino acid patterns of four typical hair proteins.

The molecular configuration of the keratins is of great importance. Harris (" Chemistry of Keratin ", *J. Soc. cosmet. Chem.*, June 1949, **1**, 223) points out that " . . . in many cases a small difference in chemical structure may determine whether a material is a rubber, plastic or a fibre. . . . For example, if the chemical structure of the molecules is such that they fit poorly into a lattice structure (in other words an amorphous state is favoured), and further if the intermolecular forces are weak, then the material should have rubber-like properties. In contrast, if the structure of the molecules is such as to provide for an easy fitting into a lattice (that is, a relatively high state of crystallinity is favoured) and the intermolecular forces are strong, the material is a fibre. In intermediate cases, plastic systems are obtained. If we now pass from the broad field of high

[1] Pincus (" The Story of a Hair Root ", *J. invest. Derm.*, 1947, p. 91) states that one single follicle, on a precisely identified spot on the back of the right hand gave rise to 12 hairs in a period of six years. While the average life span of each hair was 180 days, the actual length of life differed considerably. Furthermore, all the hairs under observation were different, each presenting highly individual characteristics.

polymers to a narrower section dealing with fibres, the same considerations are found to be applicable. . . . If the molecules fit poorly into a lattice

Amino Acids in Hair Keratins

	G. per 16 g. of N.			
	Human hair	*Chimpanzee hair*	*Swine hair*	*Lamb's wool*
Arginine	9·6	8·1	10·5	10·1
Histidine	0·9	0·6	1·1	0·9
Lysine	2·6	2·0	3·7	2·8
Tyrosine	3·1	3·3	3·4	5·5
Tryptophan	0·7	1·4	—	0·7
Phenylalanine	2·7	—	2·6	4·0
Cystine	16·0	15·5	13·9	13·6
Methionine	1·0	—	0·5	0·7
Serine	7·6	—	—	9·0
Threonine	7·2	—	6·1	6·5
Leucine	—	—	8·0	7·8
Isoleucine	—	—	4·5	4·2
Valine	—	—	5·7	5·1
Glutamic acid	14·8	—	17·2	15·4
Aspartic acid	8·0	—	7·7	7·1
Proline	—	—	9·3	8·0

and the intermolecular forces are weak, a fibre of low strength but greater extensibility results; further if the molecules are flexible the fibre can exhibit relatively long range elasticity (wool, elastic, nylon). . . ."

(The structure of keratin and its importance in the permanent waving of hair is discussed in Chapter 23.)

Mineral Constituents of Hair

Dutcher and Rothman (*J. invest. Derm.*, Aug. 1951, **2**, 65) have continued the work of the latter investigator (Rothman and Flesch, *Annu. Rev. Physiol.*, 1944, **6**, 195; *J. invest. Derm.*, 1945, **6**, 257) into the pigments present in hair and summarises their results as follows:

(i) Red hair contains greater amounts of iron than hair of any other shade. The presence of an iron pigment does not account for the whole difference. It is assumed that in the hair, iron is split off from the organic pigment complex.

(i) No relationship between the copper content and the colour shade of human hair could be found.

(iii) The ash content of red hair is significantly higher than that of hair of other colours.

Bagchi and Ganguly (*Ann. Biochem.*, 1941, **1**, 84) give the following analytical figures for the mineral constituents of human hair:

	European girl Brown hair	*Hindu woman Black hair*	*Mixed hair of thirty male adults—from a hair cutting saloon*
	per cent.	*per cent.*	*per cent.*
Carbon	44·03	44·20	44·60
Nitrogen	13·70	13·68	14·60
Hydrogen	5·58	5·60	5·40
Sulphur	3·80	1·50	3·80
Phosphorus	0·065	0·096	0·08
Chlorine	1·98	2·00	2·00
Water	3·96	4·20	4·10
		Milligrams per kilo.	
Lead	21·0	284·0	47·7
Copper	64·0	62·8	108·0
Arsenic	2·4	2·2	2·2
Zinc	116·0	182·0	212·0
Iron	133·0	126·0	141·0
Manganese	28·4	25·0	38·0
Cobalt	14·2	16·0	18·1
Nickel	5·4	5·5	8·2
Calcium	212·0	188·0	208·4
Aluminium	26·0	26·0	32·0
Silicon	188·0	178·6	150·4
Bismuth	nil	nil	nil
Silver	nil	nil	nil
Antimony	nil	nil	nil
Mercury	nil	nil	nil

(Magnesium, Iodine and Tin were also present but their quantities could not be determined because of insufficient materials.)

These authors point out, from the table above, that the amounts of carbon, hydrogen, nitrogen, sulphur and phosphorus present in hair are approximately of the same magnitude, irrespective of age, sex, and nationality.

Grey Hair

True grey hair is comparatively rare. What is usually termed grey hair consists of a sprinkling of white hairs among dark ones. Several theories have been advanced to account for such greyness but none of them has as yet been completely substantiated. These include the following conceptions :

(*a*) Grey hair has a deficiency of pigment while in white hair there is no pigment at all.

(*b*) There is a loss of pigment by wandering cells which absorb and take the pigment from hair to the skin.

(*c*) Neurotropic causes may produce a change in the hair colour. It is not yet known whether the pigment is bleached by a chemical change or the hair looks white owing to the production of gas bubbles in the shaft which reflect the light.

(*d*) Animal inheritance factors of colouring may affect the disposition and colour of the hair.

The first two theories and the last have not been proved, although some observations of Gerrit S. Miller (*see* Human Hair and Primate Patterning) suggest the latter. There appears to be some evidence in favour of a neurotropic influence ; for example, greying of hair has resulted from very severe nervous strain and possibly from severe forms of neuralgia. At the same time it appears most unlikely that sudden bleaching of the hair can occur almost ***overnight***, and it is a curious fact that while there were numerous references to it in the years 1860–84, since then, claims for such a phenomenon have not been substantiated. Statements that the hair of Marie Antoinette and Sir Thomas More, etc. turned from dark to white overnight would appear to be a case of poet's license (more dramatic than truthful). If nervous tension can produce such a ***rapid*** change it is remarkable that this fact has not been noticed.

> "My hair is grey but not with years,
> Nor grew it white
> In a single night
> As men's have grown from sudden fears."

Byron's quotation (*The Prisoner of Chillon*) should be taken with a pinch of salt. Galewsky stated that in his extensive experience he had never seen genuine cases of sudden blanching of the hair (" Canities ", *Handbuch der Haut u. Geschlechtsk.*, 1932) and considers it strange that no such cases were reported during the First World War. Hair washes and dyes have been known since the earliest days. In the case of political and other prisoners, it is *more than likely*, that those incarcerated no longer had access to their favourite dye. Uncharitable, but possibly a much more likely scientific explanation of any such occurrence.

Lutati (*Policlinico*, 1918, **25**, 680) claimed to have seen several cases among Italian troops, but I have no knowledge of any overnight blanchings of the hair occasioned by the extreme nervous tension under concentrated air raids in the war of 1939–1945.

Green and Spencer Patterson (*Lancet*, 7 Aug., 1943, p. 158) records the case of an engine-driver who slipped and fell from a stationary engine, and from the time of the accident became a feeble old man. His hair came out on the day of the accident, at first in a round patch, diagnosed as alopecia. Eventually it spread, until in four months he was completely bald. Two months later a few white downy hairs appeared. The writers point out that the literature concerning sudden greying of hair does not mention whether total alopecia preceded the pigmentary change. They add that the omission may have been due to wilful suppression of an unromantic transitional phase. (F. Spiedler, *Wien. klin. Woch.*, 1918, **31**, 1087; F. Stern, *Z. ges. Neurol Psychiat.*, **79**, 1087; W. A. Pusey, *Arch. Derm. Syph., Chicago*, 1928, **17**, 201; A. P. Thompson, *Lancet*, 1938, p. 135.)

The role of diet in grey hair, if any, has not yet been completely elucidated.

In response to a reader's inquiry the *J. Amer. med. Ass.*, 1942, **119**, 18, succinctly summed up the then present state of our knowledge regarding vitamin concentrates and grey hair as follows:

. . . . "The vitamin studies which produce greying in animals and then cure it by correction of the diet have been made on mice, rats, dogs, and silver foxes. By shaking the watery solution of liver extract, yeast or rice bran with fullers' earth the thiamin, riboflavin and pyridoxine are removed, leaving a solution of the *filtrate factor*. Animals fed with a diet containing the other vitamins but lacking this factor soon show patches of fur that has become grey and thinned, ulcers sometimes appear on the tail or hind legs, the animal's skin becomes wrinkled as in old age, it becomes feeble and it often dies within a few months if kept on the deficient diet. On adding the *filtrate factor* to the diet these symptons clear up in most cases.

"It is known that this factor contains pantothenic acid and para-aminobenzoic acid; but the effort to determine which of these is responsible for the prevention of greying has not been successful as yet, for there is disagreement among the research workers engaged in the problem. Ansbacher and his associates find that the lack of para-aminobenzoic acid causes the greying, and that adding this vitamin to the diet restores the colour of the depigmented patches ("Role of Para-Aminobenzoic Acid in the Vitamin B Complex—Studies with Mice", *Proc. Soc. exp. Biol., N.Y.*, Oct. 1941, **48**, 118. Others (G. A. Emerson, "Failure to Cure or Prevent Greying of Rats with Para-Aminobenzoic Acid", June 1941, **47**, 448; Unna, Klaus, Richards,

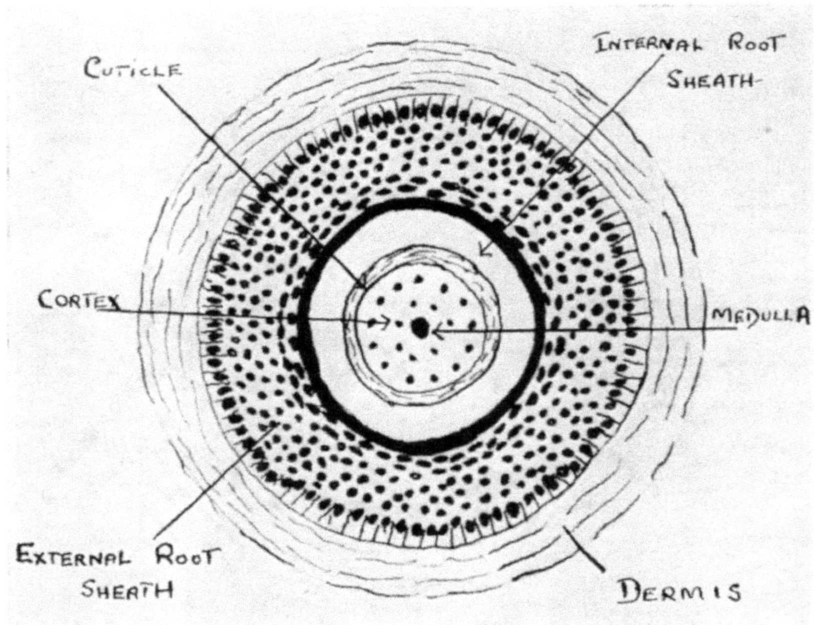

FIG. 56.—Structure of hair in transverse section (Diagrammatic).

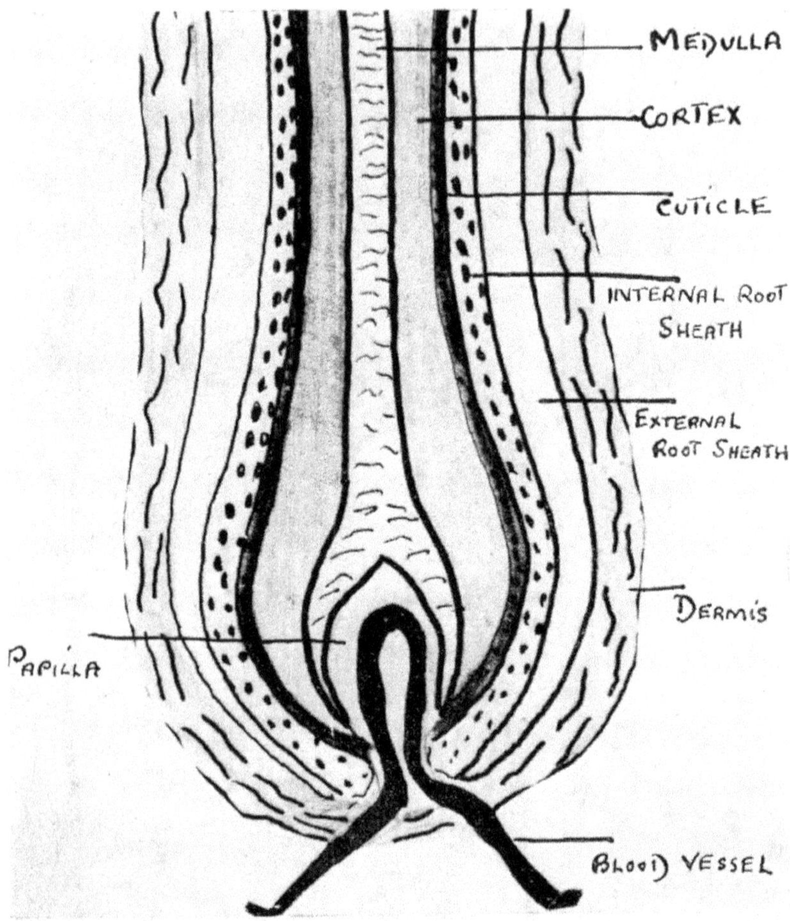

FIG. 57.—Structure of the hair in vertical section (Diagrammatic).

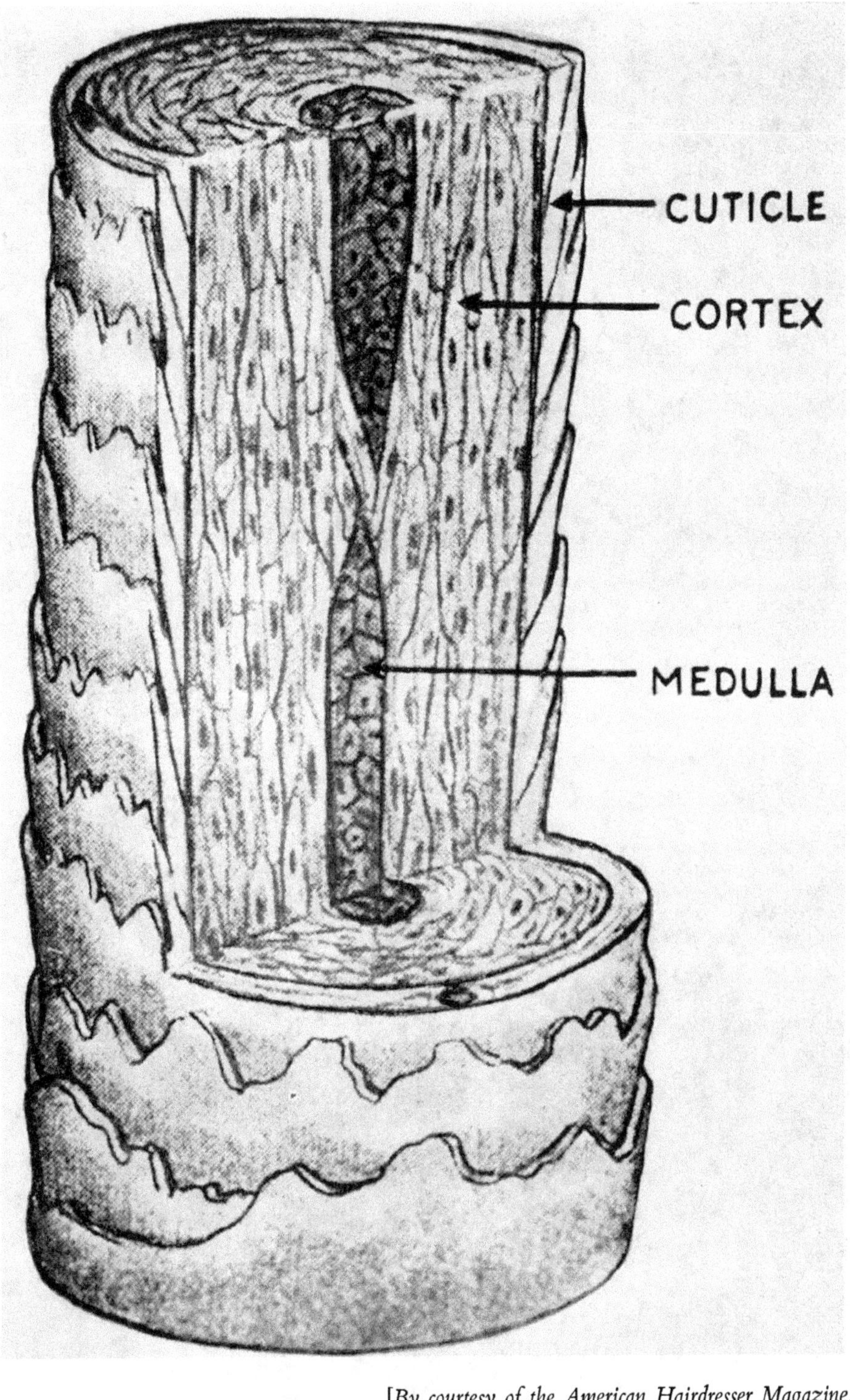

[*By courtesy of the American Hairdresser Magazine.*

FIG. 58.—Diagrammatic sketch of a section of a hair fibre.

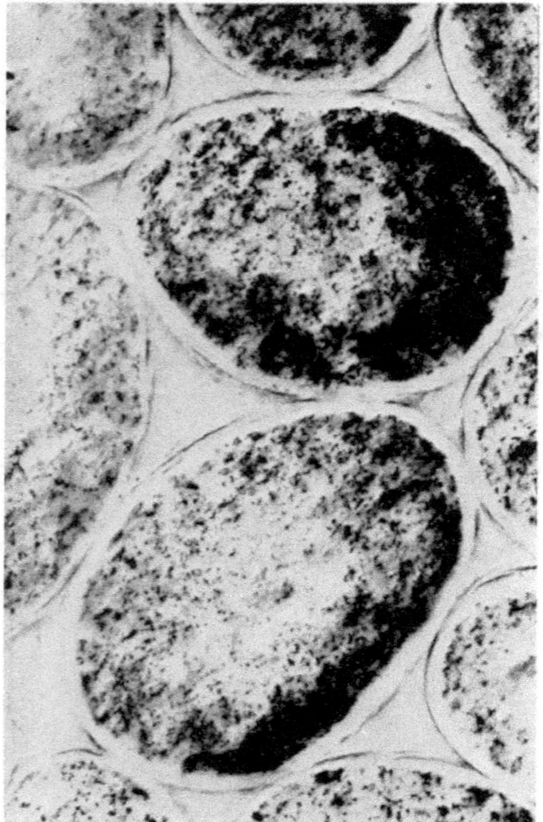

[*By courtesy of the Toilet Goods Association, U.S.A.*

FIG. 59.—Cross-section of hair showing pigment granules. (× 670.)

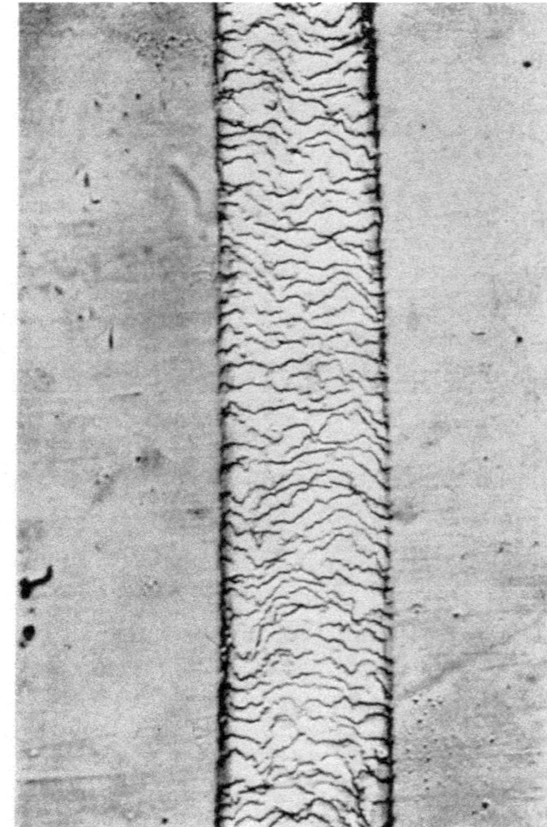

FIG. 60.—Collodion imprint of hair, showing imbrications. (× 360.)

V. Grace andW. L. Sampson, "Studies on Nutritional Achromotrichia in Rats", *J. Nutr.*, Dec. 1941, **22**, 553) have succeeded in producing the grey spots by depriving the animals of pantothenic acid and have then cured the animals by adding this vitamin to their diet. It has been suggested that there may be other vitamins, as yet undiscovered, in the *filtrate factor*.

"Apparently there are only two articles in the medical literature dealing with the effects of vitamin B complex and para-aminobenzoic acid on human hair. They are both by B. F. Sieve ("Clinical Achromotrichia", *Science*, 12 Sept. 1941, **94**, 257, "The Clinical Effects of a New B Complex Factor, Para-Aminobenzoic Acid, on Pigmentation and Fertility", *Sth. Med. Surg.*, March 1942, **104**, 135). When vitamin B complex was administered to nine patients who were under treatment for endocrine dysplasias the grey hair of all, he reports, became noticeably darker. He then began the use of para-aminobenzoic acid for the same purpose, giving it to those on treatment with endocrine preparations and also to many who were on no other treatment. In his second paper he reports over 800 cases treated in this way. Within three to eight weeks of treatment with the vitamin the grey hair became dirty yellowish and then *dark dusty grey*. . . ."

These reports justify scepticism. As far as his articles show, Sieve's only evidence of colour changes was his visual impressions. Those who have tried to judge slight colour changes in the skin or hair realise how easily one can be deceived.

The question of the possible harmful action of para-aminobenzoic acid in large doses must be considered. Several investigators have shown that this substance interferes *in vitro* with the bacteriostatic action of the sulphonamide drugs on pneumococci and staphylococci and that it promotes the growth of Streptococcus progenes (W. W. Spink and Jean Jermsta, "Effect of Sulphonamide Compounds on Growth or Staphylococci in Presence and Absence of Para-Aminobenzoic Acid", *Proc. Soc. exp. Biol., N.Y.*, June 1931, **47**, 395). Recently Hawkings (*Brit. med. J.*, 20 Feb., 1954, 425) has pointed out that the body fluids of animals contain very little para-aminobenzoic acid (otherwise sulphonamides would not be therapeutically effective) and has shown that when this substance is ingested it renders them susceptible to malarial parasites. Hawkings further suggests that the relative immunity to malaria shown by infants under 6 months in the tropics is due to a deficiency of para-aminobenzoic acid in their diet of mothers' milk. So far as calcium pantothenate is concerned, Kerland and Herwick (through *Mfg. Chemist*, July 1944, 265), after administering 20 mgm. daily for 6 months to 27 patients, found no significant changes in the colour of the hair.

Diet and Hair Health

Diet necessarily exerts an influence upon the general health of both the skin and the hair and in the absence of certain *necessary* elements, pathological changes may occur. The skin and the hair derive their nourishment from the blood supply (*see* Chapter 1), and the blood supply depends for certain elements upon diet (*see* Chapter 3), but we do not know at present whether any *specific elements* in the diet are of particular or unique importance in respect of *hair growth*.

Keratin contains a higher proportion of cystine than is found in most other proteins. Loeper (*Le Soufre*, ed. Masson, Paris, 1943; through Fridenson (*Perfum. essent. Oil Rec.*, 1951, **42**, 42)) states that the human body contains about 100 g. of sulphur, the majority of which, it is stated, is localised in the skin, nails and hair. Organic sulphur in the keratin molecule is chiefly in the form of combined cystine, as is shown in the following table which is taken principally from the work of Block and Bolling (*The Amino Acids Composition of Proteins and Foods*, Ed. Chas. C. Thomas, Springfield, Ill., 1945).

	Sulphur	*Cystine*
Human hair	3·92 - 5·47	
Blonde		17·2
Brown		17·0
Red		13·6
Children		16·4–19·6
Adults		18·3
Male		15·3–17·4
Female		14·1–16·2
Human nails . . .		10·0–12·9
Human skin (pseudo-keratin) .		2·3–4·3

[*For the typical amino acid pattern of hair see earlier discussion on keratin.*] Fridenson (*Perfum. essent. Oil. Rec.*, 1951) refers to the work of Rose (*Physiol. Rev.* 1938, 18, 109) who showed that the addition of cystine to a diet entirely devoid of sulphur-containing amino acids did not arrest the loss of weight, whilst growth was promptly resumed on the addition of methionine. The faculty possessed by methionine of replacing completely cystine in the diet of an animal has, so Fridenson states, been demonstrated not only for growth but also for the formation of hair and that administration to rats of a diet rich in methionine and poor in cystine caused an increase in the formation of hair and its content cystine. According to the reports of Jausion and Benard (*Bull. Soc. franc. Derm. Syph.*, 1949, **5**, 462) the regrowth of hair was stimulated in six of their patients, two of whom had alopecia and four seborrhoea, by the administration of methionine.

Care must be taken not to read too much import into the above claims. In the first place, cognisance must be taken of the fact that experiments on animals are not always directly relateable to man. For example, Rose (" Half-Century of Amino Acid Investigations ", *Chem. Eng. News*, June 1952, p. 2385) found that histidine and arginine—which are indispensable for the rat—are not required for the maintenance of nitrogen equilibrium in normal human adults. In the other case reported it must be remembered that cure in alopecia *may* be spontaneous without treatment (*see* Alopecia).

Rose has carefully determined the minimum and recommended intakes of a number of amino acids in man, when the diet furnishes sufficient nitrogen for the synthesis of the non-essentials. The significance of his findings are brought out by the following conclusion " . . . During the spring of 1942, the U.S. Department of Agriculture made a survey or the amounts and kinds of food purchased by different economic groups in the country. Using these figures and the best analytical data available Block and Bolling (*The Amino Acids Composition of Proteins and Foods*) calculated the average daily *per capita* consumption of the essential amino acids. The findings show that even the lowest income group consumed the eight essentials (tryptophan, phenylalanine, lysine, threonine, valine, methionine, leucine and isoleucine) that year, in amounts which exceeded the recommended intakes by factors of 1·4 to 3. . . ." It is added that the possibilities of anyone in the U.S.A. experiencing an amino acid deficiency are very remote.

So far as the author is aware, the U.S.A. has just as many—if not more—bald or balding heads than the United Kingdom, so that it does not appear as if baldness can be ascribed to methionine, cystine or any other known amino acid deficiency!

(Changes in the skin due to vitamin A and other deficiencies are discussed in Chapter 3.)

The Effect of Cutting, Shaving, and Singeing the Hair

The hair is a *dead* structure so far as that portion in view is concerned. Cutting and shaving does not affect its general rate of growth or its thickness, neither does singeing confer any benefits upon it.

Bulliard (*Ann. Derm. Syph., Paris,* June 1923, p. 386) carried out independent experiments which proved that cutting does *not* stimulate hair growth. Dr. M. Trotter (*Amer. Arch. Derm.*, 1923, vii, 93) showed that shaving did not cause any increase in the rate of growth, nor in the type of hair that grew, and that the use of greasy preparations (petroleum jelly) did not cause short downy hairs to become longer or coarser.

The different outcome of the experiments of R. Seymour (*Amer. J. Physiol.*, 1926, **78**, 281), in which cutting of the hair appeared to stimulate growth, is due to the short intervals between the times of cutting, only 12–48 hours, as compared to weeks and months in the former case.

Actually, the hair growth *is faster immediately after cutting.* This accounts for the necessity of frequently shaving to keep the face free from beard. However, it rapidly slows down as the length of hair increases; ultimately the *final length and texture of the hair are not altered.* Experiments by D. H. Strangeways (*J. Agric. Sci.*, July 1933) confirm these facts.

Singeing the hair apparently is based upon the crude belief that the hair shaft contains some crude kind of canal from which the hair draws nourishment and which has to be sealed up, *to prevent the juice running out*, when the hair is cut. This, of course, is quite wrong. Singeing is actually of harm since it dries the higher portions of the hair and destroys it.

SEBUM. The hair is kept lubricated along its shaft by sebum, the secretion of the sebaceous glands. Sebum consists of fats (olein, palmitin and stearin), fatty acids (oleic, palmitic and stearic acids), cholesterol, chlorides and phosphates of the alkaline earths, organic salts, albuminoids, water, and occasionally butyric and caproic acids. Mixed up with these are epidermal nuclei debris of cells and a few horn cells.

Schmidt gives the following analysis of the contents of a sebaceous cyst:

	per cent.
Water	31·70
Epithelium or proteins	61·75
Fat	4·16
Fatty acids	1·21
Ash	1·18

(through J. M. H. MacLeod and I. Muende, *Practical Handbook of the Pathology of the Skin*, London: H. K. Lewis & Co. Ltd., 1940). It is often stated that sebum is derived from the fatty degeneration of the epithelial cells lining the sebaceous glands. A. Policard and Y. Tritchkovitch (*Lyon Méd.*, 1922, **131**, 981), however, show that sebum is not a produce of cell degeneration but rather of fat secretion. By feeding an oil-soluble dye they showed that the cells were capable of directly fixing the fats circulating in the blood, particularly after digestion. This confirms the fact that the character of the secretion is influenced by the diet. Kuznitsky (*Arch. Derm. Syph., Wien*, 1913, **114**, 691) found more fat was secreted in the case of a carbohydrate diet than with a fatty one.

A number of investigations have been carried out in respect of the composition and rate of excretion of human sebum. Butcher and Parnell (*J. invest. Derm.*, 1947, **9**, 67) carried out experiments on four individuals who possessed the following characteristics :

(*a*) sparse hair and much dandruff ;
(*b*) little hair on the vertex and a very oily scalp ;
(*c*) had lost a little hair on the forehead ;
(*d*) had an unusually good head of hair.

To determine the quantity and contents of the sebum, collections were made once weekly usually on a Wednesday. All the individuals shampooed their heads on Friday of each week. All refrained from wearing hats and touching their foreheads as much as possible. The following were the conclusions reached :

The individual with good hair and a small amount of dandruff was found to average 0·160 mg. of fat and 0·0119 mg. of cholesterol per sq. cm. at the hairline when the collections were taken once weekly over an interval of eight weeks, the cholesterol amounting to 7 per cent. of the total sebum. When taken daily over a period of three weeks the fat averaged 0·114 mg. and the cholesterol 0·0107 mg. per sq. cm., the cholesterol amounting to 8·6 per cent. of the total sebum.

The individual with an apparently oily scalp and sparse hair was found to average 0·219 mg. of fat and 0·0149 mg. of cholesterol per sq. cm. once weekly, the cholesterol amounting to 6·3 per cent. of the total sebum. Taken daily the fat averaged 0·163 mg. and the cholesterol 0·0123 mg. per sq. cm., the cholesterol amounting to 7 per cent. of the total sebum.

Associated with a scalp containing much dandruff and thin hair was 0·168 mg. of fat and 0·0171 mg. of cholesterol when the collections were made once weekly, the cholesterol making up 9·4 per cent. of the total sebum. When taken daily the fat averaged 0·145 mg. and the cholesterol 0·0162 mg. per sq. cm., the cholesterol amounting to 10 per cent. of the total sebum.

There was no evidence that frequent removal of the sebum induced increased oiliness of the scalp.

There was considerable variation in the amount of sebum which was collected at various times.

These investigators also discovered that the sebum was not confined entirely to conical masses at the orifices of the glands but spread along the sulci between the orifices.

MacKenna, Wheatley and Wormall (*J. invest. Derm.*, July 1950, **15**, 33) pointed out that whilst an appreciable amount of information was available concerning the fat of ovarian dermoid cysts (in many cases this appeared to show close resemblance to sebum and had been assumed by many persons to be identical with it) information about the composition of human surface skin fat was scattered and was not readily correlated largely because of the varying methods used for the collection of the material. These investigators obtained the sebum by immersing the forearm in acetone followed by removal of the acetone and examination of the chloroform-soluble portion of the residue. MacKenna *et al.* suggest that average sebum contains about 20 per cent. of free unsaturated fatty acids, 25 per cent. triglycerides, 25 per cent. fatty acid esters other than glycerides, 5 per cent. cholesterol (free and combined) and 15 per cent. hydrocarbons (including 5 per cent. squalene). These investigators draw special attention to the (not previously reported) presence of identified squalene and vitamin E (tocopherols).

Jones, Spencer and Sanchez (*J. invest. Derm.*, Oct. 1951, p. 213) estimated the *rate of secretion* of sebum in man and arrived at the following conclusions:

(*a*) "... a comparison between absorption methods, scrubbing methods and direct solvent action shows that the absorption method is inadequate, the scrubbing method effective but irritating and the solvent method non-irritating and adequate if combined with gentle rubbing;

(*b*) the amount of fat on the skin of the forearm of a single individual was found to be $45{\cdot}18 \pm 2{\cdot}73$ μg. per sq. cm. initially;

(*c*) the removal of fat from the skin requires repeated washings. This removal follows a logarithmic curve. After three washings, the amount being secreted affects the readings;

(*d*) the interval of time between determinations affects the amount of fat removed and the apparent rate of secretion. Over extended intervals the rate of secretion tended to fall. A hyperbolic curve could be fitted to these rates obtained over intervals of increasing duration ... this indicated that a steady rate of secretion was of the order of 0·1 μg. *per sq. cm. per minute*. ..."

Nicolaides and Rothman ("Studies on the chemical composition of human hair fat—The squalene-cholesterol relationship in children and adults", *J. invest. Derm.*, Dec. 1952, p. 389) point out that "... surprisingly little attention has been paid to the early data of Eckstein (*J. Biol. Chem.*, 1927, **73**, 363) on the relatively high cholesterol content of children's hair fat (9–12 per cent.) as compared to that of adults (1–5 per cent.). Since squalene has been demonstrated to be present in skin

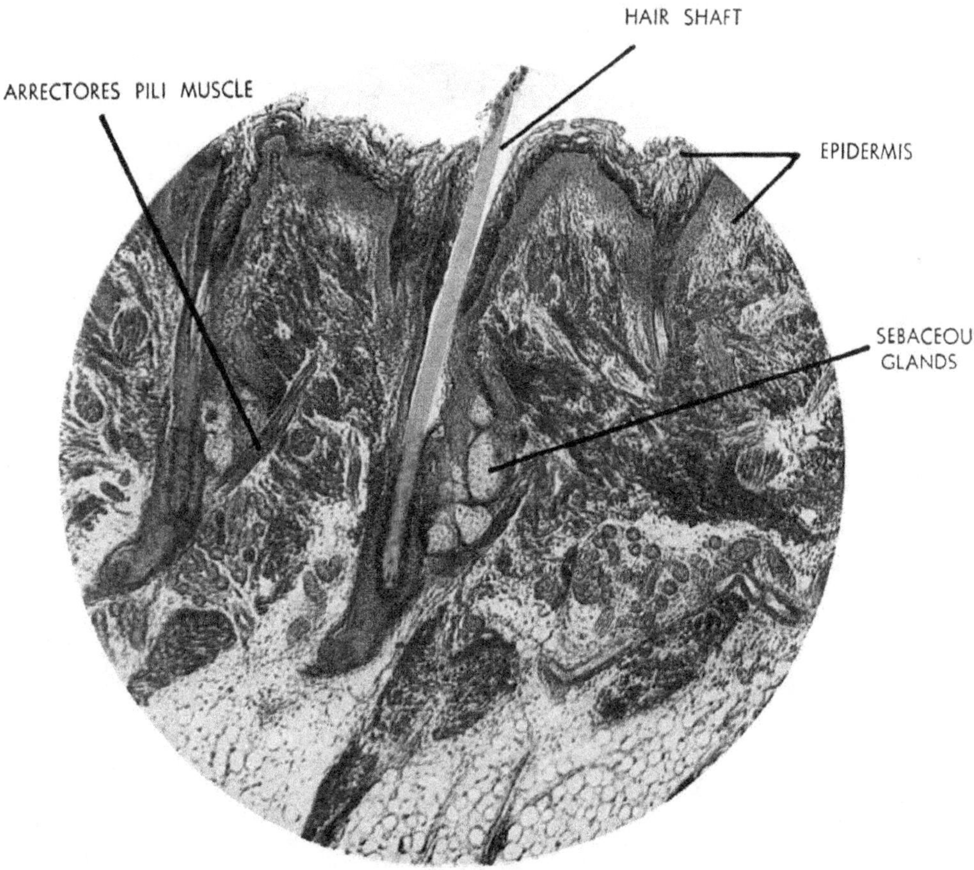

FIG. 61.—Vertical section of the scalp.
(From the Author's collection. × 50.)

surface fat and since it was shown recently that squalene is converted into cholesterol in the animal body (Langdon and Bloch, " Biosynthesis of Squalene and Cholesterol ", *J. Amer. chem. Soc.*, 1952, **74**, 1869, etc.), it was thought that some relationship might exist between these two substances as they occur in hair fat of children and of adults. . . ."

Squalene when applied locally to the skin of rabbits and guinea pigs causes temporary hair loss (Flesch and Goldstone, " Local depilatory action of unsaturated compound ; the effect of human sebum on hair growth ", *J. invest. Derm.*, 1952, **18**, 267). Nicolaides and Rothman (*J. invest. Derm.*), referring to this, add " . . . It is not yet certain whether the difference found in squalene content in male and female hair fat is significant. In any case it seems improbable that squalene . . . could play any role in the development of early male baldness, because, if anything, the squalene content of female hair fat is higher than that of male hair fat. . . ."

The most conspicuous difference is seen when the hair fat of adults is compared with that of boys. The cholesterol content of the hair fat of boys is nearly $3\frac{1}{2}$ times as great as that of either men or women. The squalene content is, on the other hand, only $\frac{1}{4}$ as great as it is for men or $\frac{1}{5}$ as great for women.

Summarising their results these investigators concluded :

(i) " . . . the average cholesterol content of the hair fat obtained from extracting pooled samples of hair from boys 6–12 years of age is 12·2 per cent., that for men is 3·8 per cent. and that for women is 3·5 per cent.

(ii) the average squalene content of the hair fat of boys 6–12 is 1·35 per cent. as compared to 5·1 per cent. for men and 7 per cent. for women ;

(iii) the ratio of moles of cholesterol per mole of squalene in the hair fat of boys is at least twelve times as large as it is for adults, thus indicating a much higher efficacy for the conversion of squalene into cholesterol by the prepubertal skin than by the skin of the adult ;

(iv) because the squalene content of the hair fat of males is not higher than that of females, squalene probably cannot be responsible for early male baldness. . . ."

H. T. Behrman (*The Scalp in Health and Disease*, London : Henry Kimpton, 1952) has drawn attention to the work carried out by Flesch mentioned above. Flesch found that squalene and a group of lipoid-soluble unsaturated compounds (with —C═C— groups) cause reversible complete baldness when applied to the skin of laboratory animals.

These compounds include the synthetic dimers of chloroprene and certain esters of allyl alcohol, naturally occurring vitamin A, oleic and linoleic acids. Flesch has postulated that the depilation is caused by the reaction between the —C=C— bonds and the sulphydryl groups of epidermal protein. Although he has not, as yet, been able to depilate human beings with any of these unsaturated depilatory agents, these findings have suggested that human sebum may have a profound influence on hair growth and keratinisation. This theory, Behrman points out, is supported by the following indirect evidence:

(1) A single application of sebum causes reversible hair loss in laboratory animals with profound changes in epidermal growth and keratinisation.

(2) Three of the depilatories (squalene, oleic and linoleic acids) are normal constituents of sebum.

(3) Since chronic exposure to two unrelated depilatory compounds (the dimers and vitamin A) cause loss of hair it is conceivable that one or several of the unsaturated components of sebum have a similar action when hair is subjected to their toxic effects over a long period of time.

(4) It is known that male sex hormones are essential for the development of common male baldness; on the other hand, male sex hormones are the most powerful known stimulants of sebaceous secretion. Additional evidence for the role of sebum in the aetiology of baldness is still in the experimental stage. . . ."

It will be noticed that the above opinions by different authorities appear to conflict. I say *appear* because I am not at all sure that they do conflict. In my opinion a few more facts are required which may provide the key to the whole problem. The fact that the squalene level in men is not higher than in women does not rule out the possibility that squalene may play an important role in man. We know that in women there is most certainly a sex-factor involved in respect of hair fall and that *women do not show the typical M-type baldness of males.* There may exist an inter-relationship between squalene and androgens; there may be incompatibility between squalene and estrogens; or there may be far more complex factors involved in the squalene-sex hormonal balance.

Sebum has been shown to differ in composition at puberty. Rothman, Smiljanic, Shapiro and Weitkamp ("Spontaneous Cure of Tinea Capitas in Puberty", *J. invest. Derm.*, Feb. 1947, p. 81) showed that with the onset of puberty the sebaceous glands of the scalp start to secrete a sebum which contains in higher concentration than before, low-boiling saturated fatty acids with selective fungistatic and fungicidal action on M. audouini. Cure of any existing ringworm infection was slow because the active acids failed to penetrate the human hair shaft. However, as the infected hair was shed, it was replaced by healthy hair since the follicles from that stage on were sterilised by the fungistatic fatty acids of the sebum.

The above investigation refers to M. audouini. It may well be that changes of a less obvious nature constantly occur in the composition of the sebum and that these changes may also be of " physiological significance ".

In Chapter 4, the importance of adequate hydration of the skin keratin has been discussed in some detail and the theory postulated that lanolin-like components in the sebum may hold water, either in the form of water-in-oil emulsions or in the form of molecular leaflets (*see* Chapter 41), and thus be of importance in helping to maintain adequate hydration.

Similar considerations apply to the sebum on the hair fibre, in that it may help to prevent the hair fibre from becoming too dry. Removal of this sebum from the hair shaft after shampooing, *may* allow the hair to become dry " by loss of moisture " (and not as is generally thought, by loss of oils). The dry hair, by combing, brushing or other forms of friction is thus very readily electrostatically charged whereupon the hair fibres repel each other and the hair is said to be " frizzy ", " fluffy ", uncontrollable and the like.

Within a couple of days or so, through the action of capillary forces and brushing, sebum becomes distributed along the hair shaft which then regains its " manageability ".

If the aqueous matter in the sebum film is held in the form of bimolecular leaflets, there is the possibility—though it may appear remote—that quite complex phenomena are involved. It is pointed out (Chapter 41) that the water-holding capacities of such leaflets are considerably influenced, and diminished, by the presence of electrolytes and it could be that when adequate moisture is supplied to the scalp and hair shaft by the process of perspiration (brought on by physical or mental exertion) the water-retentive capacities of the sebum-coated hair fibres is thus, deliberately, reduced by the presence of electrolytes from perspiration. Similarly, when the hair is " mopped ", washed, or treated in any way that removes *sebum and perspiration,* then, for a while afterwards the water-holding capacity of the freshly secreted sebum is at a maximum until such time as an adequate supply of moisture, as evidence by electrolyte from perspiration, is present.

The Endocrine Glands and Hair Growth and Health

The effect of estrogens in skin health and the cosmetic effects obtained by the use of estrogen-containing creams are discussed in Chapter 4. In view of the role which their secretions have been found to play in respect of the skin, it might be expected that some such effect would be demonstrated in the case of the hair.

Behrman (*The Scalp in Health and Disease*) points out that " . . . at the present stage of our knowledge, the following glands, as well as these natural and synthetic hormones are probably concerned with hair growth:

(i) GONADS

(*a*) *Ovaries*

(1) *Oestrogens* (natural-oestradiol, oestrone, oestriol, equilin, hippulin), (synthetic-benzoestrol, dienoestrol, diethylstilboestrol, diethylstilboestrol dipropionate, ethinyl oestradiol).

(2) *Progesterone.*

(*b*) *Testes*

(1) *Natural* (testosterone).

(2) *Synthetic* (testosterone propionate, methyl testosterone).

(ii) ADRENAL CORTEX

Twenty-five steroid hormones have so far been isolated from the adrenal cortex. Of these the following six have been shown to have important physiologic properties with regard to electrolyte metabolism: desoxycorticosterone, corticosterone, dehydrocorticosterone, 17-hydroxycorticosterone, 17-hydroxy-11-dehydrocorticosterone, 17-hydroxy-11-desoxycorticosterone. Furthermore, there is evidence indicating that some adrenal cortex hormones have estromimetic and andromimetic properties.

(iii) PITUITARY (*anterior lobe*)

(*a*) *Gonadotropic hormones* (follicle-stimulating, luteinizing).

(*b*) *Growth hormone.*

(*c*) *Thyrotropic hormone.*

(*d*) *Adrenocorticotropic hormone.*

(iv) THYROID . . . ."

Of the above complicated, and as yet only partially sketched picture, attention in this chapter is only given to the estrogens and androgens with a passing reference only to those of the adrenal cortex, and a brief mention of the recently obtained dermatotropic hormone.

Barber (*Modern Trends in Dermatology*, edited by R. M. B. MacKenna) points out that, in so far as the influence of sex hormones on the skin and pilo-sebaceous system is concerned, two essential facts have been established :

(i) that androgens stimulate the surface epithelium and the sebaceous glands tending to produce hyperkeratosis and seborrhoea ;

(ii) oestrogens have a contrary action in that they diminish keratinisation and the activity of the sebaceous glands.

Barber mentions that favourable results have been obtained by inunctions with an ointment containing an oestrogen in *female* cases of male *alopecia*, considerable re-growth of hair being obtained even in advanced cases.

Reiss and Cellis (*J. invest. Derm.*, March 1949, p. 159) have reported that percutaneous application of oestrogens in rabbits causes a reduction in the size of the sebaceous glands and a stimulation of the hair papillae with an increase in the rate of growth of the hair. With percutaneously applied testosterone there was noted hyperplasia of the sebaceous glands and reduced activity of the hair papillae (less mitotic figures) with a decrease in the rate of growth of hair. These investigators point out that during administration obvious changes occurred in the cortex of the adrenal glands.

Rony and Zakon (*Arch. Derm. Syph., Chicago*, 1943, **48**, 601) administered testosterone propionate to boys aged 8–9 years and examined biopsy specimens histologically before and after treatment. A considerable increase in the number and size of the sebaceous glands was noted in all subjects after treatment. Hamilton (*J. invest. Derm.*, 1942, **5**, 473) drew attention to the essential *maleness* of baldness, and (*J. clin. Endocrin.*, 1941, p. 570) pointed out that eunuchoid and castrate men do not develop seborrhoea, acne or common baldness, but the administration of male hormone in the majority of cases led to the development of seborrhoea and comedones. This observer also reported (*Sci. News Lett.*, 11 April, 1942) that in a group of fifty-four men who had been demasculised through accident or injury, or who had otherwise failed to mature sexually, not one case of baldness had appeared, but when male sex hormones were administered—thus changing the hormonal balance so that the female sex hormones no longer had the field to themselves—many of these men did begin to lose their hair. [*See* subsequent discussion on M-type Baldness.]

As pointed out in Chapter 14 (Acne Preparations), the administration of female sex hormones to males involves unjustifiable risks especially since the level required to produce results is very much higher than that normally used in the female.

The evidence available indicates that the circulation of male hormones leads to increased sebum production and as already discussed under sebum, the experiments of Flesch suggest that unsaturates in sebum may play a role in baldness. In this connection the presence of vitamin E, tocopherols in human sebum is of interest since they are very effective *anti*oxidants.

PROGESTERONE. The influence if any, of this hormone on hair growth has not to date been established but the greatly increased excretion of progesterone in pregnancy and the changes which often occur in the skin and hair at such times suggest that this hormone *may* play a role.

ADRENAL CORTEX. Evidence has accumulated to suggest that the adrenal cortex may act as an inhibitor of hair growth. Whitaker and Baker (*Science*, 1948, **108**, 207) carried out a series of experiments to determine whether or not various adreno-cortical preparations might exert an inhibitory influence on hair growth when applied directly to the skin. From their studies on rats it appeared that at least one of the 11-oxysteroid hormones of the adrenal cortex (11-dihydro-17-hydroxy-corticosterone) is able to exert a direct depressing effect on the growth of hair *in the rat*. This action appeared to be accomplished by some local mechanism in the tissue to which the compound was applied, since it did not depend upon the intermediary action of any recognised endocrine gland, nor in the dosage employed did it appear to affect any hair follicles not directly treated.

PITUITARY. As already mentioned, a number of factors are associated with the action of the pituitary (anterior lobe) ; these factors include one which brings about the maturation of the ovarian follicle which produces oestrus ; other so far unidentified factors are probably present. One of these has been isolated and termed by T. H. Roberts (" A Study of the Effects of Hormones on Hair Growth ", *Proc. Sci. Sect. T.G.A.*, Dec. 1952, p. 40), the *dermatotropic hormone*. It is claimed that this hormone controls the growth of hair and the action of this hormone is to bring about a resumption of the function of the papilla and follicles which no longer function. Roberts states that experiments were first conducted on hypophysectomised rats, the hormone being applied in a cream base by inunction and that effects on the hair of the treated areas were beginning to be visible after only four days' treatment. As a consequence of the success of these animal experiments, experiments were conducted on human cases. It is stated that " Reports from more than fifty doctors have shown a growth of head hair on their patients. The colour and texture of the new hair was the same as that on the patient's head at the time of treatment . . . there have been some negative

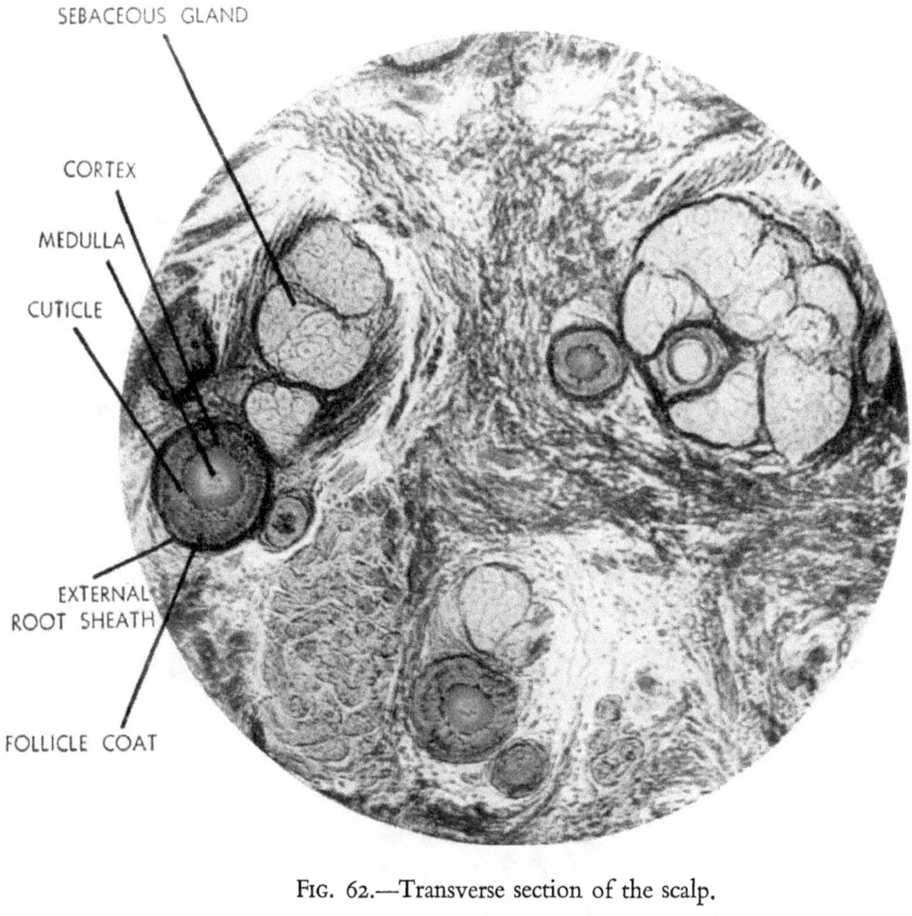

FIG. 62.—Transverse section of the scalp.
(From the Author's collection. × 100.)

results but most of these can be attributed to improper dose levels used in individual cases. The minimum amount suggested for use has been 300 mg. but this total dose level varies greatly in individual cases. Further studies planned for the dermatotropic hormone include the formation of it in a radioactive form for research studies. . . ."

The claims made for this preparation are too recent for the author to assess the credence to be accorded to this preparation. If the preparation behaves as claimed it will indeed be a remarkable development, though in view of the tremendous influence which derivatives of the anterior lobe of the pituitary exert on the body, long-term investigations will be necessary in order to assess whether its long-term usage involves any serious potential hazard.

The problem of human baldness is discussed further in this chapter under Affections of the Hair, Heredity, and also Human Hair and Primate Patterning.

There is no doubt that we are at present faced with a number of "loose ends", the key to which is still awaited; none of them are necessarily conflicting. Heredity and the fact that characteristic M-type baldness is undoubtedly a sex-linked characteristic is not necessarily antagonistic to a hair-growth hormone: for example, heredity may result in the transmission of factors responsible either (i) for the non-development of an adequate supply of the hormone (if any needed) or alternatively (ii) for the development of a damaged or inferior pituitary gland or adrenal-cortex lacking certain necessary characteristics. Similarly, there is a definite relationship between the adrenal cortex and certain sex hormones and the results obtained with either of these may depend upon a delicate balance of both in the body, the balance being different in the case of the male and female organism.

Affections of the Hair

Before considering the formulation of suitable lotions for the hair it is necessary to consider briefly those affections which occur commonly enough to be of general interest to manufacturers of hair preparations, as without having some idea of their clinical aspect it is not possible to formulate adequate remedies. Moreover, a study of this subject would cause the majority of manufacturers to modify their claims.

The whole subject is complicated because multifarious designations, sometimes apparently unrelated to one another, have in the past been applied by dermatologists and histologists to conditions exhibiting the same clinical and histological picture.

Pityriasis Simplex Capitis (*Pityriasis sicca*) ("Dandruff")

Pityriasis simplex capitis, commonly termed *dandruff,* is evidenced by the accumulation of bran-like scales on the scalp and affects both sexes. These scales are the flaking off of the outer horny layer of the scalp skin and are often termed *scurf.* These scales accumulate in patches until they are shed by brushing, combing, or scratching. Pruritis (itching) may be an accompanying symptom and the scalp may show the presence of reddening (erythema) or excoriations due to scratching. In general, however, the scalp shows no evidence of inflammatory changes. Dandruff *per se* does not produce any true or permanent loss of hair.

The Role of Pityrosporum ovale in Dandruff

On microscopical examination of the scales, dandruff is found to be accompanied by large numbers of a flask-like, shaped organism, which Unna termed the bottle bacillus, on account of its shape; later it was known as the Pityrosporum of Malassez (after Malassez who first recognised it in 1873), and today is called pityrospon ovale.

Because its culture has proved difficult, and few people have been able to reproduce the disease by means of this organism in man or laboratory animals, there are some workers who still regard it as a harmless saprophyte, i.e. a vegetable organism living upon dead or dying organic matter.

H. J. Templeton (*Arch. Derm. Syph., Chicago,* 1926, **14,** 270) stated that over half (69 per cent.) of all clinically normal scalps can be said to be in a state of sub-infection, and O. L. Levin (*Your Hair and Your Health,* New York, 1926, p. 44) considered that a normal scalp was extremely rare and that, practically speaking, there was no scalp which was not infected in some way, to some degree. It is obvious that, since this organism is so commonly found on the scalp and so infrequently grown in the laboratory, it is the investigator who lacks the requisite media and conditions; these given, the organism would probably flourish. The achievement of such conditions is not easy, since the scalp contains both sebum and sweat (which in themselves are a complex mixture) together, possibly with products produced by enzymes and carbohydrates. MacLeod and Dowling ("An Experimental Study of the Pityrosporum of Malassez; its Morphology, Cultivation and Pathogenicity", *Brit. J. Derm.,* 1928, **40,** 139), however, succeeded in causing this organism to grow on laboratory media after numerous other investigators had failed. This fungus grows very poorly on all laboratory media, the most satisfactory to the present being glucose agar.

In 1944, stated : " Attempts to transmit dandruff by this organism have not proved satisfactory. To my mind, this proves nothing, as it is perfectly obvious that, if this organism is present in three out of every four scalps and *doesn't* produce dandruff, some other factors in addition to the organism are necessary for its formation. Transmission of dandruff by the Pityrosporum will *not* occur until conditions *are* favourable." . . . If conditions *are* favourable, it might well occur *spontaneously*.

The role of Pityrosporum ovale in infectious dandruff is still the subject of controversy. Rocha, Silva, Lima and Goto (*J. invest. Derm.*, Oct. 1952) found :

(i) that no pathogenic properties of Pityrosporum ovale could be demonstrated on incubation experiments in fifty adult individuals ;

(ii) no positive reactions with intracutaneous tests performed in 200 individuals, employing two different kinds of antigens derived from this organism,

and hence concluded that P. ovale was a saprophyte without any aetiological significance at all. Whittock (*Brit. med. J.*, i. 484, 1953) examined 200 normal scalps and correlated the degree of infection with the degree of dandruff present. On the basis of this study, Whittock concluded that there was no evidence to justify the theory that Pityrosporum ovale caused the dandruff and he concluded that this was a harmless organism on the scalp which thrived best in the medium provided by a heavy flow of sebum. Reddish (*J. Soc. cosmet. Chem.*, May 1952), however, states that : " . . . *The aetiology of infectious dandruff has been proved by Koch's postulates, a reliable and time-tested method for proving the cause of infectious disease.* . . . Pityrosporum ovale conforms to the requirements of Koch's postulates because :

(i) it is present in every case of infectious dandruff ;

(ii) it has been isolated from infectious dandruff and grown in pure culture ;

(iii) in pure culture when inoculated into the skin of rabbits and the scalps of humans it has caused infectious dandruff ;

(iv) it was observed in recovered pure cultures from such experimentally produced infectious dandruff. "

Reddish states, " *This is conclusive proof that Pityrosporum is the cause of infectious dandruff*".

In assessing what credence should be given to purely " negative " results and to assumptions that " because an organism is found on a great many apparently normal human heads, it cannot be responsible for any particular pathogenic condition", two facts must be borne in mind:

(i) a positive result is more important than thousands of negative ones, providing that positive results can be repeated just sufficiently to indicate that they weren't "unique". Negative results are non-commital.

(ii) The healthy scalp may have present a protective agency, which for a while (or whilst the scalp is in a healthy condition—or during a particular period of age) may inhibit the growth of the organism. One has only to consider the investigations of Rothman, Smiljanic, Shapiro and Weitkamp into the spontaneous cure of Tinea Capitis in Puberty (*J. invest. Derm.*, Feb. 1947, p. 81) to realise the truth of this. These investigators showed that with the onset of puberty the sebaceous glands of the scalp start to secrete a sebum which contains in higher concentration than before, low boiling saturated fatty acids with selective fungistatic and fungicidal action on M. audouini.

The secretions of the scalp and skin probably contain many other selective bactericidal and fungistatic fractions of which we as yet know little. On the basis of this argument one cannot infer that because certain strains of micro-organisms do not produce pathogenic changes on all heads on which they are present, that they are non-pathogenic. The majority of persons have immunity to some strains of micro-organisms, although the specificity of this immunity varies from individual to individual.

As mentioned earlier, dandruff is a non-inflammatory disease of the scalp and does *not* produce any true or permanent loss of hair. It does, however, appear to reduce the natural protective qualities of the corneous layer so that if the dandruff is not eliminated or controlled, then at puberty—when the secretion of the male androgens causes the sebaceous glands to become very active—a secondary infection of the scaly condition (which has now become a greasy scaliness) occurs, this time with the Staphylococcus albus (formerly termed, in this connection, the polymorphous coccus of Cederkreuz). This secondary infection alters the clinical picture in that serious exudation may occur. Not everyone who has dandruff develops this oily inflammatory condition since individual immunity must play a considerable part in the pathological occurrence.

SEBORRHOEA OLEOSA (OILY SEBORRHOEA). This is a true seborrhoea, the picture being one of excessive oiliness of the scalp and face, though other parts of the skin may be involved. It is a non-inflammatory condition. Typical cases will often be found to have had dandruff in their early youth and to have accompanying bacterial infection. The causative agency in this condition is due to the production of male hormone which in some way is more effective in such individuals. It could possibly be some slight alteration in androgen constituents or more probably in the amounts. As mentioned under acne preparations, it is known that the male hormone is responsible for the production of seborrhoea, hyperkeratosis and acne.

Hormonal influences thus provide the " seborrhoeic soil " but it is no longer believed that " seborrhoea oleosa ", in itself, is in any way a *causative* factor in typical M-type human baldness.

M-TYPE BALDNESS. Baldness, particularly of the M-type, which affects a large proportion of the male population of the world, has been with us since the days of Hippocrates. The title M-type, or M-pattern, is apt, since in the balding process the hair recedes over the temples forming the outline of the letter " M " initially. Subsequently the hairfall may—and often does—extend to cover a large proportion of the scalp.

The course of this disease is often rapid, distinct evidence of the receding process being present between 18-21 years of age, whilst by 30 the area partially or completely denuded of hair may be extensive.

Such hair loss—at a period when man is in his prime, the observation that eunuchs do not go bald and that M-type baldness has never convincingly been shown to occur in a woman—are undoubtedly sex characteristics. Goodman's observation (*Treatment of Common Skin Diseases*, U.S.A., Hermes Publishing Co. Inc.) that persons who have been brought up as girls because they evidenced external genitalia of the female sex have disclosed their true endocrinologic make-up as males by evidencing the male (M) pattern baldness, is suggestive.

Sex, of course, may be influential in at least three ways : as a sexual characteristic, i.e. hormonal influences, or alternatively from the aspect of heredity, or both. It is known that baldness of this intractable type tends to run in families though the exact manner of its inheritance has never been satisfactorily determined. Osborne (" Inheritance of Baldness ", *J. Hered.*, 1916, **7**, 347), on the basis of a study of twenty-two families, advanced the view that baldness is inherited as a simple Mendelian dominant in the male and as a recessive in the female. The number of families studied was small and the results were not examined statistically. Fantham (*S. Afr. J. Sci.*, 1942, **21**, 498) suggested that inheritance might be due to a gene on the γ-chromosome but gives only one family tree, containing fourteen individuals to support his theory.

Hamilton (" Male hormone stimulation is prerequisite and incitant in common baldness ", *Amer. J. Anat.*, 1942, **71**, 451) suggested that the hereditary tendency to baldness may only manifest itself in the presence of an adequate level of androgenic hormone secretion in the body; that this level is only occasionally reached in women but is present in all normal adult men. Hamilton's evidence for the above hypothesis may be summarised thus:

(*a*) Baldness does not develop before puberty or adolescence.

(*b*) Adult eunuchs who were castrated prior to adolescence do not become bald. (Sabouraud in 1914 quoted 400 cases in support of this; Hamilton adds a further fifty-four.)

(*c*) Hamilton lists twelve persons who were beginning to go bald prior to castration. Subsequent to castration, none of these persons showed any further extension of the balding process.

(*d*) Hamilton describes twelve prepubertal castrates who were subsequently treated with a course of testosterone injections. Four of these began to go bald; these four came from families in which baldness among the normal males was a fairly frequent occurrence, the other eight (who did not go bald) came from families showing no tendency to balding.

(*e*) Baldness is not an infrequent event in women who develop masculinising tumours, e.g. of the ovary or adrenal cortex.

(*f*) The examination of family pedigrees supports the view that a man may inherit the condition through his mother, though she herself does not show it.

It appears to me that the evidence for at least two factors, viz. a hormonal influence plus the influence of heredity are overwhelming and that the outstanding investigation required is to determine what hormonal influence is involved.

As already discussed [*see* The Endocrine Glands, Hair Growth and Hair Health, above] Roberts, very recently (*Proc. Sci. Sect. T.G.A.*, Dec., p. 40), claims to have isolated a hormone from the anterior lobe of the pituitary which he has termed the *dermatotropic* hormone and which, it is claimed, controls the growth of the hair by bringing about a resumption of the function of the papilla and follicle which, in baldness, are no longer functioning correctly. Roberts states "... that reports from more than fifty doctors have shown a growth of head hair on their patients. The colour and texture of the new hair was the same as that on the patient's head at the time of treatment. It is mentioned that there have been some negative results but that these were due to improper levels of hormone, the minimum dose suggested for use of which is 300 mg. though it is stated that this total dose level varies in individual cases. . . ."

As already mentioned in an earlier discussion, the claims made for this preparation are too recent for the author to assess its value. If this preparation behaves generally as claimed, it will indeed be a remarkable development in the *treatment* of hair poverty though very careful long-term studies will be necessary to assess whether its long term and continued use will involve any potential hazard to the body (since the pituitary gland hormones exert such an important function in health and when they run wild can be so disastrous. The hormonal preparation used in all probability will have been separated from accompanying hormones which might act adversely in this manner, nevertheless it will be necessary to proceed with caution until more is known about this matter). Roberts has pointed out that extensive researches involving the hormone in a radioactive form are planned in order to be able to map out its mode of action.

Even the isolation of such a dermatotropic hormone does not invalidate the influence of heredity, since in families who have balding tendencies there may be an heredity factor which suppresses or damages in some way the secretory mechanism which should normally supply this hormone. Similarly the relationship between the sex hormones and baldness is still existent. It is hoped that this new hormone may provide a valuable key to the balding mechanism.

Human Hair and Primate Patterning

Most of the theories of hair baldness have considered the subject from the view-point that these peculiarities must have originated from conditions (pathological or cultural) or needs (physiological or aesthetic) that pertain *exclusively to man.*

Gerrit S. Miller, Jr., Curator, Division of Mammals, U.S. National Museum, has taken into consideration the zoological possibility that many features of the human hair system may be generalised primate traits instead of specifically human developments, i.e. that they may be characteristics that are forced on man because they are common property of the primates, the animal group to which man belongs. Each one of man's primate relatives has modified his portion of his heritage in such a way as to make it his own, for example, each one of the 800-odd kinds of living apes, monkeys and lemurs has developed *specific* characters by which it can be distinguished from all the others while remaining none the less a primate among primates.

That man should also have done the same is not unusual. Patterning is familiar to the zoologists because it is seen in every group of animals; but on no part of the primate form is patterning so conspicuously developed as on the head, where strikingly marked colour designs of both hair and skin are profusely exhibited and where tufts, beards, moustaches, whiskers, and crests are brought into varied contrast with areas of short hair and bare skin.

With arrival at full maturity a considerable percentage of human males undergo a modification of their hair pattern that serves to differentiate them still further from the females. The forehead begins to rise, either uniformly along its entire extent, or more commonly, by pushing back a blunt re-entrant wedge on each side (Fig. 64(4)). Frequently a bare spot begins to form at the same time on top of the crown (Fig. 64(6)) and the hair of the entire median part of the crown becomes sparse. These changes may continue until the bald forehead area has been carried back over the dome of the head, leaving a well-haired border extending around the sides and across the nape (Fig. 64(8)).

This series of maturity changes in the hair covering of the human male head has been the subject of endless speculation. The examination of many hundreds of photographs makes it appear probable that *the males of races with strong beards tend to show the highest percentage of baldness, thus differentiating themselves most fully from the females.* These observations are in accordance with the observations made by Hamilton in respect of maleness, hormones and baldness, discussed earlier in this chapter.

The types of human baldness and corresponding conditions in other primates illustrated in the accompanying Fig. 64 are as follows: Hair relationship between man and other primates is shown also in the greying of hair. When grey hairs begin to replace pigmented ones they do not appear uniformly all over the body. " A vigorous man just beginning to show a touch of grey on the temples " is an often-heard phrase that unconsciously recognises the fact. As the grey hairs increase in number they tend to form patterns, illustrated in Fig. 65 in which Nos. 7 and 8 show white locks on the human forehead line as compared with white stripes along the forehead lines in a South American spider monkey (*Ateles hybridus*), and Nos. 9 and 10 a grey area extending downward from head to middle of chest in man, and the same grey area in an Asiatic monkey (*Macaca albibarbata*).

The last conspicuous hair pattern feature of man is the tuft in the arm-pit. This, perhaps, comes the nearest of all patterns to being an exclusively human trait. Gerrit Miller, however, has observed that in several adult chimpanzees, these animals had a definitely specialised axillary tuft confined to the region of greatest glandular activity and that to produce the human condition it would merely be necessary to suppress the long surrounding hair.

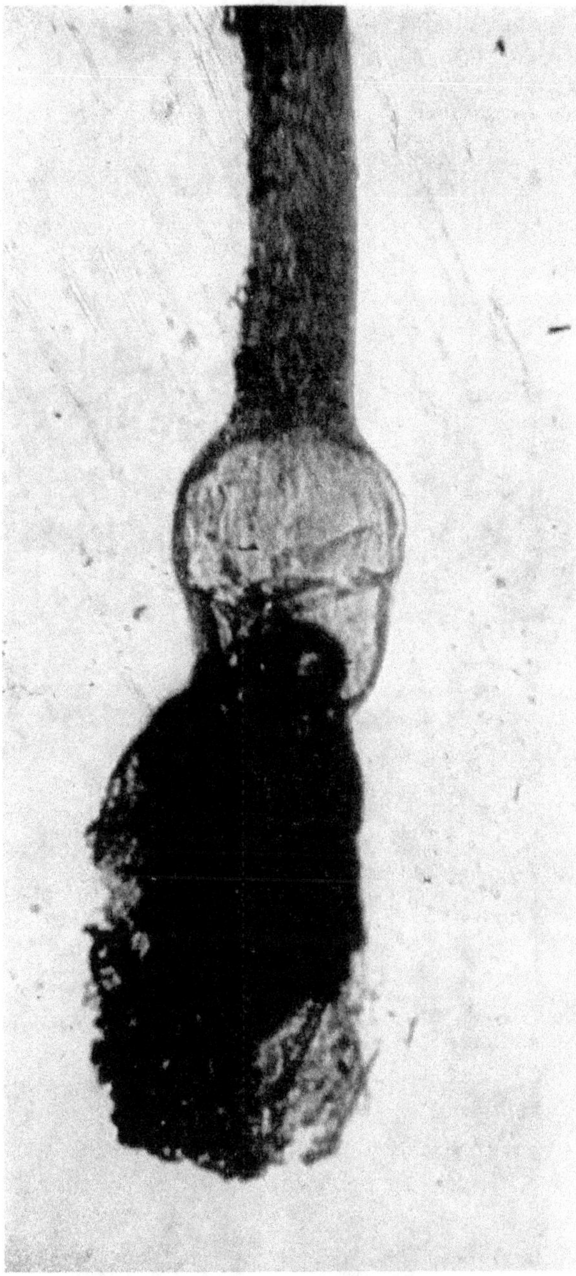

[*Illustration by the Author.*

FIG. 63.—Damaging effect of singeing the hair.

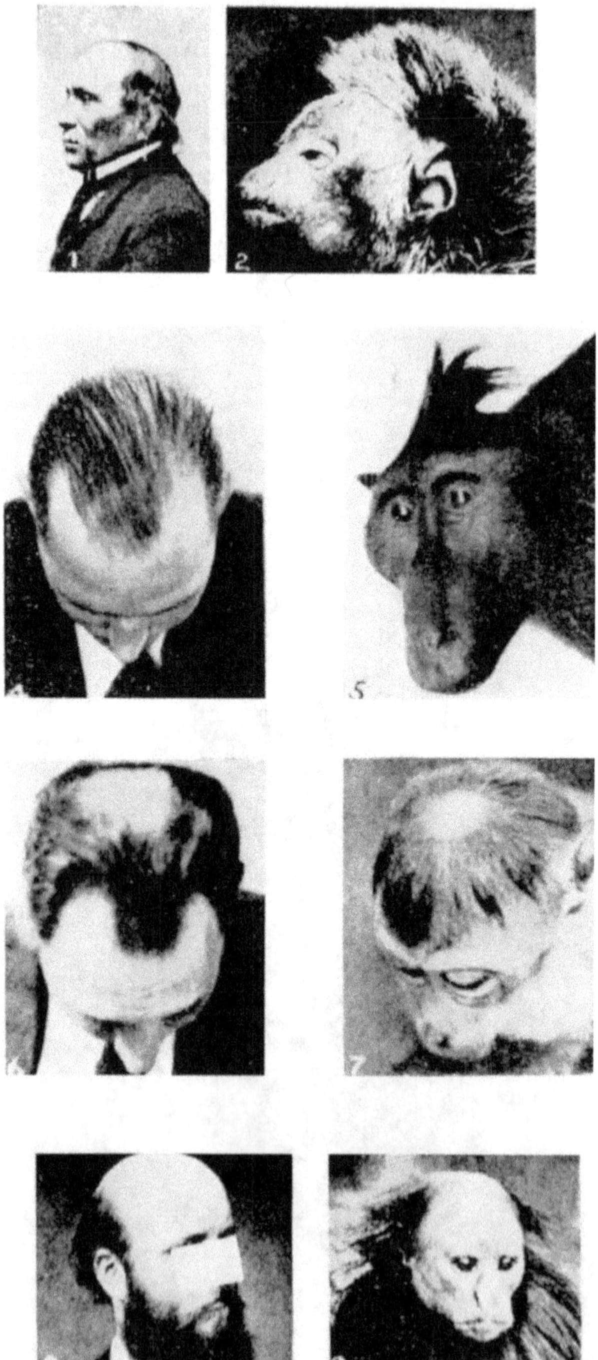

[*By courtesy of G. S. Miller (Curator of Mammals, U.S. National Museum) and the Smithsonian Institution, Washington.*

FIG. 64.—Human baldness patterns compared with the analogous patterns of four kinds of primates.

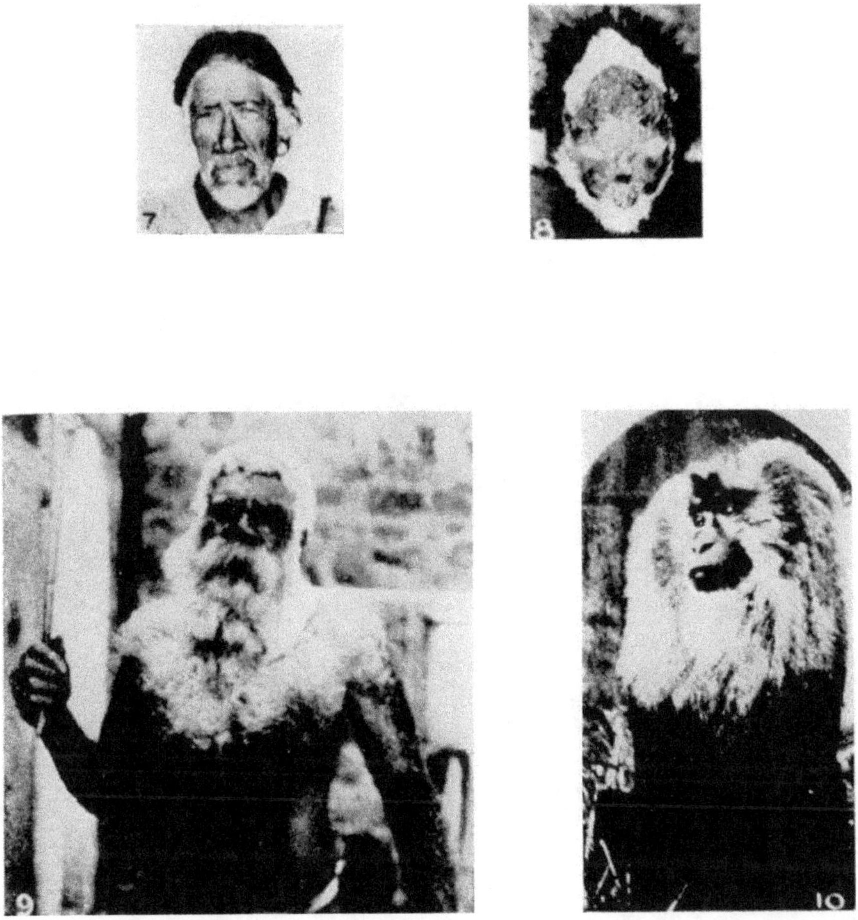

[By courtesy of G. S. Miller (Curator of Mammals, U.S. National Museum) and the Smithsonian Institution, Washington.

FIG. 65.—Human greyness patterns compared with analogous patterns of two kinds of non-human primates.

Gerrit Miller concluded that the above peculiarities in human hair are common property of the great group of mammals to which man pertains, and that neither he nor any other member of this group can wholly escape from the tendency imposed on all of them by their primate heritage.[1]

ALOPECIA AREATA (PATCHY BALDNESS). This condition is characterised by circular patches devoid of hair. Hence its title, which is derived from the Greek word for fox—the connection apparently being that foxes often have bare patches in their fur.

The number of suggested causes are legion but can be in general reduced to two, viz. :

(*a*) the condition is of psychogenic origin ;
(*b*) micro-organisms are involved.

There is strong evidence in favour of the *psychogenic* origin, for alopecia areata has been observed in cases of students after sitting their final examinations ; after parturition ; following war wounds and in other conditions of nervous tension. It often follows severe illnesses such as typhoid and scarlet fevers.

Robinson and Tasker (*Urol. cutan. Rev.*, 1948, **52**, 467) draw attention to the association of such clinical descriptions as " worry ", " anxiety ", " fear ", " fatigue ", " emotional strain ", in connection with many of the cases of alopecia areata. A study of the literature reveals psychogenic factors as the precipitating causes of an attack.

Anderson (" Alopecia areata ; a clinical study ", *Brit. med. J.*, 1950, **2**, 1250) considers that alopecia areata is a reaction of the body to stress, with the hair as the target area and probably occurs in 2–3 per cent. of the general population. Anderson observed an incidence of 2 per cent. among 15,000 hospital out-patients over a five-year period. In his series, the most frequent precipitating factor was either mental shock or acute anxiety, which in almost 25 per cent. of the cases preceded the onset of alopecia by a few weeks.

There are, however, still proponents of a theory that a parasitic agent is involved. Walker and Rothman (" Alopecia areata : statistical study and consideration of endocrine influences ", *J. invest. Derm.*, 1950, **14**, 403) have considered the possibility of a micro-organism and point out (as does Montgomery [*J. cutan. Dis.*, 1903, **21**, 529]), that those cases which begin as small coin-shaped areas of baldness spreading

[1] The author is greatly indebted to Gerrit S. Miller, Jr., Curator Division of Mammals, U.S. National Museum, and to The Smithsonian Institution, Washington, for permission to reproduce the subject-matter and illustrations dealing with Human Hair and Primate Patterning originally published by the Smithsonian Institution. (*Smithsonian Miscellaneous Collections*, Vol. 85, Number 10, Publication 3130.)

peripherally, resemble parasitic action. Walker and Rothman postulate that the micro-organism involved might be one of the many unknown virus infections. Reports of epidemics in schools, etc., would appear to support this assumption if, as Behrman (*The Scalp in Health and Disease*, London: Henry Kimpton, 1952) points out, such outbreaks have been *correctly diagnosed.*

Other factors which have been held responsible are heredity and that of a toxic focus; neither so far received extensive support. In as far as a worrying parent may induce a similar state in her children and thus implant the seeds of anxiety, fear or inferiority, the influence of the parent is to be expected; but evidence for heredity *per se* as an important factor is lacking. There is no convincing evidence of any influence of toxicity.

Against the influence of micro-organisms is the statement by Behrman that the onset of the disease "is so rapid that the completely denuded plaque may appear overnight with the lost hairs found in a heap on the pillow in the morning". Behrman points out that the course of the disease is very variable and that either the "... hair loss is instantaneous or it extends peripherally from a coin-sized patch for two or more weeks until it reaches maximum involvement ..." and that it may never progress beyond the boundaries of the original plaque, or several areas may develop simultaneously, or at irregular intervals on distant or adjacent sites. The denuded patches may touch at the borders but they never actually coalesce, being individually defined.

It is pointed out that cases of peripheral expansion, however, may involve the confluence of several patches.

So far as the duration of the disease is concerned, Walker and Rothman (*J. invest. Derm.*, 1950) studied its course in 120 patients who suffered from alopecia areata for periods of from 5 to 36 years. Walker and Rothman were able to follow the course of the condition for an average of 14 years and found that the duration of the initial attack was under 6 months for $\frac{1}{3}$ of their patients and less than a year for $\frac{1}{2}$ but that the incidence of relapse was high, being 86 per cent. over all the patients observed and 100 per cent. in patients observed over a period of 20 years or more.

Hair Tonics and Lotions

In the above brief discussion, the three major hair affections with which the cosmetic chemist comes into contact have been discussed; these conditions are of such importance that it is probably true to state that if they could be completely banished the term baldness, as we use it today, would lose its meaning.

In the light of what has been stated above can it be said that hair tonics or friction lotions play any useful role and, if so, how should they be formulated ?

The author is of the opinion that whilst the use of such tonics or lotions will *not* lead to *hair growth* (unless and until some new hormonal secretion is discovered which achieves this effect), *nevertheless the use of such preparations is of value for the following reasons* :

(i) *Therapeutics.* (*a*) In *dandruff* there is reason to suppose that bacterial organisms may be involved; in *alopecia areata*, as mentioned, some authorities still feel that micro-organisms are involved ; in M-pattern baldness there is often accompanying *oiliness* of the skin which may predispose to secondary bacterial infections of the Staphylococcal albus type (though it should be clearly recognised that bacteria *per se* are not directly or indirectly responsible for M-pattern balding) ; in *oily seborrhoea* there is present oiliness of the skin with accompanying bacteria.

(*b*) *Antiseptic, spirituous, or detergent preparations are of benefit in all the above cases, in that providing they are antiseptic then they inhibit bacterial development and if spirituous or detergent then their application, followed by friction and brushing, helps to remove excessive greasiness and thus tends to minimise the seborrhoeic soil.* To deny they grow hair is true ; to deny they are of any value is a *biased and specious* argument unsupported by any direct evidence and completely contrary to the known behaviour of antiseptic and detergent preparations.

(ii) *Psychological.* Whilst the author would not like to stress the psychogenic value of such preparations, nevertheless if alopecia is due to psychogenic causes, then in some instances they *might* be helpful, especially if such measures are combined with good diet and good psychology.

(iii) *Aesthetic.* Well-groomed hair looks better than untidy, unkempt hair. If a person bothers to use a lotion, he is interested in his appearance. We know that it is not true to claim that a clean tooth never decays (it *may* even decay more quickly than one protected by the natural enamel pellicle which forms if a tooth is not cleaned) but it looks better and so people clean their teeth.

Finally, although up to the present, no hair lotion or cream has been found that definitely " grows hair ", increasing scientific developments may possibly lead to the development of such a preparation or, more likely, to the development of a lotion, the use of which *prevents* the process of balding commencing.

CHAPTER 21

HAIR "TONICS" AND LOTIONS

NO toilet preparation has aroused such derision as the so-called hair "tonic"; the use of the word "tonic" is unfortunate in this respect; even in therapeutics the word "tonic" is viewed with grave suspicion. Much of this scepticism is the result of the claims made by the manufacturers of such preparations in the past, coupled with the experience of the user.

In point of fact, the use of a hair lotion (as pointed out in Chapter 20) is often justified and is of value for the following reasons:

THERAPEUTIC. In *dandruff* there is reason to suppose (although it has not been indisputably proved), that bacterial organisms may be involved. In *alopecia areata* (although the general belief is that psychogenic factors are involved) a number of leading dermatologists still feel that micro-organisms may be incriminated and play a role. In *M-pattern baldness* there is often accompanying *oiliness of the skin* which may predispose to bacterial infection of the skin (although it should be clearly recognised that bacteria *per se* are not directly, nor indirectly, responsible for M-pattern baldness). Of interest is the recent work of Flesch [*J. invest. Derm.*, Nov. 1952, p. 353—also discussed in Chapter 20] in which some evidence was obtained of the inhibition of keratin formation by the application of certain unsaturated substances such as sebum, vitamin A, etc. Again, the use of a spirituous preparation, whilst it may not effect the cause of the affection, may well reduce the oiliness of the skin temporarily and thus act along rational lines; if bacterial infection is encouraged by the sebum, it will also help to reduce such infection.

In *oily seborrhoea* the position regarding the presence of excessive oil and the favourable soil which it provides for invasion by micro-organisms, which then predispose to pathological changes, is similar to that already described. Spirituous preparations can reduce oiliness and minimise the danger of bacterial growth, *providing they are used regularly*, since their action is only temporary.

PSYCHOLOGICAL. Whilst the author would not like to infer any psychogenic value in such preparations, because there is no adequate scientific evidence which would provide confirmatory proof, nevertheless, if alopecia areata is entirely due to psychogenic causes, then (apart from any reasons discussed under "therapeutics" above), the mere fact of using a preparation on the head at all *might*, in itself, be of some help to persons open to " auto-suggestion ", especially if this were combined with good diet and " good psychology ". At the moment the psychogenic factor in certain affectations and infections of the body is imperfectly understood. Whilst we no longer consider it the complete answer to all ills ; neither is it considered of no importance. Evidence of psychological value from such preparations is better classed as " very doubtful ".

AESTHETIC. Well-groomed hair looks better than untidy, unkempt hair. The tendency of modern life is to have the hair either set in a more or less elaborate coiffure which it is not desired to disturb, or—in the male—it is often plastered down with a greasy or oily dressing. Hair lotions instruct the user *to massage the scalp* with the contents of the bottle. Whilst massage does stimulate the flow of blood, there is no evidence that, by such stimulation, *hair growth* is assisted. The hair lotion in this respect does play a valuable role in getting the user to massage the hair and thus temporarily remove loose dandruff scales, excessive oiliness, etc.

It will be noted that none of the above properties includes " the growth of hair ". *So far as is known, at present, there is no substance known to science, which when applied externally to the human head will cause—in a statistically significant number of cases—the regrowth of normal hair on heads which have become bald.*

The above statement includes the term *at present known*, because, as discussed in the previous chapter, there are a number of interesting avenues of exploration in connection with baldness, some of which appear to offer some promise but to which at present medical science does not hold the master key.

In the first place, Roberts (*Proc. Sci. Sect. T.G.A.*, Dec. 1952, p. 40) claims to have isolated a hormone from the anterior lobe of the pituitary which he has termed the " dermatotropic " hormone. It is claimed that this hormone controls the growth of the hair and Roberts states that reports from more than fifty doctors have shown a growth of head hair on their patients. The colour and texture of the new hair being the same as that on the patients' heads at the time of treatment. Some failures were reported, but it is stated that these were due to incorrect dosage.

This reported discovery is too recent for the author to have had the opportunity of studying the evidence available. If the preparation *does* behave as claimed it will indeed be a remarkable discovery. It is of interest that the regrowth of hair is " . . . of the colour and texture of that existing on the patient's head ", since so many of the claims made in the past seem to relate to faint downy growth, or fluff, which patients take as evidence of new hair growth but which in fact, rarely—if ever—becomes thickened and pigmented like ordinary hair fibres. As pointed out, the existence of such a hormone would *not conflict* with the present theories of baldness; it would be rather a development of the sex-hormonal relationship theory which might provide a valuable key to the " balding " mechanism. If the apparent discovery proves to be effective and safe then, after adequate physiological tests, a lotion that " will grow hair " *might* become available. At present the author preserves an open mind on this subject with a hint of scepticism!

PILOCARPINE. In 1944 (R. G. Harry, *Modern Cosmeticology*, London: Leonard Hill Ltd., 1944) attention was drawn to the claim that pilocarpine exerted a stimulating growth upon the hair and that hair growth obtained by the use of jaborandi leaves, or its alkaloid pilocarpine, is darker and coarser than that formerly. Saville (Agnes Saville, *The Hair and Scalp*, London: Edward Arnold & Co., 1944) several times mentions the use of pilocarpine internally in not unfavourable terms as regards its effect on the hair, although when given internally attention is drawn to the perspiration and profuse salivation produced. She also quotes references to the literature in which the internal use of pilocarpine had resulted in darkening of the hair. (Many of these references are dated around 1880-90 and had this substance really possessed any influence, it is assumed that further definite information would be available on this point.) An observation by Meltzer and Deme (*Arch. Derm. Syph., Chicago*, 1942, **183**, 388) is, however, of interest. These investigators made the remarkable observation that pilocarpine greatly enhances the first phase of sebum formation, i.e. a histochemically demonstrable formation of a fatty pre-substance. (*See also* Meltzer, *Derm. Wochschr.*, 1943, **116**, 121.) As already discussed under the histology of the hair, it would appear that sebum plays some role in hair health although this role is not yet understood. It has been shown that at puberty in the male the composition of the sebum changes and so does its fungicidal action against ringworm infection. At puberty also, the secretion of androgens cause the amount of sebum produced to be greatly increased. Recently it has been shown that sebum, vitamin A, and other unsaturated compounds, when applied to the hair, inhibit keratin formation. It thus appears that either favourably or unfavourably *sebum can influence the growth of the hair and also its resistance to infection.* If pilocarpine can effect the production of a fatty pre-substance akin to sebum then again, favourably or unfavourably, it may quite well influence the hair. The importance of this observation at this stage is that it points to the possibility that some of the substances applied to the scalp are not as " inert " as was at one time thought. Before one can answer the question as to whether a high secretion of sebum is an undesirable thing, it will be necessary to know more of the chemical composition and changes that occur in sebum.

Maybe the sebum of a woman, with high oestrogen secretion is in some way conducive to a good head of hair, whereas the male secretion of androgen, while it increases the amount, alters it in a way that is undesirable from the aspect of maintaining a good head of hair. We want to know if there is a beneficial "fatty secretion" (call it sebum or what you will) and an unfavourable "sebum" which differ in composition, fungicidal and bactericidal properties; these answers must be awaited. The formulations of hair lotions given below deal with those designed merely as antiseptic, spirituous and aesthetic: arguments for the use of which have been given at the beginning of this chapter.

It may be of interest to refer to Chapter I (section dealing with the hydration of the skin) where evidence has been produced to show that skin dryness, as might be expected, appears to be due in general to loss of moisture and that hence humectants such as glycerin, sorbitol, etc., are effective in alleviating this condition. For this reason the inclusion of a little glycerin in hair lotions may be of considerable assistance in alleviating dry branny conditions of the scalp. The fact that cationics adsorb on the hair shaft, improving its "handle" or "feel", and are also bactericidal, would suggest their use in low concentrations in hair lotions. (*See also* Hair Rinses in Chapter 22.)

	per cent.
Alcohol	60·0
Glycerin	5·0
Cationic (from about ½–1 per cent.)	*q.s.*
Water to	100·0
Colour	*q.s.*
Perfume	*q.s.*

Cationic Agents

Quaternary ammonium compounds are synthetic cationic surfactants, of general structure:

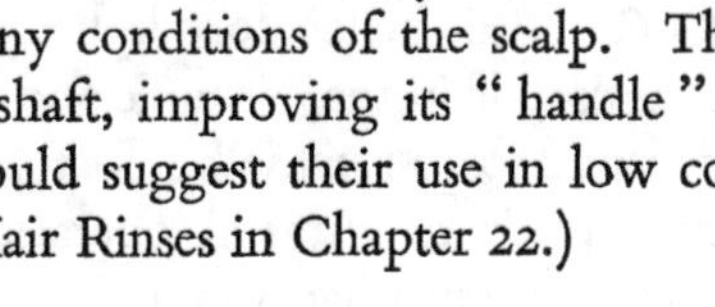

where $[X]^-$ the anion is usually chloride or bromide. R_1 an alkyl, alkenyl, alkylaryl or alkaryloxy group, having from 8 to 20 carbon atoms. R_2, R_3 and R_4 are generally methyl, ethyl or benzyl groups though in certain compounds derived from heterocyclic amines the latter groups are replaced by a ring structure (W. E. Botwright, *J. Soc. cosmet. Chem.*, Aug. 1952, p. 118). Although thousands of such compounds have been described in the literature, those most commonly employed are "Cetab" (Cetavlon) (cetyl trimethyl ammonium bromide); "Ceepryn" (Cetyl pyridinium chloride); "Hyamine" 10-X (di-isobutyl-cresoxy-ethoxy-ethyl-dimethyl-benzyl ammonium chloride), and Benzalkonium chloride, i.e. "Zephiran". A more complete list with their trade names will be found in a monograph by Lawrence (*Quaternary Ammonium Germicides*, 1950). Botwright points out that these quaternaries are not irritant to the skin *at the low concentrations necessary for achieving antiseptic action,* and that, so far as eye irritation is concerned (*see* Shampoos, Potential Hazard to the Eyes), it may be concluded from the experiments of Draize and Kelly that concentrations ranging from 0·5 per cent. to 1·0 per cent. are not injurious to the eye. Benzalkonium chloride is stated to be useful in seborrhoea of the scalp and has been incorporated in several preparations designed to clear the head of scales or scurf.

G-11 (Hexachlorophene); 2·2′-methylenebis 3,4,6-trichlorophenol, or 2·2′-dihydroxy-3,5,6,3′,5′,6′-hexachlorodiphenylmethane, has found wide acceptance as an antiseptic in the cosmetic and toilet industry and in the preparation of antiseptic soaps for use by doctors and surgeons in the "pre-scrub technique" prior to surgical operations. The following formulation exemplifies its use in a hair lotion:

	per cent.
Oleyl alcohol (best)	15·00
G-11	0·25
Industrial alcohol (for toilet purposes)	84·00
Perfume (Cologne)	0·75
Colour	*q.s.*

Apart from these newer formulations, parachlormetacresol—first recommended for use as an antiseptic in cosmetic preparations by the author in R. G. Harry, *Mfg. Chemist.*, Aug. 1936, **7**, 269, may be employed in concentrations of around 0·05 to 0·1 per cent.

More recently "Actamer" (Monsanto Chemical Co.) chemically, 2,2′-Thiobis (4,6-Dichlorophenol) has been introduced. This compound has many similarities in structure to G-11 and is stated to be effective and innocuous. Although only slightly soluble in water, it is soluble to a sufficient extent in organic solvents to allow of its use in cosmetics (a little over 2 per cent. in 95 per cent. ethyl alcohol). The properties of this, and other antiseptics, are discussed in a subsequent chapter.

The following formulae illustrate the use of the older and perhaps at present more commonly used ingredients in hair lotions:

QUININE LOTIONS. The stimulant properties of such preparations have been questioned. Quinine is a general protoplasmic poison and paralyses all forms of living matter (such as amoeba, sperms) and inhibits the action of oxydases, etc.

For this reason it may be of some value in keeping the hair in a moderately sterile condition, while the alcoholic solution itself and the friction may act as a stimulant.

	per cent.
Quinine hydrochloride[1]	0·01 to 0·2
Alcohol	30·0
Water	69·0
Perfume	*q.s.*
Colour	*q.s.*

RESORCINOL (*m*-DIHYDROXYBENZENE)

Because resorcinol is a more powerful antiseptic, and apparently less poisonous and irritant than phenol, it (and its acetate) has been widely used as a constituent of antiseptic preparations for the hair, dandruff lotions, etc. The following formulation is typical:

	per cent.
Resorcinol	5·0
Tincture of capsicum	5·0
Castor oil	5·0
Alcohol, 90 per cent.	85·0
Perfume	*q.s.*

Large doses of resorcinol are, however, known to be toxic and collapse has been reported following extensive external use due to the production of methaemoglobin. Death has followed ingestion. *More recently it has been discovered that its prolonged use may produce myxoedema due to a specific anti-thyroid action of this substance.* (G. M. Bull and R. Fraser, *Lancet*, 1950, 851; Q. J. G. Hobson, *Proc. R. Soc. Med.*, 5191, **44**, 164.) In this connection it should be remembered that resorcinol may be absorbed through the skin, particularly from injured or raw surfaces, and in my opinion, *there is no longer any justification for its inclusion in a cosmetic preparation.* (Resorcinol, in the presence of soap, discolours fair hair, and following its use soap and alkaline shampoos should be avoided.)

OIL OF CADE

Oil of cade (synonym Juniper Tar Oil), obtained by the destructive distillation of the wood and branches of *Juniperus Oxycedrus* (Linn.), is a dark brown to nearly black oily liquid, partly soluble in cold alcohol,

[1] Most of the leading quinine tonics have 0·01–0·02 per cent. quinine hydrochloride. In the U.S. the use of the term *Quinine* may be considered misbranding under the F.D. & C. Act in that it may be claimed that (*a*) quinine is present only in insignificant quantity and (*b*) even if present would be of no value.

used in the treatment of various affectations of the scalp—in particular Pityriasis simplex capitas.

From 1–10 per cent. may be incorporated in an oil or ointment base either as a simple oily mixture or as an oil-in-water emulsion. Its odour and colour militate against its wider toilet use. If included in ordinary proprietary hair preparations it is my opinion that only low concentrations, say from ½–2 per cent., should be included in order to restrict the possibility of irritation arising through its indiscriminate use in high concentration.

Beta-Naphthol (Beta-Hydroxynaphthalene)

Possesses more powerful antiseptic and germicidal action than phenol but is far less toxic. It is only slightly soluble in water (0·1 per cent.); boric acid increases this solubility somewhat. It may be combined with "salicylic acid".

	per cent.
Beta-naphthol	½–2·0
Alcohol, 90 per cent.	50·0
Water	48·0
Glycerin	*q.s.*
Perfume	*q.s.*

Capsicum

Consists of the dried ripe fruits of *Capsicum minimum,* and contains a crystalline colourless pungent principle—capsaicin. Sierra Leone capsicum is regarded today as the most pungent. It is used in hair lotions in the form of its tincture (5 per cent. in 60 per cent. alcohol).

Pilocarpine

This is the alkaloid contained in jaborandi leaves.

It is claimed to exert stimulating effects on hair growth, and is often used in proportions of up to 0·4 per cent., either alone or with cantharidin or quinine. It is soluble 1 : 8 in water. It is stated that hair growth obtained by the use of pilocarpine is coarser and darker than formerly, but scientific proof of this claim is lacking. (*See* Pilocarpine earlier in this chapter.)

Cantharides (Spanish Fly; Blistering Beetle)

This consists of the dried cantharis vesicatoria and contains a crystalline lactone cantharidin.

Cantharidin is very irritating, and must be used with great care.

It is incorporated in hair lotions on account of its supposed stimulating properties:

	per cent.
Cantharidin	0·002
Alcohol	30·000
Acetic acid (glacial)	0·600
Water	69·398

5 per cent. glycerin may be included if desired.

Isopropyl alcohol diluted with water forms a suitable basis for the preparation of stimulating hair lotions. A 35 per cent. solution has proved of value in the treatment of acne of the face complicated with severe seborrhoea, and also in cases of pityriasis and seborrhoea of the head. (*B.M.J.E.*, 11/21, 85.)

(*Note*: The above remark applies to isopropyl alcohol which is non-irritant. The isomeric normal propyl alcohol is more toxic and is unsuitable for such purposes.)

	per cent.
Isopropyl alcohol	50·0
Water	49·6
β-Naphthol	0·2
Salicylic acid	0·2
Perfume	*q.s.*

	per cent.
Industrial methylated spirit	80·0
Castor oil	19·7
Salicylic acid	0·3
Green colouring	*q.s.*
Perfume	*q.s.*

	per cent.
Ti-tree oil	1·0
Isopropyl alcohol	55·0
Water	40·0
Glycerin	4·0
Eau-de-Cologne	*q.s.*

The above preparations are of particular value where the head is greasy. However, in the case of normal hair they tend to be too drying when used over long periods. In such cases, oily preparations may be used intermediately, or in the case of dry hair, may replace them entirely. (*See also* Hair Rinses and Conditioners.)

It will be observed that all of the above preparations are either stimulating [1] or antiseptic. In conjunction with a proper friction, they

[1] The word stimulant applied to a hair lotion in this chapter refers only to the stimulating feeling or glowing of the scalp occasioned by the presence of small amounts of a rubefacient and should not be taken to imply that any preparation actually stimulates the growth of the hair.

help to keep the hair temporarily free from dandruff, and to reduce bacterial infection to a minimum. They may be used regularly by persons with very greasy scalps, but usually prove too drying for normal hair. In such cases their use may be interspersed, with advantage, with applications of a brilliantine or other emollient hair dressing. In cases of dry hair it may be advisable to restrict their application to twice a week, with regular intermediate applications of a brilliantine.

It must be remembered that antiseptic and stimulant dressings such as the above may prove irritant to some scalps, and it is well to include with such products a warning that if they produce irritant effects, soreness, or itching *after* application, their use should be discontinued.

Preparations similar to those supplied by dermatologists and containing sulphur, tar extract, salicylic acid in *relatively large concentration* should not be sold as cosmetic or toilet products. Their regular use without adequate supervision may produce a dermatitis.

In addition to the above products, lotions may be prepared from various oil-in-water emulsions, in which may be incorporated one of the active stimulants or antiseptics already discussed. Representative types are discussed under hair fixatives, complexion milks and acid milks and lotions. The chapters on skin nutrition, *p*H of the skin, and skin respiration, on so-called skin foods or lubricating creams, and histology of the hair and hair affections may be studied with advantage in selecting a suitable formula.

Many manufacturers are convinced of the efficacy of their own particular product in which the active constituent may range from lanolin, lanolin extracts or the sterols, to various vitamin preparations or unsaturated fatty acids. Such preparations will be effective only in cases in which the hair poverty was caused by general ill-health or nervous strain. Any success will mainly be due to improvement in the general bodily tone, the removal of excess sebum, a temporary bacteriostatic effect, or the stimulating effect of friction on the blood supply to the scalp. It must be borne in mind that following severe nervous strain or illness recuperation is delayed for some months and the tonic may get the credit when actually improvement in bodily tone is responsible.

The truth, unpalatable as it may be, is that although such preparations may reduce or eliminate dandruff and bacterial infection temporarily, and in conjunction with friction will increase the blood circulation of the scalp, *there is as yet no known preparation which can be relied upon to grow new hair.* Many fallacies in this connection are discussed elsewhere. (*See* Histology of the Hair.)

The *necessity* of hair as a protective covering for the human body has vanished, and so has the majority of our bodily hair. It may be that what we are trying to fight is not an affliction at all, but a part of our continual process of evolution. Hair now regarded by some as an ornament (by others not so fortunate as a *sign of brains* on the principle that "one does not often see a hairless donkey"), may one day, in the not so distant future, be regarded with as much derision as the long locks of the ancients or the furry coats of our ancestors. (*See* Heredity and Primate Patterning in Baldness; Histology of the Hair.)

Until this happens, however, man will continue to endeavour to cultivate the growth of scalp hair and the manufacturer will seek to satisfy the demand.

CHAPTER 22

HAIR SHAMPOOS, RINSES AND CONDITIONERS

Definition of "Shampoo"—Mechanism of Detergent Action—Detergents of Cosmetic Interest—Performance Tests on Detergents—Surface Tension—Interfacial Tension—Wetting Test—Foam—Evaluation of Hair Shampoos—"Scroop"—Detergents as Potential Eye Hazards—Toxicological Properties of Detergents—Formulation of Shampoos—Sequestrants and Chelate-Forming Compounds—"Builders"—Powder Shampoos—Liquid Shampoos—Liquid Cream Shampoos—Cream Shampoos—Soaps *v.* Syndets—Oil Shampoos—Conditioning Agents in Shampoos—Hair Rinses—Hair Tints—Hair Reconditioning (Conditioning) Creams.

A SHAMPOO consists of a suitable detergent [1] for the washing of hair, packaged in a form convenient for use.

I would *define* a shampoo as . . . *a preparation of a surfactant (i.e. surface active material) in suitable form—liquid, solid, or powder—which when used under the conditions specified will remove surface grease, dirt and skin debris from the hair shaft and scalp without affecting adversely the hair, scalp or health of the user.* (The word health is here used in its widest sense to cover injury to any bodily organ, as for example, the eye, as well as dermatological or physiological effects. The statement "without adversely affecting the hair" is taken to cover the health and physical condition of the hair fibres including manageability.)

The best known and cheapest of the detergents, though not the oldest,[2] is soap. It is believed that soap was used, though on a very limited scale, as early as A.D. 200. By A.D. 700, soap-makers' guilds were formed in Italy, and by 1700, the use of soap had extended throughout Europe.

Soap, whilst possessing many valuable properties as a detergent, possesses also certain disadvantages, which will be discussed later. These disadvantages have led to the development of a very large number of synthetic detergents which do not suffer from such drawbacks.

All these compounds, including soaps, have one feature in common, namely, their molecules contain a hydrophobic and a hydrophilic portion, the former portion comprising the hydrocarbon chain and the latter the water-solubilising portion. Soaps consist of the alkali salts etc., of the higher fatty acids, and hence sodium stearate $C_{17}H_{35}COONa$

[1] A "detergent" is defined by the American Society for Testing Materials as "any material which cleans".

[2] Potash obtained from the ashes of burnt vegetable matter was used several centuries B.C. for the degreasing of wool, etc.

may be taken as an illustration of the above statement. Here the hydrophobic portion of the molecule is represented by the hydrocarbon chain $C_{17}H_{35}$—— and the hydrophilic portion of the molecule by ——COONa.[1]

To appreciate the importance of this hydrophobic-hydrophilic design of a detergent molecule it is necessary to have some idea of the modern concept of the mechanism of detergent action.

Mechanism of Detergent Action

Although the mechanism of detergent action involves a number of complex physical phenomena, many of which are but imperfectly understood, it appears evident that detergency, i.e. the removal of dirt, involves the following processes. *Firstly*, the ability of the detergent solution to wet both the dirt and the fabric which in the case of a shampoo is the keratinised hair fibre; hence it must lower the surface tension. *Secondly*, the interfacial tension must be reduced to an extent where it will allow the dirt or oil particles to be displaced by the detergent solution. *Thirdly*, the dirt particles must be kept dispersed in order that they may readily be washed away.

Recent work has shown that solubilisation of the oily portion of the dirt is accomplished by the orientation of the hydrophobic portion of the detergent molecules such that their non-polar heads bury themselves within the oily dirt whilst the polar portion of the detergent molecule is orientated outwards into the water. (*See* Chapter 41, Emulsions and Dispersions.)

Such solubilisation of oil may be a major factor in those cases where the dirt is oily in character. Such an action may also account in part for the drying action of detergents on skin (formerly attributed incorrectly to the alkalinity of soap when hydrolysed by water) also, as discussed later in this chapter, "scroop" may play a role in the characteristics called "dry skin".

For solid dirt particles to be removed it is necessary not only to separate, or disperse, the particles of soil from the fabric—in this case the hair shaft—but also to keep the dirt suspended, otherwise it would merely re-deposit and would not be rinsed away.

Dispersion is believed to be achieved by the formation of a stable monolayer at the solid-liquid interface (Lomas, *Jour. Soc. Chem. Ind.*, 1949, **68**, 37 *et seq.*). In the presence of free ions, the dirt particles become

[1] A more detailed discussion of the structure and behaviour of surface active molecules will be found in Chapter 41, Emulsions and Dispersions. Here too will be evidenced the relationship between transparent oil dispersions and the process of solubilising oil which occurs in detergency.

electrically charged and thus repel one another (in a manner analogous to the repulsion of electrically charged droplets in an oil-in-water emulsion).

DETERGENCY STUDIED BY PHOTOMICROGRAPHIC MOVIE TECHNIQUE. In their investigations, Procter and Gamble, technicians (1946), developed an apparatus for taking photomicrographs on a movie camera of human hair being washed in order to study what actually happens when detergent solutions come into contact with dirt. The fibre to be washed is mounted securely in a metal holder placed in position over the detergency cell. At one side of the cell is a reservoir in which a stirring mechanism causes the circulation of the detergent solution at any desired speed. (*Soap and Sanitary Chemicals*, June 1946, p. 53.)

The accompanying illustration (from *Soap and Sanitary Chemicals*, by courtesy of the publishers and of the Procter and Gamble Co.) shows the action of suds on a single strand of hair. The churning detergent action of the cleaning solution is clearly shown, as the millions of tiny bubbles keep up a continuous pulling and pushing bombardment until the hair fibre is clean.

Colloids assist dispersion by their protective action, i.e. by coating the individual particles with colloidal material. This action is well illustrated by lampblack. In the absence of a colloid this may be removed from suspension in water by filtration but, in the presence of soap, the filtrate will be found to be coloured. McBain has pointed out that whilst protective action may be brought about by non-electrolytes, suspending action requires free ions.

McBain (*Advances in Colloid Science*, 1942, **1**, 99, Interscience Publishers Inc.) has drawn attention, amongst other factors, to the role which may be played in detergency by base exchange. To illustrate such action he points out that, if a glass flask be wetted with methylene blue solution and then rinsed with water until the washings are colourless, then if a further rinsing be given with either soap solution, sodium chloride solution, or any other ordinary electrolyte a bright blue solution will be obtained. McBain adds that such ion exchange is a real factor in removing dirt that is in itself electrolytic or is derived from ionisable material and that both cation-active and anion-active substances are capable of ion exchange. Commercial detergents that are non-electrolytes may produce ion-exchange by virtue of their contamination or dilution with electrolytes. It is pointed out, however, that such exchange is not "cleansing", in the sense of absolute removal of all material from the surface, but is rather a process of substitution. Many of the salts most commonly used as soap builders,

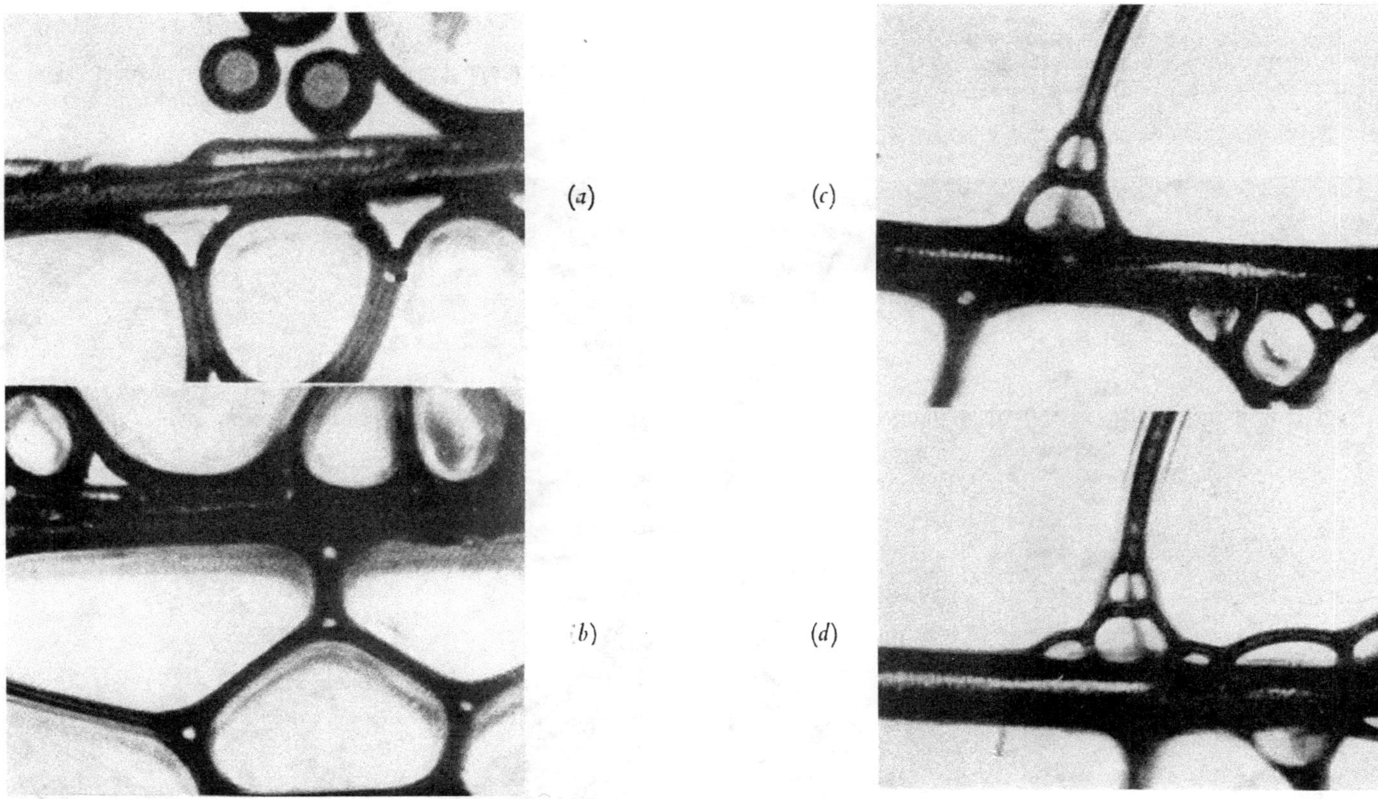

(a) (b) (c) (d)

[*By courtesy of Soap and Sanitary Chemicals and Procter & Gamble Co.*

Fig. 66.—Detergency studied by photo-micrographic movie technique. (*a*)–(*d*) The four photo-micrographs show the action of suds on a single strand of hair. The churning detergent action of the cleaning solution is clearly shown, as the millions of tiny bubbles keep up a continuous pulling and pushing and bombardment until the hair fibre is clean.

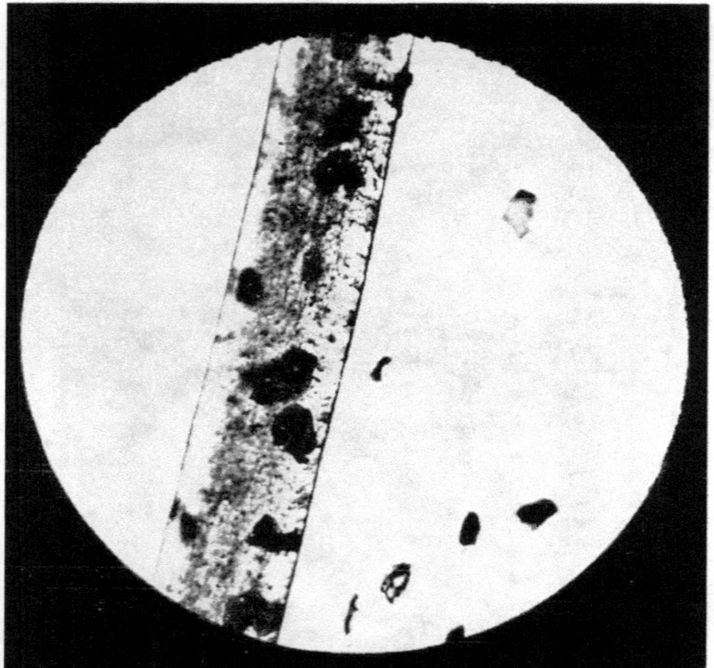

FIG. 67.—Hair fibre photo-micrographed prior to shampoo, showing loose dandruff scales. (× 55.) Basic Fuchsin stain.

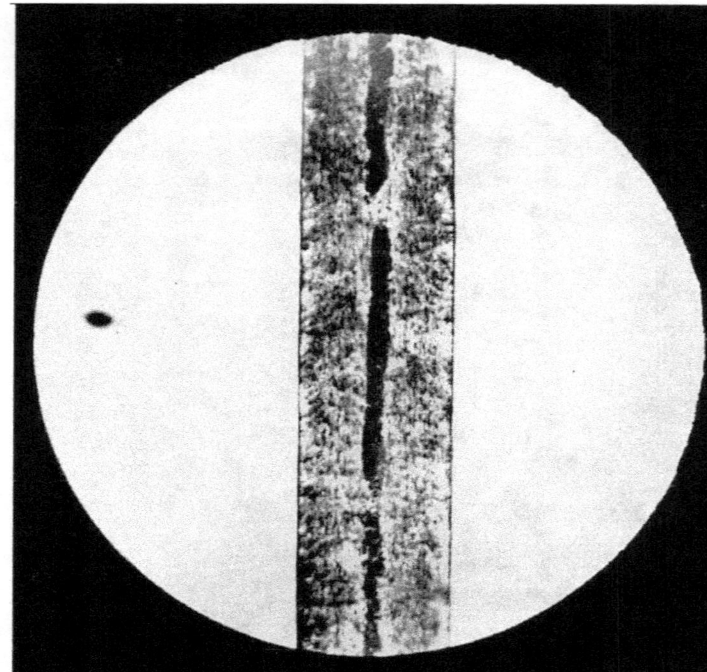

[*By courtesy of Reed, Denbeste & Humoller, Jour. Soc. Cos. Chem.*

FIG. 68.—Hair fibre taken after a shampoo from the same individual as that in Fig. 67. In this particular fibre the medulla is quite pronounced. (× 160.)

although themselves devoid of solubilising powder, are very effective in the process of ion-exchange.

Although the public commonly associate " foam " with detergency these terms are by no means synonymous and many very effective detergents do not foam well. Foam, or lather, however, is of psychological importance in the choice of a detergent for a shampoo.

Foam. For a detailed discussion on the complex physical phenomena of foams, reference should be made to standard works on this subject.[1] However, it may be stated that the fundamental condition for the formation of a foam is that a difference of concentration shall exist between the surface layer of the dissolved substance as compared with the concentration of this substance in the bulk of the solution. If the material employed is either too soluble or too insoluble it will not produce a copious foam. Foams are necessarily labile since their production involves a large increase in surface area which is opposed by thermodynamical forces acting to bring the system to a stable state, by reducing this increase in area to a minimum. No foam is produced in a homogeneous liquid, since foam formation requires a heterogeneous interface layer. Berkman and Egloff (*Emulsions and Foam*) define foam as a " formation in which macroscopic, microscopic and/or ultramicroscopic gas bubbles are separated by micronic or submicronic layers (i.e. skins) ".[2]

As already discussed under Emulsions, detergents differ markedly in their ability to wet, deterge, foam and disperse, etc., and hence, many of the synthetic detergents available have been designed and " tailored " for a specific purpose.

In selecting a detergent for any particular purpose, the following characteristics have to be taken into account :

(i) the efficacy of the detergent at an economic concentration ;
(ii) the effect of the detergent upon the surface to be cleansed ;
(iii) the stability of the detergent under the conditions which are likely to exist in use.

Factor (i) although, naturally, of importance is perhaps of less interest to the cosmetician than say for example, to the launderer, since the ratio of cost to selling price in the case of a shampoo allows great latitude. Factor (ii) is of considerable interest to the cosmetician, since, not only must the detergent be non-toxic and dermatologically innocuous but the " handle " of the hair afterwards must be satisfactory. So far as factor (iii) is concerned, the cosmetician is interested chiefly in the behaviour of the detergent in soft and hard water respectively.

[1] *See* S. Berkman and G. Egloff, *Emulsions and Foams*, Reinhold Publishing Co., New York.
[2] The measurement of foam is discussed later in this chapter.

In the light of the above discussion, it is now possible to consider the relative merits of soap versus synthetic detergents in shampoos.

Soap is defined strictly (R. G. Harry, *Cosmetic Materials*, 1948, p. 285, London: Leonard Hill Ltd.) as " the product of the reaction occurring between a fatty acid and a base ". Such a definition would include also the insoluble metallic soaps and hence by common consent the term " soap ", without any qualification, is taken to mean, the " water-soluble compounds of fatty acids of C_{12} and upwards, having a detergent action and the characteristic psychological and physiological action associated with ' soap ' ". In the case of sodium stearate, which was considered earlier in this chapter as an illustration of a soap, the hydrophilic or water-loving portion of the molecule, i.e. —COONa is insufficiently powerful to confer adequate solubility upon the hydrocarbon portion $C_{17}H_{35}$— in cold water. To overcome this disadvantage one may increase the solubilising action by shortening the $C_{17}H_{35}$— portion of the chain to, for example, $C_{11}H_{22}$—, in which case we obtain the soap, sodium laurate, which is quite soluble in cold water. In fact, this shortening of the hydrophobic portion of the molecule is virtually what the cosmetician accomplishes when he uses sodium (and potassium) laurate in part replacement of sodium (or potassium) stearate in a shaving cream or shaving stick where high solubility and lathering power is a desirable feature. However, the hydrophilic portion of the molecule cannot be shortened very much without losing the characteristic psychological and physiological properties associated with the term " soap ". For example, going to extremes, we would arrive at CH_3COONa, which is sodium acetate, a salt having no surface-active properties !

However we may vary the fatty portion of the soap molecule, we still have present the terminal alkali carboxylate (—COONa) group. It is this group which reacts with water containing dissolved calcium or magnesium salts with the precipitation of the insoluble calcium and/or magnesium soaps. These exhibit no detergent properties, and hence represent a loss in detergent efficacy, and also produce an insoluble scum which is deposited on the washbasin and upon the hair shaft with consequent loss in the lustre of the latter.

Synthetic detergents have been developed with a view to removing the limitations of the —COONa terminal group in soap, by blocking this group, so that the formation of salts is impossible ; for example, it may be blocked by forming an ester or an amide and so on.

In a book such as this, it is not possible to list more than a fraction of the multifarious surfactant materials now available to the cosmetician throughout the world. Many of these substances have various proprietary trade names and qualifying numbers (which may from time to time change) so that, in some cases, one material may be available under a number of trade descriptions. For this reason, the following brief list of detergents of possible interest to the *cosmetician* is confined to the generic name of products handled by a supplier, from whom further information can be obtained. The same general name with varying qualifying numerals, usually covers a range of detergents of often, but not invariably, the same or similar " family tree " :

Aerosols (*see also* Manoxol)	American Cyanamid Co.
Alropons	Alrose Chemical Co.
Alrosols	Alrose Chemical Co.
Aquacol	Bernard Keegan Ltd.
Arctic syntex	Colgate-Palmolive-Peet.
Duponols	E. I. du Pont de Nemours & Co.
Emcols	Emulsol Corporation.
Empicols	Marchon Products Ltd.
Empilans	Marchon Products Ltd.
Igepons	General Dyestuff Corporation.
Intramines	Synthetic Chemicals Inc.
Iranopol	Anglo-Iranian Co.
Lissapols	Imperial Chemical Industries Ltd.
Manoxol	Hardman and Holden Ltd.
Maypons	Maywood Chemical Co.
Miranols	Miranol Chemical Co.
Nacconols	National Aniline Division, Allied Chemical and Dye Corp.
Ninols	Ninol Laboratories.
Orvus pastes	Proctor and Gamble Co.
Pluronics	Wyandotte Chemicals Corp.
Santomerse	Monsanto Chemical Co.
Sipons	American Alcolac Corporation.
Sulphonated Lorol	Ronsheim and Moore.
Teepol	Shell Chemicals Ltd.
Tergitols	Carbide and Carbon Chemical Corp.
Tritons	Rohm and Haas Co.
Ultrawets	Atlantic Refining Co.

The range of materials available for general industrial and domestic detergent uses is very much larger as the criteria of colour and odour are, in such case, of somewhat less importance.

With such a range of materials at his disposal (because apart from the " proprietary " names, a number of firms supply detergent materials under their general chemical nomenclature), it is sometimes a little difficult to choose the one most suited to the job in hand. Qualities desired, such as effective lowering of surface and interfacial tension, have been mentioned under detergency. In addition it must be dermatologically innocuous; and for psychological reasons should foam well—for manufacturers interested in studying the pressurised-dispensing of shampoos, the corrosion aspect will be very important (*see* Chapter 29, Shaving Creams, Pressurised Dispensing of); from the economic aspect it should be inexpensive and from the sales and consumer angle it must be capable of being attractively perfumed and coloured.

In a very instructive article, H. L. Sanders (Ninol Laboratories, "Surfactant Performance", *Soap, N.Y.*, Dec. 1951; paper presented at 38th annual meeting C.S.M.A., Washington) has listed in tabular form some of the important characteristics of well known surfactant materials; some of these are reproduced below:

FOAMING POWER OF SURFACTANTS (ROSS-MILES TEST)

Surfactant	*per cent. Activity as marketed*	*Type*	*Foam height (mm.)* Distilled water 0 min.	Distilled water 5 min.	350 p.p.m. Hard water 0 min.	350 p.p.m. Hard water 5 min.
Miranol HM	40	Lauroyl imidazoline	220	215	120	110
Duponal WA paste	31	Sod. lorol sulphate	200	200	125	120
Ultrawet K	85	Sod. alkaryl sulphonate	200	195	225	220
Arctic syntex M	32	Sod. monoglyceride sulphate	205	195	205	200
Antaron K460	60	Sod. alkaryl polyglycol sulphate	190	185	220	215
Igepon T H.C.	72	Sod. oleyl taurate	195	195	170	170
Maypon 4C	35	Oleic-Protein condensate	175	170	155	145
Ninol 128	100	Amine condensate	170	165	45	35
Pot. Coconut soap	15		160	150	15	10
Onyx BTC	50	Quaternary	190	70	190	20
Aerosol OT	100	Sod. dioctyl sulphosuccinate	180	15	50	15
Brij 35	100	Lorol polyglycol ether	120	110	95	85
Nekal BX H.C.	80	Sod. dibutyl naphthalene sulphonate	105	25	180	15
Triton X100	100	Alkyl phenol polyglycol ether	125	75	115	60
Tergitol 4	25	Sod. *sec*-alcohol sulphate	110	5	90	5
Tween 20	100	Sorbitan monolaurate polyglycol ether	85	75	80	70
Monosulph	68	Sulphonated castor oil	90	30	20	0
Sterox CD	100	Tall oil polyglycol ester	35	30	35	30

Note: Run at 0·1 per cent. active ingredient at 30° C.

SURFACE ACTIVITIES OF SURFACTANTS

Surfactant	*Surface tension*	*Interfacial tension*	*Spreading coefficient*
Ninol 128	26·6	0·3	+ 3·1
Ultrawet K	26·8	1·2	+ 2·0
Triton X100	29·1	1·6	− 0·7
Miranol HM	24·0	7·0	− 1·0
Arctic syntex	27·6	4·0	− 1·6
Aerosol OT	28·5	5·2	− 3·7
Igepon T H.C.	28·0	7·4	− 5·4
Duponol WA	25·2	11·8	− 7·0

Hair Shampoos, Rinses and Conditioners

Surfactant	*Surface tension*	*Interfacial tension*	*Spreading coefficient*
Onyx BTC	37·1	1·6	− 8·7
Coconut soap	24·4	14·9	− 9·3
Sterox CD	36·0	6·0	−12·0
Tween 20	35·8	6·6	−12·4
Brij 35	37·0	7·4	−14·4
Monosulph	38·1	10·4	−18·5
Nekal BX H.C.	42·0	12·3	−24·3
Tergitol 4	38·8	28·6	−37·4

Note : Measured at 0·05 per cent. active detergent in distilled water at 30° C.

Corrosiveness of Surfactant Solutions

Surfactant	*Rusting*
Ninol 128	None
Monosulph	None
Coconut soap	None
Sterox CD	Slight
Miranol HM	Slight
Ultrawet K	Considerable
Triton X100	Considerable
Duponol WA	Considerable
Nekal BX H.C.	Considerable
Onyx BTC	Considerable
Aerosol OT	Considerable
Tween 20	Considerable
Brij 35	Considerable
Igepon T H.C.	Considerable
Arctic syntex M	Considerable
(Water)	Considerable

Note : Steel strips in 10 per cent. active detergent in distilled water for 2 weeks.

Acute Oral Toxicity of Surfactants

Surfactant	*Type*	*Woodward* LD 50 (*g./Kg.*)	*Hopper* LD 50 (*g./Kg.*)
Zephiran	Alkyl dimethyl benzyl ammonium chloride	0·35	
Roccal	Alkyl dimethyl benzyl ammonium chloride		0·34
Emcol 888	Alkyl naphthalene pyridinium chloride		0·47
CDEA	Cetyl dimethyl ethyl ammonium bromide		0·60
Tergitol 4	*Sec.* alcohol sulphate	1·3	
Nacconol NRSF	Alkylaryl sulphonate	1·4	
Tergitol 7	*Sec.* alcohol sulphate	1·4	
Aerosol OT	Dioctyl sulphosuccinate	1·5	4·8
Tetrosan	Alkyl dimethyl chlorobenzyl amm. chloride		2·0
Santomerse D	Decyl benzene sulphonate	2·0	2·1
Aresklene 400	Dibutyl phenyl phenol sulphonate		2·2
Emulsept	Ester of colaminoformyl methyl pyridinium chloride		2·5
Duponol C	Sod. lauryl sulphate	2·7	

Surfactant	*Type*	*Woodward* LD 50 (*g./Kg.*)	*Hopper* LD 50 (*g./Kg.*)
Igepal CA	Alkyl phenol polyglycol ether		3·5
Tergitol 08	*Sec.* alcohol sulphate	4·0	
Igepon T	Sulphonated methyl oleylamide	4 +	6·6
Nopcogen 14-L	Amine condensate		9·7
Triton 720	Alkaryl polyglycol sulphonate	12·6	
Soap	. . .	16 +	
Tween 20	Sorbitan monolaurate polyglycol ether		25 +
Monosulph.	Sulphonated castor oil		25 +
Nopalcol 6-0	Polyglycol oleate		25 +

Wetting Speeds of Common Surfactants (Draves Test)

Surfactant	*Wetting time (sec.)*
Aerosol OT	7
Triton X100	28
Ultrawet K	37
Ninol 128	41
Igepon T H.C.	45
Miranol HM	50
Tergitol 4	118
Duponol WA	118
Pot. coconut soap	Over 180
Arctic syntex M	Over 180
Brij 35	Over 180
Nekal BX H.C.	Over 180
Sterox CD	Over 180
Monosulph	Over 180
Tween 20	Over 180
Onyx BTC	Over 180

Note: Run at 0·05 per cent. active in distilled water at 30° C., using 1·5 g. hook. Average of three runs.

Much useful information in comparing the properties of certain materials in the laboratory may be obtained by measurement of surface and interfacial tensions, wetting-out speeds, etc.

SURFACE TENSION. The popular method of measuring surface tension is by use of the DuNouy Tensiometer in which the force, in dynes per centimetre, required to lift a suspended platinum ring of standardised dimensions out of the liquid, from a position of rest at the immediate surface, is noted.

INTERFACIAL TENSION. In surface tension, the force required to break the surface between liquid and air is measured. In interfacial tension, the force necessary to break the interface between immiscible liquids such as oil and water is determined. Again the DuNouy Tensiometer is used, but in this case a layer of oil is carefully floated on the aqueous surface, through which the platinum ring is pulled and the interfacial tension in dynes per centimetre again recorded.

WETTING TEST (DRAVES METHOD). In this method, the time required to sink a standard weighted cotton skein to the bottom of the solution to be tested (in a standard cylinder) is noted. In water alone, the time required is more than 8 hours ; with a powerful wetting agent the skein may sink in a few seconds.

DISPERSION TESTS. There is no generally accepted test, and data obtained by one laboratory cannot therefore be readily compared with those obtained by another using a different technique.

The results of measurements such as the above, whilst of laboratory interest, must be applied with extreme caution to judging the suitability of a detergent for a shampoo.

In the first place, the conditions of the interfacial test, though useful for comparative purposes are quite artificial, for one thing, the result obtained indicates the ability of the detergent to emulsify the particular oil under test ; it may be a poor emulsifier for other oils or for brilliantines, hair creams, or even human skin fat. Moreover in practice, the surface active agent may well be distributed both through the water and the oil phases.

Foam. Whilst the lathering power of a detergent is not necessarily a guide to its detergency, the public *expect a good lather* and psychologically, the better the lather the better the product is considered to be by the consumer.

Various methods have been suggested from time to time for the measurement of foam : many of them being simple tests in which a solution of known strength is placed in a standard cylinder. Alongside the solution to be tested is the " control " detergent with which the test detergent is to be compared. By inverting the cylinders a known number of times, or by a standardised shaking procedure, the solution is agitated with air, and the volume of the resulting foam measured together with the drainage from the foam and the rate at which it collapses.

In other methods a perforated plunger may be mechanically worked up and down in a cylinder containing a standardised solution of detergent, and again the volume of lather and rate of collapse compared with a control. Zussman (*Soap, N.Y.*, 1948, **24**, 57) has described the use of a special mechanical mixer with a disc blade rotating close to the bottom of a large glass jar to produce a shearing force. After standardised mixing, the lather formed is examined for appearance, for height and for stability.

Matalon ("Foam Formation and Foam Stability", *J. Soc. Cosmet. Chem.*, Nov. 1952, **3**, 216) has described a new technique which he has developed in order to follow the significant properties in a foam.

The most widely used practical test for the determination of foaming properties is that described by Ross and Miles (Colgate-Palmolive Peet Co.; *Oil and Soap*, May 1941, **18**, 99) in which the test solution is allowed to fall from a dropping funnel into a supply of the same test solution: the height of the fall being standardised and the test conducted in a long glass column, maintained at constant temperature. Air introduced below the surface of the liquid by the falling drops, produces foam. When the dropping funnel is empty, the height of the foam is measured and a second measurement is taken after a suitable interval of time.

Although the above test is useful for comparing, in the laboratory, the foam-producing properties of various surfactants, the results cannot necessarily be applied directly in practice. For example, H. L. Sanders (*Soap, N.Y.*, Dec. 1951) has pointed out that whilst a low height of foam in the Ross-Miles test is a fairly reliable indication of poor foam, the converse does not necessarily apply and a high foam may be misleading, particularly if a considerable amount of soil is present. Sanders states that "... a series of dishwashing tests was carried out with some of the better foamers (in the table, Foaming Power of Surfactants) in order to illustrate this point. The tests were made by soiling dishes with 'Crisco' and then washing them in a 0·1 per cent. active solution of detergent in tap water of known hardness until the foam had largely subsided; the number of dishes washed was taken as a measure of the foam stability. The results were as follows: ..."

Detergent	*Number of Dishes*
Miranol HM	20
Duponol WA	16
Ultrawet K	14
Igepon T H.C.	8
Arctic syntex M	7

Sanders remarks "... Obviously the last two perform much more poorly than might be expected from the Ross-Miles results. ..."

Whilst these tests refer to "dish washing", it must be remembered that male heads are often smothered with hair oil and hair cream and that this aspect of the effect of grease must be kept well to the fore.

Evaluation of the Efficacy of a Detergent or Shampoo Formulation as a "Hair Shampoo"

In practice, hair shampooing is carried out in two stages, the shampoo being divided in half and about half applied to the head, worked into a lather, rinsed off and then the remaining half of the shampoo added. *There is very good reason for this two-stage technique.* In the first application, the shampoo emulsifies and loosens the surface grease which is then washed away under the tap. The second portion of the shampoo is then applied to a " cleaned " wetted fibre and the detergent is available for building up a lather or foam. If one tries to use the same amount of shampoo (as that which has produced an excellent foam on an individual in two stages) in one stage, then in most cases the result is an " utter flop ". The grease, most of which should have been removed in Stage 1, is still present and this grease knocks back the lather to an astonishing extent.

Many years of experimental work with a number of detergents has convinced me that there is no substitute at present for actual head tests on shampoos.

In the soap and detergent industries, the limitations of tests based purely on physical chemistry have been realised and it is the custom to judge washing efficiency by means of a practical launderometer test, though even here the " soil " used is of necessity an arbitrary one.

When we come to the hair, we are faced not only with the same problems as those of the laundry industry, but with additional problems which are unique to shampoos. In the first place, it is known that the diameter of the fibre used to produce a lather has a considerable effect on the lather, and that certain types of " wiry " hair can be " lathered " only with difficulty ; in the second place, there is a very wide range indeed of artificial soil on human hair, varying from gums and mucilages left on female hair by the use of setting lotions and lacquers, to hair creams of the oil-in-water and water-in-oil type, often containing fatty acids, sometimes containing calcium salts and sometimes insoluble metallic soaps. Apart from the diameter of the hair fibre, the type of hair, and the artificial soil there are big variations in the " natural " soil-" sebum ", both in amount and probably in composition. It is known that (i) at puberty the composition of the sebum changes and (ii) that with the secretion of androgens in the male at that time, the amount of sebum is increased (*see* Chapter 20).

A further complication is that, in comparing the detergent actions of shampoos, even on heads, one cannot go on diluting shampoo A and compare the dilutions with shampoo B. In detergent solutions there is a critical micelle concentration at which the detergent properties increase very sharply, but above which further increases in concentration have very much less effect. It is therefore imperative that in comparing dilutions of two different shampoos, they should both be within the critical micelle concentration. To dilute shampoo A for example, ten times, and then say that because it needs twenty times as much of this dilution as of shampoo B, shampoo A is " only half as good ", might well prove to be an absurdity when used at the correct strength.

Finally, the function of a shampoo as defined at the beginning of this chapter is to " remove surface dirt, skin debris, etc. . . . without adversely affecting the hair . . . etc.".

This means that providing the hair *looks clean,* or shall we say *does not* " look dirty ", and providing it has a *gloss or sheen*—and so long as it is not " frizzy "; " fuzzy " *or* " unmanageable " (i.e. without adversely affecting the health or *physical* properties of the hair) then the shampoo has done its job.

There is no justification whatsoever for judging a shampoo on the amount of degreasing of the hair shaft (or of a wool fibre) *which it can accomplish.*

Barnett and Powers (" A Quantitative Method for the Evaluation and Study of Shampoos ", *J. Soc. Cosmet. Chem.*, May 1951, p. 219) have reported results on a test in which they judged the efficacy of a shampoo on its cleansing properties. A greasy wool yarn (of standardised grease content) was scoured in a definite concentration of shampoo or detergent in a known volume of water under standardised conditions. The scoured wool, after washing and drying, was extracted with petroleum ether. They reported that they were " forced to the conclusion that many of the successful shampoos are relatively ineffective as cleansing and scouring agents ".

In the author's opinion, shampoos should *not* be sufficiently good detergents to remove the *majority of the sebum* in the hair shaft. *Only surface cleansing is required* and the nearer we can get to that the better. We only want the hair to *look* and *feel clean.*

The test of Barnett and Powers did not take into account the " two-stage cleansing " which should be a " must " in shampooing. Neither, of course, was it meant to cover the very important properties of " appearance or lustre ", handle (i.e. feel) or the psychological angle of " foam ".

LUSTRE (GLOSS) is usually judged visually. By suitable choice of hair from a sufficiently large panel of heads it should be possible to build-up a set of standards of glossiness, from low to high gloss for each colour of hair. Such a method is, however, tedious, though it would probably give a more accurate representation of the findings when compared with an " observer panel " (*see* Lustre of Teeth, Chapter 16, where the physical and psychological implications of lustre measurement are discussed in some detail).

Thompson and Mills (" An Instrument for Measuring the Lustre of Hair ", *Proc. Sci. Sect., T.G.A.*, May, 1951, p. 12) have described an apparatus for measuring the lustre of hair along the lines of that used for measuring the gloss of a polished surface.

" Handle " (" Feel ") of Hair and " Scroop "

Zussman (" Shampoo Formulation ", *J. Soc. Cosmet. Chem.*, Dec. 1949, p. 335), points out that if the hands are washed with a relatively concentrated solution of purified neutral C_{12} alkyl aryl sulphonate, a copious lather with good lubricant properties is first obtained but that, as the hands are rinsed, one becomes aware of the abrupt development of a high coefficient of friction, making it difficult to pass one palm over the other ; a peculiar crackle is also produced. On towelling the hands a tackiness may be noted, but this disappears on complete drying. If the hands are rewetted, the high coefficient of friction on the skin is again noted. It is generally thought, Zussman states, that this sensation is typical of the ultra-clean skin but he points out that the reasons given below make it difficult to explain on such grounds :

(i) because short chain alkyl naphthalene sulphonates (which are notoriously poor detergents and fat emulsifiers) produce the same effects as the high molecular weight alkyl aryl sulphonates, whilst oleic acid soaps, which are generally conceded to be excellent emulsifiers do not " dry " the skin ;

(ii) genuine defatting of the skin with organic solvents does not produce this effect ;

(iii) the skin of the palms of the hands, where this effect is most noticeable, is notably lacking in sebaceous, i.e. oil-secreting glands.

The above facts make it unlikely that the effect observed is one of defatting of the skin and Zussman has pointed out that these effects may be described in terms of " scroop "—a term borrowed from the textile industry. This is a finish imparted to silk by treating it with a dilute organic acid. It is characterised by a high coefficient of friction and the silk crackles when rubbed against itself.

Zussman goes on to state, that it may be inferred (from some experiments one can carry out, and from what we know about the adsorption of detergents on wool) that the sensation of an ultra-clean skin surface (" scroop "), as described, is produced by an absorbed film of surface-active agent, and goes on to suggest methods by which the problem of " scroop " produced by the use of certain detergents, may be modified.

Here again, practical trials on volunteers in the laboratory will soon determine whether the formulation possesses the undesirable property of conferring "scroop", and making the wet hair feel very harsh to handle.

Detergent Shampoos as Hazards to the Eyes

Throughout this book, the question of the dermatological harmlessness of the preparation formulated has been reiterated; shampoos, however, need more than to be just *dermatologically* innocuous, essential though this is. In the process of shampooing the hair, it is not unusual for some of the shampoo to trickle down the face and gain access to the eye. When diluted adequately on the head, this is not usually harmful, but in many cases it has recently been found that the access of any of the undiluted shampoo to the eyeball may (depending upon the type of detergent employed, its concentration and the formulation) involve a very serious hazard and even lead to scarring and opacity of the cornea of the eye.

The attention of the industry in the United States has been particularly directed to this question by a recent announcement by the U.S. Federal Food and Drug Administration, of the existence of a group of shampoos on the market which were found to be capable of causing permanent injury, if accidentally introduced into the eye during the shampooing process. At least three brands of shampoo were seized on the grounds that they were a potential hazard to the eyes. The shampoo material consisted of a non-ionic detergent described as a polyethylene-oxide-alkyl-phenol-ether in combination with a quaternary ammonium salt. Consumers had complained that the shampoo produced eye irritation; this was confirmed by tests on animals in the laboratories of the Food and Drug Administration. Contact with the detergent mixture caused clouding of the cornea, the "glass-like" portion of the coat of the eyeball, thus impairing vision.

In many cases, if one judges from the technical literature, many of the surfactants have been released for use on the basis of dermatological and toxicological tests without the toxicity of these substances to the eye mucosa having been determined. However, some data are available in the case of those detergents which have been tested for eye-irritation in connection with the clinical and ophthalmic uses of such materials as in the use of sulpha drugs in the eyeball.

Several studies have comparatively recently appeared in the literature, dealing with the relation of surface-active properties to corneal irritation and toxicity, and some of these are summarised below.

Whilst various modifications may be made by different observers, a number of investigators have employed the technique of Draize *et*

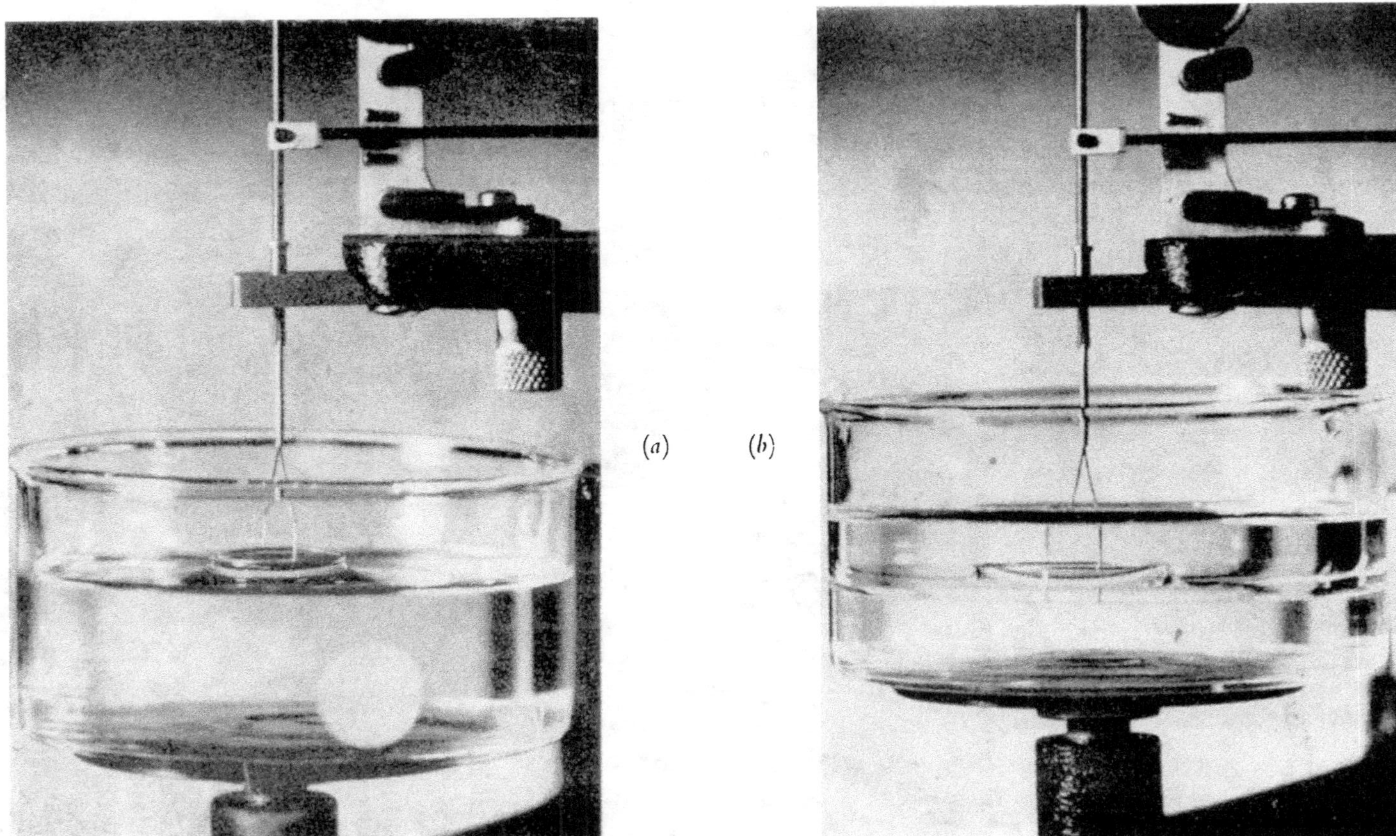

(a) (b)

[*By courtesy of Atlas Powder Co., U.S.A.*

FIG. 69.—Surface tension measurements by Du Nuoy Tensiometer. Surface tension is the force in dynes per centimetre required to lift the suspended platinum ring out of the liquid from a position of rest at the immediate surface. Interfacial tension measurement. Oil is laid over water in which the ring is immersed. Measurements are made of the force required to lift the ring through the oil-water surface

FIG. 70.—(*a*) Figure made three days after instillation of 0·1 cc. of a 10 per cent. water solution of a common household soap. Cornea and iris normal, slight congestion of blood vessels of conjunctivae. (This is considered an insignificant reaction.)

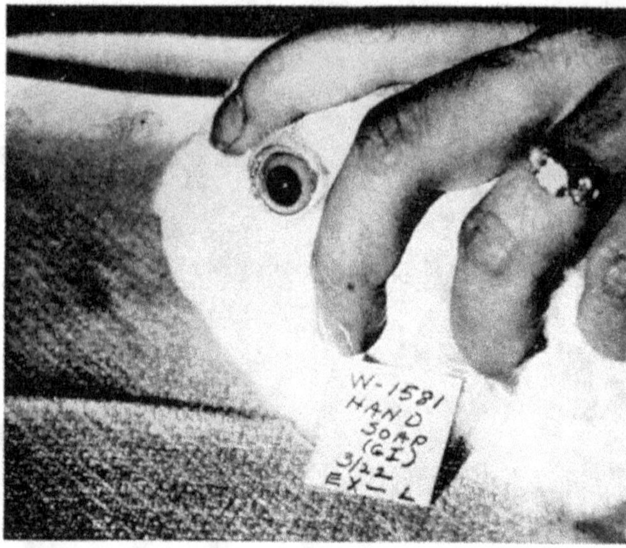

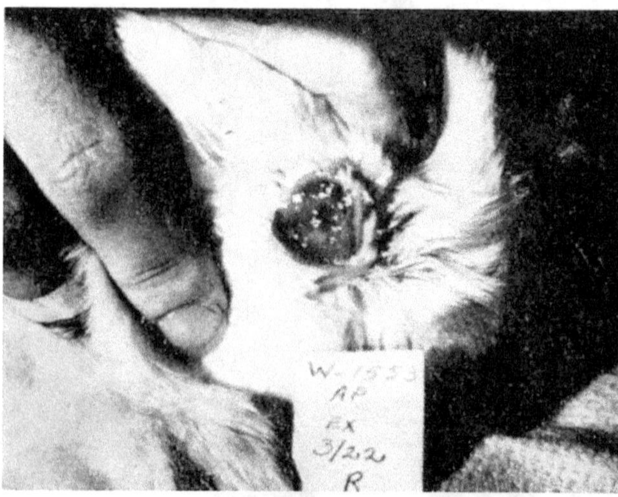

(*b*) Picture taken three days after instillation of a bubble bath preparation consisting of 96 per cent. non-ionic surface-active agent. Illustrates an acute severe reaction—almost complete opacity of entire cornea, severe iritis, severe chemosis and redness of conjunctivae, moderate purulent discharge.

(*c*) Picture taken 105 days after the instillation of 0·1 cc. of a shampoo preparation containing 18 per cent. non-ionic agent with 2 per cent. of a cationic agent. Illustrates permanent or semi-permanent eye injury, connective tissue scarring of cornea with invasion of the cornea by blood vessels—the aftermath of a severe pannus and a chronic conjunctivitis.

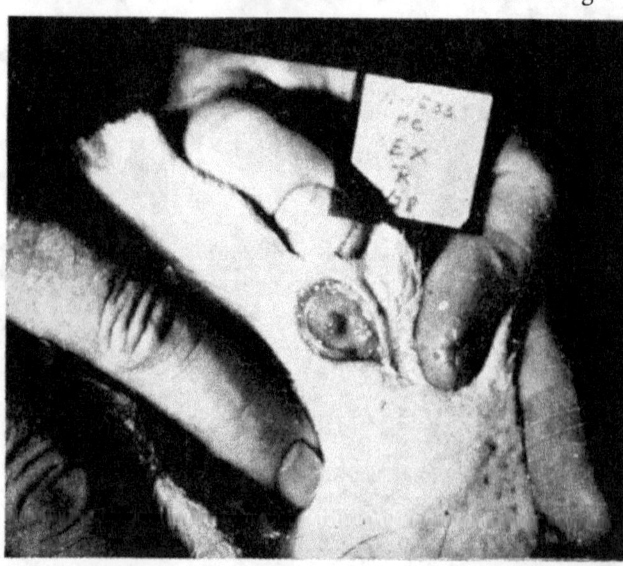

[*By courtesy of J. H. Draize.*

al. (J. H. Draize, G. Woodward, and H. O. Calvery, *J. Pharmacol.*, Dec. 1944, **82**, 377). In this method a 0·1 ml. portion of the preparation under test is instilled into the conjunctival sac of an albino rabbit with the left eye being allowed to serve as a normal control. After a four-second period of contact both the treated and control eyes are flushed with 25–30 cc. of physiological saline to remove the test solution. Observations for pathological symptoms are made 1 hour after installation, again after 2 hours, and thence daily for 35 days.

Draize and Kelly (Division of Pharmacology, Food and Drug Administration, Federal Security Agency, Washington D,C.. ; "Toxicity to Eye Mucosa of Certain Cosmetic Preparations containing Surface-Active Agents, *Proc. Sci. Sect. T.G.A.*, May 1952, p. 1) have examined a number of cationic, anionic and nonionic surface active agents used in cosmetic preparations for eye mucosa irritation. The "maximal tolerated concentrations", as given in the following table, are, Draize points out, not to be interpreted as the concentration of these agents producing no eye reactions, but were the concentrations at which no corneal or iris lesions were evident by the reading after seven days.

EYE IRRITATION STUDIES WITH SURFACE-ACTIVE AGENTS

Trade name	*Chemical designation*	*Maximal tolerated concentrations of active ingredients per cent.*
	A. CATIONICS	
BTC®	Lauryldimethylbenzylammonium chloride	0·5
Hyamine 1622®	*p*-Diisobutylphenoxyethoxyethyldimethylbenzylammonium chloride	0·5
Roccal®	Alkyldimethylbenzylammonium chloride	0·5
Isothane Q-15®	Laurylisoquinolinium bromide	0·8
Ethyl Cetab®	Cetylethyldimethylammonium bromide	1·0
Triton X-400®	Stearyldimethylbenzylammonium chloride	1·0
	B. ANIONICS	
Nacconol NRSFO.	Alkylaryl sulphonate	5·0
Miranol SM®	Capryl imidazolene derivative	10·0
Aerosol OT®	Dioctylester of sodium sulphosuccinic acid	15·0
Duponol WA®	Sodium lauryl sulphate	20·0
Orvus WA®	Sodium lauryl sulphate	20·0
Triton X-200®	Sodium salt of alkylated aryl polyether sulphonate	28·0

Trade name	Chemical designation	Maximal tolerated concentrations of active ingredients per cent.
	C. NONIONICS	
Triton X-100®	Alkylated aryl polyether alcohol	5·0
Nonic 218®	Polyethylene glycol tertdodecyl thioether	10·0
Alrosol®	Fatty acid amide condensate	10·0
Neutronyx 600®	Aromatic polyglycol ether condensate	15·0
Detergent 1011®	Secondary amide of lauric acid	15·0
Ninol 2012®	Fatty acid alkanolamine condensate	20·0
Span 20®	Sorbitan monolaurate	100·0
Tween 20®	Sorbitan monolaurate polyoxyethylene derivative	100·0
Span 80®	Sorbitan mono-oleate	100·0
Tween 80®	Sorbitan mono-oleate polyoxyethylene derivative	100·0
Arlacel A.®	Mannide mono-oleate	100·0

(*Courtesy, Draize and Kelly.*)

Smyth *et al.* (*J. industr. Hyg.*, 1941, **23**, 478) tested the effects of the Tergitol penetrants on the eyes of rabbits against soaps, any damage to the cornea being observed by staining with fluorescein. (An area of necrosis is visible readily because it takes up the colour of the fluorescein whilst the normal cornea does not.) The minimum concentrations of these substances causing injury to the cornea, according to Smyth *et al.*, are shown below.

	Minimum concentration causing injury per cent.[1]
Tergitol 08 (sodium 2-ethylhexanol sulphate	3
Tergitol 4 (sodium 7-ethyl-2-methyl-4-undecanol sulphate)	1
Tergitol 7 (sodium 3, 9-diethyl-6-tridecanol sulphate)	2
Green soap	5·00
White soap	1·00
Sodium lauryl sulphate	0·03

The above figures show that the Tergitols are more irritating to the eyes than green soap. However, Tergitols 7 and 08 are less irritating than ordinary white soap.

Hazleton (*Relation of Surface-Active Properties to Irritation of the Rabbit Eye Proc. Sci. Sect. T.G.A. May* 1952) points out that " . . . for quite a number of years materials having potential industrial hazard have been

[1] Per cent. active ingredient.

" screened " on the basis of their irritant potential for eyes. This test was used to predict the possible hazard which plant employees might suffer from exposure to dusts or vapours of the various chemicals in the plant. . . . There has been, however, rather recently, a renewed interest in this field as it applies to the evaluation of cosmetic preparations and the estimate of their potential hazard to the public. . . ."

After pointing out that a wide variety of materials has been tested in routine manner for evaluation of hazard under different conditions of use and additional numbers in the process of product development, Hazleton lists a number of detergents together with information concerning their chemical nature and continues : " . . . In general, the method of evaluating injury involved local application to the eyes of rabbits and periodic observation for signs of injury. These signs include

(1) erythema and oedema of the eyelids ;
(2) erythema and oedema of the nicitating membrane ;
(3) lachrymation ;
(4) signs of pain response ;
(5) the incidence of opacity ;
(6) vascularisation of the sclera and of the cornea.

" A wide variety of materials has been tested in routine manner for evaluation of hazard under different use conditions, and additional numbers have been carefully investigated.

" For some time it has been realised that in general the eye irritant potential of surface active agents follows the order of cationics >anionics >nonionics. There are, however, exceptions to this order which suggest that factors other than this classification by chemical nature might be involved, or that there may be a correlation between eye irritation and some more specific property of these agents. The results to be presented are essentially those arrived at in attempts to reveal such a correlation. The materials tested and their physical properties are summarised in Table 2.

METHODS

" With this in mind, certain physical and chemical properties were studied for correlation with *capacity* to produce eye injury, as well as *potency* in such activity. To confine the survey to general trends, no attempt has been made to review the minimum exposures required to produce injury. In turn, injury has been interpreted broadly rather than strictly. As outlined elsewhere, eye injury may involve generalised erythema, oedema, necrosis, vascularisation of the sclera and/or cornea, and opacity. Also, injury may vary in onset, severity, and duration.

TABLE I

"CHEMICAL NATURE OF CATIONICS, ANIONICS, AND NONIONICS

Commercial name or Laboratory No.	*per cent. active*	*Chemical nature*
		CATIONICS
G-271®	35	N-soya-N-ethyl morpholinium ethosulphate
Hyamine 1622 ®	100	Di-isobutyl phenoxy ethoxy ethyl dimethyl benzyl ammonium chloride monohydrate
Ceepryn®	100	cetylpyridinium chloride
Emcol E607®	100	N(acyl colamino formyl-methyl) pyridinium chloride
Roccal®	50	Mixture of high-molecular weight alkyl - dimethyl - benzyl - ammonium chlorides
Hyamine 2389®	50–52	Alkyl (C_9H_{19} to $C_{15}H_{31}$) cetyl methyl trimethyl ammonium chlorides
Isothane Q-15®	20	lauryl isoquinolinium bromide
		ANIONICS
Duponol WAT®	50	Triethanolamine salt of lauryl sulphate
Ultrawet 60L®	60	Triethanolamine salt of alkyl aryl sulphonate
Armour's —600		
KOP Soap®	100	Potassium coconut oil soap
Ivory Soap®	100	
		NONIONICS
Span 20®	100	Sorbitan monolaurate
Span 80®	100	Sorbitan mono-oleate
Tween 20®	100	Polyoxyethylene sorbitan monolaurate
Tween 40®	100	Polyoxyethylene sorbitan monopalmitate
Tween 60®	100	Polyoxyethylene sorbitan monostearate
Tween 65®	100	Polyoxyethylene sorbitan tristearate
Tween 80®	100	Polyoxyethylene sorbitan mono-oleate
G-7569J®	100	Polyoxyethylene sorbitan monolaurate
Myrj 45®	100	Polyoxyethylene monostearate
Myrj 52®	100	Polyoxyethylene monostearate
Brij 30®	100	Polyoxyethylene lauryl ether
Brij 35®	100	Polyoxyethylene lauryl ether
G-2132®	100	Polyoxyethylene lauryl ether
G-3721®	100	Polyoxyethylene 2 butyl octanol
Renex®	100	Polyoxyethylene esters of mixed resin and fatty acids
G-1690®	100	Polyoxyethylene ether of alkyl phenol
G-1790®	100	Polyoxyethylene lanolin condensate
G-1441®	100	Polyoxyethylene sorbitol lanolin derivative

" Criteria for injury evaluated were adopted on the basis of moderate to severe degree and duration of several days following application to the eye. Additional weighting included certain more hazardous injuries such as prolonged opacity and incidence of pannus. For quantitative comparison the maximum concentration, in per cent. of active ingredient in aqueous solution, which will produce only moderate irritation is used if available. Exceptions are those agents used undiluted and designated as 100 per cent., but which did not necessarily produce injury. This capacity to induce injury is the irritant potential for a specific material. Potentials of 1 per cent. to 10 per cent. may be considered as severe irritants, 10 per cent. to 20 per cent. as moderate, and above 20 per cent. as mild. Without these generalised groupings, such a correlation study would become buried in minutia and the details would be endless.

" On the basis of available data the observations as shown on page 410 appear to be justified.

1. Surface Activity

" Of the materials included in this report the maximum variation in surface tension of the 1 per cent. solution is from 27 to 46 dynes per cm. Determinations were made on the Cenco-du-Nuoy Tensiometer at 25° C. In view of the wide variations in irritant potential there appears to be very little possibility of a correlation between this and surface activity.

2. *p*H

" The *p*H of aqueous solutions of the surface active agent is not necessarily characteristic of the chemical, but is influenced by manufacturing process. The *p*H of various dilutions of the test materials used was determined on the Beckman Model G *p*H Meter. The range of the *p*H was from 3·93 to 9·52, with most of the values falling at approximately *p*H 6·0 to 7·0. Experience with other classes of compounds and lack of correlation within the present series eliminates the significance of *p*H *per se* as the cause of eye irritation. Examples of this are as follows :

	*p*H	*Irritant potential per cent.*
Soap	9·5	10·0
G-1790 ®	5·8	100·0
Roccal ®	7·0	1·0
Isothane Q-15 ®	4·8	1·0

TABLE 2

"SURFACE ACTIVE AGENTS AND THEIR PHYSICAL PROPERTIES. WETTING POWER WAS DETERMINED BY THE DRAVES METHOD AND FOAM HEIGHT BY THE ROSS-MILES METHOD. C = CATIONIC, A = ANIONIC, N = NONIONIC.

Trade Name	*Class*	pH 10 *per cent.*	*Surface tension dynes/cm. at* 10 *per cent.*	*Wetting power sec. at* 0·1 *per cent.*	*Foam height mm. at* 1·0 *per. cent.*	*Protein PPT* 1 *per cent. or* 10 *per cent.*	*Irritation potential*	*Opacity*
G-271 ®	C	7·11	33	>300	217	+	1	+
Hyamine 1622 ®	C	7·01	36	142	268	+	1	+
Ceepryn ®	C	4·79	41	258	240	*	1	+
Emcol E607 ®	C	3·48	37	300	213	*	1	+
Roccal ®	C	7·28	33	234	110	*	1	+
Hyamine 2389 ®	C	7·30	31	85	292	+	1	+
Isothane Q-15 ®	C	3·93	34	300	150	+	1	+
Duponol WAT ®	A	7·11	32	31	273	—	20	+
Ultrawet 60L ®	A	7·10	30	10	302	—	10	+
Armour's 600 KOP Soap ®	A	9·52	27	>300	375	—	10	+
Ivory Soap ®	A						>10	+
Span 20 ®	N		28	>300	14		100	—
Span 80 ®	N		30	>300	13		100	—
Tween 20 ®	N	6·81	36	203	173	—	100	(—)
Tween 40 ®	N		40	>300	87	—	100	(—)
Tween 60 ®	N		43	>300	81		100	—
Tween 65 ®	N		31	>300	27		100	—
Tween 80 ○	N	6·46	40	>300	59		100	—
G-7596J ®	N		33	203	162		100	—
Myrj 45 ®	N		33	>300	15		100	—
Myrj 52 ®	N		44	>300	26		100	—
Brij 30 ®	N	4·70	28	51	18	—	20	+
Brij 35 ®	N	6·02	42	174	220		100	—
G-2132 ®	N	5·98	28	13	247	—	20	10
G-3721 ®	N	4·39	27	7	287	—	<20	+
Renex ®	N	6·95	39	>300	77	—	100	—
G-1690 ®	N		31	8	235	—	<10	++
G-1790 ®	N	5·83	46	>300	23	o	100	—
G-1441 ®	N		43	>300	31		100	—

* Precipitated in alkaline solution only.

3. Wetting Power (Draves Method) at 0·1 Per Cent.

"Within the group of materials tested six were moderately good wetters with values below 51 seconds, and the balance were 85 or above. When all the materials are compared there appears to be very poor correlation between wetting power and irritation, for example :

	Seconds	*Irritant potential per cent.*
Tween 40, 60, 80 ®	>300	100·0
Brij 30 ®	51	20·0
Isothane Q-15 ®	300	1·0
Alkyl aryl sulphonate	10	10·0

"Among the nonionics only there appears to be a correlation between the wetting properties and the relative degree of irritant potential. None of the group having a value of 174 seconds or longer exhibited irritation either undiluted or in solution. Four of the nonionics had values of 51 seconds or less, and each was rated for irritation at 20 per cent. or less. No such correlation could be established within either the limited anionic or cationic groups studied.

4. Foaming Power (Ross-Miles Test) at 1·0 Per Cent.

"Foam heights for non-injurious, undiluted materials ranged from 13 to 220 mm., and even higher for material with an irritant potential rating of 20 per cent. or above. Therefore, good foamers are not necessarily irritant, but there is some evidence that most of the irritant chemicals are good foamers. Of these irritant at 1·0 per cent., Roccal ® has the lowest foam value, 110 mm.

5. Wetting and Foaming

"Since it is indicated that there might be some slight correlation between wetting power or foaming power and eye irritation, the combination of these two properties is obviously suggested. The data here suggest that good wetting plus good foaming may be an irritant combination. For example :

	Wetting secs.	*Foaming mm.*	*Irritant potential per cent.*
alkyl aryl sulphonate	10	302	10·0
G-3721 ®	7	287	<20·0
G-1690 ®	8	235	<10·0

"That these two properties are not essential to highly irritant material is adequately indicated by:

	Wetting secs.	*Foaming mm.*	*Irritant potential per cent.*
Hyamine 1662 ®	142	268	1·0
G-271 ®	>300	217	1·0

"Unfortunately the series does not include a really good wetter which is a poor foamer. . . ."

Hopper, Hulpieu and Cole (*J. Amer. pharm. Ass., Sci. edn.*, 1949, **38**, 428) have tested a number of commercial detergents for corneal irritation in rabbits. These investigators, however, used solutions of 1 per cent. concentration only, and these are very much weaker than those which might enter the eye during shampooing. Nevertheless, according to these investigators, Aresket 300 (butyl diphenyl sodium sulphonate), Santomerse 3 (dodecyl benzene sodium sulphonate) and Santomerse D (decyl benzene sodium sulphonate) produced severe inflammation of the cornea.

In the above tests, Aerosol O.T. did not come out very favourably, though Bellows and Gutman (*Arch. Ophthalmol.*, 1943, **30**, 352) found solutions containing 1 per cent. or less of Aerosol O.S. harmless to the conjunctiva and cornea (2 per cent. Aerosol O.S., however, produced inflammation).

Quaternary Ammonium Salts

The shampoos seized by the U.S. Food and Drug Administration contained a quaternary ammonium salt as an antiseptic.

Hopper *et al.* (*J. Amer. pharm. Ass.*, 1949) showed that some of the quaternaries are capable of producing serious injury to the eyes at a concentration of 1 per cent. Severe inflammation and clouding of the cornea were observed in rabbits' eyes after the instillation of 1 per cent. solutions of cetyl-dimethyl-ethyl-ammonium-bromide; Emcol 888 (polyalkylnaphthalene pyridinium chloride) and Roccal—the technical grade of alkyl-dimethyl-benzyl-ammonium chloride of "Zephiram".

A 0·005 per cent. of Roccal was found by Whitehill (*J. Amer. pharm. Ass., Sci. edn.*, 1945, **34**, 219) to be the strongest which could be applied to the eyes of rabbits and guinea pigs without causing irritation. However, the *pure* grade of the same material (viz. "Zephiram") produced no irritation when used in concentrations up to 0·033 per cent. Note that, even so, this is a very *low concentration.*

In concluding the above brief discussion on the potential hazards of detergent solutions to the eyes, attention should be drawn to the warning of Dr. A. J. Lehman, Chief of the Division of Pharmacology of the U.S. Food and Drug Administration that *mixtures of surface-active agents may be more irritating to the eyes than could be predicted from the ocular toxicity of the individual components.*

The only way to *ensure the safety* of a given shampoo formulation, in the opinion of the author, is to have the *finished formulation, including any antiseptics, perfumes,* etc., tested for corneal irritation and toxicity, by instillation into the eyes of animals ; the albino rabbit is a suitable experimental laboratory animal. To save unnecessary pain to such animals, the formulation should be examined in the light of a knowledge of the components therein and formulations *known* to be " risky " from this aspect reformulated before trial.

Toxicological Properties of Surface-Active Agents

In the above discussion, attention has been confined to toxicity of such preparations to the eye. Because of the concentration at which some detergent preparations are retailed, the question of general toxicity also arises. Adelson and Sunshine (*Amer. J. clin. Path.*, 1952, **22,** 656, through *Brit. Med. J.*, 20 Dec. 1952, p. 1348) record the case of a middle-aged woman who died some 30 minutes after taking a drink which she believed was " whisky and ginger ale " but which in fact was " whisky and a 10 per cent. solution of a cationic detergent " (methyl dodecyl benzyl trimethyl ammonium bromide) sold for domestic cleaning purposes. Although, it is stated, she only swallowed about a mouthful and vomited within a few minutes, she collapsed soon after walking across the road to hospital and died shortly after admission. Chemical tests on the stomach contents demonstrated the presence of quaternary ammonium compounds. Within a few moments of Adelson and Sunshine giving some of the same material to rats (equivalent to 370 mg. per kilo body-weight), the animals had violent convulsions and were dead.

It is pointed out that whilst the mode of action of these substances is unknown they exert a general toxic effect on living cells such as leucocytes.

Whilst it is rather unlikely that shampoo manufacturers will put up solutions of quaternary ammonium compounds at such strengths, nevertheless, in view of the possibility of children using such compounds for " blowing bubbles " and such like, it behoves manufacturers to exercise every care in their formulations. Some toxicity figures on certain surface-active agents have been published by Woodward and Calvery [1] (*Proc. Sci. Sect. T.G.A.*, June 1945). In addition many of the leading detergent manufacturers have information on the toxicities of their materials.

The tables of toxicities on pages 415 and 416 are from the report by Woodward and Calvery by courtesy of the authors, and the U.S. Toilet Goods Association who state:

"... *Oral and parenteral administration.* Of the studies on wetting agents, those on toxicities by oral administration seem to be the most extensive. We have attempted to summarise in Table 3 the results of single-dose administration of those reported in the literature in addition to data obtained in this laboratory.

"Of the agents listed, the one cationic detergent, alkyl dimethyl benzyl ammonium chloride, is considerably the most toxic. Within one species (rat), it is also apparent that the anionic and non-ionic agents give LD 50s of the same order of magnitude.

"A number of surface-active agents have also been studied for toxicity by subacute or chronic administration in the drinking water or mixed with the diet. A summary of the available published data and a limited amount of data from this laboratory are presented in Table 4. In this table the 'effects' are referred to by a letter which designates a short paragraph describing them. The paragraphs follow:

"(*a*) Epstein *et al.* noted that animals on 5 and 10 per cent. concentrations died within 5 days. Four of 11 animals survived 160 days on 1 per cent. No effect on growth was noted on the 0·1 per cent. but at 0·25 per cent. or above, growth was diminished; the primary effect was local irritation of the gastrointestinal tract.

"(*b*) The experiments on the 'Tergitols' by Smyth *et al.* revealed no changes in blood counts and no death during the experiment caused by the agents fed. Sixteen of 55 kidneys and 4 of 50 livers showed slight damage. Other tissues were normal.

"(*c*) In the experiments reported by Benaglia *et al.* the rat actually consumed approximately 75 per cent. of the desired dosages given in Table 4. No deaths were noted. Growth curves for all levels were slightly lower than for the controls. Total red and white cell counts remained normal but a transient shift in neutrophil-lymphocyte ratio was noted. No foreign blood pigments were observed. Dogs and monkeys showed little or no effect of this regimen and no pathology at the end of the experiment. In the rabbits, the death of three animals

[1] Division of Pharmacology, Food and Drug Administration, Federal Security Agency, Washington, D.C.

TABLE 3

SINGLE DOSE TOXICITIES OF SOME SURFACE-ACTIVE AGENTS

Surface-active agent	*Animal*	*Route*	*Approx. LD 50 g./kg.*	*Inves-tigator*
Sodium lauryl sulphate	rats	I.P.	0·21	(6)
	"	oral	2·7	(5)
	"	"	1·0	—[1]
Alkyl aryl sulphonate	"	"	1·4	(5)
	"	"	1·5	—
	mice	"	2·8	—
Sodium lauryl sulphoacetate	rats	I.P.	0·3	(6)
Soap	"	"	0·98	(6)
	"	oral	16+	(5)
Sodium 2-ethyl hexanol sulphate	rats	"	4·0	(5)
	guinea pigs	"	1·5	(5)
Sodium 7-ethyl-2-methyl undecanol-4 sulphate	rats	"	1·3	(5)
	"	"	2·0 (purified)	(5)
	guinea pigs	"	0·6	(5)
Sodium 3, 9-diethyl tridecanol-6 sulphate	rats	"	1·4	(5)
	guinea pigs	"	0·4	(5)
Sodium lauryl and myristyl collamide sulphonate	mice	"	2·0	—
	rats	"	3·5	—
Sodium hydrocarbon sulphonate	"	"	4·0+	—
Sodium monethyl phenyl phenol monosulphonate	"	"	2·0	—
Sodium dioctyl sulphosuccinate	mice	"	1·5	(7)
N-(sodium sulphoethyl) oleamide	rats	"	4·0+	—
	mice	"	6·3	—
Sodium decyl benzene sulphonate	"	"	2·0	—
Alkyl aryl amine sulphonate	"	"	2·8	—
Sodium aryl alkyl polyether sulphonate	"	"	12·6 (comm. sol. not 100 per cent.)	—
Alkyl dimethyl benzyl ammonium chloride	rats	oral	0·35	—
	"	I.P.	0·05	—
Aryl alkyl polyether alcohol	mice	"	3·1	—

[1] The agents used in the studies in this laboratory were unpurified commercial preparations. References below refer to table 4 on next page as well.

(5) *J. indust. Hyg.*, 1941, **23**, 478.
(6) *J. Amer. dent. Ass.*, 1939, **26**, 1461.
(7) *J. nat. Cancer. Inst.*, 1940, **1**, 355.

TABLE 4

REPEATED DOSE TOXICITIES OF SOME SURFACE-ACTIVE AGENTS

Surface-active agent	*Animal*	*Medium*	*Level per cent.*	*Duration days*	*Effects*
Sodium alkyl sulphate	rats	water	0·1	160	*a*
			0·25	160	*a*
			0·5	160	*a*
			1·0	160	*a*
			5·0	5	*a*
			10·0	5	*a*
	guinea pigs	,,	0·2	180	*d*
" Tergitol 08 "	rats	,,	0·25	30	*b*
			0·5	30	*b*
			1·0	30	*b*
			2·0	30	*b*
			4·0	30	*b*
" Tergitol 4 "	,,	,,	same	same	same
" Tergitol 7 "	,,	,,	same	same	same
Sodium dioctyl sulpho-succinate	,,	diet	0·25 g./kg./day	160	*c*
			0·5	160	*c*
			0·75	160	*c*
			1·0	160	*c*
			1·25	160	*c*
	rabbits		0·5	160	*c*
	monkeys		0·125	160	*c*
	dogs		0·25	160	*c*
			0·1	160	*c*
	guinea pigs	water	0·2	180	*d*
Sodium isopropyl naphthylene sulphonate	,,	,,	0·2	180	*d*
Sodium alkyl aryl sulphonate	,,	,,	0·2	180	*d*
Lorol meta sodium sulphobenzoate	,,	,,	2·0	180	*d*
Sodium decyl benzene sulphonate	,,	,,	0·2	180	*d*
N-(sodium sulphoethyl) oleamide	,,	,,	0·2	180	*d*
Mono butyl phenyl phenol sodium mono-sulphonate	,,	,,	0·2	180	*d*
Aryl alkyl polyether alcohol	,,	,,	0·2	180	*d*
Alkyl dimethyl benzyl ammonium chloride	,,	,,	0·2	40	*d*

out of seven on experiment was attributed to sodium dioctyl sulphosuccinate.

" (*d*) Of the ten surface-active agents fed to guinea pigs in this laboratory the cationic alkyl dimethyl benzyl ammonium chloride was by far the least tolerated with none of twelve animals started, surviving over forty days. The sodium lauryl sulphate was slightly more toxic than the other eight agents. Microscopic examination of lungs, heart, liver, gall bladder, spleen, pancreas, stomach, small intestine, colon, kidney, adrenal, testes, lymph nodes, thyroid, bones, and muscles, showed no damage directly attributable to the materials fed but showed varying degrees of damage typical of inanition."

The mechanism of detergent action, some of the detergents available, properties of some detergents and their potential hazard to the eyes when used as shampoo, etc., have been briefly discussed. Before considering the actual formulae of such preparations there is one other aspect that applies to many types of formulae and that is, the need for preservation.

Preservation of Shampoos

Attention has been drawn to the fact (*Mfg. Chem.*, July 1951, p. 281) that the possibility of certain types of cosmetic preparations developing a mould growth is an ever present danger. It is therefore of special significance and importance that certain non-ionic detergent and emulsifying agents have been reported to possess mould-stimulating properties. Apart from " moulds " there is good reason to suppose that certain bacteria can grow and flourish in shampoos, particularly those of the paste and cream variety. This fact should be borne in mind. The question of preservatives in toilet preparations in general is discussed in Chapter 42, Antiseptics and Preservatives.

Formulation of Shampoos

Shampoos may be classified in general into three groups, with subdivisions in each group :

(1) LIQUID SHAMPOOS. Clear " transparent " liquid ; Opaque liquid " Liquid Cream ".

(2) PASTE SHAMPOOS. Clear transparent gel. ; Opaque solid (" Solid Cream ").

(3) POWDER SHAMPOOS.

There exists a possible fourth group, " bar or tablet form ", e.g. soap (and detergent blocks) ; but in this country at any rate, apart from the use of toilet soap, the above three groups can be considered as covering the general market.

Before discussing shampoo formulae under the above headings there is a problem which is common to all types, especially to clear transparent liquids or gels; a problem which applies to both soap and soapless shampoos though perhaps more particularly to the former. That is the addition of substances to "sequester" unwanted metal ions. The question of "sequestrants" will therefore be considered first.

Sequestering Agents ("Sequestrants")

Such materials are usually complex-forming substances which can remove certain metal ions from solution and prevent themfrom reacting in the normal manner. Certain phosphates are able to do this, and, indeed, sodium metaphosphates of the "Calgon" type have been used for many years for this purpose. Two other well-known members of these "condensed phosphates" are tetrasodium pyrophosphate and sodium tripolyphosphate (more correctly sodium triphosphate). The structural relationship between these phosphates is shown in the detailed formulae below (*Sodium Tripolyphosphate*, Albright and Wilson Ltd.):

Tetrasodium pyrophosphate ($Na_4P_2O_7$)

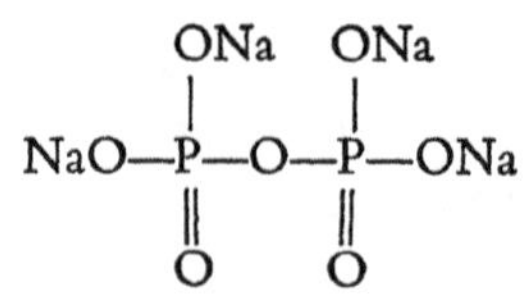

Sodium tripolyphosphate ($Na_5P_3O_{10}$)

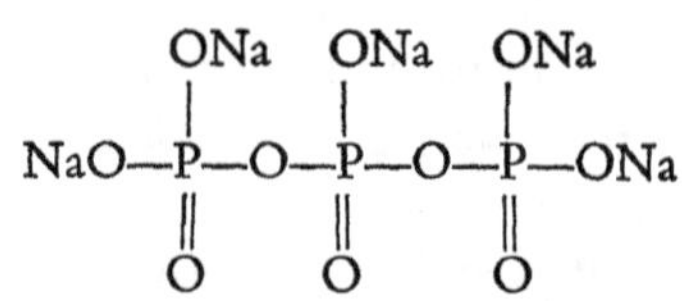

Sodium metaphosphates including glassy sodium phosphates (e.g. Calgon) and Kurrol salt

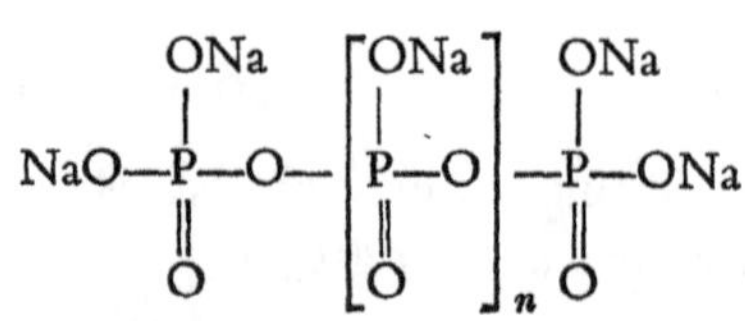

The value of *n* may be quite high, of the order of 1,000 or more in Kurrol salt, which is a body of asbestos-like appearance, dissolving slowly in water, but more quickly in solutions of potassium or ammonium salts, to give viscous solutions.

Whilst tetrasodium pyrophosphate possesses considerably less sequestering action for calcium salts than does "Calgon" (sodium hexametaphosphate), it is slightly better than "Calgon" in respect of sequestering magnesium salts. Advantages of the pyrophosphate are its greater dispersing power and, so far as laundering is concerned, the fact that it is very much more stable at boiling water temperatures than is " Calgon ". Tripolyphosphate possesses better sequestering properties for calcium salts than does the pyrophosphate, but not as good as Calgon. Tripolyphosphate, unlike " Calgon ", only picks up moisture slowly and is relatively stable.

A number of synthetic amino acids have been found to possess the property of sequestering ions by forming chelate compounds with metals. The most important of these substances is ethylenediamine tetra acetic acid (also known as ethylene bis-iminodiacetic acid), A. E. Martell and F. C. Bersworth, "Amino Acids as Chelating Agents," *Proc. Sci. Sect. T.G.A.*, Dec. 1948.

Martell and Bersworth state that the formula of the tetrasodium salt of this substance may be represented thus :

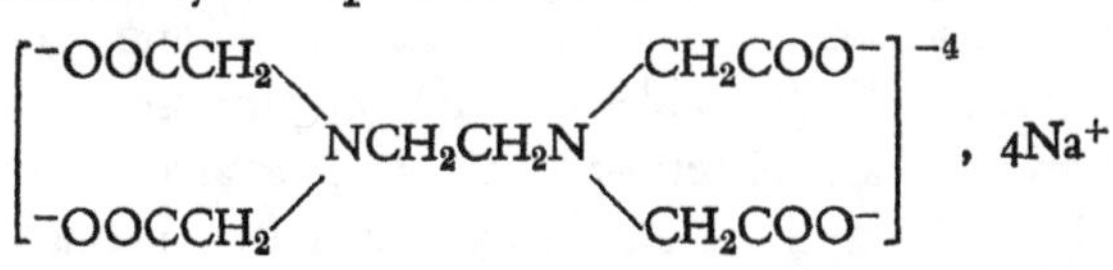

and point out that ". . . in general a chelating compound may be considered as a ' complex ' type of substance in which an ion is bonded simultaneously to two or more positions in a molecule, forming one or

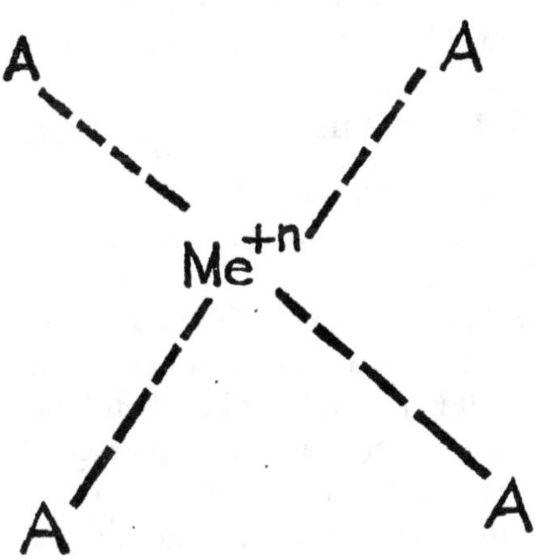

(2)

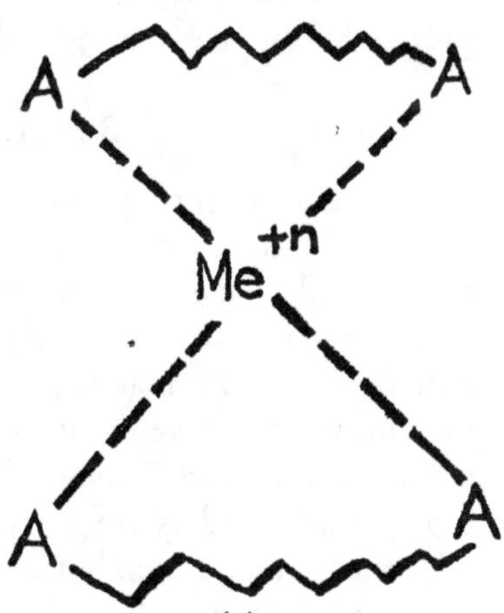

(3)

(After Martell and Bersworth, *loc. cit.*)

more chelate rings. The only difference therefore, between a chelate compound and a complex compound lies in the formation of such ring structures. An important consideration, however, is the fact that chelate compounds are usually much more stable and a metal or hydrogen ion is bound into a chelate ring much more firmly than would be the case with ordinary complexes. Formulae (2) and (3) represent schematically this fundamental distinction between metal chelates and metal complexes. . . ."

It is claimed that chelate-forming substances are in general more effective sequestrants than ordinary complex-forming agents. At present the amino acid sequestering agent most generally used is ethylenediaminetetra-acetic-acid (synonym ethylene bis-iminodiacetic acid), which was manufactured by I. G. Farbenindustrie under the title Trilon B. This substance is made by the Alrose Chemical Co. in the United States under the proprietary name of "Sequestrene", under U.S. Pat. 2,130,505 and 2,240,957. The technical pure acid, and the di, tri and tetra sodium salts are available under the titles "Sequestrene" AA, NA2, NA3 and NA_4, respectively. The name "Versene" is the registered trade mark of the Bersworth Chemical Co. (U.S.A.) used in connection with certain powerful amino acids and their salts, used as complexing agents; again, a range of "Versenes" is available for different purposes. In the United Kingdom, ethylenediamine-tetra-acetic acid is available under the title "Irgalon B.T."[1] (Geigy Ltd.) and as a 30 per cent. aqueous solution of its tetrasodium salt under the name "Tetralon S" (Allied Colloids Ltd.).

Because certain detergents as purchased are "built", or "boosted" by the addition of various builders by the manufacturers, the actual benefit gained by the addition of a sequestrant to a "bought proprietary product" can be evaluated only by actual laboratory and "head" tests.

"Builders" for Detergents

Because many proprietary detergents are already, at least partially, "built" by their manufacturers it is of interest to consider the function of a "builder" and of what these "builders" consist.

Kramer (*J. Amer. Oil. Chem. Soc.*, Nov. 1952, p. 529) has defined a builder as ". . . a material which, when added to a synthetic detergent or soap, will improve its performance. It is not a diluent but contributes to the over-all effectiveness of the cleaning operation. The more commonly used builders are inorganic compounds which have little or no inherent cleaning action but which greatly improve the cleaning effectiveness of a detergent. . . ."

Kramer classifies examples of the more widely used compounds for such purposes under the following headings:

(1) *Alkali salts of weak organic acids.*

(*a*) Carbonates (soda ash, modified soda, sodium sesquicarbonate).

[1] Now termed "Sequestrol"

(*b*) Silicates (meta-, sesqui- and orthosilicate).
(*c*) Phosphates (trisodium orthophosphate, sodium hexametaphosphate, tetrasodium pyrophosphate, sodium tripolyphosphate, sodium tetraphosphate).
(*d*) Borates (sodium tetraborate).

(2) *Alkali hydroxides* (sodium hydroxide).

(3) *Neutral inorganic salts* (sodium sulphate, sodium chloride).

(4) *Colloidal additives* (bentonite and other clays, water glass of 1 : 2 to 1 : 4 $Na_2O : SiO_2$ ratio, sodium carboxymethyl cellulose, proteins, amino acids, methyl, ethyl and hydroxyl ethyl celluloses, water soluble cellulose ethers, sodium starch glycolate, lecithin, peptides).

(5) *Solvents* (pine oil, aliphatic and aromatic solvents, hexalin, tetralin).

(6) *Sequestering agents* (sodium salts of polyaminocarboxylic acids).

(7) *Proprietary mixtures.*

Though the above description applies to the use of detergent mixtures generally, much of it can be applied to shampoos. There are of course certain exceptions, in that sodium hydroxide (2) would not be present, at least, in the free state. Apart from this, the majority of the other substances quoted may be encountered. In the above table only the amino derivatives have been classified as sequestrants, actually the phosphates are also sequestrants.

Shampoo Preparations

Powder Shampoos (Saponaceous Type)

	per cent.
Powdered soap	60·0
Sodium sesquicarbonate	40·0
Perfume	*q.s.*

The above formula is a simple soap-sesquicarbonate formulation to which may be added one of the " builders " or sequestrants described above. The addition of sequestrants in a soap-powder shampoo is not, however, the complete answer because of the large volume of (possibly hard) water used in the shampooing and rinsing. In such cases a better effect is obtained by using the sequestrant separately as a hair rinse subsequent to the shampoo. (*See* Hair Rinses.)

The proportion of soap-powder and sesquicarbonate may be varied to suit costing or other purposes; builders other than sesquicarbonate may be added and/or sesquestrants included.

Liquid Shampoos (Saponaceous)

Before quoting some examples of liquid soap shampoos, attention should be drawn to the common misconception that "soap" shampoos are antique and now quite démodé, and that synthetic detergents or "syndets" are infinitely superior. Such is by no means the case. Foster Dee Snell has pointed out (*Soap and Sanitary Chemicals*, Feb. 1950) in a discussion on synthetic detergents and soap, that ". . . Effective surface-agents in solution reduce surface tension from 72 dynes per cm. for plain water to a range of 25-35 dynes per cm. They will reduce interfacial tension against benzene containing 0·1 per cent. oleic acid from about 29 dynes per cm. for plain water to about 5 dynes per cm. or less. . . . In terms of *surface tension* value at 0·1 per cent. they are in order of decreasing effectiveness. . . .":

SURFACE TENSION

	dynes
Coconut tallow soap	22·8
Sodium lauryl sulphate	27·9
a "non-ionic"	28·7
an alkyl-aryl	30·6

Values over 30 dynes are not very good.

INTERFACIAL TENSION

	dynes
Coconut tallow soap	2·0
Alkyl-aryl	2·5
Sodium lauryl sulphate	2·7
Non-ionic	16·0

Values should be under 5 dynes to be effective.

DISPERSING POWER

	dynes
Coconut-tallow	37·0
Alkyl-aryl	7·4
Non-ionic	7·1
Sodium lauryl sulphate	5·7

Good values are $>$10.

(*After Foster Dee Snell.*)

The above tables show the efficacy of soap. In soft waters soap has most of the properties desirable in a detergent and approaches most nearly to the ideal cleanser. For the reasons discussed at the beginning of this chapter, soaps are in general very susceptible to calcium and magnesium salts; even here by suitable choice, such as by the use of a coconut oil soap and by the subsequent use of a rinse, excellent results may be obtained.

Zussman (*J. Soc. cosmet. Chem.*, Dec. 1949, p. 355) points out "... Another common misconception is that soap is not suitable for formulation of hard water shampoos. There is no question that soap, especially coconut oil soap, has many desirable properties not easily duplicated by synthetics. Aside from the fact that soap produces the conventional feel of skin and hair, the lather produced by coconut soaps is excellent. It is copious, viscous and stable in soft water. In hard water, the volume and viscosity of the lather fall and during the rinsing operation, the dilution of soap with large quantities of water containing calcium and magnesium results in the precipitation of the corresponding alkali earth soaps on the hair. . . ."

Zussman continues, "... It is now possible to manufacture liquid soaps which often do not require refrigeration or filtering, and which will not cloud in glass containers. The addition of a few per cent. of ethylenediamine-tetraacetate to a soap shampoo will prevent the decrease in lather volume and viscosity in hard water. . . . It is not adequate, however, to neutralise the hardness of all the rinse water used. . . ." He adds, "... the precipitation of calcium and magnesium soap on the hair during dilution may be prevented by the addition to the soap of a lime-soap dispersant. . . ."

The following formulation for a non-alcoholic liquid soap shampoo is from the *Drug and Cosmetic Industry* (Oct. 1949, **65**, 455):

	per cent.
Coconut oil	10·00
Potassium hydroxide 85 per cent.	5·38
Sodium hydroxide 95 per cent.	0·50
Glycerin	12·65
Oleic acid	14·00
Water	56·72
Perfume	0·75

Procedure

Melt the potassium hydroxide in a third of the water. Melt the coconut oil and add the alkali solution in a thin stream with continuous stirring until saponified. Allow the coconut soap to become cold, stand overnight before proceeding with the batch. Mix the glycerin with half the remaining water and bring it to the boil, then add the coconut oil soap in small portions and stir until dissolved. Dissolve the sodium hydroxide in the rest of the water and add to the soap solution immediately after the coconut soap has dissolved. Add the oleic acid and stir slowly until completely saponified, then perfume. Age, chill to 32° F. and filter.

Various other mixtures of oils and fats may be used in such formulations, for example, about 25 per cent. coconut oil and 5 per cent. castor oil; 20 per cent. coconut and 8 per cen olive oil and so on. Small amounts of sodium soap along with the potassium soap are prepared to obtain a suitable viscosity. A modern method of achieving this effect is by the use of certain surface active additives, such as those of the fatty acid amide type, of which an example is "Alrosol" (Alrose Chemical Co., U.S.A.). Increased viscosity effects may also be obtained by the use of certain colloids and by some of the cellulose derivatives. An example of the use of a sequestrant and of a wetting agent of the fatty amide type is given by the following formulation (*courtesy* Alrose Chemical Co. from the booklet "Sesquestrene"):

	per cent.
Potassium coconut soap	20·0
Sequestrene AA (potassium salt)	0·5
Alrosol	2·0
Water	77·5

The actual amounts of alkali required for neutralisation in any particular formulation may be obtained from the analytical figures on the oils by calculation, it being remembered that if a mixture of potassium and sodium hydroxides is being used, the sodium hydroxide should be calculated "in terms of potassium hydroxide" (i.e. 56 parts KOH ≡ 40 NaOH so that every 1 part of NaOH ≡ 56/40 ≡ 1·4 KOH and the total amount of alkali to neutralise the mixed fat charge calculated in terms of one of the alkali, preferably the KOH). Another method is by titrating a portion of the actual fat charge with the mixed lye it is proposed to employ.

With the commercial availability of fatty acids, the manufacture of liquid shampoos has been considerably simplified, in that neutralisation is rapid and mild alkalis such as triethanolamine may be employed. The following example is quoted in the literature ("Emulsions and Detergents", Carbide and Carbon Chemicals Corporation, New York, p. 61):

	parts
Coconut oil fatty acids	42
Oleic acid	56
Propylene glycol	55
Triethanolamine	58

Procedure

Mix the fatty acids, add the amine and then the propylene glycol. Stir until a clear solution is obtained. No heating is required. Dilute with water to any desired consistency. When the water is first added, the shampoo concentrate assumes a petrolatum-like consistency and gradually changes to a clear, very slightly viscous solution of pale amber colour. If the water becomes cloudy, stir in more amine, a little at a time, until it becomes clear. A solution of 1 part with 3 parts by weight of water before use makes, it is stated, an excellent shampoo (*p*H about 7·93).

Builders, sequestrants, antiseptics, perfumes and any " speciality " ingredients can, of course, be included in the above " type " formulations with a view to imparting character to the shampoo.

Shampoo Powders (Soapless)

These preparations still enjoy a large sale, since, when properly formulated, they are effective cleansers, economical and very easy to pack and carry about. Because the " appearance " of the product in respect of volume is important, such formulae must either be bulked with diluents or " puffed " or " beaded " by putting the detergent, or in some cases the finished formulation (apart from perfume), down a spray tower; this is carried out usually by the detergent manufacturers. In considering such formulations it must again be remembered that manufacturers sometimes " build " their detergents with tetrasodium pyrophosphate and other builders and/or sequestrants and that such correctly built preparations in many instances require only the addition of perfume, followed by packing.

The sulphated fatty alcohols are excellent materials for the preparation of powder shampoos. (The title " sulphonated fatty alcohols " sometimes given to these products is a misnomer; they are not the true sulphonic derivatives of these alcohols, but merely the sulphuric acid esters of fatty alcohols of the formula $R . CH_2 . O . SO_2O . Na$ in which the sulphur is not linked directly to the adjacent carbon but only through the oxygen atom.)

Sodium lauryl sulphate is widely used in these preparations, and is available commercially under various proprietary designations such as " Sulphonated Lorol " (Ronsheim and Moore) " Empicol P " and " Empicol LZ " (Marchon Products), etc. About one-fifth of an ounce of the detergent powder is sufficient for a shampoo, but from a sales and psychological aspect this would appear " poor value for money ", unless a powder of light density, such as Empicol LZ or similar product were employed.

In choosing a diluent, consideration must be given to the solubility of the diluent in the amount of water which is likely to be employed in dissolving the shampoo. The following exemplify such preparations:

	per cent.
" Empicol L.Z." powder	40·0
Tetrasodium pyrophosphate	6·0
Sodium bicarbonate	54·0
Perfume	*q.s.*

Here a large bulk has been obtained by the use of a light density grade of sodium alkyl sulphate, bulked still more with a cheap, readily soluble and innocuous diluent-sodium bicarbonate. The addition of tetra-sodium pyrophosphate acts as a " builder " and as an excellent peptising and dispersing medium. The ratio of these substances may be varied to suit cost and bulking properties required.

(Instead of " Empicol LZ ", a suitable grade of " Sulphonated Lorol " or other proprietary sulphated lauryl alcohol may be used.)

Another example is :

	per cent.
" Sulphonated Lorol " powder	35·0
Sodium sulphate	10·0
Disodium phosphate	5·0
Sodium bicarbonate	50·0
Perfume	*q.s.*

By omitting alkaline builders and including some adipic, boric, tartaric or other suitable mild organic acids, shampoos having a mildly acid reaction may be prepared.

Mixed soap-soapless shampoos may also be prepared, if desired along the following lines :

	per cent.
Sodium lauryl sulphate (powdered)	40·0
Soap powder	30·0
Sodium bicarbonate	20·0
Tetrasodium pyrophosphate	10·0

Liquid Shampoo (Transparent Type)

Triethanolamine lauryl sulphate forms an excellent basis for liquid shampoos and is available under such names as " Sipon " LT/5 and " Sipon " LT/6, " Sulphonated Lorol ", Liquid TA ; " Empicol " TA.

The first formulation instances the use of triethanolamine lauryl sulphate alone :

	per cent.
Triethanolamine lauryl sulphate	40·0
Water	60·0
Colour (green)	*q.s.*
Perfume (Cologne)	*q.s.*

The following formulation is based upon the use of " Sipon " LT/6 and also represents an inexpensive formulation :

	per cent.
" Sipon " LT/6	49·0
T.E.A. Oleate 50 per cent. [1]	9·8
Octylene glycol	2·0
Oleyl alcohol	1·0
Distilled water	38·2

T.E.A. Oleate 50 *per cent.* [1]	*per cent.*
Oleic acid	32·7
Triethanolamine	17·4
Distilled water	49·9
	100·0

(Personal Communication, J. E. Andre, American Alcolac Corporation.)

" Alrosol ", a wetting agent of the fatty acid amide type already mentioned, can be used in lauryl sulphate shampoos as a foam stabiliser and viscosity builder. It is pointed out that whilst triethanolamine lauryl sulphate solutions are fairly commonly used in the United States, they suffer from the handicap of producing rather thin solutions. The addition of Alrosol [1] with a small amount of acetic acid gives a satisfactory viscosity and at the same time lowers its cloud point (Personal Communication, H. W. Zussman, Alrose Chemical Co., U.S.A.), viz. :

	per cent.
Triethanolamine lauryl sulphate	30·0
" Alrosol "	10·0
Acetic acid	1·8
Water	58·2

(*Courtesy H. W. Zussman.*)

Shampoos utilising " Aerosol " O.T. (Manoxol O.T.—Hardman and Holden Ltd., England) may also be prepared. The following formula is reproduced from the " *Manoxol* " *Technical Bulletin*, Aug. 1952 :

	per cent.
" Manoxol " O.T. 20 per cent. solution	80·0
Liquid paraffin (70 cps.)	5·0
Cetyl alcohol	5·0
Lecithin	1·0
Water	9·0

By sulphonation of olefines derived from petroleum cracking, detergents of the type

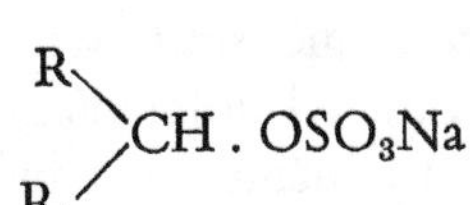

where R_1 usually consists of CH_3 and R may be from C_{12} to C_{16} with an average of C_{14} have been developed.

[1] Detergents of the type mixed fatty amides, RCON $(C_2H_{11}OH)_2$ plus amine soaps and excess amine are sold under the proprietary trade names of " Alrosol ", " Ninol ", " Emcol " 5100, etc. These substances besides thickening the product contribute to its overall effectiveness.

"Teepol" (Shell Chemicals Ltd.) is of this type, and during the Second World War became widely used in liquid and other shampoos. Because of odour and other characteristics there has been rather a swing back towards the sodium and ethanolamine derivatives of lauryl sulphate. However, the following formulation instances the use of "Teepol" in a liquid preparation:

	per cent.
"Teepol" (20–22 per cent. active detergent)	70·0
Glycerin	3·0
Ammonium chloride	2·0
Water	25·0
Colour	*q.s.*
Perfume	*q.s.*

A rather similar product to "Teepol" is "Iranopol" (Anglo-Iranian Oil Co.).

A small quantity of glycerin is sometimes included with a view to minimising dryness of the residual hair though it is, to say the least, doubtful whether under the conditions of use, it can exert any such effect.

"Ultrawet" 60L (Atlantic Refining Co., U.S.A.) is claimed to be neither a primary irritant nor a sensitiser and it is said solutions of this material up to 25 per cent. are safe in so far as eye irritation is concerned. (Personal communication, J. E. McCullen, Atlantic Refining Co.)

The following formulation (Glyco Products Co. Inc.) has been suggested as a starting point formulation for a clear liquid shampoo utilising "Ultrawet" 60L:

	per cent.
"Ultrawet" 60L	33·0
Glyceryl Mono Laureate S-1062	2·0
Water	65·0

It is stated that although "Ultrawet" 60L is not nearly as harsh as the sodium alkyl aryl sulphonates, a conditioning agent is often desirable to leave the hair and scalp with a pleasant feeling. Two products are suggested for use; lanolin in amounts of 0·5 per cent. or less (above this amount, lanolin substantially reduces the foam) or a maximum (for the same reason) of 2 per cent. lecithin.

(*Note.—Because the ultimate feel or handle of the hair is so intimately bound up with the suitability of a particular shampoo and because this "feel" or handle can be also brought about by the subsequent use of a rinse or conditioner, the problem of hair rinses and conditioning creams is discussed later in this chapter.*)

Liquid Cream Shampoos

These preparations have developed from the so-called cream (actually paste) shampoos, and may logically be considered as a compromise between clear liquid shampoos and paste shampoos. The following example (by courtesy American Alcolac Corporation) instances the use of "Sipon" LS (sodium lauryl sulphate):

	per cent.
"Sipon" LS	25·0
Polyethylene glycol 400 distearate	5·0
Magnesium stearate	2·0
Distilled water	68·0
"Ninol" AB 21	*q.s.*
Oleyl alcohol	*q.s.*
Perfume	*q.s.*

(Addition of the "Ninol" and Oleyl alcohol compounds is for thickening and "conditioning" purposes, respectively.)

Discussing the formulation of liquid cream shampoos, deNavarre (*Amer. Perfum.*, Aug. 1950, p. 109) states, quite correctly, that ". . . the best foaming agent continues to be fatty alcohol sulphate paste constituting anything from 25-45 per cent. of the finished cream shampoo. A permanent opacifier such as magnesium stearate is very desirable although whitening or opacifying of the liquid can be obtained with the higher alcohols, spermaceti or other higher alcohol esters. In view of the inclusion of a metal stearate, a mucilaginous thickener such as a solution of polyvinyl alcohol; methyl cellulose, solubilised methacrylate, gum alginate, Irish moss or carboxy methyl cellulose should be used to the extent of from ½ per cent. upwards depending on the thickening agent used. . . ."

deNavarre continues, ". . . It is the custom to use 1 per cent. lanolin and either a glycol or glyceryl laurate or stearate to the tune of 1 or 2 per cent. to further opacify and thicken the emulsion. . . ."

Pantaleoni, Shanks and Valentine (Fine Chemicals Division, E. I. du Pont de Nemours and Co.) have given examples of various shampoo formulations incorporating fatty alcohol sulphates (*Proc. Sci. Sect. T.G.A.*, Dec. 1949, p. 9) including one along the lines discussed above, viz.:

	per cent.
Fatty alcohol sulphate paste A[1]	30·0
Magnesium stearate	1·0
Polyvinyl alcohol, 10 per cent. solution	20·5
Methyl cellulose, 3 per cent. solution	9·0
Water	38·0
Lanolin	0·5
Glyceryl monolaurate	1·0

[The method of preparation given is applicable to all formulations of this type. It is as follows: "The magnesium stearate is pasted with the fatty alcohol sulphate, then the polyvinyl alcohol, methyl cellulose and water are each added separately to make the water phase. The mixture is agitated while heating to 71° C. The oil phase is brought to the same temperature and the water phase is added with agitation.]

(The fatty alcohol sulphate paste A[1] in the above formulation refers to Duponol ® WA Paste. Other sulphated alcohol pastes may be investigated in this formula.)

A liquid cream formulation employing "Veegum" as thickening agent and utilising "Alropon". Concentrate mixed with "Duponol" WA as detergents is recommended by R. T. Vanderbilt, viz.:

	parts
"Alropon" concentrate	13·0
"Duponol" WA	17·0
Lauric acid	2·0
Triethanolamine	0·14
"Veegum" 5 per cent.	21·0
Water	47·0

The following is a suggested starting point formulation for the use of "Ultrawet" 60L., viz.:

	per cent.
"Ultrawet" 60L. (Atlantic Refining Co.)	33·0
"Aldo" 33 (Non self-emulsifying Glyceryl monostearate (Glyco Ltd.))	2·0
Magnesium stearate	1·0
Water	64·0

Paste or "Cream" Shampoos (Solid)

The formulation of these preparations is very similar to those of the liquid cream shampoos discussed; the main difference being in the fluidity of the latter type of preparations. The following is an example of the use of Sipon LS:

	per cent.
"Sipon" LS	50·0
Stearic acid	5·0
Sodium hydroxide	0·75
Lanolin	1·0
Distilled water	43·25

(*Courtesy American Alcolate Corporation.*)

The following formulation utilises "Empicol LA7 paste (Marchon Products Ltd., England). This is one of a series of lauryl sulphate pastes prepared to meet the varying needs of the user. "Empicol" L special paste is a narrow-cut lauryl alcohol paste of medium active matter content ; " Empicol " LA7 paste is a medium-cut lauryl alcohol paste of medium active matter content ; " Empicol " LM paste is a medium-cut lauryl alcohol paste of high active matter content. Empilan TN is a trade name for a product specially developed by Marchon Products, in England, as a thickening agent, etc., for shampoos and other detergents :

	per cent.
" Empicol " LA 7 paste	50·0
" Empilan " TN	2·0
Sodium hydroxide	*q.s.* *
Triethanolamine	*q.s.* *
Stearic acid	8·0 to 12·0
Water to	100·0

* Equal molecular parts, sufficient to saponify the fatty acid.

The following exemplifies the use of a glyceryl monostearate stabilised for use on the acid side, viz. " Tegacid " Special (Goldschmidt Chemical Corporation, New York) :

	per cent.
" Tegacid " special	8·0
Lanolin	1·0
Detergent paste	75·0
Water	16·0

" Tegacid " Special is stated to be used intensively as a stabiliser in cream shampoos, and to maintain the correct degree of creamy viscosity veen at low temperatures.

The use of neutral salts, together with a hydrophilic colloid for producing detergent gels which may be used as shampoos, has been patented by Marriott (Brit. Pat. 590,839). The broad basis of the claim is as follows : . . . detergent creams and pastes of uniform consistency are prepared from sulphuric esters of higher fatty alcohols, a hydrophilic colloid such as cellulose ethers or salts of cellulose glycollic acid and a neutral salt such as sodium chloride or sulphate which are instrumental in maintaining the consistency. . . .

Apart from soapless cream shampoos of the above type, clear gel shampoos have been popular. These may be formulated either as soapless shampoos or as a mixture of soap and soapless detergent, the following formulation exemplifies a preparation of the latter type :

	per cent.
Triethanolamine lauryl sulphate	20·0
Sodium lauryl sulphate	10·0
Coconut oil fatty acids	15·0
Triethanolamine (technical)	10·0

	per cent.
Sequestrant	1·0
Water	44·0
Perfume	q.s.
Colour	q.s.

By varying the amounts of triethanolamine-coconut soap, triethanolamine lauryl sulphate and sodium lauryl sulphate, preparations of different consistencies and textures may be obtained. By variation in the type and amount of sequestrant the properties of this gel may be modified.

Oil Shampoos

The development of sulphonated oils (i.e. oils which have been treated with sulphuric acid or other sulphonating agents under the influence of heat and then neutralised, and in which the sulphur atom is linked directly to the adjacent carbon atom) led to their introduction, some years ago, as hair shampoos. They were effective detergents in that they removed dirt and oil from the hair but lacked "foaming" properties. For this reason they never really "made the grade" as competitors to the ever increasing number of surfactant materials which were becoming available.

However, there has been a tendency to use them in the formulation of "oil shampoos" in which the head is treated with a mixture of sulphonated oil and a conditioning oil, which is allowed to remain on the head for a short time and is then rinsed off.

As discussed under skin cleansers, certain sulphonated oils have been found useful as detergents for persons who suffer from certain skin affections and cannot use soaps; the fact that owing to the configuration of the castor oil molecule, even the sulphonated oil contains a considerable amount of unchanged glycerides, probably reduces the degreasing effect of this material. So far as conditioning the hair in respect of "handle", or "feel" is concerned, there are now methods which utilise cationic agents (*see* Hair Rinses and Conditioning Creams); nevertheless, sulphonated oil shampoos, with suitable adjustment to *p*H to be on the acid side, can also act in this manner.

The first example is that of a sulphonated oil detergent preparation; sulphonated castor oil alone is apt to be too sticky whilst sulphonated olive oil lacks body—hence the blend:

	per cent.
Sulphonated olive oil	16·0
Sulphonated castor oil	16·0
Water	68·0
Colour	q.s.
Perfume	q.s.

The second example contains some mineral oil and a little glycerin. A little lanolin derivative (grades of both oil and water-soluble lanolin derivatives are now available) or other emollient substance may be added, in place of either the mineral oil or oleyl alcohol :

	per cent.
Sulphonated castor oil	77·0
Mineral oil (light grade)	3·0
Oleyl alcohol	3·0
Glycerin	3·0
Water (distilled or softened by ion exchange)	14·0

This is more of the " oil " conditioning type shampoo.

Additives in Shampoo Formulation (Conditioning Agents)

Detergent solutions in general do not distinguish between extraneous greasy dirt and the normal skin fat—sebum—of the scalp and hair shaft. (*See* Sebum, Chapter 20.) The cult of sun and sea bathing and also bleaching and tinting tends to increase dryness.

Dry hair is not only dull, and prone to split, but also because of its lack of oil along the hair shaft, appears dry and lifeless. With a view to minimising such tendencies, certain additions have, from time to time, been made to shampoos. Hollenberg (*Proc. Sci. Sect. T.G.A.*, May 1952) has pointed out that if a cleansing solution does not foam, it is thought by the public that it will not clean, and that to obtain an adequate lather, it is frequently necessary to employ an amount of detergent *in excess* of that actually required for cleansing, which often results in the removal of all fatty substances from the hair. This factor is recognised in general by the detergent industry, and Foster Dee Snell, giving the Medallist's Address (" Detergents and Detergency ", Annual Meeting, Society of Chemical Industry, 13 July 1949), states that the frequent dryness and harshness of the skin, caused by reduction in its content of sebaceous matters, regardless of whether the detergent is soap or a synthetic, is in his opinion explained by the observations of McBain, and of Harkins, that the water-insoluble matter is dissolved in the detergent micelli. (*See also* Emulsions and Dispersions, Chapter 41.) In Dr. Snell's opinion, reducing the detergent efficiency of soap by adding certain fatty and other matters, reduces the drying effect of the solution on the skin.[1]

These additions may take the form of fatty alcohols, such as oleyl, cetyl, etc., lanolin, fatty acids and so forth ; in brief an attempt is made to condition the hair in one operation, instead of using a shampoo followed by a conditioning rinse or conditioning cream. Whilst

[1] The effect of "scroop" in such dryness must also be kept in mind.

convincing evidence of the value of such additions is lacking, such additives *may* be of value both in reducing the efficacy of a shampoo in respect of its " degreasing " action, and secondly, in actually depositing some of the additive on the hair shaft. At first sight it might appear impossible that a shampoo can both *cleanse* by removal of oil and dirt, and yet *condition* by depositing the oily conditioning agent. Such is not necessarily the case, because if, in the first stage of cleansing, the shampoo is kept in a fairly *concentrated solution* and then rinsed *quickly* from the scalp, the amount of detergent and sequestrant is sufficient to keep the soil, together with the conditioning agent incorporated in the shampoo, dispersed. After rinsing the hair quickly (when the soil is washed away), a second application of shampoo is made, and this time the user deliberately dilutes the shampoo lather on the head, making the lather as *dilute* as possible. Under these conditions, the concentration of detergent and dispersant in the diluted shampoo can fall to a level below that necessary to keep the conditioning agent " dispersed ". Under these conditions the conditioning agent would be largely deposited, in Stage 2 of the shampoo process, namely on " cleaned " hair.

Other additives, such as " egg ", have been suggested for use in shampoos. Apart from the aspect of " feminine psychology ", I can see no advantage for such additives to modern synthetic detergents. If egg yolk or dried egg is used for this purpose, from 1 per cent. to 1·5 per cent. may be used, viz.: enough to be evident, but not too much to inhibit the foaming properties of the preparation. (Other conditioners: *see* effect of cationic agents in the next paragraph.)

CATIONIC DETERGENTS IN SHAMPOOS. Although cationic surface-active agents are very briefly described in Chapter 41 (Emulsions and Dispersions), it will be observed that they have not been included in the shampoo formulations discussed. The reason for this lies in the fact that the majority of cationics are poor detergents and are strongly absorbed on hair and wool; they are in general ineffective as " hair shampoos ".

Hair Rinses

Various rinses, based upon the use of sequestrants, may be used to remove any calcium and magnesium soaps from the hair shaft following the use of a soap, or soap-soapless shampoo, in hard water areas. For example, the rinse may consist of a 1 per cent. solution of " Calgon ", or of the amino acid chelating compound, ethylenediamine tetra-acetic acid sodium salt, as for example, " Sequestrene ", " Versene ", " Irgalon " B.T., etc. These latter rinses not only solubilise the insoluble soaps of calcium and magnesium, but are capable of removing traces of metals from the hair, and have been recommended for use for this purpose as rinses, prior and subsequent to, cold waving or hair tinting.

Although, as mentioned earlier, quaternary ammonium salts are in general ineffective as hair shampoos because of their tendency to adsorb on fibres, this property may be utilised with advantage in the formulation of hair rinses. It is claimed (*Parfum. mod.*, Dec. 1948, p. 47) that on rinsing dull-looking and brittle hair in a solution of a quaternary ammonium compound the hair is left silky and manageable.

Apart from simple solutions, there are on the market a number of " cream " hair rinses (in other words, " opaque hair rinses ").

The following formulae will serve as examples of this type of preparation :

	per cent.
Quaternary ammonium compound	4·0
Glyceryl monostearate	3·0
Water	93·0

Other opacifying agents may be used in place of the monostearate. (*Drug Cosmet. Ind.*, 1952, p. 705.) The use of Cetavlon as a cationic might be considered for this purpose.

	per cent.
" Alromine " RA (Alrose Chemical Co.)	4·0
" Triton " K-60 (Rohm and Haas)	4·0
" Rhotex " GS (Rohm and Haas)	0·5
Water	91·5

This preparation may be diluted with 2 or 4 volumes of water prior to use.

Remarks given under shampoos, that the potential hazard to the cornea of the eye must be evaluated, also apply to hair rinses. Some information on certain materials, in respect of such hazard has already been given under that section dealing with detergents earlier in this chapter.

Hair Tinting Solutions (Colour Rinses)

Apart from genuine hair rinses, given as mentioned above, to condition the hair and improve its sheen and " handle ", the nomenclature of " hair rinses " has become confused because of the apparent sensitivity of some persons to the term hair " dyes ". Subsequent to shampooing the hair, so-called " rinses " are given to " bring up the highlights ". In point of fact these are very often dyes such as henna, bleaches (such as peroxide or perborate) or water-soluble colours (dyes) which are not as strong as those normally employed in hair dying. In addition, particularly in the United States, so-called " coloured rinses " are used to dye the hair, some natural, others to exotic or bizarre shades for a party or for a " night out ". These dyes are merely temporary and can subsequently be washed out.

Colour Rinses

The conditions for dyeing the hair by means of henna are described in the chapter on Hair Dyes. As used in shampoos, the strength of powdered henna employed is not sufficiently strong, and the period of contact too short, to achieve very marked effects. Liquid extracts of henna that are more powerful are available: these consist of a saturated solution of Lawsone—it is claimed—in a solvent. To achieve tinting from a henna solution, the *p*H of the shampoo should be on the acid side, i.e. about 5·5.

Camomile rinses, used to " brighten " fair hair, may contain an amount of Infusum Anthemidis Conc. (Brit. Pharmacopœia 1923) equivalent to 5 per cent. of the camomile flowers in the finished rinse. In point of fact, because of the cost and trouble of preparing such products, in many cases the brightening rinses for fair hair contain a substance capable of yielding active oxygen as a mild bleach.

In the U.S.A. the newer colour rinses, applied after a shampoo, consist of acidified aqueous solutions of certified colours.

The theory of tinting the hair in this manner involves making the dyestuffs employed substantive to the hair. As we have discussed (Chapter 20) the hair is a protein, containing an active amino group and a carboxy group and is amphoteric in character; that is to say, under suitable conditions, the hair protein can react with either anionic or cationic groupings. In the dyes under present discussion, the tinting process is carried out from an acid solution and combination occurs between the carboxy group of the hair protein molecule and a positively charged dyestuff ion. These colour rinses are meant to be temporary, and are removed on washing the hair. The dyestuffs most frequently employed are (according to *Amer. Perfum.*, 1948, p. 523):

F. D. and C. Red	1, 2, 3 and 4
F. D. and C. Yellow	5 and 6
F. D. and C. Blue	1 and 2
D. and C. Violet	1
D. and C. Black	1
Ext. D. and C. Red	1
Ext. D. and C. Green	1

The acid employed in such preparations is usually tartaric as it is far less hygroscopic than many other acids. More recently the use of sulphamic acid for this purpose has been patented (Brit. Pat. 593,314). It is claimed that this acid is non-hygroscopic and that less of the acid is required to achieve the desired purpose.

It is stated (*Drug Cosmet. Ind.*, April 1952, p. 523) that in general, up to about 20 per cent. of dye is mixed in the dry organic carrier and the dry mixture then packed in glassine or similar water-resistant envelopes containing about 30 grains of the mixture per envelope. Instructions are to add the contents to a gallon of water for use as a rinse. A typical preparation of this sort for a jet black hair rinse consists of:

	parts
D. and C. Black No. 1	80
D. and C. Red. No. 13	12
D. and C. Brown No. 1	8
Tartaric Acid U.S. Pharmacopœia	400

It will be noticed that to obtain suitable shades, a *blend* of these colours is employed. From the single dyestuff colours given above, by employing mixtures, a wide range of colourings may be obtained. [The composition and general characteristics of these dyestuffs will be found in *Cosmetic Materials*, pp. 392-479, R. G. Harry, London: Leonard Hill Ltd., 1948. In many instances English *equivalents* may be obtained from the leading dyestuff manufacturers, though the actual content of certain organic and metallic impurities in such dyes may, in some instances, fall outside the U.S.A. Regulations.]

Hair Reconditioning ("Conditioning") Creams

In order to deposit a film of the conditioning agent upon the hair fibre it is necessary to (i) utilise a cationic agent, or (ii) if an anionic emulsifier is employed it should be adjusted so that its pH is on the acid side. The following formulae illustrate the use of such emulsifiers:

	per cent.
Empiwax SK (Marchon Products)	15·0
Cholesterol	0·5
Lanolin	0·5
Lactic acid	1·0
Water	83·0

(*Courtesy, Marchon Products.*)

A straightforward conditioning cream may be prepared along the following lines:

	per cent.
Lanette wax SX (Ronsheim and Moore)	15·0
Mineral oil	3·5
Lanolin	1·5
Citric acid	0·8
Water	79·2

or, employing a cationic conditioner, and therefore replacing Lanette wax SX (an ionic) by Cetyl alcohol:

	per cent.
Cetyl/Stearyl alcohols	15·0
Mineral oil	3·5
Lanolin	1·5
Cationic agent	*q.s.*
Water to	100·0

If an additional emulsifier is required to stabilise the cream with the particular cationic chosen, a non-ionic emulsifier may be used. The amount of cationic active material will vary according to the substance used; in general, between ¾-2 per cent. should be sufficient.

The above types of preparations are applied to the hair and distributed thoroughly over the fibres, allowed to remain in contact for a short while and then washed out. *They may be applied to hair which has just been shampooed and rinsed, the conditioning cream being left on the wetted hair fibre for a short while* and then rinsed off with water.

CHAPTER 23

PERMANENT WAVING

From the time the earliest Egyptian woman curled her hair by means of wet mud, and through the Roman and Grecian era, up to the present day, the desire of all women has been to possess an attractive and beautiful coiffure.

Since curly hair is more attractive than straight hair, and at the same time provides more opportunities for rearrangement in suitable and fashionable styles, any process by which curls could be " artificially " produced was bound to affect to a very marked degree the trend of modern hairdressing.

Suter (*J. Soc. cosmet. Chem.*, March 1948, p. 103) has pointed out that " . . . until around 1910, hair was always curled by means of a curling iron or by boiling it in water. This, however, never resulted in a lasting wave. . . . Three pioneers, Charles Nessler, E. Frederics and Eugene Suter, each working independently, found that the addition of chemicals such as borax to water under the influence of heat would curl hair so that it would survive several washings. Around 1924 ammonium hydroxide first came into use in connection with borax. . . ."

Subsequently " chemical methods of heating " and the " cold wave " have been developed ; these are discussed at greater length in this chapter. First of all, it is necessary to consider the molecular structure and elastic properties of hair in order to see how these agents are believed to act.

The statement that naturally curly hair is observed to be oval or flattened when examined microscopically while straight hair is usually circular is incorrect. Many naturally curly hairs are oval, but many others cannot be differentiated from ordinary straight hair. Kneberg (*Amer. J. phys. Anthrop.*, 1935, **20,** 51) has shown that hairs of widely varying cross-sectional form may or may not curl, while Danforth of the Department of Anatomy, Stanford University (*Physiol. Rev.*, Jan. 1939, **19,** 99), states that there would seem to be no reason why a shaft that is uniform in structure should curl merely because its cross-section is elliptical in outline, and it frequently does not. If, however, the upper and lower sides of the shaft were of different density, or if the transverse axis did not bisect the vertical, a differential would be provided which might be expected readily to induce curling.

The Molecular Structure and Elastic Properties of Hair[1]

The histology of hair has already been discussed. Chemically it is composed of keratin, a protein which occurs naturally in nails, hoofs and hair, and is characterised by its high proportion of sulphur (4-5 per cent.).

Proteins may be defined as naturally occurring substances of high molecular weight (ranging from a few thousands to many millions) and composed of "polypeptide chains". A polypeptide chain may be represented by the general formula:

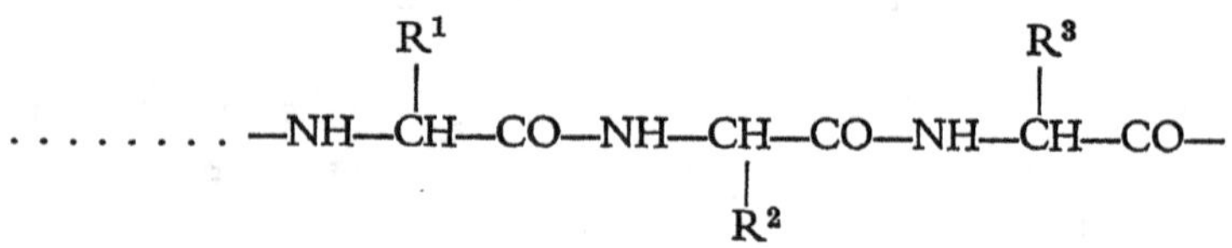

etc. . . . MAIN-CHAIN

← . . . . *Direction of Fibre-axis* . . . . →

in which R^1, R^2, R^3, stand for various univalent radicles, such as —H, —CH_3, —CH_2—CH_2—COOH, etc.—only about two dozen types—which function as "side-chains" to the "main-chains"—are used in the whole of protein chemistry and serve to distinguish one protein from another. In the case of hair keratin, such polypeptide chains, probably hundreds of times as long as they are thick, lie along the length of the hair fibre and attach themselves to one another by combinations between their "side-chains" for example:

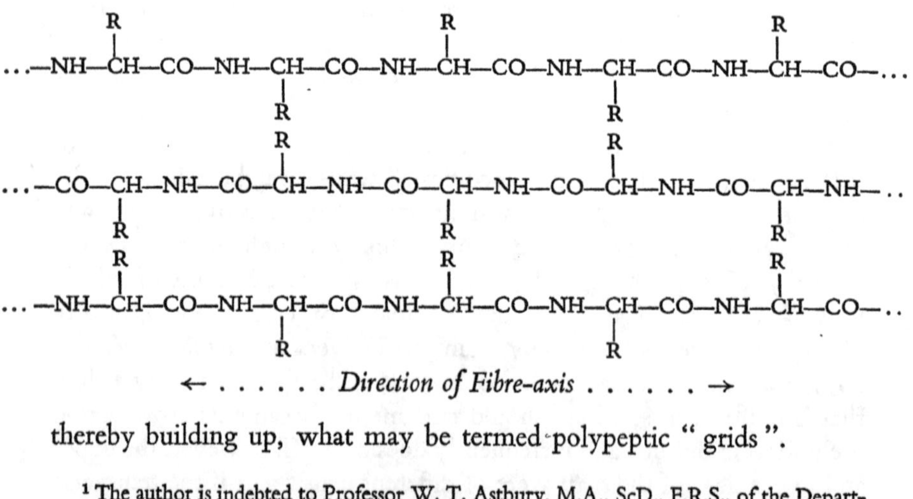

← . . . . . . *Direction of Fibre-axis* . . . . . . →

thereby building up, what may be termed polypeptic "grids".

[1] The author is indebted to Professor W. T. Astbury, M.A., ScD., F.R.S., of the Department of Bimolecular Structure, Leeds University, and to Edward Arnold, Ltd., for permission to reproduce the illustrations (The Hair and Scalp), etc., dealing with the molecular structure and elastic properties of keratin.

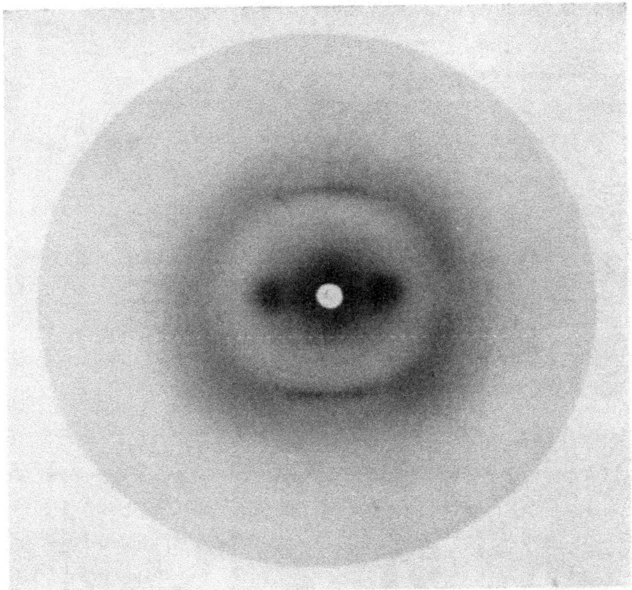

Fig. 71.—X-ray diffraction photograph of a small parallel bundle of unstretched human hairs (α-keratin).

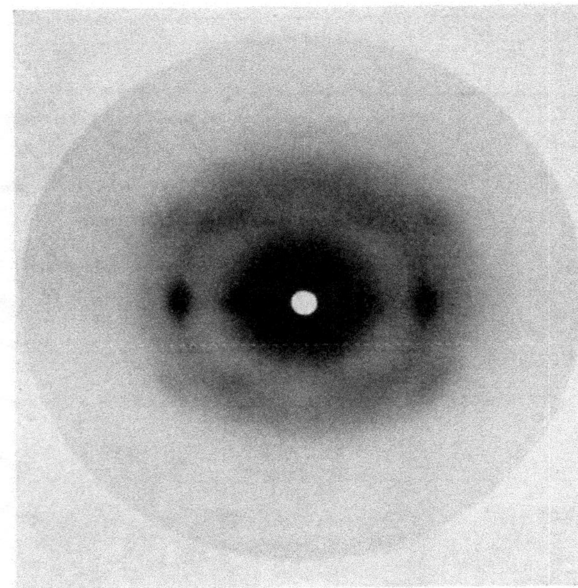

[*By courtesy of Edward Arnold Ltd.*

Fig. 72.—X-ray diffraction photograph of a small parallel bundle of human hairs stretched in steam to twice their original length (" steam-set " β-keratin).

Fig. 73.—Diagrammatic representation of secondary fold (unstretched hair).

Diagrammatic representation of primary fold (stretched hair).

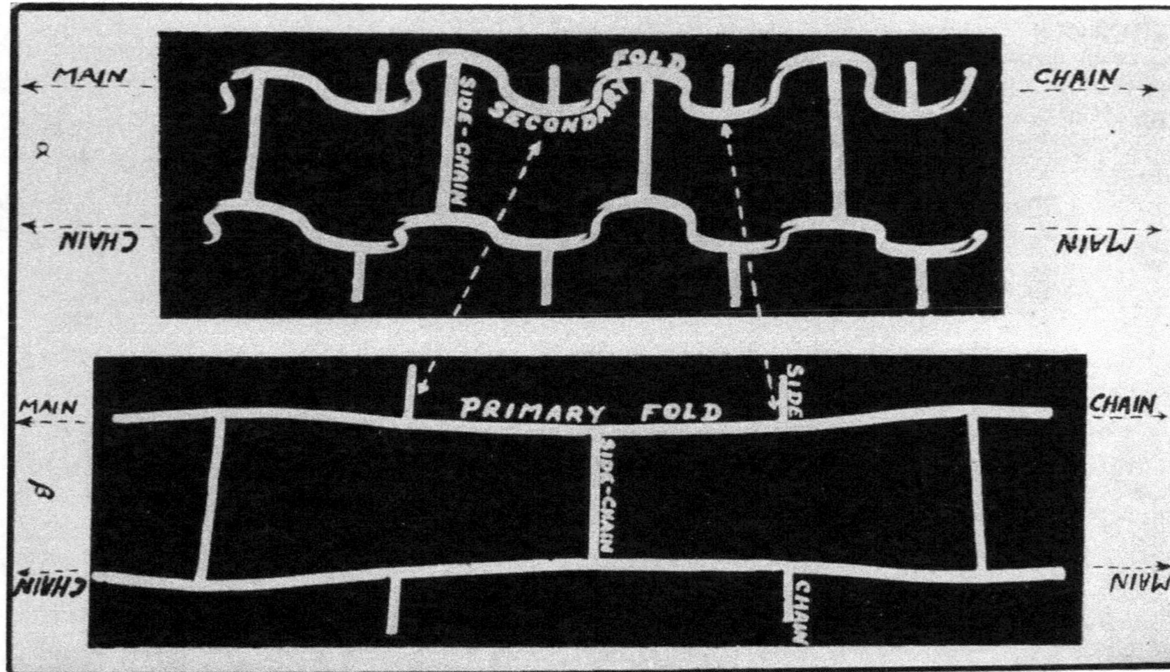

[*By courtesy of Edward Arnold Ltd.*

X-ray diffraction patterns show that these grids are not flat, as represented above but in ordinary unstretched hair are " buckled " represented graphically again. When hair is stretched, however, X-ray studies show that the grids (previously " buckled ") are pulled out flat (Fig. 72). When the hair is allowed to contract, it returns once more to its original " buckled " form. So far we have discussed this stretching of hair without reference to moisture. In point of fact, in the absence of water, certain parts of the keratin molecule cling so tightly to one another, that the transformation from the alpha-keratin to beta-keratin does not occur, and the hair fibre cannot be stretched. Water appears to act as an " intramolecular " lubricant however, and in its presence the intramolecular transformation illustrated readily takes place.

Astbury has pointed out that as alpha-keratin is pulled out into the beta-configuration, stresses pile up in the linked side-chains of the keratin molecule, and thus accumulate energy for the spontaneous contraction which will occur if the stretched fibre is afterwards released in water. This recovery force is dissipated however, if it should happen that the cross-linkages collapse under the stress—and the results of X-ray examination show definitely that they do so collapse under the continued action of water, and at a rate which increases as the temperature of the water is raised, or if, for example, it is made alkaline.

This is the basic principle of the permanent wave, in which the hair is wound around a suitable rod, thus producing a strain on one side of the hair shaft. The hair is then subjected to the action of moisture and alkali ; a chemical reaction termed hydrolysis occurs and certain cross-linkages in the polypeptide chains are broken down, and new, somewhat unstable links are formed which tend to maintain the hair in its new position. Finally, a stage is reached when the set becomes permanent and can no longer be reversed. This is the so-called permanent wave, and on wetting the hair it will now always strive to return to this new configuration. Astbury has summarised the steps in the process as follows :

(i) The continued action of water or alkalis on the strained keratin molecule leads to hydrolytic breakdown in the cross-linkages between the main chains (" relaxation "), which dissipates the stresses that are the driving force of elastic recovery in cold water.

(ii) New, but relatively unstable, linkages then build up which tend to fix the molecule in the stretched state (" temporary set ").

(iii) On raising the temperature of the water in which the fibre is held stretched, relaxation is accelerated and the new linkages become more and more stable (" permanent set ").

(iv) The degree of permanence of set depends on the temperature of the water in which the fibre was held stretched, the time for which it was held stretched and the temperature of the water to which it is afterwards submitted in order to reverse the set.[1]

So far we have been referring to hair keratin. However, Astbury (*Brit. J. Derm.*, Jan. 1950, **62**, 1-15) has pointed out that the elastic properties of mammalian hairs apply also to horn nails, hedgehog spines and porcupine quills and that in these substances, the keratin exists in the unstretched (i.e. alpha-keratin form); whilst in the case of feather keratin (and X-ray diagrams of essentially the same type are given also by birds' beaks and claws, snakes' scales, etc.) the structure is analogous to that present in stretched human hair (i.e. beta-keratin).

This remarkable relationship turns out to be only the foreshadowing of a much wider and deeper master plan. X-ray diagrams of essentially the keratin type are found also with the other fibrous proteins of the epidermis, the chief muscle protein myosin, and two other recently discovered muscle components, paramyosin, and tropomyosin, the bloodclotting proteins, fibrinogen and fibrin and most recently—

[1] It is believed that cystine (*See* Histology of Hair, Chapter 20) is of vital importance in the waving process and that the cystine forms a bridge between parallel peptide chains (*See* Speakman, *J. Soc. chem. Ind., London*, 1931, IT; *Nature*, 1933, **132**, 930) thus:

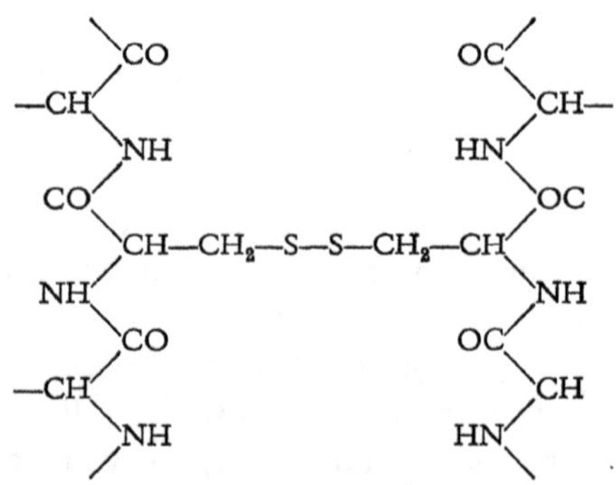

Speakman considers that hydrolysis of the cystine disulphide linkages occurs:

$$R.S.S.R. + H_2O \rightarrow R.SH + R.SOH$$

whilst rebuilding is thought to occur by the condensation of sulphenic and amino groups:

$$R.SOH + R.NH_2 \rightarrow R.S.NH.R + H_2O.$$

This reaction, as mentioned, is accelerated by steam and alkali. It is believed that once hair is unable to form R . SOH groups, permanent waving is impossible.

More recently Blackburn and Lindley (*J. Soc. Dy. Col.*, 1948, **64**, 305) consider that a major role is played by hydrogen bonds. In this scheme, stretching of hair causes the polypeptide chains to uncoil and take up the beta-configuration. At the same time main chains are orientated in the direction of the fibre axis. Reduction of adhesion between chains by the hydrating action of steam on hydrogen bonds and polar groups of side chains, allows the polypeptide chains to slip past one another (J. L. Stoves, *Perf. essent. Oil. Rec.*, July, 1952, p. 232).

bacterial flagella. All these differ considerably in detail, nevertheless X-rays show that in the last resort they are all derived from a single master plan which Astbury and his co-workers have called the keratin-myosin-epidermis-fibrinogen (k-m-e-f) group. The molecular plan common to all of them when they are in the unstretched state, is the folded alpha-structure and likewise, when they are stretched, they pass into a common beta-structure form.

Permanent waving may be broadly subdivided into two classes, namely:

(*a*) The hot method, in which the hair is treated with an alkaline sulphite solution and then wrapped around a rod of small diameter. Heat is then applied to produce a permanent wave. (Originally the heat was supplied by means of electrical heaters ; more recently chemical mixtures which develop exothermic heat of reaction have largely replaced the former type, particularly in the U.S.A.)

(*b*) The cold process, in which the hair is similarly wrapped around a rod of suitable diameter either prior to or after treatment with an alkaline reducing agent such as ammonium thioglycollate. In this method the hair is transformed from its straight form into the desired undulating form, without the application of external heat. When this has been achieved, as determined by the inspection of test curls, the undulations are fixed in the hair by the application of a suitable oxidising agent. More recently it has been found possible to omit this final neutralising process (*See* pp. 461-2).

These methods will now be discussed in greater detail, but first it is of interest to consider (i) the effect of shampooing the hair prior to waving it, (ii) the effect of the physical process of " wrapping " the hair, and the effect of the diameter of the rod on the resultant wave, and (iii) the effect of the fineness or coarseness of the hair to be waved, i.e. the diameter of the hair shaft.

The effect of these factors has been discussed in an excellent paper by Reed, DenBeste and Humoller (*J. Soc. cosmet. Chem.*, March 1948, p. 109), and the author is indebted to these investigators for permission to reproduce *in extenso* the following information dealing with the above.

. . . Prior to giving any permanent wave, but particularly prior to giving a successful cold wave, it is essential that the hair be effectively cleansed. A good shampoo will obviously remove surface dirt and epidermal debris, and it will also remove to a greater or lesser degree the surface coating of oil or sebum from the hair ; this is well shown in the illustrations of a hair fibre taken before and after shampooing. (*See* Hair Shampoos, Rinses and Conditioning Creams, Chapter 22.) But modern synthetic detergents do more than this. Hair consists of keratin, as we have seen, and keratin is not chemically inert but contains many polar groups which can react with anions or cations. For example, Neville and Harris (*J. Res. nat. Bur. Stand.*, 1951, **14**, 765) have demonstrated that when samples of wool (which is also keratin) are soaked in soap solutions there is a greater absorption of cations than there is of anions. Furthermore, Steinhardt *et al.* (*J. Res. nat. Bur. Stand.*, 1940, **25**, 519) have demonstrated in their studies on the combination of wool protein with acid and base, that this is not a simple physical adsorption, but rather that keratins react with anions and cations chemically. Similar conclusions were reached by Speakman and Elliott (*Proc. Symp. Fibrous Proteins*, Univ. Leeds, May 1946) in their studies on the combination of wool with acids and acid dyes.

It is evident, therefore, that the action of detergents on hair goes far beyond that of surface cleansing in that they may combine with and modify the polar groups of the keratin, and thus influence the subsequent action of the chemicals used in the actual waving process.

In the cold permanent waving process the hair is divided into, approximately, fifty rectangular sections and the hair from each of these sections is wrapped around a plastic rod. The diameter of these rods may vary from $\frac{1}{8}$ in. to $\frac{3}{8}$ in. or more. A little reflection will show that the diameter of the rod may influence the type of undulations produced in the permanent waving process, taking into consideration, of course, the fact that as the hair is wound around the rod, the effective diameter will increase with each turn and the curvature will decrease. The following table lists some interesting calculations; these data indicate that the per cent. differential elongation is inversely proportional to the diameter of the curvature, either of rod, or of rod plus hair, if more than one turn of hair is placed around the rod, and directly proportional to the diameter of the hair fibre.

Diameter (Inner periphery wrapped fibre), inch	*per cent. Differential extension fibre diameter*	
	0·001 *inch*	0·005 *inch*
0·125	1·60	8·00
0·250	0·80	4·00
0·500	0·40	2·00

(The above considerations show that the physical process of wrapping does, or can influence, the subsequent wave pattern.)

In the systems of cold waving as currently practised, the waving lotion is applied to the hair before it is wrapped around the rod. In practical terms, the degree of alteration of reduction of hair in the cold wave process depends upon the amount of thioglycollate which diffuses into the hair, and upon the rate with which this is accomplished. The amount of thioglycollate which is available for diffusion into a hair fibre is a function of the capillary air space between the fibres wrapped around the rod during the waving process. The following diagram illustrates a cross-section of a tress of fibres in close-packed relationship.

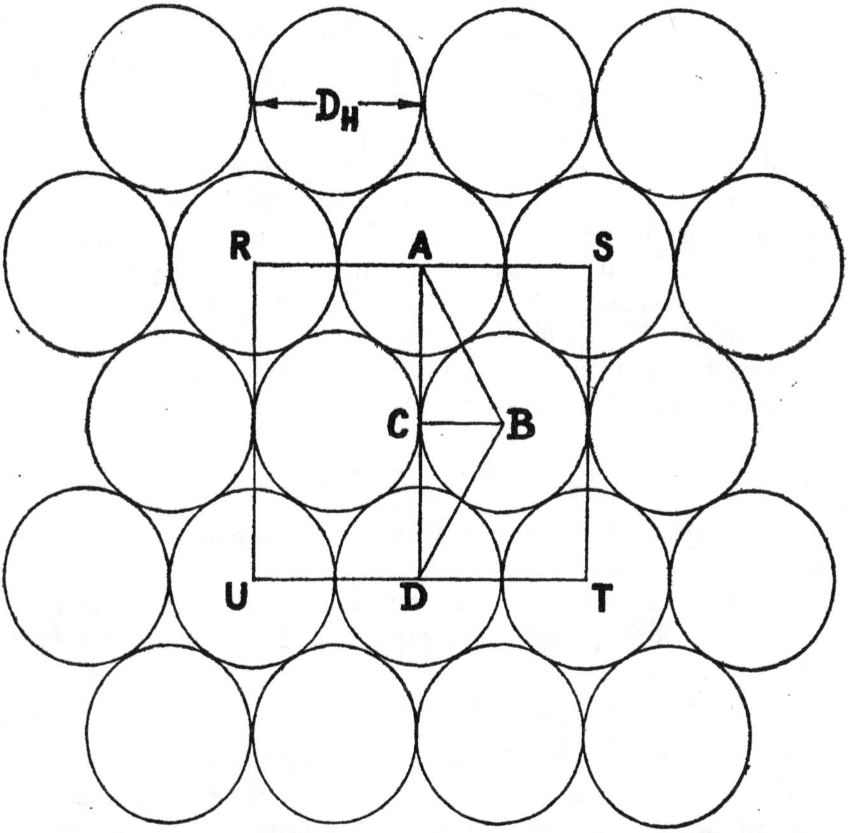

FIG. 74—Diagrammatic representation of a cross-secton of a tress of hair fibres in close-packed relationship.

In the particular case illustrated, hair fibres of uniform diameter are assumed to form a rectangle (*RSTU*) with one side equivalent to a total of two hair fibre diameters ($2D_H$). Due to close packing the second dimension is somewhat less than this amount, and it can be shown readily that it is equivalent to $\sqrt{3}\,(D_H)$. Therefore the area of the rectangle *RSTU* equals

$$A = 2(D_H) \times \sqrt{3}\,(D_H).$$

Since the equivalent of four fibres is inscribed in this rectangle the cross-sectional area of these hair fibres is given by the expression:

$$A' = \pi(D_H)^2.$$

The ratio of the area of the rectangle to the area of the fibres included within the rectangle is given by the following equation:

$$\frac{A}{A'} = \frac{2\sqrt{3}(D_H)^2}{\pi(D_H)^2} = \frac{2\sqrt{3}}{\pi} = 1{\cdot}1 \qquad (1)$$

It can readily be visualised that a tress of hair is made up of n rectangles each containing four fibres. Introducing n in equation 1, it will be found that it appears both in the numerator and denominator and hence will cancel out. Equation 1 is therefore of general nature, applicable to any number of fibres. A consideration of the equation for the value of A' indicates that in a given cross-sectional area this value must remain constant regardless of fibre diameter. If this be true then it follows that the volume of air space must also remain constant. In any tress of hair therefore, the capacity of the curl for permanent waving lotion—if it is assumed that all air will be dispelled—is constant.

Assigning the term N to the total number of hair fibres in any cross-section, the following relationship is arrived at:

$$N = \frac{A'}{\pi(D_H/2)^2} \qquad (2)$$

where A' equals the cross-sectional area of the hair fibres and D_H equals the diameter of each fibre.

A relationship between the reactive keratin surface (S) in terms of N, L (length of fibres) and D_H may then be established by the following equation:

$$S = \pi D_H \times L \times N \qquad (3)$$

In as much as the value for N varies inversely with the square of the radius of the hair fibres, it will be seen that the reactive keratin surface in a tress will be profoundly affected by the fibre diameter. For example, if the hair diameter is doubled, the number of fibres in a given cross-section will be reduced to one-fourth the previous numbers. Accordingly the keratin surface would be reduced by 50 per cent.

In deriving these equations it was assumed that all hair fibres are of uniform diameter and are wrapped in a uniform close-packed arrangement. It need not be emphasised that these conditions are idealised and are seldom realised under actual waving conditions.

In hair undergoing a cold wave treatment in which the tress is saturated with ammonium thioglycollate, the following reaction takes place:

$$\text{Hair—S—S—Hair} + 2HSCH_2COONH_4 \leftrightharpoons$$
$$2\ \text{Hair-SH} + NH_4OOCCH_2\text{—S—S—}CH_2COONH_4.$$

In the above equation Hair—S—S—Hair is used to represent a normal segment of a keratin molecule as shown in the figure below.

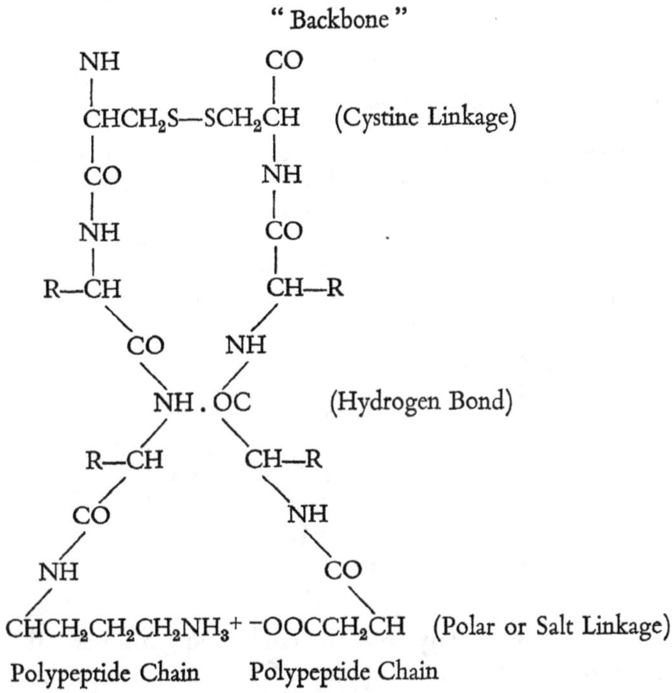

Hair—SH is used to indicate this segment after the reductive splitting of the disulphide bonds. Several methods have been used to follow the reduction of the disulphide bonds in hair undergoing a cold waving treatment. Reed, DenBeste, and Humoller (*J. Soc. Cosmet. Chem.*, March 1948) have used the Sullivan cystine method [*Publ. Hlth. Rep.*, *U.S.P.H.S.*, 1926, **41**, 1030 ; 1929, **44**, 1421] as modified in their laboratory, for following the action of thioglycollates on hair. The table on p. 448 shows the results obtained in one of these investigations.

It should be pointed out that in these studies small tresses of hair (about 1 g.) were reduced for the time stated by immersing them in a beaker containing a commercial cold wave lotion (—SH = 0·72 N ; pH = 9·2, at room temperature). The results show that under these rather drastic conditions the reduction is practically complete within four minutes and further treatment has very little effect upon the residual disulphide linkages. It should not be concluded from this experiment, however, that the same degree of reduction is obtained during the process of cold waving, for in this particular experiment a huge excess of ammonium thioglycollate was available whereas under normal waving conditions the amount of thioglycollate is limited by the ratio of capillary air space to the amount of hair on the curling rod, as previously discussed. It should also be realised that this amount of reduction is not necessary or even desirable in actual practice. One-fourth the amount of reduction quoted in the table is, so Reed *et al.* state, the degree of reduction obtained in an average cold wave. . . .

EFFECT OF TIME ON THE DEGREE OF REDUCTION OF HUMAN HAIR USING A COMMERCIAL COLD WAVING SOLUTION (DCR-3) AT ROOM TEMPERATURE

Reduction time Min.	*Cystine found per cent.*	*Average*
0—Control	17·0	
0—Control	16·0	16·5
4	3·0	
4	2·9	3·0
8	2·6	
8	2·6	2·6
14	2·4	
14	2·6	2·5
20	2·5	
20	2·4	2·5

". . . The final step in any process of cold waving consists of fixing the undulation produced by the wrapping of the hair around the curling rod and the subsequent action of the alkaline thioglycollate solution. Offhand, this would seem to be a very simple step since the oxidation of the sulphydryl groups alone may produce the desired effect. In actual practice this reoxidation is produced by the so-called neutralising or fixing lotions. Essentially these are dilute solutions of oxidising agents such as potassium bromate, hydrogen peroxide, potassium iodate, etc. If the fundamental aspects of this step are examined carefully, it soon becomes evident that it is far from being simple, and in fact it is as involved as the other steps in cold waving. One purpose of this step is to reorient the amino acid side chains in positions comparable to those which they had had before the ammonium thioglycollate was applied. Then, too, the swelling of the hair fibre must be reversed, the sulphydryl groups of the hair must not only be oxidised but re-oxidised to disulphides, and salt linkages and hydrogen bonds must be reformed in such a manner that the hair will retain its curled state even when exposed to the action of repeated shampoos and the elements.

"As was pointed out before, keratin, which has been swelled and reduced by the action of ammonium thioglycollate, shows a good deal more randomness in the arrangement of the amino acid side chains than untreated hair. When such hair is treated with an oxidising agent such as bromate or peroxide, disulphide bonds will be reformed. The amount of rebuilding of these bonds will be a function of several variables such as concentration of the oxidising agent, time of contact, and temperature. . . .

" . . . Considerable work has been done on the oxidation of sulphydryl compounds and disulphides by various workers. Thus Stoves (*Trans. Faraday Soc.*, 1942, **38**, 501) has contended that cystine links of keratin fibres are first hydrolysed by aqueous solutions of oxidising agents and the sulphur is then oxidised to sulphuric and sulphonic acid residues. Rutherford and Harris (*J. Res. nat. Bur. Stand.*, 1938, **20**, 559), working with wool, came to the conclusion that the action of hydrogen peroxide on keratin consists of the oxidation of the disulphides with the formation of disulphoxides and similar compounds. In another paper (*ibid.*, 1938, **20**, 563) these authors suggest that the disulphide sulphur of wool, exposed to the irradiation of a carbon arc, even in an atmosphere of nitrogen, will be oxidised in part to sulphuric acids. Lemin and Vickerstaff (*Proc. Symp. Fibrous Proteins*, Univ. Leeds, May 1946) also agree with Harris and co-workers that the action of hydrogen peroxide on keratin leads to the oxidation of disulphide bonds. It seems, therefore, that oxidation of hair or keratin does not necessarily stop at the cystine stage but will frequently go beyond it. This is a point which should be remembered when evaluating the efficacy of fixative or 'neutralising' agents."

Experimentally, as Reed *et al.* have pointed out, "it is possible to follow the oxidation of sulphydryl groups in hair quantitatively much more easily than to follow the other changes which occur in hair as a result of the oxidation step. One of the actions of ammonium thioglycollate is to swell the hair. In such hair it would seem that some of the pairs of sulphydryl groups are separated too far to allow their reoxidation to disulphides. The work of Phillips *et al.* (*Nature*, 1942, **150**, 57) on the oxidation of thioglycollate-reduced wool by oxygen also indicates that oxidation of sulphydryl groups to disulphides may not be as smooth a process as is generally conceived.

"It can be visualised that when reduced hair is treated with an excess of oxidising agent, be it hydrogen peroxide, bromate, or iodate, some of the sulphydryl groups will be in a fortuitous position so that they can be oxidised immediately to disulphides. Others will not be so situated and either will not be oxidised at all or will be oxidised to sulphuric or sulphonic residues. The number of disulphide bonds formed may be sufficient to give the hair a more or less permanent set. Yet, due to insufficiency of —S—S— bonds formed and the effect of the secondary valence bonds which eventually will be re-established in the fibre plus the tendency to a higher state of entropy, considerable strain is placed on the reformed disulphide bonds and it is therefore not surprising that in actual beauty-shop practice the relaxation of a 'permanent' wave is not uncommon."

Reed and his co-workers have drawn attention to the fact that "certain commercial waving processes have been designed to overcome this difficulty. In these processes an absorbent pad is placed around each curl after the waving lotion (ammonium thioglycollate) has acted sufficiently long and before the fixative (oxidising) solution is applied; these pads withdraw the excess waving lotion from the spaces between the fibres by capillary action. By removing the excess thioglycollate from the outside of the fibre without removing significant amounts of solution from within the fibre, they tend to reverse the action of the reducing agent. A little reflection will readily show that at the end of the reducing step the ratio of dithiodiglycollate to thioglycollate is higher within the fibre than it is outside of the fibre. Going back to the equation showing the reaction of hair with thioglycollates given at the beginning of this paper, it can certainly be expected that the reaction will not go any further to the right, but since it is an equilibrium reaction and it so happens that the Redox potentials of cysteine/cystine and thioglycollic acid/dithioglycollic acid systems are the same (Rykland and Schmidt, *Univ. Calif. Publ. Physiol.*, 1944, **8**, 257) it may be reversed.

"Under the influence of the absorbent pads we thus may have a partial reoxidation, which under optimum conditions may be sufficient to give some permanent set to the hair. The contribution of the absorbent pad to the success of the cold wave is more than inducing the reoxidation of sulphydryl group. By withdrawing the waving lotion from the air spaces surrounding the hair fibres and rebuilding some disulphide linkages, the absorbent pads initiate the deswelling of the hair fibres. Since this is a gradual and controllable process, it allows the amino acid side chains to reorient themselves in positions which are more favourable to the formation of desirable salt linkages and hydrogen bonds. But beyond this, the slow deswelling action of the absorbent pads permits the sulphydryl groups, which were spacially too far separated to be oxidised to disulphides, to be brought into juxtaposition so that they can be thus oxidised.

"Briefly stated, the function of the absorbent pad is therefore the initiation of the rebuilding of the covalent —S—S— bonds, the gradual deswelling of the hair fibres thus allowing the establishing of desirable co-ordinate valence bonds, and the bringing together spacially—SH groups, which would otherwise be resistant to oxidation to disulphides.

"In the discussion of the chemistry of the cold wave process the picture has been intentionally oversimplified. In the treatment of various steps it has been assumed that the hair fibre possesses a homogeneous structure. This obviously is not true. As yet, little is known as to what role the cuticle, the cortex, and the medulla play in the process of cold waving. The papers of Phillips [*Proc. Symp. Fibrous Proteins*, Leeds Univ., May 1946], Stoves [*Trans. Faraday Soc.*, 1942, **38**, 501 ; *Proc. Roy. Soc. Edinb., B*, 1945, **62**, 132], Lehmann [*Kol. Zeitsch.*, 1944, **108**, 6], Mercer and Rees [*Aust. J. exp. Biol. Med. Sci.*, 1946, **24**, 147], Hock and McMurdie [*J. Res. Nat. Bur. Stand.*, 1943, **31**, 229] and others indicate that the problem of the structure of keratin fibres, as related to their chemical reactivity, is receiving more and more attention."

The theoretical aspect of permanent waving having been discussed above, the rest of this chapter is devoted to the chemical and practical aspects of such waving.

Procedure (Methods involving Heat)

The professional procedure in hair waving is first to remove any grease from the hair by the application of a shampoo. The hair is then divided and wound around a suitable roller under slight tension. A sachet or absorbent strip dipped in a suitable solution is wound over the hair and the whole encased in an electric heater, and the hair *steamed* for the required period. It must be understood that the above description is modified somewhat according to whether the *sachet* or *oil* waving is being employed and according to the particular type of wave desired. Usually heat is supplied to the rollers by means of an electric current ; in the wireless system the heaters are previously heated and allowed to cool for the desired period. More recently chemical heating methods have been introduced which avoid the necessity of electrical heating with its attached wires. In these, moisture from the wrapper induces an exothermic, i.e. heat-evolving chemical reaction in contact with a suitable mixture. The advantages claimed for this latter system are that there is no risk of electric shock and the individual has freedom of head movement.

Permanent waving demands, in addition to suitable reagents, considerable professional skill and experience.

The selection of suitable methods of winding and of strengths and types of reagents, times of steaming, etc. (according to the type and condition of hair treated), is of paramount importance.

Claims are often made that (1) permanent waves are not so successfully given to a pregnant person as to one who is not pregnant, (2) that they are not so successfully given within four weeks of an ether anaesthetic as prior to the anaesthetic, and (3) that permanent waves are not successfully given when the menses are present.

These claims were discussed in "Queries and Minor Notes" (*J. Amer. med. Ass.*, 1943, **122**, 14) in answer to an inquiry when it was pointed out that with regard to statements (1) and (3) it has been shown by Baslet (*Med. Klin.*, 1930, **35**, 1111) by careful measurements of the pull needed to epilate hairs on the forearm and other parts of the skin, that the force necessary varies during the menstrual cycle—the hair becoming more firmly fixed in the skin just before the flow and less and less firmly fixed as menstruation began. After the menstrual flow ceased, the firmness of the hair in the skin returned to normal. *There is no definite proof, but it is possible that claims made by the hairdressers are correct.* Our knowledge of the changes in the skin and hair during menstruation and pregnancy and following parturition and surgical operations, in which ether anaesthesia was used, is very meagre.

Goodwin (*ibid.*, 1943, **123**, 11) however, considers that hair keratinised and erupted beyond the limits of the hair follicle is outside the sphere of influence of anything taking place inside the body and that only the freshly growing part of the hair within the follicle—the part not yet keratinised—is under the influence of the body. He points out that hairdressers have successful salons in hospitals and that the actual causes of failure are (1) taking too large a section of hair, (2) taking too small a section of hair, (3) too much alkali, (4) too little alkali, (5) too tight winding, (6) too loose winding, (7) too much time of steaming, (8) too little time of steaming. Studies on rubber ribbon have been supplemented by control experiments of permanent waving of human hair which has been removed from the head and in conclusion he points out that such suggestions provide excuses for the careless hairdresser, the hurried technician and the cut-rate shop operator who does not make a test curl.

The following formulae are illustrative of those used in permanent waving of the "heated" type; either electrically heated or chemically heated (the so-called "wireless type").

Permanent Waving Solutions

These are almost invariably strongly alkaline in reaction, since the presence of alkalis considerably shortens the time necessary to produce a satisfactory wave. Those recommended for such purposes include ammonium hydroxide, morpholine, triethanolamine, monoethanolamine, as well as borax and sodium and potassium carbonates and bicarbonates.

In view of the paucity of information concerning such preparations, the following examples may be of interest.[1] In my opinion the most satisfactory concentration is 0·88 ammonium hydroxide, in combination with a proportion of borax and/or sodium or potassium carbonate. The following formulae give good results on average hair in about 10 minutes' steaming time. (This being adjusted to suit the type of hair):

	per cent.
Ammonium hydroxide (s.p. 0·88)	20·0
Sodium carbonate	4·0
Potassium sulphite	2·0
Water	74·0

	per cent.
Ammonium hydroxide (s.p. 0·88)	14·0
Borax	4·0
Potassium sulphite	2·0
Water	80·0

The former formula gives somewhat better results and approaches a well-known proprietary product. The latter may be preferred, however, in some cases.

The use of an inorganic salt, usually an alkali such as borax, or the alkali carbonates, results in the production of a somewhat firmer wave, due possibly to the deposition of a film of the inorganic substance with consequent increase in the temperature attained by the hair shaft.

The interaction of the alkali in the waving solution with metallic salts present in the hair, either as a result of the application of a hair dye, or the ingestion of a medicinal preparation, may result in discoloration in some cases. To avoid this, a reducing agent, such as a few per cent. of an alkali sulphite, may be included.

Monoethanolamine (2-Hydroxyethyl amine)

This amine has many of the properties of triethanolamine but has a much greater alkalinity, being somewhat stronger even than ammonia. It is colourless, but has a distinctly ammoniacal odour, although this is

[1] It was essential that these solutions should be tried out by an expert in actual practice if these formulae were to be of any service as a basic guide for manufacturers, and the author acknowledges with thanks the assistance of Mr. A. T. Wardley, Professor of La Société de la Coiffure and International Hairdressers Society, London, in testing out the formulae quoted.

not too obvious in the diluted solution. The strengths usually recommended for this amine have been in the neighbourhood of 5 per cent. I find these too dilute to obtain results comparable with the more usual solutions. The following solution may be considered a basic guide for further experiments :

	per cent.
Monoethanolamine	14·0
Borax	4·0
Potassium sulphite	2·0
Water	80·0

If desired, the ammonia in permanent waving solutions may be partially replaced by ammonium carbonate, with the result of a more constant evolution of ammonia gas throughout the heating process.

More recently the sulphites of the amino compounds have been introduced commercially for permanent waving, for example, triethanolamine sulphite containing about 10-11½ per cent. SO_2 and monoethanolamine sulphite containing about 18–19 per cent. SO_2. Both these are equivalent to about 60 per cent. of the amino sulphite itself.

Recently three new amino compounds have been introduced in the United States, each of which is representative of a whole series of similar compounds, e.g. 2-methyl-2-amino propanol ; 2-methyl-2-amino-1,3-propanediol and trimethylaminomethane. These products are being advertised for the cosmetic industry, and it is likely that they may enter into the composition of permanent waving fluids of the future. In general, however, the chief proprietary preparations rely on ammoniacal preparations, which are efficient and cheap.

Ralph Auch (*Soap Perfum. Cosm.*, Jan. 1937, p. 43) has quoted a preparation which contains no ammonia as such but which has, he states, proved quite popular, and is indicated especially for hair that has been dyed, viz. :

	per cent.
Potassium sulphite	5·50
Borax	2·65
Sodium carbonate	0·45
Ammonium carbonate	0·25
Perfume	*q.s.*
Distilled water to	100·00

Paul Sorensen (*Drug Cosmet. Ind.*, 1938, **43**, 2, 161) states that the following formula is practically a universal solution which should give results with any hair and any operator, adding, that should this solution be too active and discolour dyed hair, some of the sulphite and the

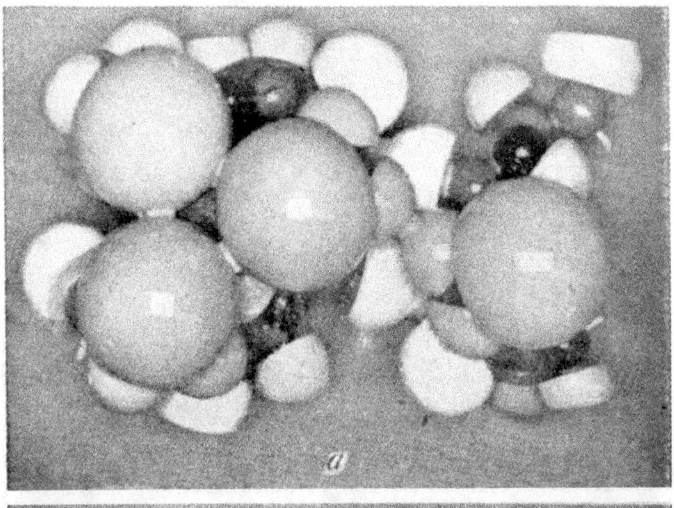

FIG. 75.—Close packing of side chains in the fold of Keratin and Myosin.

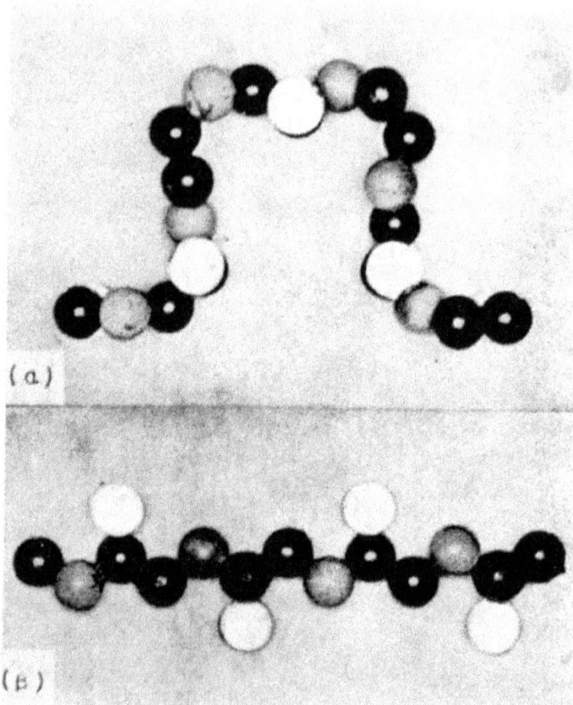

FIG. 76.—Skeleton models of a polypeptide chain in the extended α-form and the same chain folded into β-form proposed for the normal state of members of the k-m-e-f group of fibrous proteins. (White balls represent the side chains in rudiment.)

carbonates may be replaced by sodium bisulphite which has a bleaching effect :

	parts
Powdered borax	6·0
Sodium carbonate monohydrate	1·0
Ammonium carbonate	8·0
Sodium sulphite	4·0
Glycerin	1·0
Sulphonated olive oil	2·0
Water	106·0

F. Wall (*Amer. Perfum.*, June 1938, p. 40) has pointed out that volatile alkalis, such as ammonia, have advantages over the fixed alkalis, sodium and potassium, in that eventually nothing is left on the hair, whereas with other compounds a solid compound is left in and on the hair which tends to make it more dry or brittle. If borates or phosphates are used, this residue is almost like glass.

Chemical Heating Methods

Chemical heating methods have been introduced, in which the necessary heat required for the normal waving process is obtained without the aid of electricity. Such methods depend upon heat evolved by the reaction of an exothermic material with a moistening medium as a result of one of the following :

(1) Oxidation and reduction.

(2) Hydration.

(3) Chemical neutralisation.

The origin of this chemical method of permanent waving was in England, the original patents being taken out in 1923 by P. Sartory who founded the firm of Va-Per-Marcel Ltd. (Brit. Patent 225,256 ; U.S. Patent 1,565,509). These patents were concerned with the use of quick lime for the purpose of generating the heat.

In 1923 (U.S. Patent 1,892,389) Ralph Evans patented a method of "... imparting a permanent wave to hair by subjecting the hair to heat generated by the reaction of an exothermic material with a moistening medium, the natural development of the heat being delayed by combining a suitable medium with the moistening medium. . . ." It was the use of a delayed medium to prevent the pad evolving heat too rapidly which marked the advance over the earlier patent.

In this patent the heating agent was quicklime and the moistening agent contained ammonium sulphate, sugar or ammonia to delay development of heat.

Since that time numerous chemical mixtures have been recommended and patented, including as active agents aluminium and its chloride and sulphate, ammonium salts of various organic acids, barium salts, copper carbonate, nitrate, iron filings and salts, etc., etc.

As an illustration of some of the more important lines along which patents have developed, I can do no better than quote from an article by McDonough ("The Development of Machineless Waving", E. G. McDonough, *J. Soc. cosmet. Chem.*, 1948, **1**, 183). McDonough, discussing Winkel's invention (U.S. Pat. 2,051,063), points out that "... this involved the use of a single moisture-absorbent element to accomplish the following functions:

(i) to supply the water to initiate and continue the exothermic chemical reaction;

(ii) to serve as a wet shield to prevent the hair from being damaged by being heated to a high dry heat;

(iii) to serve as a fast heat conductant.

A second element in Winkel's invention involved the use of a flexible impervious envelope one face of which was perforated allowing water to be pressed through to the chemical reactant.

"In the very first stages of work on the Winkel machineless pad, it was recognised by Evans and McDonough that other exothermic chemical reactions would better serve to generate the heat than the hydration of lime, which Winkel's patent mentions as a suitable example of an exothermic reaction.

"Among the many reactions studied, the oxidation-reduction type of reaction involving the oxidation of a metal like aluminium with an oxidiser like a chlorate offered the most possibilities. The explosive violence with which aluminium combined with an oxidiser to generate a very intense heat and high temperature had been put to use in the metal thermit welding units of Goldschmidt.

$$Al + Fe_2O_3 \longrightarrow Al_2O_3 + Fe + \Delta$$

How to control this type of reaction became the subject of a research programme, giving rise to the invention specified in the Evans and McDonough patent U.S. Patent Re 22,660.

"Compositions utilising the oxidation of a metal, e.g. aluminium to generate heat for the permanent waving of hair have been disclosed in the Racen U.S. Patent, 2,183,587 and Reed's U.S. Patent 2,208,815.

"Apart from development of patents along the above lines, a second group of improvements was directed at pad construction to effect certain types of chemical reaction.

"Most basic of this group is the U.S. Patent 2,431,220 to Evans and McDonough. The broad concept of this patent is shown by the fact that before issuing it became involved in no less than seven interferences.

"That this pad covers the 'oil-fired' pad idea as well as the oxidation of sheet metal is shown by the following claim. Claim 5 states: A heating pad for the permanent waving of hair having ingredients, certain of which are unmixed but which when in sufficiently intimate contact with each other react to generate heat, certain of said ingredients when treated with a solvent passing into sufficiently intimate contact with the remainder of said ingredients to generate heat.

"U.S. Patent 2,239,410 to Bonat covered one specific composition of the so-called oil-fired pad. All the claims are directed towards a composition containing glycerine, whose oily feel in the absorbent gave rise to the term 'oil' pads.

"Similarly U.S. Patent 2,350,926 to Reed covers, as is shown in the following claim, the use of hexahydric alcohols such as sorbitol, mannitol, and dulcitol. A typical claim, 3, reads: A chemical composition capable of generating heat upon the addition of water thereto, said composition including a hexahydric alcohol and an oxidising agent comprising a permanganate which is sufficiently soluble in water to effect the heat-generating reaction upon addition of water to the composition.

"Various patents (2,132,681 to Davis, 2,133,115 to Reynolds, 2,144,811 to Reynolds, 2,153,671 to Markel and Reynolds, 2,153,676 to Reynolds, 2,153,677 to Reynolds, Reissue 21,276 to original 2,153,678 to Reynolds) have been issued on the use of oxidising of a sheet or sheets of aluminium foil. As stated above, the more important of these were losers in interferences with the Evans and McDonough U.S. Patent 2,431,220. . . ."

Whilst the above discussion has touched upon some of the more important patents, it does not cover all the patents involved in chemical methods of heating. The situation in respect of patents is very involved and intending manufacturers should make very careful enquiries as to the patent situation in their own country and the possibilities of infringements.

Cold Waving of Hair

The so-called cold waving of hair does not differ very much in basic principle from the methods already described. Instead of using a heated alkaline solution, however, it was found that by the use of certain reducing agents a break-down of the disulphide linkages of the keratin molecule could be achieved without the external application of any heating.

Some of these early preparations marketed for home use consisted of mixtures of sodium bisulphite or sodium sulphite together with added alkali such as sodium carbonate or sodium sesquicarbonate; for example, mixtures along the following lines:

	per cent.
Anhydrous sodium sulphite	50·0
Sodium carbonate	25·0
Sodium bicarbonate	25·0

about 15 g. of this mixture being dissolved in a sufficiency of water prior to use.

However, the development of cold waving based upon the use of neutralised, i.e. salts of thioglycollic acid, or allied mercaptans has resulted in the capture of the world markets by such products. It is stated (A. E. Bell, "Cold Waving and Other Industrial Uses of Thioglycollic Acid", *Mfg. Chemist*, July 1948, p. 295) that the possibilities of cold waving, especially in the form of a "home-kit", were considered so enormous that the Gillette Razor Co. in the U.S.A. were reported to have *then* paid £4,000,000 for the world rights of the Toni home-permanent-waving system.

The patent position has been the subject of considerable legal battles. The two basic patents involved in the battle of the machineless wave were U.S. Patent 2,051,063 and U.S. Patent Re 22,660; these two patents together covering every presently marketed means and method of machineless permanent waving [apart from the Sartory process which, as mentioned under "chemical heating methods" has apparently been successfully operated only by that firm]. Patent 2,051,063, the invention of Fred Winkel, is a basic pioneering patent of the machineless art whilst U.S. Patent Re 22,660, inventors Ralph L. Evans and E. G. McDonough, overcame some of the impractical aspects of the Winkel invention.

U.S. Patent 2,577,710 covers solutions for permanent waving, especially cold waving. While covering a group of chemical compounds and solutions for such purposes, the examples specifically recommended in the patent include compositions of the type used in the cold waving industry today. The types of mercaptan solutions covered include thioglycollic acid between 1 and 10 per cent. in which the *p*H is adjusted by ammonia to be higher than *p*H 7·0 and not higher than *p*H 9·5 preferably at about *p*H 9·2.

U.S. Patent 2,577,711 covers more specifically one class of mercaptans which, it is claimed, have unique qualities, namely the non-polar compounds of the hydroxyl type. Among these is the compound glyceryl monomercaptan (thioglycerol).

The following formula, illustrating the use of thioglycollate in a hair waving preparation, appeared in *Modern Cosmeticology*, R. G. Harry, Brooklyn, N.Y., 1947, Chemical Publishing Co. Inc., p. 310:

	per cent.
Ammonium thioglycollate	6·0
Distilled water (free from traces of copper or iron) . .	94·0
Adjusted to a pH *of* 9·5 *at* 20° C.	

A neutraliser is of course necessary with this formulation. One suggested formula for such a preparation is hydrogen peroxide (6 per cent. 50 cc., Tartaric acid 3 g., distilled water to make 100 cc. (*Drug Cosmet. Ind.*, Aug. 1952, p. 223).

Such solutions are not very stable. When sodium perborate monohydrate is used, stabilisers such as magnesium sulphate, sodium silicate and sodium pyrophosphate may be used. It is understood that at least some of these stabilisers are patented for use in this connection.

In waving with thioglycollate solutions the hair is first given a shampoo in the usual manner and is then wound upon rollers or curlers made of material which will not react with the thioglycollate. The hair is moistened thoroughly with the waving solution and, at the end of the required period, which may vary from 30 minutes to an hour, and before the hair is unwound from the curlers, it is treated with the arresting or "neutralising" agent which contains an oxidising compound, the function of which is to arrest the action of the thioglycollate. This stopping solution may consist of an acidified solution of hydrogen peroxide or other oxidising agent and it should be left on the hair for a time sufficient for it to penetrate the hair shaft and check the reducing action of the thioglycollate. This period of time should not be less than 5 minutes and when hydrogen peroxide is used as the arresting solution, the excess of thioglycollate should be rinsed off with water before applying the acid peroxide solution. (Theory—cf. pp. 443-451).

Owing to the reactivity of the thioglycollic acid molecule and the materials from which thioglycollic acid is prepared commercially,[1] various by-products are present in the commercial acid, the most important being dithioglycollic acid and thiodiglycollic acid. The complex nature of the sulphur bodies present in aqueous solutions of such thioglycollates is shown by the following analysis of a commercial

[1] *Manufacturing Note.*

The decomposition of thioglycollates is catalytically accelerated by minute traces of manganese, iron or copper and solutions of thioglycollates should be prepared in suitable vessels such as glass, porcelain or certain plastics. Traces of iron in the water will produce a red-violet coloration in the solution; this colour reaction is employed analytically in the determination of iron.

waving preparation quoted by Dahle and Newburger (*Amer. Perfum.*, Feb. 1945, p. 35):

	per cent.
Sodium thioglycollate	6·6
Sodium dithiodiglycollate	1·6
Sodium thiodiglycollate	3·0
Sodium chloride	8·0
Ammonia	1·0
Water	79·3
Undetermined	0·5

The analysis of the waving solution assumed that all of the sulphur not present as thioglycollic acid or as thiodiglycollic acid was present as the thioether, whereas it has been shown more recently that this is not strictly correct in that there may be large quantities of thioglycollide present which were previously assumed to be thioether (J. F. Mulvaney, "Chemical and Physical Properties of Thioglycollic Acid", *Proc. Sci. Sect. T.G.A.*, May 1946, p. 38).

Mulvaney has drawn attention to the fact that Bersin and Steudel (*Ber.*, 1938, **71**, B, 1015–1024) in a polarimetric study of the system

$$\text{1-Cystine} + 2\ \text{Thioglycollic Acid} \rightleftharpoons 2\text{1-Cysteine} + \text{Dithiodiglycollic Acid}$$

showed that this reaction was reversible and established the equilibrium at 50 per cent. conversion. Because of the competing reactions, an increase of the concentration of dithiodiglycollic acid should lower the effect of the reducing agent. This conclusion, Mulvaney states, has been verified in practice. Experiments have shown that the waving action of thioglycollic acid lotions decreases markedly as the concentration of the dithio acid increases. If more than 1 per cent. of dithiodiglycollic acid is present, the quality of the resulting wave is noticeably inferior.

Martin (U.S. Patent 2,350,178) claimed to overcome the disadvantage of older methods of permanent waving and to facilitate the cold wave procedure by the use of hydroxylamine sulphate as a cold waving agent, using thioglycollic acid as an accelerator. Thus the following solution is applied to the hair after it has been wound on rods:

Thioglycollic acid	10·0 g.
Sodium hydroxide	7·0 g.
Hydroxylamine sulphate	10·0 g.
Water	100 cc.

At the end of 15 minutes, the hair is treated with the following solution:

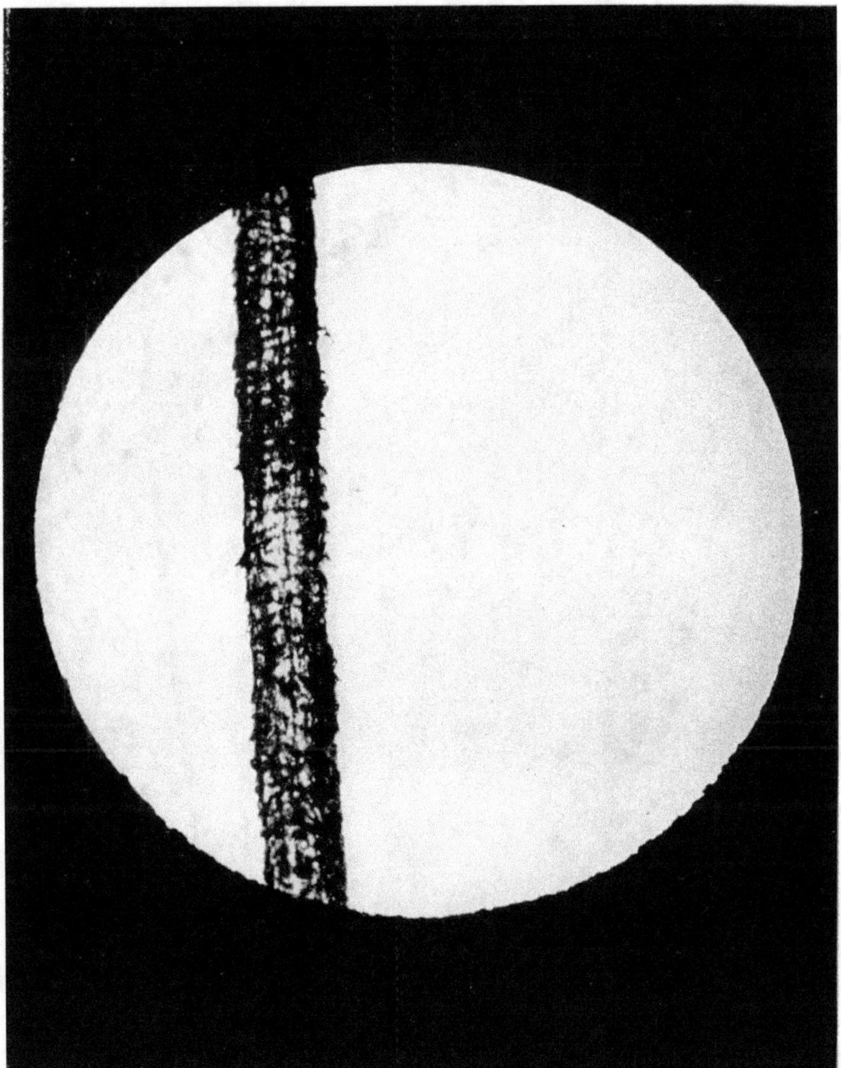

[*By courtesy of Reed, DenBeste and Humoller.*

FIG. 77.—Hair fibre showing physical damage to the cuticle. Fibres such as this will not " hold " a wave satisfactorily. (× 55) Basic Fuchsin.

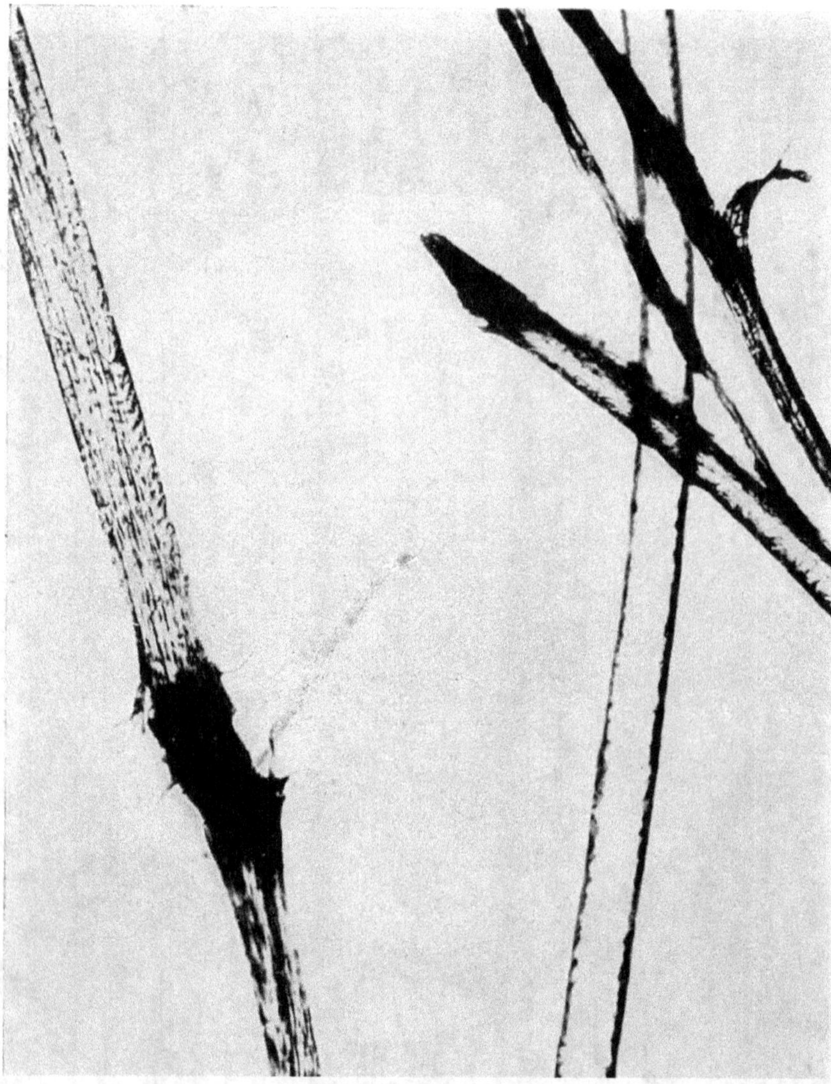

[*By courtesy of Reed, DenBeste and Humoller.*

FIG. 78.—Hair Fibre showing physical damage to the cuticle. Fibres such as this will not "hold" a wave satisfactorily. (× 55) Basic Fuchsin.

Water	500 cc.
Hydrogen peroxide (20 vol.)	500 cc.
Tartaric acid	30 g.

Cream Lotions for Cold Waving

According to U.S. Patent 2,464,280, stable cold-wave lotions having a creamy appearance and suitable viscosity may be prepared with the aid of wetting agents such as Triton 720. A typical cold-waving lotion is said to be made from thioglycollic acid (0·9 fl. oz.), ammonium hydroxide (1·66 fl. oz.), water (13·44 fl. oz.) and Triton 720 paste (3·0 fl. oz.). This lotion is said not to separate on standing and to be taken up rapidly by the air. If desired, a portion of the Triton paste may be replaced by Rhoplex, a water dispersion of acrylic acid copolymers (U.S. Patent 2,464,281).

Mace (U.S. Patent 2,479,382) claims that unusually stable ammonium thioglycollate emulsions, based upon the use of sorbitan mono-oleate, an oil-soluble non-ionic emulsifier known as Arlacel 80 in conjunction with a water-soluble derivative of sorbitan mono-oleate may be prepared. The following formula gives a stable emulsion of medium viscosity containing 8 per cent. by weight of ammonium thioglycollate. Examples of the types and proportions of constituents employed are given in the patent specification and one of these is quoted below :

	parts
Mineral oil	2·0
Lanolin	6·0
Chlorinated paraffin	15·0
Sorbitan mono-oleate	7·5
Sorbitan mono-oleate polyoxyalkylene derivative	15·0
Gelatin	0·5
Borax	40·0
Ammonium thioglycollate	40·0
Ammonia (as NH_3)	8·0
Water	to make 500

In the above formula, which is quoted as a "heavy" emulsion, the chlorinated paraffin is described as having 25 carbon atoms and 43 per cent. chlorine.

The Neutraliser in Cold Waving

The role of the neutraliser in cold waving has been discussed in earlier theoretical considerations given at the beginning of this chapter. Amongst the substances suggested for this purpose have been peroxides, bromates and perborates, etc. Peroxides are rather unstable and difficult to handle; bromates, whilst satisfactory in other respects, are very toxic and hence introduce potential hazards in the home particularly where young children may be about. Attention has been drawn recently (Soc. Cos. Chem. Meeting, June 1952, through *Amer. Perfum.*, June 1952) to the use of sodium perborate stabilised with sodium hexametaphosphate which is considered to be non-toxic and but mildly irritant if taken by the stomach or splashed in the eye.

The use of organic acids having an alpha-keto group as neutralisers for thioglycollate waving solutions has been patented by Halmos and Kollonitsch (Hungarian Patent 139,973); examples of such acids are pyruvic acid and benzylformic acid.

Recently Whitman (*Proc. Sci. Sect. T.G.A.*, Dec. 1952, p. 27) has discussed the role of the neutraliser in cold waving. *See also* Hamburger and Morgan (*loc. cit.* p. 44).

Cold Waving without an Oxidising Rinse

A patent covering the use of a " self-neutralising " cold wave, has been granted to Beste and Reed (Canadian Patent 465,446; U.S. Patent 2,564,722). In the customary procedure, the hair is treated with an oxidising rinse as mentioned above, in order to arrest the action of the waving solution and to restore the hair fibres to their original strength by the regeneration of the cystine linkages. In the new procedure, these oxidising reactions still take place but are effected by means of the oxygen of the air acting under the influence of a catalyst contained in the waving solution. It is claimed that by this process, a better control of the reducing reaction is obtained, and that the risk of injury to the hair and scalp is diminished. Moreover, the bleaching effect of peroxide rinses is said to be avoided.

As previously mentioned under thioglycollate cold waving, traces of metallic soluble salts, particularly of manganese, copper or iron have been, up to the present, considered as undesirable impurities, since, as pointed out by Mulvaney (*Proc. Sci. Sect. T.G.A.*, May 1946), the presence of 100 parts per million of copper in a thioglycollate lotion resulted in a loss of nearly half the thioglycollic acid content in one day when the solution was exposed to the air in a beaker.

In the patented self-neutralising cold wave, the auto-oxidation reaction is deliberately utilised as a means of limiting the action of the waving solution on the hair. If a manganese salt is incorporated in the waving lotion for this purpose, the recommended concentration is 100 to 300 p.p.m. of manganese.

A waving solution containing such addition might have the following composition :

Ammonium thioglycollate	0·7 normal
Ammonium hydroxide	0·7 normal
Hydrated manganous chloride	720 p.p.m.
Aerosol AY	0·6 per cent.
Water	to 100 per cent.

The Use of Amino-Sulphides as Cold Waving Agents

Schwarzkopf (Austrian Patent 166,240, June 1950) describes the application of substituted ammonium sulphides in which monoethanolamine, or some other alkanolamine, is reacted with hydrogen sulphide. Monoethanolamine sulphide is said to give the most satisfactory results. This substance, it is stated, may be prepared by dissolving 5 parts of monoethanolamine in 45 parts of water and saturating the solution with hydrogen sulphide. The solution is adjusted to a *p*H of between 9·0 and 11·0 by the addition of excess monoethanolamine or of concentrated ammonia. The range of concentration of monoethanolamine sulphide covered for use in such preparations is 5–15 per cent. A neutralising rinse is required and the oxidising agents recommended are those usually employed in connection with thioglycollate cold-wave solutions, e.g. hydrogen peroxide, potassium bromate, etc.

Dermatological Action of Cold-Waving Solutions

Used with due care the sulphite-carbonate home-wave kits do not appear to involve any dermatological hazard, providing the material is employed at the specified strength and for the specified time and is not splashed carelessly on the scalp of an individual who is hypersensitive to alkali.

The safety of the thioglycollic waving preparations has given rise to much controversy but it is now generally conceded by leading authorities that their use by normal healthy individuals, according to the directions given by the manufacturer, does not involve hazard.

Cotter (*J. Amer. med. Ass.*, 15 June 1946) reported five cases, which he said were selected from a large group (number not stated) showing the damaging effects of thioglycollates. McCord (*ibid.*, 29 June) stated that thioglycollic acid or its alkaline salts, in concentrations below 8 per cent., did not produce primary skin irritation, and that he had not seen evidence of sensitisation or allergic responses to solutions prepared with properly purified materials. The formation of hydrogen sulphide in the solution on keeping could be controlled by stabilisers.

Cappel and Cappel (*Amer. Perfum.*, Aug. 1946, p. 43) have also reported a limited number of tests with thioglycollates, as a result of which they consider that from 4-7 per cent. of ammonium thioglycollate at a *p*H from 9·0 to 9·6 may be applied to normal healthy human skin without reddening or blistering, and that contact periods of up to 24 hours are without danger. They should not, however, in their opinion, be applied to abraded or broken skin.

H. T. Behrman has pointed out (*The Scalp in Health and Disease*, p. 139, London: Henry Kimpton, 1952) that on perusal of the case histories reported by Cotter, the latter was not justified in drawing such a definite inference regarding the effect of thioglycollates. Behrman reports the results of studies by himself and colleagues on ". . . normal subjects and on subjects with various skin diseases; on persons with no known contact with cold wave solutions; and on many in intimate and prolonged contact, in order to delineate fully and critically the part played by cold-wave lotions on the health of that part of the population most likely to come in contact with these materials. Over 1,200 persons in varying degree of contact with such preparations were used as subjects. . . ." Patch tests and physical examinations were performed on 931 individuals many of them engaged in the manufacture of cold-wave preparations; examinations were also made of the scalps of 174 women undergoing actual waves with commercial waving solutions—each of these women had had from one to twenty cold waves.

The composite conclusions reached showed that cold-wave preparations of the type investigated, exhibited only a very low level of skin irritation and a low sensitising potential and that cutaneous reactions from contact or exposure to these materials are of negligible incidence. No evidence of systemic toxicity from frequent exposure to cold-wave solutions was found and it was concluded that cold-wave lotions of the composition used in this study were safe for general use. [In order that the test might have "practical" value the material employed was a commercial home cold wave rather than an empirical solution of a salt of thioglycollic acid; *see* Behrman, Coombes, Weissberg, Mulinos and Hurwitz, "The Cold Permanent Hair-Waving Process", *J. Amer. med. Ass.*, 1949, **140**, 1208; also Siegel and Meltzer, "Patch Tests Versus Usage Tests with Special Reference to Volatile Ingredients", *Arch. Derm. Syph.*, 1948, **57**, 660.]

Behrman points out that thioglycollates probably owe their hair-waving activity to the sulphydryl group, a group that is of great physiological importance and one that can act as a detoxifying agent. In this connection he illustrates the success of dimercaprol [the British

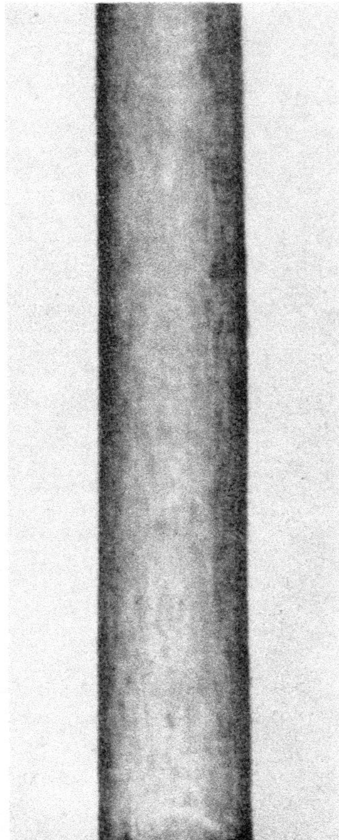

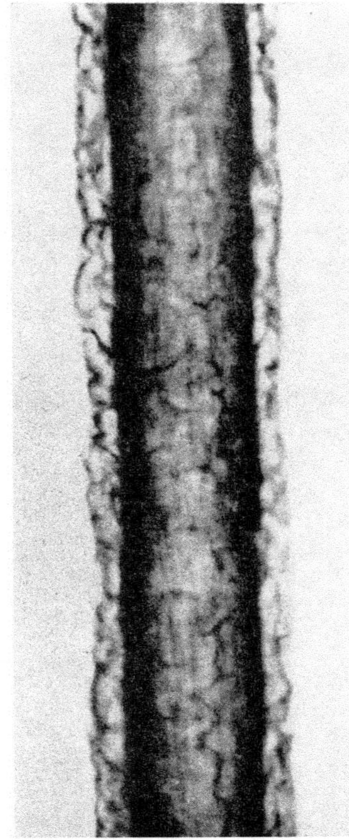

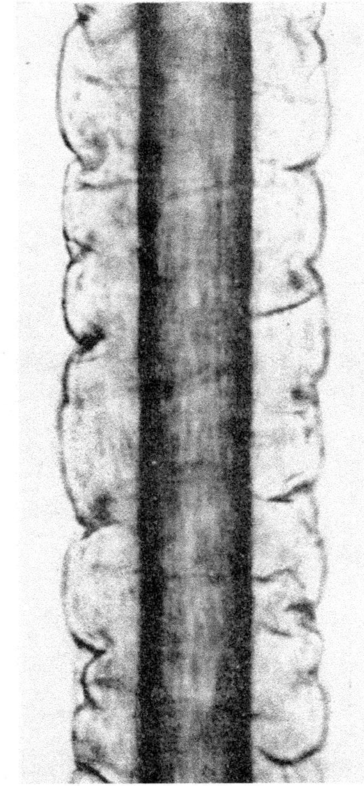

[*By courtesy of R. L. Evans* (*Proc. Sci. Sect. T.G.A., Dec.* 1948.)

FIG. 79.—Raw hair in solution of glycerol and water (× 280).

Hair after $1\frac{3}{4}$ minutes in 3 per cent. Thioglycollate solution of *p*H 12·5 (× 280).

Hair after $2\frac{3}{4}$ minutes in 3 per cent. Thioglycollate solution of *p*H 12·5 (× 280).

Anti-Lewisite (BAL), a dimercaptopropanol] in the treatment of heavy metal poisoning.

In my opinion there is no doubt that ammonium thioglycollate waving preparations, prepared along the lines specified in the Evans-McDonough patents, are safe when used according to the directions given in the home-wave kits and represent no undue dermatological hazard.

CHAPTER 24

HAIR-SETTING LOTIONS AND LACQUERS

Hair-setting lotions, also known as finger wave lotions, wave sets, etc., are used periodically by ladies to keep the waves in the hair *set*, and consist of vegetable mucilages, together with a little alcohol, suitably preserved.

A little alkali is sometimes included since it tends to soften the cuticle, and renders the hair shaft more amenable to setting.

This appears to be the only field in cosmetics and toilet preparations which has not undergone any revolutionary changes. Cellulose preparations in general have not as yet been very successful owing to the residue which they leave on the hair shaft. Certain hexitol derivatives offer important possibilities.

Gum Tragacanth

This is commonly used not only for setting lotions for ladies but also for fixative lotions for men. The following is an example of its use for the former :

	per cent.
Gum tragacanth	1·2
Alcohol	10·0
Glycerin	5·0
Water	83·8
Preservative	*q.s.*

Gum Karaya

This may be used in place of gum tragacanth. It has the advantage of forming a clear solution, but on the other hand such mucilages occasionally appear to thin on standing.

	per cent.
Gum karaya	1·5
Borax	1·5
Alcohol	10·0
Water	82·0
Glycerin	5·0
Preservative	*q.s.*

Quince Seeds

About 2·5 per cent. of the seeds produce a suitable mucilage which requires only the addition of alcohol and preservative. Alternatively, a stock of 4 per cent. mucilage of quince may be diluted as required, but this must be well preserved as it is very prone to mould growth.

	per cent.
2 per cent. quince seed mucilage in water	90·0
Alcohol	10·0
Preservative	*q.s.*
Colour	*q.s.*
Perfume	*q.s.*

Irish Moss

Irish moss makes a very satisfactory hair setting preparation :

	per cent.
Irish moss	2·0
Water	98·0
Preservative	*q.s.*
Colour	*q.s.*
Perfume	*q.s.*

Water-soluble mucilages extracted from Irish moss are available commercially in powdered form under various trade names ; these consist of calcium carragheen sulphate. Part of the water, about 10 per cent. in the above formulation, may be replaced by alcohol to speed up drying.

Sodium Alginate

The following formulation is claimed to hold curls effectively in position and to be cheap and easy to make :

	parts
Manutex SA/KP (Alginate Industries Ltd.)	5·0
Industrial alcohol	28·0
Preservative (Nipagin M)	0·6
Colour	0·002
Perfume (Cologne)	3·0
Water to	600·0

(*Courtesy Alginate Industries Ltd.*)

Other substances used for this purpose are Psyllium seed, and synthetic cellulose derivatives such as carboxymethylcellulose derivatives at a level of about 1 per cent. Carob gum at a level of about 0·5 per cent.

has also been recommended by Janowitz (*Soap Perfum. Cosm.*, Feb. 1945, p. 134).

Wave-Set Powders for Home Use

These may be prepared by mixing the powdered gum with any other powdered constituents in the formulation. Karaya gum is readily soluble in water and may conveniently be used for such products, as may also sodium alginate. Gum acacia may also be used but weight for weight gives a much thinner mucilage than karaya or tragacanth:

	per cent.
Gum karaya powder	30·0
Gum acacia powder	47·0
Borax	15·0
Sodium carbonate	8·0
Perfume	*q.s.*

[10 g. of the above mixture are sufficient for about 1 pint of water.] The powdered constituents are given a dry mix and the perfume, in a little alcohol, sprayed into the mix. The alginates lend themselves to similar preparations.

Apart from straight setting lotions, there was a temporary vogue about the year 1949 for something "different" in this field and gelatin capsules containing iron in solution were sold as "Curl Capsules" under various proprietary names. Preparations containing metal salts such as the above, involve hazard in two ways. In the first place any iron salts in the hair may react with ammonium thioglycollate waving solutions giving "off-colours" and in the second case, if hydrogen peroxide is applied in alkaline solution (either for home or professional bleaching, prior to re-tinting or platinum-blonding, or even in the application of an oxygenating neutraliser in the cold wave) the iron salts may act catalytically to yield oxygen at very high reaction speeds with damage to the hair fibre.

A rather different type of hair-wave capsule, containing gums, borax, sodium sulphite and boric acid was quoted in the *Chem. & Drugg.*, 10 Dec. 1949, p. 806, viz.:

	per cent.
Gum acacia	15·0
Gum tragacanth	10·0
Borax	20·0
Sodium sulphite	10·0
Boric acid	45·0
Perfume	*q.s.*

[It is stated that the above mixture is encapsulated, 2 g. per dose. One capsule is dissolved in a small cupful of water and the solution combed into the hair and allowed to dry without further treatment.]

Hair Lacquers

The development of the upswept coiffure led to a demand for a quick-drying preparation which would impart just sufficient rigidity to the " set " to keep it in place, would control loose ends and would not detract from the natural sheen of the hair.

During the war, shortage of shellac led to the use of various substitutes but it appears that these were not all as innocuous as they should have been. Schwartz (" An outbreak of dermatitis from Hair Lacquer ", *Publ. Hlth. Rep., Wash.*, 1943, 29 Oct., **5**, 1623) drew attention to the fact that before the war shellac was a constituent of hair lacquers but when supplies became scanty, substitutes were used. Two substitutes were synthetic resins ; these were obtained by the manufacturers from widely different sources but each contained resin and maleic anhydride. Complaints of dermatitis were received from many people who had used lacquers containing these resins, and patch tests showed that the lacquers were the cause of the dermatitis, which was apparently due to *sensitisation* rather than to primary irritation. The alkalinity of one of the products (*p*H 9·0), and the strong acidity of the other, aided the penetration of the resin into the skin. Lacquers containing genuine shellac but rarely cause dermatitis.

deNavarre (*Amer. Perfum.*, Aug. 1948, p. 117) has pointed out that hair lacquers are essentially 8–15 per cent. solutions of solubilised shellac, the shellac having been rendered soluble by the use of soda, or borax with or without ammonia. These fixed alkalis render the lacquer readily removable by washing the hair. The following formula appeared in the *American Perfumer*, July 1950 :

	lb.
Shellac (bleached, dewaxed)	3·5
Ammonium hydroxide (28 per cent.)	0·5
Water	32·0

Procedure

Add the ammonia and about half the water to the shellac and warm with constant stirring until solution is obtained. Add the rest of the water ; the solution should be clear (if not, more ammonia should be added), filter and cool. (This solubilised-shellac may then be diluted for use.)

It is a *sine qua non* that excess alkali be avoided, otherwise skin irritation due to the alkali itself and not to the shellac may result.

If proprietary shellac derivatives are employed in such lacquers, the manufacturer should take steps to see that the finished preparation is neither a primary irritant nor a sensitiser before marketing. Even in the absence of such derivatives, the alkalinity of such preparations should be checked in the laboratory (and by skin tests prior to marketing) because of the possible influence of other factors, e.g. perfume which may be included in the formulation.

A rather different type of lacquer is produced by the use of "non-solubilised" gums and resins as, for example:

	per cent.
Rosin	1·0
Gum Benzoin	2·0
Alcohol	97·0

The author is not in favour of such non-solubilised products.

CHAPTER 25

HAIR BRILLIANTINES, CREAMS AND FIXATIVES

THESE are used to impart a lustrous sheen to the hair, and in the case of the heavier types, as fixatives. Their use is by no means confined to the mere male. Preparations of lighter viscosity, particularly of the petroleum oil type, when delicately perfumed, form an essential part of feminine cosmetics.

Excessive or unskilled hair bleaching and dyeing, or continued exposure to sunlight (particularly after immersion in sea water), make the hair dull and brittle. Warm brilliantine is often applied to the head to overcome these defects in the hair.

Single solution, or non-separable brilliantines, usually consist of light white mineral oil, with or without the addition of vegetable oils. A typical formula for a simple preparation being :

	per cent.
Light mineral oil	99·0
Perfume	1·0
Dye (oil-soluble)	*q.s.*

The perfume must be specially compounded otherwise cloudiness may result, owing to the relative insolubility of the majority of perfume constituents in mineral oil. Alternatively, olive oil may be included in the formulae as described below.

Often a little vegetable oil is incorporated with the mineral oil. This serves a useful purpose in that many perfumes which are practically insoluble in liquid petroleum may be incorporated by previously dissolving them in a vegetable oil, this being then mixed with the mineral oil. Now that olive oil is obtainable in a deodorized perfumery quality, this is pre-eminently the best medium for such a purpose, and a stock solution containing about 10 per cent. of the perfume may be prepared, allowed to mature, and added to the main bulk as desired.

Numerous other oils may be included to suit any particular purpose, including almond, apricot kernel, deodorised olive, arachis, grape-seed, avocado, castor, turtle, etc. There appears little justification for the use of the more expensive almond oil, when apricot oil may replace it. (R. G. Harry, " The Chemical and Physical Examination of Almond and Apricot Kernel Oils ", *Pharm. J.*, 22 Feb. 1936 ; also R. G. Harry, " Skin Penetration ", *Brit. J. Derm.*, March 1941).

The day of the heavy brilliantine has waned. The modern aim is to secure a glossy sheen and light fixative action without the suggestion that it has been plastered down. Formerly, it was not possible to incorporate a suitable volatile oil in a mineral oil base, but by the use of deodorised kerosene, or esters such as isopropyl myristate, a fine film of the oil may now be deposited on the hair shaft.

The addition of an antioxidant is useful in checking rancidity in vegetable oils. (*See* Antioxidants.)

Numerous oil-soluble dyes are obtainable for colouring purposes. By the addition of deodorised kerosene, the viscosity of light petroleum oil may be further reduced ; such preparations lend themselves to spraying on the hair :

	per cent.
Light mineral oil	60·0
Deodorised kerosene	40·0
Colour	*q.s.*
Perfume	*q.s.*

If it is desired to add vegetable oils, olive, avocado, apricot kernel, or sesame may replace part of the mineral oil. Because of the tendency of the majority of vegetable oils to rancidity, the addition of a suitable antioxidant to such preparations is necessary.

Alternatively isopropyl myristate may be employed together with, if desired, a small proportion of lanolin, viz. :

	per cent.
Isopropyl myristate	24·0
Lanolin	1·0
Light mineral oil	75·0
Colour	*q.s.*
Perfume	*q.s.*

Alcoholic or Spirituous Brilliantines

These are solutions of castor oil in alcohol (occasionally in rectified spirit) suitably coloured and perfumed. They do not possess very marked fixative properties although, *if the hair is combed with a damp comb immediately after application*, the precipitation of the castor oil in a finely dispersed form gives sufficient body to act as a fixative for hair that is not very dense:

	per cent.
Castor oil	20·0
Industrial alcohol	80·0
Perfume	*q.s.*
Colour	*q.s.*

Preparations such as the above, with or without the addition of an antiseptic, have enjoyed, and do enjoy, a fair sale in different countries. The greatest drawback to castor oil brilliantines is their distinctive odour on ageing. Although *the solution in alcohol*, when suitably perfumed, may not smell of castor oil, in use the oil is deposited in the wad of the bottle, and particularly along the threads of the bottle neck ; this develops a distinctive castor oil odour in time. Unless the hair is washed fairly frequently, a slight castor oil smell may also develop on the heads of the users.

The substitution of oleyl alcohol provides an alternative formulation, viz. :

	per cent.
Oleyl alcohol (best)	18·0
Alcohol	82·0
Colour	*q.s.*
Perfume	*q.s.*

Such a preparation does in time develop a somewhat fatty odour around the bottle neck and on brushes, etc., but is not as objectionable as castor oil. The introduction of isopropyl myristate allows for an even more satisfactory product in respect of odour. Unfortunately both of these preparations lack fixative properties though they are useful, with suitable additions of perfume and antiseptics (if desired), as a friction lotion or as a dressing by the older man with thinning hair :

	per cent.
Isopropyl myristate	20·0
Cetyl alcohol	2·0
Alcohol	78·0
Colour	*q.s.*
Perfume	*q.s.*

The development of hydrophilic derivatives of beeswax and lanolin respectively, has opened a wide field for cosmetic development along such lines. Formerly the cosmetician was handicapped in that, to obtain solubility of certain ingredients, a high alcohol concentration was necessary and in this concentration other desirable ingredients were sometimes insoluble. The development of hydrophilic " tailored " molecules of widely used cosmetic substances considerably extends the scope of development in such fields.

Methods of producing transparent dispersions of certain oily and fatty materials in water have been patented by Cordero (U.S. Patent 2,402,373). The surfactants employed are the lauric acid monoesters of the sorbitol anhydrides (sorbitans) or mannitol anhydrides (mannitans) and condensation products of these esters with ethylene oxide. As an example of such formulation is mentioned . . . a solution of modified mannitan monolaurate (19 parts), in water (19 parts), is added to a mixture of sorbitan monolaurate (12 parts), deodorised light petroleum distillate (45 parts), and light mineral oil (5 parts). As the aqueous solution is mixed with the oils, the mixture, it is stated, becomes first thin and cloudy and then thick and clear. Additional ingredients, if soluble in either the oil fraction or the aqueous fraction, may be dissolved in a mixture of this kind without affecting the transparency.

Other transparent preparations, this time of the polyalkylene glycols, have been patented for use as hair dressings, Wilkes and Wassell (U.S. Patent 2,309,722). The following claim is illustrative ". . . A toilet preparation for dermal application containing as an essential ingredient a polyoxyalkylene glycol of the 1,2 series containing not more than 3 carbon atoms in each oxyalkylene radicle, said polyoxyalkylene glycol having an average molecular weight not less than about 400. . . ."

It is claimed that hair dressings with these glycols impart a well groomed appearance without excessive stickiness or oily appearance, and that further, because of their complete solubility in water, these dressings can be applied and distributed evenly without the use of organic solvents.

Solid Brilliantines

These consist of suitably hardened, tinted and perfumed petroleum jelly. For the purpose of hardening the jelly, paraffin wax, ozokerite, beeswax, ceresin, carnauba wax or one of the synthetic waxes may be employed. A simple mixture which is satisfactory is:

	per cent.
Petroleum jelly	90·0
Paraffin wax (uncrystallisable)	10·0
Colour	*q.s.*
Perfume	*q.s.*

or a slightly more complex mixture:

	per cent.
Carnauba wax	5·0
Paraffin wax	5·0
Petroleum jelly	70·0
Mineral oil	20·0

Lourie (*Soap Perfum. Cosmet.*, April 1940) has suggested the following:

	parts
Mineral oil	150
Rosin (WW)	60
Paraffin wax	30
Petroleum jelly (pale yellow)	20

Lourie states that the above composition "... congeals very slowly but gives a stable, brilliant, easily spread and perfectly satisfactory hair-grooming fixative. The addition of paraffin wax is necessary, because rosin, though very hard at ordinary temperatures, does not yield a solid composition on cooling, after having been incorporated in hot oil ... too high a proportion of rosin should be avoided as it tends to give a fixative that is too sticky in character. The addition of petroleum jelly is intended to inhibit exudation of oil; it also adds considerably to the plasticity and general appearance of the finished preparation. Rosin tends to improve the consistency and gloss. ..."

Two-Solution or Separable Brilliantines

These may be prepared by adding a solution of the desired perfume in the requisite amount of alcohol to light mineral oil. It is usual to colour both the oily and alcoholic layers a similar colour:

	per cent.
Industrial alcohol	60·0
Light mineral oil	40·0
Spirit-soluble yellow dye	*q.s.*
Oil-soluble yellow dye	*q.s.*
Perfume	*q.s.*

The product may be varied by altering the ratio of the alcoholic to oily phases, and may be cheapened by using a diluted alcohol (providing the strength is sufficient to dissolve the desired perfume or alternatively that the perfume is formulated so that it is soluble either in the oil phase or in the diluted aqueous-alcohol phase).

Rider and Gershon (U.S. Patent 2,543,061) have patented a two-layer brilliantine which emulsifies rapidly on shaking the bottle, but rapidly separates into two layers when not in use. It is claimed that by this means, the bulk of the oil (which is vegetable oil) is removed from contact with the water with, consequently, less tendency to rancidity. Olive oil is the vegetable oil employed in the formulation, and a combination of an oil-soluble and water-soluble emulsifier is employed. The oil-soluble emulsifier is Atlas Emulsifier G-1165 (*see* Emulsions and Dispersions), which is described as the tetraoleate of a polyoxyethylene derivative of propylene glycol glucoside, whilst the water-soluble emulsifier is a quaternary ammonium salt, especially of the "Emulsept" type.

The quaternary ammonium compound confers some antiseptic action upon the preparation. Tocopherol (vitamin E) is incorporated in the oil phase and sodium bitartrate in the water phase to protect the oil against rancidity:

Hair Dressing

Oil Phase	*per cent.*
Olive oil	7·64
Atlas G-1165 emulsifier	0·33
Tocopherol concentrate (34 per cent.)	0·08
Perfume	0·21
Water Phase	
Ethyl alcohol	40·50
Water	49·80
"Emulsept"	0·34
Sodium chloride	1·07
Sodium bitartrate	0·03

NON-OILY FIXATIVES, MUCILAGES, ETC.

As contrast to the oily types of fixatives discussed above, mucilages, chiefly based upon gum tragacanth, became popular. These possess vastly improved fixative properties and do not produce greasy stains on hats, etc. On brushing the hair, this setting is lost, and the particles of gum which flake off tend to accumulate on scalp and clothes. Moreover, the resultant hair may acquire a dull appearance, although this difficulty can be sometimes overcome by the addition of a proportion (up to 15 per cent.) of coloured and perfumed oils.

GUM TRAGACANTH. Gum tragacanth varies enormously in its mucilaginous properties, and a source of supply should be standardised and a check kept on the viscosity of its resultant mucilage.

Occasionally these products lose their opacity. In order to reduce this tendency to a minimum, a good quality gum should be used and a small proportion of castor oil and up to 10 per cent. of alcohol should be included, e.g.:

	per cent.
Gum tragacanth (powdered)	1·0
Alcohol	6·0
Castor oil	2·0
Water	90·0
Glycerin	1·0
Preservative	*q.s.*

If desired, about 10 per cent. oil may be added to this cream. In its manufacture, the gum should be dispersed in the alcohol, the perfume and any oils added, and the aqueous solution run in with continuous agitation. The cream is allowed to stand to thicken, re-stirred, filtered through muslin and bottled. The addition of a little tincture of benzoin, tolu, or styrax assists in increasing the whiteness of the product.

GUM KARAYA. Gum karaya may be employed instead of gum tragacanth, and it is claimed that if a good clean grade is employed, and alkali rigidly excluded, such preparations have little tendency to flake on the hair.

	per cent.
Gum karaya	2·0
Alcohol	5·0
Water	93·0
Perfume	*q.s.*
Preservative	*q.s.*

The method of preparation is similar to the above, and oil may be similarly added.

Hair Creams (Oil-in-Water Type)

Stable oil-in-water creams of varying viscosities may be obtained by the use of triethanolamine stearate, together with, if higher viscosity is desired, some fatty alcohol, such as cetyl alcohol. The following exemplifies a simple formulation along these lines:

	per cent.
White mineral oil	45·0
Stearic acid	3·5
Triethanolamine	1·5
Water	50·0
Preservative	*q.s.*
Perfume	*q.s.*

By addition of 1 to 3 per cent, cetyl alcohol the viscosity may be increased.

Druce (*Mfg. Chemist*, Nov. 1949, p. 11) has described the formulation of a hair cream incorporating triethanolamine and borax as alkalis and stearic acid and beeswax as the source of fatty acids, viz.:

	parts
Mineral oil	33·00
Beeswax	3·00
Stearic acid	0·50
Cetyl alcohol	1·30
Borax	0·25
Triethanolamine	1·85
Water	59·80
Chlorocresol	0·10
Perfume	*q.s.*

Procedure

The oils, fats and waxes are melted at 60°-65° C. and added to the aqueous phase containing the triethanolamine and borax at the same temperature. The cream is then stirred and cooled.

[It is stated that the above cream was shelf-tested over a period of two years in the laboratory without separation.]

Glyceryl monostearate, self-emulsifying grade, may also be employed for the manufacture of hair creams; the following formula exemplifies the use of "Tegin" in this connection (Courtesy Goldschmidt Chemical Corporation, New York):

	per cent.
Tegin (Goldschmidt Corp.)	3·0
Mineral oil	8·0
Petrolatum	3·0
Propylene glycol	5·0
Paraffin wax	1·5
Stearic acid	1·0
Water	78·4
Preservative (Tegosept P.)	0·1

By the use of Diglycol laurate, stable emulsions may be obtained in the cold:

	per cent.
Diglycol laurate (Glyco Inc.)	14·0
White mineral oil	36·0
Water	50·0
Preservative	*q.s.*
Perfume	*q.s.*

A simple formulation utilising Diglycol stearate has also been suggested (*Drug Cosmet. Ind.*, Jan. 1949, p. 125):

	parts
Diglycol stearate	12·0
Liquid petrolatum	35·0
Water	120·0
Perfume	*q.s.*
Preservative	*q.s.*

The following two formulations of the oil-in-water type exemplify the use of the more recently introduced non-ionic emulsifiers.

		per cent.
A	Petrolatum	6·0
A	Mineral oil 65/75	37·5
A	Lanolin (anhydrous)	3·0
A	Beeswax	12·0
A	"Arlacel" C. (sorbitan sesquioleate)	3·0
A	Span 20 (Sorbitan monolaurate)	1·0
A	Tween 20 (Polyoxyethylene sorbitan monolaurate)	2·0

		per cent.
B	Borax	0·5
	Water	35·0
	Preservative	*q.s.*
C	Perfume	*q.s.*

Procedure

Heat (A) to 70° C. and (B) to 75° C. Add (B) to (A) slowly with agitation. Perfume at 45° C. and stir till cold.

		per cent.
A	Petrolatum	7·5
	Mineral oil 65/75	37·5
	Beeswax	2·0
	Atlas G-1425 modified lanolin	4·5
	"Arlacel" 83	2·0
B	Water	46·5
	Preservative	*q.s.*
C	Perfume	*q.s.*

Procedure

Bring (A) to 75° C. Bring (B) to 75° C. Add (B) to (A) slowly with moderate but thorough agitation. Perfume at 45° C. and agitate until cold.

(*Courtesy, Atlas Powder Co., Wilmington.*)

WATER-IN-OIL CREAMS

Water-in-oil creams have considerable popularity and in the United Kingdom are the largest-selling hair dressing. It is claimed that they possess greater fixative properties, in relation to their oil content, than do similar creams of the oil-in-water type and that they impart a better gloss to the hair.

Such creams are usually prepared from mixtures of calcium hydroxide with fatty acids as the emulsifying agent. Alternatively mannide mono-oleate and other hexitan derivatives, ursolic acid, cholesterol and lanolin, etc., may be employed in their formulation. The following is a typical formula of the calcium oleate type :

	per cent.
Beeswax	1·50
Calcium hydroxide	0·07
Oleic acid	1·00
Petroleum oil	40·60
Perfume	1·00
Water	53·83
25 per cent. aqueous solution of magnesium sulphate crystals [1]	2·00

[1] Deakers (Pfaff, *Soap Perfum. Cosm.*, July 1939, p. 604) found that small proportions of magnesium salts, such as magnesium sulphate, assisted very considerably in the stabilisation of water-in-oil emulsions.

It is convenient to incorporate the calcium hydroxide in the form of limewater which contains approximately 0·14 per cent. of calcium hydroxide. By the use of sugar solutions, higher amounts of calcium salts may be rendered soluble in the form of calcium saccharate.

If the calcium hydroxide is added in form of limewater, it should be subjected to a simple titration before use to establish its content of calcium hydroxide.

The beeswax, oleic acid, and oil are warmed to 70°–75° C., and the limewater is added with constant stirring. Finally the solution of magnesium sulphate crystals is added, followed by the addition of the perfume. The mixture should be kept in continuous agitation until it has cooled down to about 20° C.

It may be added that the manufacture of a stable water-in-oil cream, which is also pourable at ordinary temperatures and suitable for use as a hair dressing, is a very difficult job and many of the preparations sold in the retail market cannot be considered, from the technical aspect, to be perfect.

Experimental formulae for preparing water-in-oil hair creams using Amerchol L–101, a lanolin-derivative emulsifier, in connection with beeswax-borax soap are given below; they cover two different grades of viscosity. (Courtesy, Amerchol Sterol Products, American Cholesterol Products, Inc., Milltown, N.J.)

	Viscosity of lotion	
	Medium parts	*Heavy parts*
"Amerchol" L–101	11·0	15·0
Lanolin	3·0	2·5
Beeswax	3·0	7·5
Mineral oil (70 vis)	31·5	25·0
Petrolatum	5·5	—
Borax	0·75	0·5
Water	46·5	49·0
Perfume and Preservative	*q.s.*	*q.s.*

Procedure

Dissolve Amerchol, lanolin, beeswax, mineral oil and petrolatum in one container and heat to 70° C. Dissolve borax in water, heat to 70° C. and add aqueous solution to the oils with rapid agitation. The emulsion forms immediately but should be mixed until cool and homogenised for best results. Perfume may be added when the emulsion temperature has fallen below 45° C.

The following formulation is based upon the use of Abracol CBB (A. Boake Roberts), a proprietary soft-jelly-like product developed, it is claimed, for the manufacture of stable water-in-oil hair creams:

	parts
"Abracol" CBB	10–15
Liquid paraffin	37·0
Distilled water	60·0
Preservative	*q.s.*
Perfume	*q.s.*

(*Courtesy, A. Boake Roberts.*)

Procedure

Heat the oil to about 40° C. stirring in the "Abracol" CBB until fully dispersed. Raise the temperature to 120° C. while stirring is continued. Allow to cool to about 60° C. and then add the water (which can be added either hot or cold) whilst stirring. Perfume at about 45° C. and homogenise.

(*Note.* Preservative is dissolved in the water phase before adding to hot oil solution.)

The following illustrates the use of another proprietary water-in-oil emulsifier "Emul" W (Polak and Schwarz):

	per cent.
"Emul" W (Polak and Schwarz)	22·0
Mineral oil	38·0
Water	40·0
Perfume	*q.s.*

Procedure

Heat "Emul" W with oil to 40° C. When dissolved add the water also at a temperature of 40° C. When an emulsion has formed add the perfume and continue to stir until cool.

The disadvantage of proprietaries such as the last example lies in the large amount of proprietary emulsifier which must be included whereas the hair cream market is highly competitive in price. Much more attractive on these grounds is the following formulation based upon the use of a comparatively small amount of a non-ionic proprietary emulsifier, viz. sorbitan sesquioleate:

	per cent.
Petroleum jelly	7·5
Mineral oil 65/75	37·5
Lanolin (anhydrous)	3·0
Arlacel C (sorbitan sesquioleate)	3·0
Beeswax	2·0
Borax	0·5
Water	46·5

(*Courtesy, Atlas Powder Co., Wilmington.*)

Procedure

The petroleum jelly, mineral oil, lanolin, sorbitan sesquioleate and beeswax are melted and the borax and water are heated separately to 75° C. The aqueous solution is then added, at 75° C., to the molten fats at the same temperature with continuous stirring. If it is desired to add magnesium salts they may be added at this stage. Perfume at 45° C., and stir until cold.

CHAPTER 26

HAIR DYES

GREY hair is associated, often erroneously, with advanced age. In these days of increasing competition the appearance of grey hair or a grey beard may jeopardise a man's future. In the case of a woman it is, at best, a shock to her vanity, an unpleasant reminder of the march of time, but more than that, it may destroy her chance of employment or ruin her chance of marriage.

It is natural, therefore, that the individual concerned should make every effort to disguise this condition by the use of a hair dye.[1]

Hair dyes are conventionally divided into three classes:

(*a*) Vegetable dyes;
(*b*) Metallic dyes;
(*c*) Synthetic organic dyes.

CHARACTERISTICS OF AN IDEAL HAIR DYE

The ideal hair dye should possess the following properties:

(1) It should be non-injurious to the hair-shaft, but should colour the shaft while the natural texture and gloss of the hair should be retained.

(2) It should possess no *systemic* toxic effect when applied to the hair or skin.

(3) It should possess no primary irritant action and be free from sensitising properties, i.e. it should not be a dermatitic agent.

(4) It should be stable on exposure to air, sunlight and salt water and should not change colour nor bleach out on the application of toilet preparations such as brilliantines, setting lotions, hair lacquers, soaps and/or soapless shampoos; neither should it discolour when the hair is exposed to alkalis, reducing agents, oxidising agents or procedures such as are employed in hair waving.

The above specification for the ideal hair due is so stringent that it is small wonder that none of the hair dyes at present known comply with all of them.

In an excellent survey of the subject R. L. Evans ("Some Technical Aspects of Colouring the Hair", *Proc. Sci. Sect., T.G.A.*, Dec. 1948, p. 9)

[1] See also Hair Colour Rinses, Chapter 22.

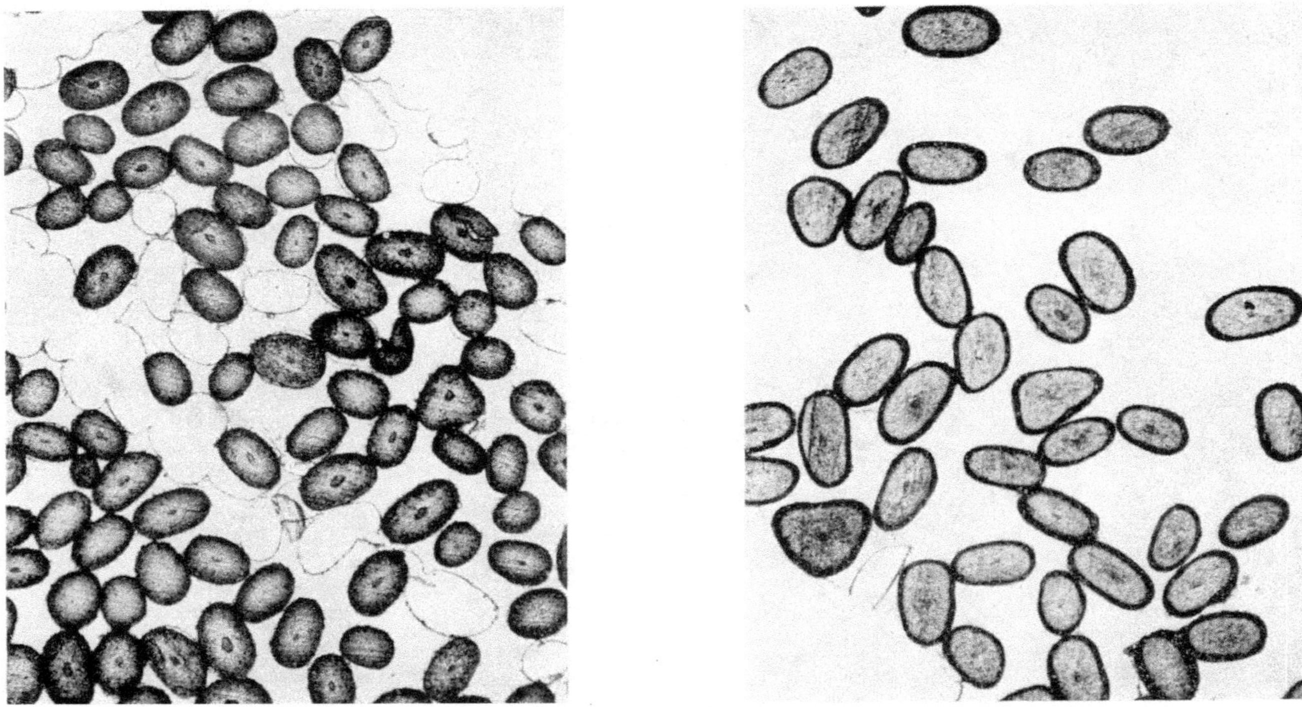

[*Illustrations by the Author.*

FIG. 80.—(*a*) Blonde hair dyed with henna. (*b*) Blonde hair dyed with silver nitrate.

The above photographs illustrate the essential difference between the action of Henna (which, like the para-phenylene diamine group of dyestuffs, *permeates the entire hair shaft*) and metallic dyes such as Silver and Copper which form a *coating around* the hair shaft, and when used continually give rise to an unpleasant metallic sheen.

has drawn attention to some of the technical difficulties involved in the formulation of the ideal hair dye. Evans points out that "... few dyestuffs lend themselves to colouring hair by penetration. X-ray measurements of the keratin lattice structure indicate that molecules much larger than ethylene glycol penetrate keratin slowly if at all. The interatomic and interchain distances in hair can be altered by causing hair to swell in aqueous solutions at high *p*H values. As is shown such swelling will promote absorption and diffusion of solute molecules into the hair shaft. But the degree of reversible swelling that may be resorted to without damage to the hair is limited and therefore the molecular size of the dyestuff that can diffuse within also is limited. . . ."

Evans continues, "... as molecular size increases, solubility, speed of diffusion and usefulness as a colouring agent all rapidly approach zero. It is interesting that in the most successful dyeing system, ammonia, water, hydroxyl ion, hydrogen peroxide, *p*-phenylenediamine and resorcinol, are all small molecules. The first four can certainly penetrate rapidly into the hair shaft. . . ."

The smallness of the phenylenediamine molecule and its rapid diffusion into the keratin molecule is undoubtedly an important factor in the popularity of this dye. (*See* Synthetic Organic Dyes.)

The dyeing of human hair differs from the problem of dyeing textile fibres in a number of important aspects, for example :

(*a*) Since the hair is attached to the human scalp, the dye employed must be *dermatologically innocuous*. Not only does this mean that the dyestuff shall not produce sensitisation but also that it shall not produce *primary irritation* either by chemical or physical means. Hence the *p*H must not be so far from neutrality as to damage the skin within the period of usage and also, to avoid *physical* damage, the temperature of the solution cannot appreciably exceed 40° C.

(*b*) The process of dyeing must be achieved rapidly, since each hair of the head must be treated at one sitting and the excess of dye washed out and the hair re-set.

(*c*) The appearance of the dyed hair fibres should be "natural". To achieve this, as pointed out, the dye molecule must penetrate the fibre and not form an "artificial" coat on the outside. (*See* Fig. 80.)

(*d*) In the process of dyeing, keratin cross-linkages in the fibres and other molecular configurations should not be affected adversely. This would rule out the prior use of powerful swelling agents, and strong oxidising agents. Metallic deposits in the air can be harmful, at least theoretically, in several ways. In the first place they may react with dyestuffs subsequently employed with adverse effect upon the resulting colour and in the second place, if the hair is subsequently bleached with hydrogen, or other peroxides, the catalytic effect of the metal on peroxide decomposition may be detrimental to the hair fibre.

Vegetable Hair Dyes

Of the vegetable hair dyes, henna is the only dye of present day importance. Henna consists of the dried powdered leaves of Lawsonia alba, Lawsonia spinosa and Lawsonia inemis, which are removed from the plants prior to flowering.

Henna owes its hair-dyeing properties to the presence of 2-hydroxy-1,4-naphthaquinone, often termed *lawsone*, which is soluble in hot water and is, in acid solution, a substantive dye for keratin. In dyeing hair with henna a paste of the powdered henna and hot water, slightly acidified with citric, adipic or other suitable acids to an optimum pH of about 5·5, is applied. The hair has previously been given a shampoo to remove all extraneous grease from the hair shaft. This henna *pack* is allowed to remain for the required period, which depends upon the shade desired, the texture and condition of the hair, the activity of the henna, the acidity of the paste, and the temperature at which it is applied and maintained by means of towels, etc. The time may vary from five to sixty minutes, after which the hair is thoroughly shampooed, rinsed, and dried.

Henna has the advantage of not possessing local or systemic toxicity. It is neither a primary irritant nor a sensitiser. The colour obtained is relatively stable and is deposited in the hair shaft, whereas metallic dyes coat the hair shaft and produce a metallic appearance. Unfortunately it suffers from the disadvantages that it is messy to use, and the range of colours produced is limited to reddish auburn shades. Contact with the nails in applying the paste must be avoided or the keratin of the nails will also be stained. *Constant* dyeing with henna tends to spoil some of the effects and produces a flat somewhat hard auburn colour.

In addition to its use as a hair dye henna, in the form of an extract, is incorporated in certain hair rinses which, as already stated, must be on the acid side. The difficulty here lies in the fact that any rinse strong enough to tint the hair is equally likely to tint the nail during application unless the nail is previously protected with nail lacquer.

HENNA RENG

By the addition of other substances to henna, shades other than auburn may be obtained; for example, a mixture of powdered indigo leaves and henna produces blue-black shades. Such mixtures known as *henna rengs* are used in the Far East, but according to Redgrove and Bari-Wooliss (*Hair Dyes and Hair Dyeing*, London: Heinemann, 1939) they are not satisfactory for use in colder climates. Mixtures of quebracho logwood, powdered senna and sage, catechu, etc., have also been suggested for use in hair dyeing, but today, in general, such mixtures may be considered obsolete.

COMPOUND HENNA

By the addition of pyrogallol and copper or other metallic salts, a wide range of shades may be obtained. The following formulae typify the use of henna and pyrogallol with copper as the only metallic salt:

	Light Brown	*Dark Brown*	*Black*
	per cent.	*per cent.*	*per cent.*
Henna (powdered)	90·0	83·0	73·0
Pyrogallol	5·0	10·0	15·0
Copper sulphate (powdered)	5·0	7·0	12·0

In general, such mixtures suffer from certain disadvantages. Pyrogallol introduces possibility of toxic results if carelessly applied on a burn or open wound and the metallic salts confer their own characteristic metallic sheen, discussed later under *metallic dyes*.

WHITE HENNA

This term is incongruous. Such mixtures usually contain alkali plus a bleaching agent, e.g. sodium perborate and magnesium carbonate. They have nothing in common with henna itself, and the term white henna is quite definitely a misrepresentation of fact.

CHAMOMILE

Apart from henna the only other vegetable dye of importance today is chamomile. Of the various species of chamomile, only Anthemis nobilis (Roman chamomile) and Matricaria chamomillae (German chamomile) are important from the cosmetic aspect and appear to be equally useful in tinting hair. The active ingredient in these flowers is 1,3,4-trihydroxyflavone, known also as "Apigenin" (Power and Browning, *J. chem. Soc.*, 1914, **105**, 1829, 2280). Either an aqueous extract or a paste of the ground flower heads may be used. To obtain substantial lightening of the hair, Redgrove and Bari-Wooliss (*Hair Dyes and Hair Dyeing*, London: Heinemann, 1939) recommend the application of a paste comprised of 2 parts chamomile and 1-2 parts powdered kaolin mixed to a thin cream with hot water and applied to the head for a period varying from 15 minutes, where a lightening rinse is required, to 60 minutes for a warm blonde tint.

Chamomile is also used as a constituent of hair-brightening rinses and shampoos. Here some confusion has arisen as to whether it is really effective. The point is that *at least 5 per cent. chamomile, or its equivalent in extract*, must be present to produce *any effect*, and much higher concentrations are desirable. Nowadays it is usual to incorporate sodium perborate or some other oxygenated bleaching agent in shampoos and rinses to obtain such effects more surely, more rapidly, and at lower cost. (*See also* Chapter 22, Hair Rinses.)

Metallic Hair Dyes

In the metallic dyes, compounds of lead are the most frequently used; compounds of silver, copper, iron, nickel and cobalt are sometimes employed, and less frequently salts of bismuth.

It is not quite certain whether the colours produced by such compounds are due to a reaction between the sulphur in the keratin and the metallic salts with the production of the sulphide of the metal, or whether the keratin acts as a reducing agent causing the precipitation of the metal as oxide. It is possible that both reactions occur to some extent.

Reaction of such dyes with the sulphur of the cysteine and cystine in hair might account for the difficulty of waving dyed hair. Whatever the mode of action, the result obtained is the deposition of a coloured metallic film along the hair shaft which, eventually, gives the hair a characteristic dull metallic appearance, renders the hair brittle and diminishes the efficacy of a subsequent permanent wave.

LEAD DYES

The active ingredient in these dyes is usually lead acetate together with some precipitated sulphur, glycerin and water. The following examples (*More Secret Remedies*, British Medical Association, 1912) are analyses of three then popular proprietary preparations:

	per cent.	*per cent.*	*per cent.*
Precipitated sulphur	1·3	1·40	3·2
Lead acetate	1·6	0·13	1·8
Glycerin	9·6	19·00	5·7
Rose-water	87·5	79·47	89·3

Sodium thiosulphate may be incorporated in place of precipitated sulphur. Such preparations have poor stability.

The action of lead dyes is slow and progressive so that some purchasers of such dyes are under the illusion that they are not using a dye at all. The shades produced in grey hair usually pass from yellow through brown to black. The shades achieved between depend upon the concentration of lead salts in the preparation, the number of applications, the original colour of the hair and the time during which the colour has been allowed to develop.

Probably due to interaction with skin proteins, such lead solutions are relatively non-toxic under normal conditions of use. However, it must be remembered that such preparations are usually sold for home use. Systemic effects may follow if lead remains on the hands, particularly under the finger nails, prior to preparing a meal and so contaminates the food. The ingestion of it by children might be fatal. Such preparations should carry adequate precautionary notices.

BISMUTH DYES

Bismuth dyes also act progressively. Winter (*Soap Perfum. Cosm.* Dec. 1938, p. 1084) gives the following formula for such a dye :

Bismuth citrate	50 g.
Distilled water	50 g.

Place these in a graduated vessel and add concentrated (25 per cent.) ammonium hydroxide until a clear solution is obtained. When dissolved, add water to bring the volume to 500 cc.

Prepare separately a solution of

Sodium thiosulphate	30 g.
Distilled water	470 g.

and add this solution to the preceding bismuth solution with thorough mixing. Keep in well-corked bottles. Bismuth dyes give colours changing from blonde to medium or dark chestnut.

SILVER DYES

With these dyes the hair, after being given a shampoo in the usual manner, is treated with an aqueous solution of silver nitrate containing ammonium nitrate and ammonium hydroxide. Ammonium hydroxide is added because alkaline solutions of silver nitrate are readily reduced. The ammonium nitrate assists in keeping the silver hydroxide in solution without using an excessive amount of ammonia. After the above solution has been allowed to remain on the hair for a short while a solution of pyrogallol is applied.

Two-Bottle Silver Dye (Black)

Solution (1)

		per cent.
Silver nitrate		5·0
Ammonium nitrate		3·0
Ammonium hydroxide (conc.)		*q.s.*
Distilled water	to	100·0

Solution (2)

	per cent.
Pyrogallol	4·0
Alcohol	46·0
Water	50·0

For lighter shades the proportion of silver nitrate may be reduced to ½–1 per cent. In place of pyrogallol the use of dilute solutions of liver of sulphur in water has been suggested.

Silver salts used alone tend to produce a greenish-black metallic appearance on the hair which may be modified by the addition of copper, cobalt, or nickel. By suitable adjustment of the concentration and relative proportion of these salts, shades from ash-blonde to black may be obtained.

Care should be taken in the application of silver salts to avoid contact with the skin because they stain the keratin black.

COPPER SALTS

The use of copper salts with henna and pyrogallol has already been described. In addition copper, either alone or with other metallic salts, e.g. ferric chloride, cobalt nitrate, silver nitrate, nickel sulphate, or nickel nitrate, is often employed in hair dyes. The following analyses (*More Secret Remedies*, British Medical Association, 1912) exemplify the use of copper and pyrogallol together, in two makes of brown dyes, which were very popular at that period:

	No. 1	*No.* 2
Pyrogallol	3·8	2·1
Copper chloride (anhydrous)	1·8	1·3
Hydrochloric acid	0·75	0·3
Sulphuric acid	0·07	—
Water to	100·0	100·0

NICKEL AND COBALT SALTS

These salts may be used in aqueous solution either alone or in the form of a mixture, the proportions varying from 0·2 to 4 per cent. In the case of nickel, chiefly the nitrate and sulphate are used; in the case of cobalt, the nitrate. They are widely used also as modifiers to modify and extend the range of other metallic salts, in particular silver salts.

In all the above cases the colours are developed by the subsequent application of a 3-5 per cent. aqueous solution of pyrogallol. Alternatively the pyrogallol may be included in the solution to produce a *one-bottle* or *single-application* dye. *In such cases a reducing agent in sufficient quantity must be present in the mixture*, sodium sulphite being usually included in proportions of about 5 per cent. for this purpose.

Redgrove and Bari-Wooliss (*Hair Dyes and Hair Dyeing*, London : Heinemann, 1939) quote the following as producing excellent chestnut colours, colours unobtainable by means of silver salts alone.

	per cent. *No.* 1	*per cent.* *No.* 2	*per cent.* *No.* 3
Silver nitrate	1·0	0·5	Nil
Cobalt nitrate	5·0	5·0	5·0
Nickel nitrate	Nil	0·5	1·0
Ammonium nitrate	3·0	3·0	3·0
Ammonium hydroxide (0·880 specific gravity)	*q.s.*	*q.s.*	*q.s.*
Water to	100·0	100·0	100·0

No. 1 is described as a rather dark chestnut, while No. 3 is a rather light chestnut shade. The colour in each case is developed by means of a second solution containing 3 per cent. pyrogallol dissolved in water or diluted alcohol.

Winter (*Soap Perfum. Cosm.*, Dec. 1938, p. 1082) quotes the following *one-solution* dye using cobalt nitrate for an ash-blonde shade :

	per cent.
Pyrogallol	2·0
Cobalt nitrate	1·0
Sodium sulphite	4·0
Water	93·0

Synthetic Organic Dyes

Solutions of synthetic organic dyestuffs comprise the vast majority of modern hair dyes since such dyes penetrate the hair shaft instead of merely coating it, and give the hair a natural appearance. Moreover, the colour range is extensive.

It is important, however, that an oxidising agent should be utilised in such dyeing to ensure proper oxidation of the dyestuff and any partially oxidised or unoxidised dyestuff must subsequently be removed from the hair by adequate washing. The most extensively used dyes of this class employed at the present time are para-phenylenediamine (1,4-diaminobenzene) commonly referred to as *para*, and para-tolylenediamine (2,5-diaminotoluene, commonly and incorrectly called para-toluylenediamine), and similar derivatives together with various other organic compounds as modifiers. Either para-phenylenediamine itself or its hydrochloride may be employed; in the latter case, alkali is added prior to use as *para* is effective only in alkaline solution. The oxidising agent necessary may take the form of a separate solution of hydrogen peroxide, or, more usually, suitable tablets of a stabilised hydrogen peroxide-urea compound are supplied to be dissolved according to the accompanying directions.

TOXICITY AND DANGERS OF *para* DYESTUFFS

Oxidation of para-phenylenediamine follows the following course:

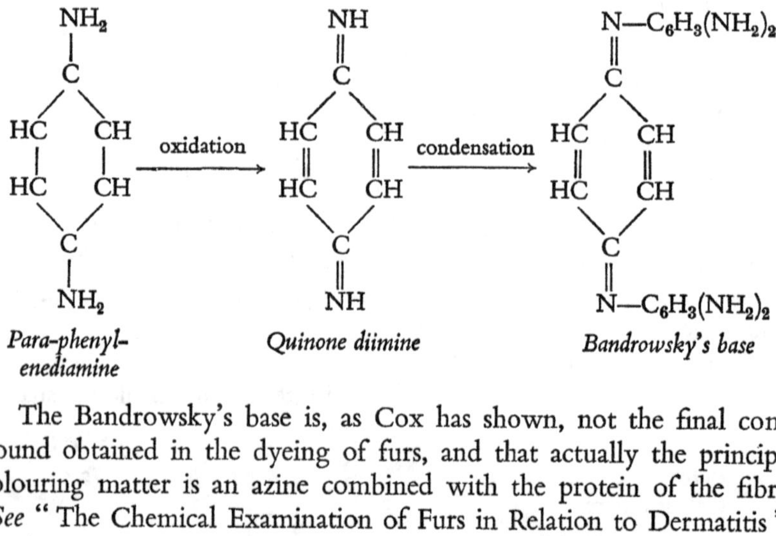

Para-phenyl-enediamine *Quinone diimine* *Bandrowsky's base*

The Bandrowsky's base is, as Cox has shown, not the final compound obtained in the dyeing of furs, and that actually the principal colouring matter is an azine combined with the protein of the fibre. (*See* "The Chemical Examination of Furs in Relation to Dermatitis", *Analyst*, Dec. 1929; Dec. 1933; Jan. 1934; June 1935; Dec. 1935.)

Previously the deleterious effects of these dyes had been attributed to the action of Bandrowsky's base but Knyvatt Gordon (*Analyst*, Dec. 1929) has shown by cutaneous tests that this substance was neither poisonous nor irritating and stated that he had applied it to scarified human skin without vesiculation or effect whatever. Sensitivity appears to be due to the *para* itself and not to any intermediate product. (Cox, *Analyst*, 1933, 3, p. 294; 1934, p. 738.) O'Donovan (*Brit. med. J.*, 1932, **II**, 294) has pointed out that a normal person may fail to react to a 10 per cent. solution of Ursol (containing para-phenylenediamine) whereas susceptible cases react to concentrations as low as 0·005 per cent. Ingram (*Brit. J. Derm.*, Aug.-Sept. 1932) conducted experiments on 1,000 persons and found 4 per cent. of apparently normal subjects were idiosyncratic to *para*; a quarter of these persons being acutely sensitive.

In 1924, the Section of Dermatology and Syphilology of the American Medical Association (H. N. Cole, *J. Amer. Ass.*, Feb. 1927, pp. 88, 397) sponsored a study concerning the number of cases of dermatitis resulting from the use of hair dyes then on the market. It was found that para-phenylenediamine was present in a large number of these preparations. In a compilation and discussion of cutaneous reactions to about 500 different substances as elicited by over 10,000 tests on approximately 1,000 patients, Rostenberg and Sulzberger (*Arch. Derm. Syph.*, Chicago, March 1937, **35**, 433) carried out 411 tests with 2 per cent. *para* in petroleum jelly. Definite positive reactions were obtained in twenty-three cases and slight positive reactions in twenty-six cases ; the percentage of persons reacting in these tests being 6·3 per cent.

PARA-TOLYLENEDIAMINE

Used as a hair dye either in conjunction with or as a replacement for *para* and is considered to be especially useful in the production of ash shades. It has been recommended as a substitute for *para* on the grounds that it is less toxic in use. Cox (*Mfg. Perfum.*, April 1938, p. 109), however, pointed out that, as it is included with *para* on the Poisons Register and was nearly as irritant, its use entailed no great advantage.

The U.S. Food, Drug and Cosmetic Administration states that it has received very definite evidence of injury from this dye and it is therefore banned, along with *para*, for use in the region of the eyes. It may be concluded that in the present state of our knowledge, the remarks made concerning the dermatological action of *para* apply also to para-tolylenediamine, the so-called para-toluylenediamine.

In an effective hair dye there is included in addition to the *para* or other diamines a quantity of a polyhydric phenol such as resorcinol, catechol or pyrogallol, together, in some cases, with a buffer salt and wetting agent. The main functions of phenols in such a mixture are to produce a range of fast colours, particularly of light brown shades. Para-phenylenediamine alone dyes the hair black to blue-black. Moreover, they give a better colour with the same amount of diamine.

Note : Legislation forbids the use of *para* in France, Germany, and Austria, though until 1939 these countries manufactured it for export to Britain and the United States.

In Great Britain the Pharmacy and Poison Act (1933) stipulated that all hair dyes containing phenylenediamines or toluenediamines or other alkylated benzene derivatives or their salts must be labelled with the words " *Caution.* This preparation may cause serious inflammation of the skin in certain persons and should be used only in accordance with expert advice."

In the United States, Sections 601 (a) and 902 (a) of the Food, Drug and Cosmetic Act require among other things that a coal tar hair dye which may be injurious to users shall bear the statement :

" *Caution.* This product contains ingredients which may cause skin irritation on certain individuals, and a preliminary test according to accompanying directions should first be made. This product must not be used for dyeing the eyelashes or eyebrows ; to do so may cause blindness."

In a notice to " Manufacturers of Hair Dye Preparations ", dated 17 Oct. 1938, the U.S. Food and Drug Administration of the United States Department of Agriculture, Washington, D.C., states " It is necessary, as provided in the caution statement that all such hair dyes bear labelling prescribing adequate preliminary tests. For the benefit and guidance of those interested, there are published herewith directions which, in the light of present knowledge and information, are regarded as acceptable. This information is given merely as a guide and does not mean that other tests may not be acceptable.

" *Directions for Making Skin Test*

" (1) The hair dye contained in this package must never be used for dyeing the hair unless a preliminary skin test has been made. The skin test must be made each and every time before the hair is to be dyed, regardless of whether or not a skin test has been made at some time previously.

" (2) The dye used for the preliminary test must be a portion of the article intended to be used for dyeing the hair.

" (3) The sample of dye to be used for the preliminary skin test should be mixed and prepared in exactly the same manner and according to the directions applicable to the actual use of the hair dye itself.

" (4) By means of a suitable applicator (clean camel's hair brush, cotton-tipped applicator or other applicator) a streak of dye not less than a quarter of an inch wide and at least one-half inch long is made on the skin and scalp behind one ear. It is *important* that the streak of dye extend into the hairy portions of the scalp as well as that portion of the skin that is hairless.

" (5) The streak of dye should be permitted to remain for at least 24 hours. The test should be read between 24 and 48 hours after application. Preferably the test area should not be covered with any type of dressing and contact with comb, hats, spectacles or any other object should be avoided.

(6) " *Warning* : If redness or burning, or itching, or small blisters, or any other type of eruption appears in the general area used for the skin test during the first 24 hours the individual is sensitive to the dye, and under no circumstances should it be used for dyeing the hair. Hair dyes should not be used when there is any disease or eruption present anywhere on the skin or on the scalp."

Section 602 (c) requires that the caution statement appear on the label in a prominent and conspicuous place. This requirement would be met if the caution statement appears conspicuously in a colour that contrasts with the background and the remainder of the printed matter. The caution statement should appear on the main panel of the label with the name of the product.

Published information on the shades attained by the use of various aniline derivatives on hair is extremely scanty. The following compilation by Dr. Winter (*Soap Perfum. Cosm.*, Dec. 1938) on the nature and application of the various aniline derivatives in hair dyes is therefore of particular interest :

PARA-PHENYLENEDIAMINE (PARA)

Readily soluble in water and alcohol. Gives very beautiful shades but is extremely dangerous. Should not be used.

SULPHO-PARA-PHENYLENEDIAMINE (*also the sulphate and hydrochloride*)

These are innocuous and permissible. (In practice the officially declared harmlessness is always relative and should be treated cautiously in view of possible idiosyncrasies.) Gives brown (chestnut) tones without a false reflex but only dyes slowly. Soluble in water and dilute alcohol.

DIMETHYL PARA-PHENYLENEDIAMINE

Reputedly innocuous but frequently causes skin irritation. Soluble in water and dilute alcohol; gives brown tones with violet reflex.

META-PHENYLENEDIAMINE AND META-TOLUYLENEDIAMINE

Soluble in water and dilute alcohol. Innocuous, give brown tones without a false reflex. Are used mainly as additional agents to obtain modified shades (nuanceurs). *See* para-aminodiphenylamine.

PARA-TOLUYLENEDIAMINE

Innocuous (*Note*: this is Dr. Winter's opinion, not the author's), readily soluble in water and dilute alcohol, produces all shades but with a most unattractive reddish-violet reflex which develops and becomes intensified as time goes on. Nevertheless, it is an excellent base for dyes if precautions are taken to avoid formation of undesirable reflexes by adding appropriate modifiers (para-aminodiphenylamine; 1,4-diaminodiphenylamine, etc.).

PARA-AMINOPHENOL (RODINAL) AND ORTHO-AMINOPHENOL

Fairly soluble in water and dilute alcohol. Give blonde-mahogany and chestnut-red shades. Pure blondes are produced with the sulphonated derivatives, the sulphate and the hydrochloride.

SULPHO-PARA-AMINO-META-CRESOL (METOL)

Also known under the name of sulpho-meta-methyl-para-aminophenol. The sulphate (Aldilol) and the hydrochloride are also in use. Soluble in water; insoluble in alcohol. Gives chestnut tones with a red reflex. Shades can be varied and the reflex eliminated mainly with the aid of para-aminodiphenylamine.

SULPHO-2, 5-DIAMINOPHENOL (AMIDOL)

Soluble in water and dilute alcohol. Gives chestnut-red tones. The toner used is para-aminodiphenylamine. The sulphate and especially the hydrochloride give brown and black tones.

SULPHO-ORTHO-AMINOPHENOL

Soluble in water and dilute alcohol and gives blonde tones.

PARA-AMINODIPHENYLAMINE

This product is almost insoluble in water, readily soluble in dilute alcohol, soluble in alkaline water. Gives blackish-grey tones. Is chiefly used as a toner (see metol, amidol and para-toluylenediamine). A whole range of shades may be obtained in combination with other aniline derivatives (meta-phenylenediamine, metol, amidol, etc.):

SULPHO-PARA-AMINODIPHENYLAMINE AND ITS SULPHATE

Soluble in water and dilute alcohol, used in alkaline solution. Forms bluish-black tints.

1,4-DIAMINODIPHENYLMETHANE

Soluble with difficulty in water, but more soluble than para-aminodiphenylamine; soluble in dilute alcohol. Grey and bluish-black tones.

SULPHO-DIAMINODIPHENYLAMINE

Soluble in water and dilute alcohol. Gives all shades but especially a very beautiful jet black. The sulphate and hydrochloride are also used.

Apart from the above principal aniline derivatives, the following are also used: 2-sulpho-1,4-diaminobenzene; 2,7-dihydroxy benzo-parathiazine; 1,4-diamino-5-methyl benzene; 1,4-diaminoanisol; 1,2-diaminonaphthol (naphthylenediamine). Derivatives of glycine (phenyl acetic acid can also be used); para-aminoglycine, for instance, for browns, para-hydroxyglycine for chestnut, and para-nitroglycine for blondes. Other nitro-derivatives which may be considered are sulpho-dinitrophenol, and sulpho-2,4-dinitro-4-hydroxydiphenylamine.

Winter states that nitro compounds should always be used in the sulphonated forms because the non-substituted compounds give rise to irritation.

Winter, in the same article, gives the following examples (amongst others) of modern synthetic dyes:

Black

Para-toluylenediamine	5 g.
Para-aminodiphenylamine	5 g.
Sodium sulphite (crystals)	10 g.
50 per cent. Aqueous alcohol	100 cc.

This is the solution of dye. A second bottle of "developer" is also supplied. The developer in the above case contains four pastilles of 0·5 g. urea peroxide. Bottle No. 1 contains 10 cc. of the dye solution.

Mode of use. Transfer the pastilles from the bottle of developer (No. 2) to a small saucer. Fill the empty bottle to the neck with water, pour this amount of water onto the pastilles, crush with a spatula and stir until all is dissolved. Add the aniline dye (Sol. 1), mix and apply. *Contact time 1 hour.*

Blonde

Para-toluylenediamine	1 g.
Sulpho-ortho-aminophenol	3 g.
Pyrogallol	0·5 g.
Sodium sulphite	4 g.
10 per cent. Ammonium hydroxide	5 g.
Alcohol	20 cc.
Water	80 cc.

Bottle No. 1 contains 10 cc. of this solution. No. 2 contains two pastilles of 0·5 g. urea peroxide. Procedure as above. *Contact time ½ hour.*

Chestnut

Para-toluylenediamine	2 g.
Para-aminophenol	2 g.
Para-aminodiphenylamine	1 g.
Sodium sulphite	5 g.
50 per cent. Aqueous-alcohol	100 cc.

Bottle No. 1 contains 10 cc. of this solution. Bottle No. 2 contains three pastilles of 0·5 g. urea peroxide. Procedure as above. *Contact time ¾ hour.*

Brown

Para-aminophenol	1 g.
Para-toluylenediamine	3 g.
Para-aminodiphenylamine	3 g.
Sodium sulphite (crystals)	6 g.
50 per cent. Aqueous-alcohol	100 cc.

Bottle No. 1 contains 10 cc. of this solution. Bottle No. 2 contains three pastilles of 0·5 urea peroxide. Procedure as above. *Contact time 1 hour.*

The following examples are taken from the patent literature and serve to illustrate the type of compounds which have been covered by patents.

J. Saphir (German Patent 119,187) using oxidising dyes together with certain specified " catalysts ", states :

" Oxidising dyestuffs are employed whose activity is increased by the addition of catalysts acting as oxygen carriers. These colouring matters which, as used hitherto in alkaline media attack the scalp, can also be used in an acid medium ; the dye bases from salts having no action on the skin. The catalysts are iodine, iodides, nitrites, bromides, heavy metal salts (principally those of higher valency), iron, copper, nickel, cobalt, manganese, chromium salts, etc., and finally, certain ferments, pancreatic ferment, diastase. The colouring matters are the hydrochlorides of *o*- or *m*-phenylenediamine, *p*-toluylenediamine, *o*- or *p*-aminophenol; the sulphates of *o*- or *m*-toluylenediamine, *p*-aminodiphenylamine, methyl-*p*-aminophenol, the pyrogallols, etc."

Example 1, *Reddish Blonde.* Apply to the hair a mixture of 5 parts of *o*-phenylenediamine hydrochloride, 0·1 part of ferric chloride, 0·5 part of sodium lauryl sulphonate and 44·4 parts of distilled water. After a few minutes apply 50 parts of 6 per cent. hydrogen peroxide, leave on the hair for 20 to 30 minutes and wash.

Example 2, *Medium Blonde.* Proceed in the same manner with 2 parts of *m*-phenylenediamine hydrochloride, 0·2 part of potassium chromate, 0·1 part of sapamine acetate, 60 parts of distilled water, 60 parts of 6 per cent. hydrogen peroxide.

Example 3, *Chestnut.* 2 parts of *p*-aminophenol hydrochloride, 0·1 part of potassium iodide, 0·5 part of Indian tragacanth, 100 parts of distilled water, 100 parts of 6 per cent. hydrogen peroxide.

Example 4, *Dark Brown.* 2 parts of *p*-toluylenediamine sulphate, 20 parts of 0·5 N caustic potash, 0·1 part of potassium iodide, 1 part of the sodium salt of the condensation product of taurine and oleic acid, 100 parts of 6 per cent. hydrogen peroxide.

Example 5, *Blonde.* 5 parts of *m*-toluylenediamine, 95 parts of 0·5 N hydrochloric acid, 0·5 part of tragacanth, 0·5 part of sodium oleyl-sulphonate, 0·1 part of ferric chloride, 100 parts of 6 per cent. hydrogen peroxide.

Brit. Patent 524,293 (Clairol, N. V., and H. H. Meyer of Holland) relates to what are claimed to be improved hair dyes of the oxidation type in solid form. The invention consists in a method of producing a preparation for the dyeing of living hair in the form of a stick, bar, cake or the like compact solid form and containing a soap and an adequate proportion of a water-soluble oxidation dye intermediate which consists in mixing the dye intermediate with an alkali such as ammonia or sodium carbonate and a small amount of water, this amount being insufficient to dissolve a substantial proportion of the dye intermediate, so as to form a thick paste, mixing the paste with partially dried soap chips, milling the mixture, plodding the milled product and cutting it into sticks, bars, cakes or the like compact solid form. The milling and plodding operations are carried out in the manner well-known in the manufacture of toilet soap.

Soapless detergents may additionally be incorporated with the preparations. These consist essentially of the sodium salts of sulphonated fatty alcohols and sulphonated fatty alkyl esters or amides, such as the methyl tauride of oleic acid. Fuller's earth, talcum powder or a similar bulky powder which when mixed with water forms a paste may be additionally incorporated with the preparations, the pasty consistency sustaining the dyeing action during the hair-dyeing operation. The finished sticks or the like may be coated with a thin layer of a paraffin or other wax, collodion, cellulose varnish or other suitable material, so as further to protect the preparations from oxidation by air. Two of the examples cited in this patent are as follows:

(1) 120 g. of para-toluylene diamine sulphate are mixed with 65 g. of ammonia (25 per cent.) and 40 g. of fuller's earth, and made up into a paste with 50 g. of water. This paste is milled with 760 g. of toilet soap chips having a fatty acid content of 75–80 per cent. and the homogeneously milled product is plodded and cut to shape. The product applied, e.g. by rubbing, to hair which has been moistened with a 2 per cent. hydrogen peroxide solution, gives a brownish-black colour.

(2) 80 g. of meta-toluylene diamine are mixed to a paste with 50 g. of ammonia (25 per cent.) and milled with 870 g. of toilet soap chips with a fatty acid content of approximately 80 per cent. The homogeneously milled product is plodded and cut to shape. The product applied, e.g. by rubbing, to hair which has been moistened with a 2 per cent. hydrogen peroxide solution, produces a blonde colour.

(An extension of this patent is referred to in British Patent Specification 531,741 which states: "The present invention offers a novel device by means of which the solid hair dyes can be applied simultaneously with the oxidising developer and which when used with such solid hair dyes is free from the defects of the hair-dyeing and bleaching appliances used hitherto. The invention consists in a device for the dyeing and bleaching of human hair comprising in combination a solid dyeing and/or bleaching stick or the like secured to a reservoir adapted to contain a liquid such as water or a solution of a bleaching agent and provided with outlet openings or channels through which when the device is inverted the liquid may pass to the free end of the dyeing and/or bleaching stick so as gradually to dissolve the latter.")

Orelup (U.S. Patent, 2,359,783) claims that by applying new pre-treatment materials to the hair it is possible to employ for hair dyeing a large class of non-toxic dyes hitherto unavailable for such application. These pre-treatments or fixative compounds consist of salts of cation-active materials which themselves possess a desired degree of cation activity and are prepared by reacting higher fatty acids with the specified compounds.

An illustrative example from the patent specification is as follows: "A reaction vessel is charged with 210 lb. of coconut fatty acids and 109 lb. of 2-amino 2-methyl 1-propanol. The reaction mixture is kept at a temperature of 175° C. for about 6 hours. Glacial acetic acid is then added until a test shows clear solubility in water at a *p*H of 6·0 to 6·3. When used in the actual dyeing treatment, as, for example, for dyeing the hair black, a 2 per cent. solution of this acetate product is shampooed through the hair at room temperature and allowed to remain for 15 minutes. The hair is then rinsed once and a 1 to 3 per cent. solution of naphthol blue-black thickened with gum tragacanth is applied and allowed to remain for 20 minutes. The hair is then rinsed with water until no colour is seen in the wash water, whereupon the process is complete." It is claimed that practically any colour may be applied to the hair by such methods, and any non-toxic dye used.

German Patent (I. Fehrmann, German Patent 541,404) refers to the addition of haematoxylin (logwood): "Hair dye consists of mixture of haematoxylin with diamines, with exception of para-phenylenediamine. Mixture may consist of 0·5 part of haematoxylin with 0·3 part of ortho-aminophenol. Striking blonde shade is obtained thereby. Mixture which contains 0·5 part of haematoxylin and 0·3 part of para-amino-diphenylamine, gives deep black shade which does not turn greenish-black. Mixture consisting of 0·5 part of haematoxylin and 0·5 part of para-aminophenol gives fine chestnut-brown shade, while mixture of 0·5 part of haematoxylin and 0·5 part of meta-phenylenediamine gives beautiful platinum-blonde shade."

For other examples the patent literature may be consulted.

Platinum Blondeing

Obviously no description of hair dyes would be complete without a reference to the method of producing platinum blondes. This is accomplished by bleaching the hair in the usual manner to the palest possible shade of blonde with ammonia and peroxide of hydrogen. The hair is afterwards given a rinse with a blue rinse containing about 1 : 100,000 of methylene blue (Ext. D & C Blue No. 1), or other suitable blue certified colour, in somewhat the same manner as people add some ultramarine or washing blue to the rinsing water in washing clothes, to make it appear " whiter " or " more bluish ", as the human eye considers a substance *very slightly* bluish as *more white.*

Bleaching of the hair must be thorough or the combination of a deep yellow hair shaft and a blue rinse may give the hair a distinctly greenish appearance.

CHAPTER 27

THE PROCESSING OF TOILET SOAP

ALTHOUGH the basic principles of soap manufacture remain unchanged, recent years have seen many innovations in the soap-making industry in particular methods of continuous soap-making utilising either fatty acids produced by continuous high temperature fat-splitting (as for example, the Colgate-Emery process), or continuous processes for the use of conventional fats such as the Sharples, Clayton, and Monsavon processes.

This brief chapter is concerned not with the ramifications of the soap industry nor with recent developments in soap-making but only with the production of toilet soap from milling base chips, such as may be practised by the medium-sized cosmetic manufacturer.

By such processing, soap chips purchased from one of the larger soap boilers, may be converted into tablets of toilet soaps of various shapes and sizes, attractively perfumed and coloured, and possessing improved solubility.

The processing involves amalgamation, milling (or alternatively pre-plodding), plodding, cutting and stamping and though in theory the processes involved seem almost automatic and fool-proof, in practice it is sometimes surprising to see the characteristics and quality of the soaps produced. These individual plant operations will be considered separately.

QUALITY OF SOAP MILLING BASE

Although incorrect processing can ruin the characteristics of a good quality toilet milling base the converse is by no means true in that processing conditions, whilst very important, cannot make a first class soap from an inferior milling base.

The *fat charge* of the base has undergone modifications since the days of the classic 25 per cent. Cochin coconut oil and 75 per cent. prime Beef Tallow, and today will include some distilled bone grease fatty acids, animal greases and the like although the greater proportion of the charge will still, in general, be composed of tallow and palm kernel oils. A few per cent. of rosin may be present. Edible oils and fats, at least in Britain, will be almost if not entirely absent. As pointed out later in this chapter, the presence of soft oils in the fat charge can influence the cracking propensities of the soap tablet in use.

According to the quality and colour of the materials used in the manufacture of the base, the milling base may be graded as a No. 1, No. 2 or No. 3 milling base.

Thickness of Chip. The chips should be of good colour, evenly dried and showing no dried soap specks and should preferably be moderately thick, since *a thin chip dries very readily* and is also to some extent more prone to rancidity.

Moisture content of milling base. If the soap chips are received in a dry condition no amount of subsequent treatment will avoid the probability, almost certainty, of dried soap specks showing up in the finished tablets, moreover, soap that is too dry will not plod satisfactorily. On the other hand, if the soap base is too wet it slows up the milling process and becomes hot and plastic; plodding is difficult and the cut billets are often too soft to handle without marking. To some extent the desirable moisture content of the soap base is related to the amount of perfume to be incorporated and, with amounts of perfume much in excess of 1 per cent. (about 18 fl. oz. per cwt.), it is often advantageous to use a base of a somewhat lower moisture content than is usually employed. In those cases in which the perfume level is about, or under, 1 per cent. and in which any added superfats are low, a moisture level of between 12–14 per cent. will usually be found satisfactory. To allow for some drying-out in storage, the moisture level of the chips as purchased should be a little higher.

The amount of salt permissible in a base as regards its influence on cracking will depend upon the titre of the fats and the fat charge; in general a level of 0·5 per cent. NaCl and below can be regarded as satisfactory. In some instances the salt may run as high as 0·75 per cent. without giving much trouble. Titres may run from 37·5°–39·0°, the lower titres tending to give a soap that is less white in colour and sometimes a little less prone to cracking than pure white soaps of higher titres. A content of free alkali (as Na_2O) of less than 0·1 per cent., and a free caustic alkali of less than 0·05 per cent. are criteria commonly employed in the industry.

Amalgamation. The soap chips, often stored in lined bags of approximately 1 cwt., but preferably stored in storage bins or in a soap silo, are transferred to the amalgamator. The best method is for the plant to be arranged either so that an elevator is employed, or better, so that the soap can be dropped by gravity. Whichever method is employed it is essential to ensure that no pocketing occurs in storage, since this would not only permit of the chips "drying out" but would also involve the possibility of deterioration in the odour of the soap chips.

Soap chips alone, particularly if plodded with perfume, would produce a product having insufficient opacity to be attractive. Opacifying ingredients are therefore added at this stage; these are either zinc oxide, titanium dioxide or a mixture of the two, which some people consider to give a better effect. Although the proportions of opacifiers added may vary, the amounts usually employed are from about $\frac{1}{2}$ to 1 per cent. zinc oxide, or approximately $\frac{1}{4}$ of this amount of titanium dioxide.

If a soap preservative is to be added (with a view to preventing the development of rancidity and therefore more correctly termed an anti-oxidant), it may be incorporated with the soap chips prior to the addition of the zinc and/or titanium oxides. (*See* Antioxidants for Soap, Chapter 43.)

At this stage are also added any soap colours which it is desired to employ, and the perfume. If the soap is to be superfatted with lanolin cold cream, petroleum jelly and the like, these are also added at this stage.

The above materials are blended for a prescribed period, usually from 10 to 20 minutes, in the amalgamator which consists of a horizontal trough mixer, preferably of stainless steel or lined with other suitably resistant metal. At the end of the prescribed period of amalgamation the mixture is dropped into the hopper of either the soap mill or the soap refiner (or pre-plodder), according to the method of "working" the soap which is to be employed.

In the older, conventional and widely used milling process the soap, mixed with the other additives, is fed to a series of mill rolls operating at different speeds so that a shearing force is exerted on the films of the soap. Modern mills are built up of a series of water-cooled steel units, since by such means the temperature of milling can be more closely controlled, and overheating, which results in deterioration and loss of perfume and also affects the physical characteristics of the finished soap, is avoided. Such mills may be either a battery of 3-roll mills, or a 5-roll mill may be employed.

It has been the author's experience that milling temperatures approximating to 31° ± 1° C. (87° F.-*c.* 90° F.) are satisfactory, it being arranged so that (as there is normally a slight rise in temperature) the milled soap leaves the last roller at or about this temperature.

It has been shown by a study of X-ray diffraction patterns that, in the process of working soap as in milling, changes in the forms of the soap molecules occur, and that certain soap "phases" are produced which have definite physical characteristics; the number of such phases has been the subject of some argument; Ferguson *et al.* [*Industr. Engng. Chem.* (Ind. Ed.), 1943, **35**, 1005] distinguished three phases which they termed, beta, delta and omega phases. The beta phase was characterised by its ready solubility and lathering characteristics; the omega phase was characterised by greater durability and its reduced lathering properties and the delta phase by a tendency to cracking, reduced hardness and lathering properties intermediate between the beta and omega phases (lathering ratios 24 : 5 : 17 respectively).

Using a commercial 80 per cent. tallow, 20 per cent. coconut oil soap, Ferguson *et al.* were able to produce all three phases by varying the conditions and temperatures of working, for example, after going through the ordinary milling and plodding operations the soap was converted practically 100 per cent. to the beta phase. The same soap heated in a sealed container to 190° F. and allowed to cool slowly to room temperatures was shown to be converted to the omega phase. A third sample mechanically worked at a temperature of 50°-60° F. (*c.* 10° C.-16° C.) was shown to have been converted to the delta phase. Many other complex factors enter this question of "mechanically working the soap" to achieve certain desirable phases; for example, moisture has an effect upon such transformation, other fats present in commercial soaps and possibly the presence of any "additives" may affect the resultant phase of the plodded soap. In fact as has been aptly stated the plain simple truth is rarely plain and never simple.

It would appear that low temperature plodding may well be associated with the delta phase, since it has been the author's experience that soaps plodded at low temperatures are particularly liable to cracking. (The problem is, however, complicated by the fact that some reversion of phases *may possibly* occur in certain soaps on ageing.)

Instead of milling, some firms pass the soap mixture through a series of pre-plodders in which the soap is worked mechanically, not by milling, but by forcing the soap by means of screw impellers through a series of fine mesh screens which are supported by perforated pressure plates. These pre-plodders are modified plodders in which the soap is *not* compressed into a billet.

Advantages claimed for this method are (i) reduction in the floor space required for milling; (ii) reduced power consumption and labour, and (iii) frequently a marked improvement in the quality of the finished soap (J. W. Bodman, *J. Amer. Oil. Chem. Soc.*, Nov. 1952, p. 521). Other features of this method of processing are that it reduces noise and removes foreign material accidentally introduced into the soap between the drying and plodding operations. In general, such methods of pre-plodding are mostly suitable for the processing of the softer soaps.

When pre-plodded or refined in this way the soap is pelletised before being fed to the plodder. When a milling process is involved, it is usual

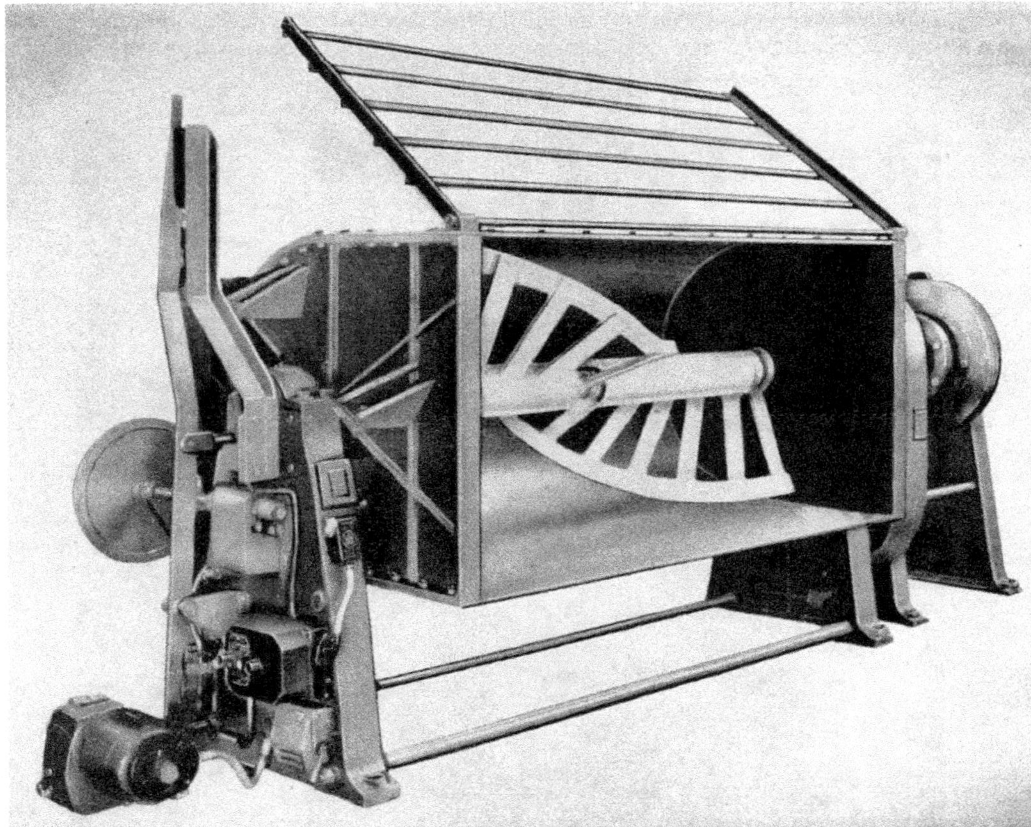

[By courtesy of Vickers-Armstrongs Ltd.

FIG. 81.—Soap Amalgamator.

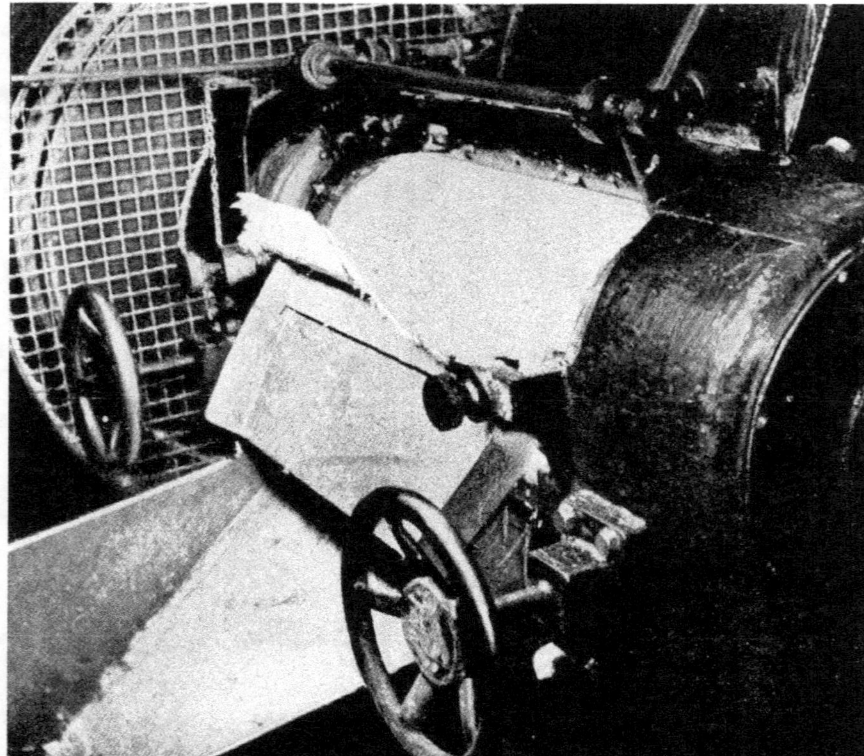

[*By courtesy of Henry Simon Ltd.*

FIG. 82.—An untouched action photograph taken instantaneously with a " micro-flash " showing a layer of soap coming off the top roll of a Simon three-roll toilet soap mill. Notice the even distribution of the soap film over the entire length of the roll.

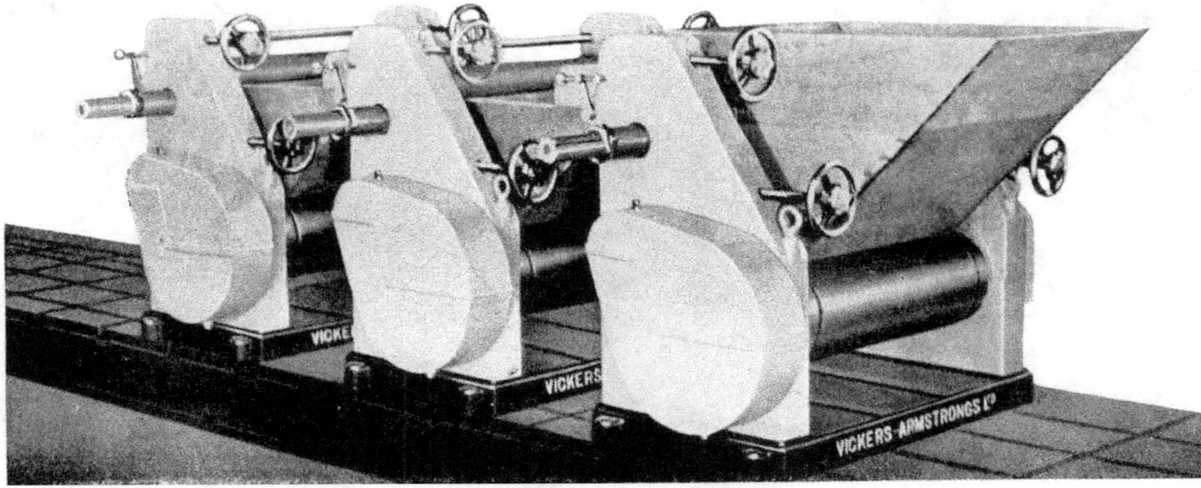

[By courtesy of Vickers-Armstrongs Ltd.

FIG. 83.—Three mills type S330 arranged with single hoppers for continuous production.

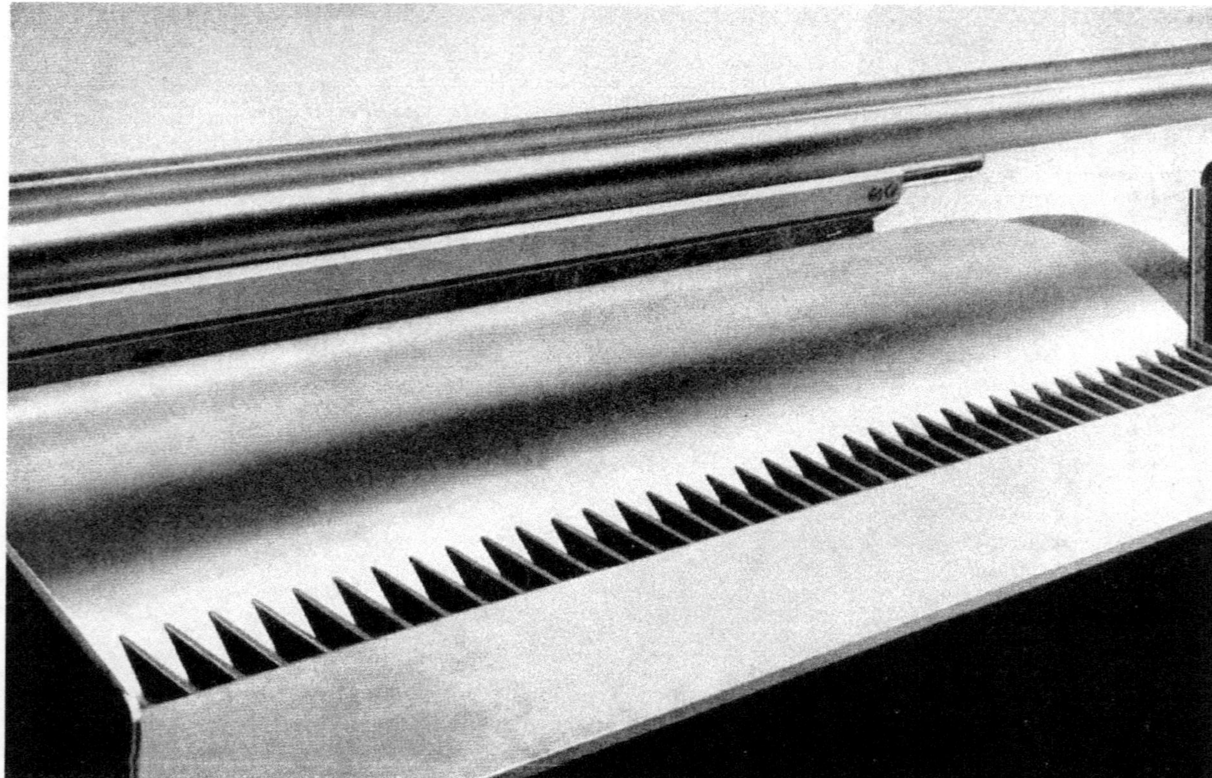

[*By courtesy of Vickers-Armstrongs Ltd.*

FIG. 84.—Special Crimping Scraper.

for the scraper blade to " crinkle " the soap coming off the last mill in order to assist in packing the plodder with a minimum amount of bridging, as such compressed pieces are more readily packed into the plodder, because of their greater bulk density than are long soap "ribbons".

As has already been mentioned, the soap coming off the last mill should be at a temperature of about 31° C. (90° F.) and should be mechanically conveyed, directly it leaves the mill, to the plodder hopper so that no cooling of the milled soap occurs.

The Plodding Operation

In the plodder the mechanically worked and pelletised or crimped soap is compressed into a smooth billet, free from air and free from surface cracks and marks. The avoidance of entraining air in the plodding operation is most important as this leads to air becoming occluded in the soap billet which then shows pronounced cracking tendencies. To achieve this, it is necessary to ensure that the worm of the plodder is always covered and that the speed of the screw is appropriate for the soap being made and the size of plodder employed. As an additional precaution a partial vacuum may be attached to the plodder feed hopper.

The temperature of plodding may be controlled by the temperature of the water in the surrounding jacket, which is usually obtained from the mains water supply and may be anything from about 14° C.–18° C. or more, depending upon the time of the year and the prevailing weather conditions. On modern plodders the temperature of the plodder nozzle is electrically controlled. McCutcheon (*Soap, N.Y.*, April 1946) has suggested a temperature of between 96° F–107° F. (i.e. about 36° C.–43° C.) ; many people prefer to operate at nearer the 50° C. mark. The optimum temperature is best judged by observing the condition of the issuing soap billet ; if it is rough, with fibres tending to curl outwards, the temperature of the nozzle is too low ; if blistered, it is obviously too high. The desirable temperature for this operation will depend upon the titre of the soap being processed, its composition and the rate of plodding ; the best guide the visual appearance of the plodded bar !

The issuing plodded billet of soap is then cut into smaller billets of the appropriate length by means of a soap cutter, the older type of piano-wire cutter has now been replaced in modern continuously-operating plants by an automatic mechanically operated cutter, in which the cutter is driven by the extrusion of the soap billet itself, so that the rate of cutting is automatically controlled by the rate of extrusion and, it is claimed, the cut pieces cannot possibly vary in weight or size (Simon Soap Cutter, Type C.9). The soap billet size and shape should be as near to that of the stamped tablet as possible as distortion of the billet encourages cracking.

The success of the soap processing operation up to this stage has been to keep the soap continuously moving, and at the appropriate temperatures. If the soap is allowed to cool at any stage in the cycle of events leading from milling to plodding the chances of the soap cracking in use are considerably increased; this means that so far as possible the operating machinery should not be stopped for luncheon breaks for personnel since this involves leaving soap to cool in the plodder, unless it is completely emptied.

Once the soap has arrived at the " cut billet " stage, however, it may be found that the soap is too warm to take a perfect impression without adhering to the dies in the stamper. To a large extent, the severity of the " die marking " of the soap will depend upon the moisture and perfume contents of the soap, and the presence of any added superfats. To overcome this difficulty it is usual to cool the surface of the soap just sufficiently to form a surface skin which may then be stamped. This may be achieved by traying the soap for up to an hour or two and then withdrawing the soaps in rotation for stamping, or by passing the tablets through a cooling tower, the speed of the conveyor through the tower and the length of the tower being adjusted to produce a suitable surface " skin ".

Soap Stamping

The cut, partially cooled billets then pass to the stamper where they receive the desired impression from the soap dies. The stamping process may be achieved either by hand or automatically; automatic stamping being particularly suitable for simple rectangular shapes and hand stamping often being employed for more fancy shapes although automatic toggle die stampers are now available for stamping all types of shapes.

To prevent the soap sticking to the die, it is usual to apply a small quantity of a lubricant (a 5 per cent. solution of sodium chloride is commonly employed for this purpose) at intervals to the surfaces of the tablets to be stamped; excessive use of brine for this purpose results in surface cracks appearing in the tablet *prior* to washing.

Soap Wrapping

The relatively low thermal conductivity of soap should be borne in mind and though it is possible to stamp tablets satisfactorily after a short period of cooling, such tablets should not be wrapped until they have been stored sufficiently to cool, a period of 24 hours being recommended. If soaps are wrapped soon after stamping they are likely to become disfigured by " sweating ".

Defects in Toilet Soap

Many defects in the finished tablets of soap are obvious by visual inspection, for example dirt, finger marks, rubbing at some stage, marks due to belt or elevators, surface cracking, incorrect colour, the presence of dried soap specks, etc. These can be remedied by taking the appropriate action; others such as entrained air may only be visible by taking sections through the soap and examining for air pockets.

"Sandiness" or roughness in the tablets and the propensity of the toilet soap tablets to cracking in use can be determined by wash-down tests in the factory or laboratory.

Cracking of Toilet Soaps

When toilet soap has been used and is then allowed to stand in a soap tray in a wetted condition, then—particularly in winter months—certain phenomena known as cracking occur. These may vary from fine hair lines running across the shorter edges of the tablets, and hardly visible on casual inspection, to deep fissures running down the surface of the soap and even to segments of the soap cracking sufficiently to break away.

Milled toilet soap is very soluble in water and, on the side in contact with the soap ledge, tends to form a sludge or gel of thickness dependent upon the amount of moisture with which it is in contact. If this tablet be turned over and allowed to dry out, cracking will very often occur. By standardising conditions of washing, time and temperature, and the drying conditions, it is possible to compare the cracking propensities of one soap against another or against a control soap. It has been the author's experience that a number of factors contribute to soap cracking. These factors may be classified as follows:

Composition of Fat Charge. The presence of certain soft oils appears to reduce the tendency to cracking. Whether this is due to the fact that unsaturates can hold water better than saturated fats is not known. (Attention has already been drawn to the water-holding capacities of lanolin in Chapter 4, The Hydration of the Skin.) Smith (*Amer. Perfum.*, Aug. 1951) has pointed out in connection with the drying of soap that "... Soaps made from oils containing highly unsaturated fatty acids are more difficult to dry than those from saturated fatty acids. ...".

The *plasticity* of the soap may be a factor in those cases in which the tablet shape deviates appreciably from a rectangular block. Rayner (*Soap Perfum. Cosm.*, Dec. 1938, p. 1086) found hardness for coconut oil and palm kernel oil soaps of 20 lb. and 15 lb. respectively as against only 2½–3 lb. for a tallow soap.

Conditions of Usage. If the tablets of soap are left to soak in water for an unduly long time or are allowed to stand in a soap trough in which the water does not completely drain away and the tablets are then exposed to drying atmospheres either in a heated bathroom or in an unheated room open to draughts and drying winds (particularly if they are used at infrequent intervals) then cracking is almost certain to occur, though it may be reduced either by the inclusion of certain additives or by the choice of a more suitable fat charge.

Processing Conditions. Since it is not possible to control the conditions of usage once the tablet has left the manufacturers' premises, and since (in the majority of cases today) the composition of the fat charge is governed by prevailing conditions of supply and the soap manufacturer has to do the best he can with the fats and oils available, this only leaves plant operating conditions in the processing of the soap [plus possibly the addition of certain superfats and/or alteration in the perfume level] with which the cracking propensities of the product can be minimised. Some outline of the processing conditions necessary to minimise cracking has been given earlier in this chapter.

The Superfatting of Soap

As pointed out in Chapters 22 and 41, it is well known that detergents, in removing grease and dirt from the skin, are not able to differentiate between extraneous soiling matter and the natural oil secretion of the skin, which (*see* Chapter 4) is believed to play a role in the maintenance of the normal hydration of the skin. Hence in cleansing the skin with soap, it tends to become dry.

The defatting action of detergents appears to be recognised in the industry generally. Dr. Foster Dee Snell, giving the Gold Medallist's Address at the 1949 Annual Meeting of the Society of Chemical Industry stated that " the frequent dryness and harshness of the skin caused by reduction in its content of sebaceous matters, regardless of whether the detergent is soap or synthetic, is explained by the observations of McBain and of Harkins that the water-insoluble material is dissolved in the detergent micelle ". Dr. Snell continued " . . . Reducing the detergent efficiency of soap by adding lanolin or other excess fatty matter reduces the drying effect of the solution on the skin. . . ."

Stillians [*Illinois med. J.*, 1923, **43**, 388]; Kesten [*New Engl. J. Med.*, 1943, **228**, 125]; Kile [*Arch. Derm. Syph., Chicago*, 1942, **45**, 377] have reported favourably upon the action of superfatted soaps from the dermatological angle, although dermatologists in general find this matter controversial. From a theoretical aspect superfatting, in appropriate amounts and with a suitable superfat, should be dermatologically

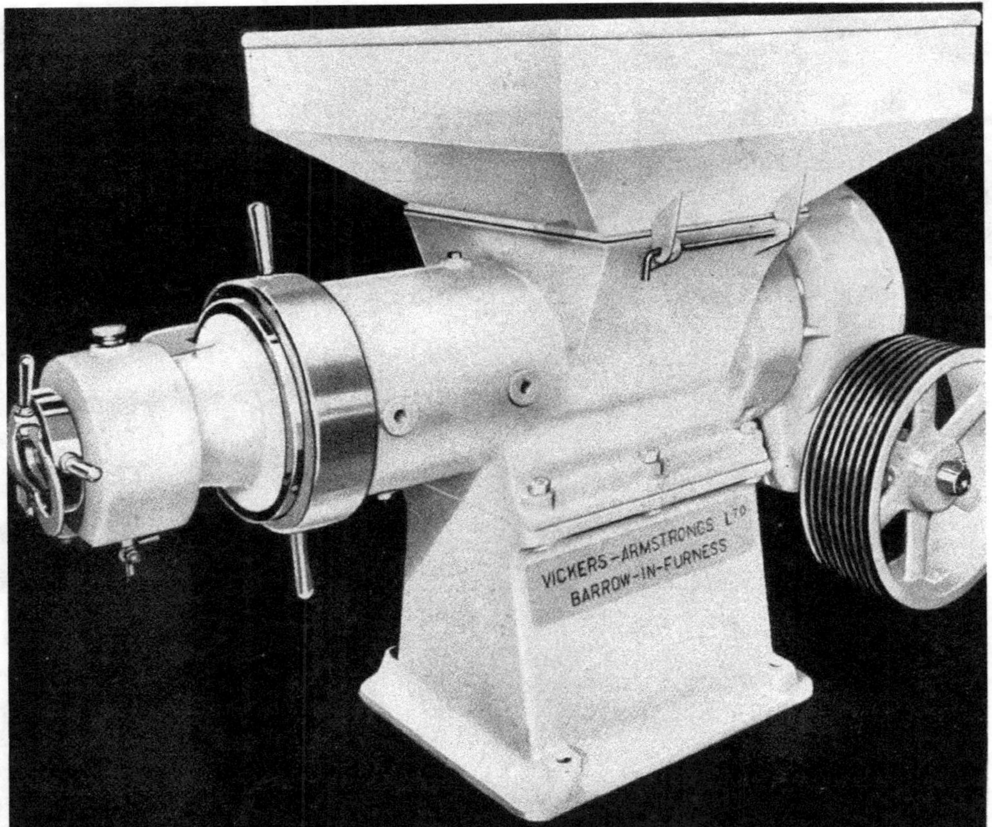

[*By courtesy of Vickers-Armstrongs Ltd.*

FIG. 85.—Toilet soap plodder (with left-hand drive).

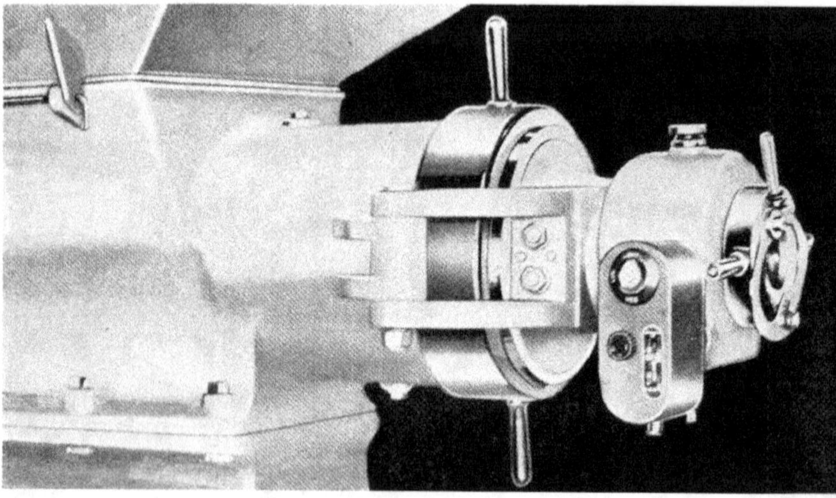

FIG. 86.—Illustration of nozzle showing coupling closed and control box of the electric immersion heater.

[*By courtesy of Vickers-Armstrongs Ltd.*

FIG. 87.—Illustration of opened nozzle showing bayonet type coupling.

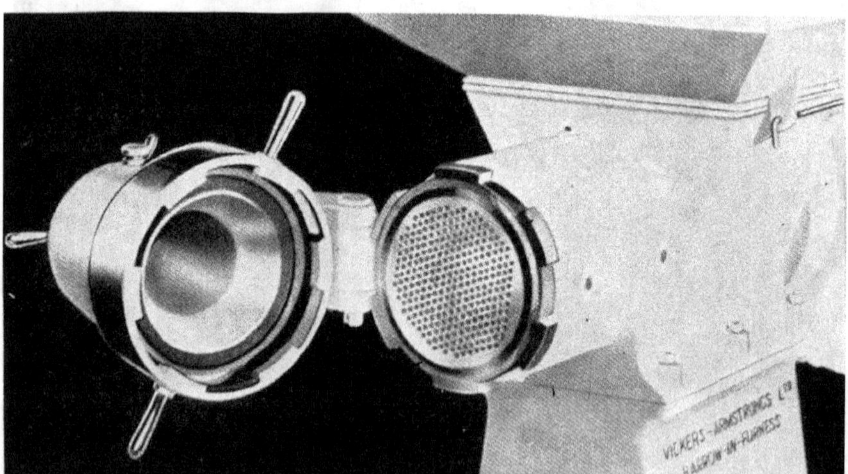

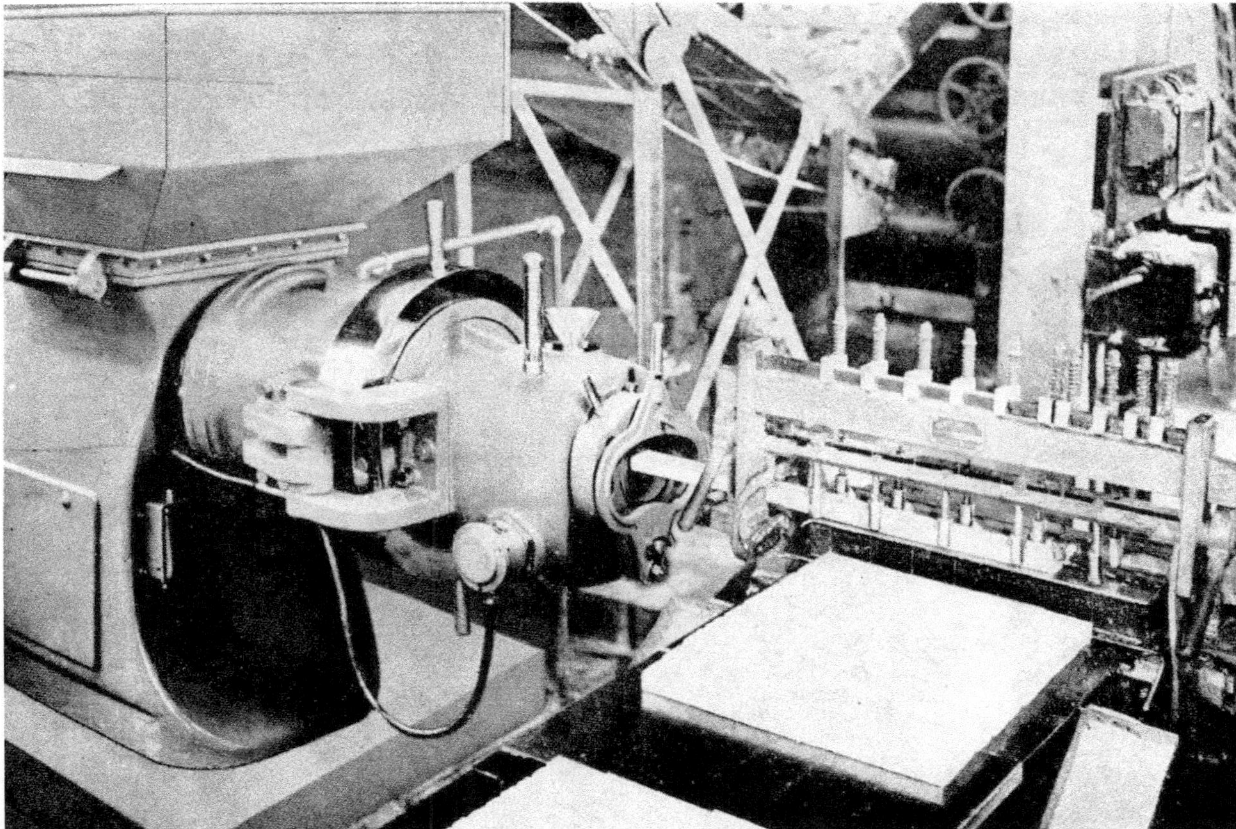

[*By courtesy of Henry Simon Ltd.*

FIG. 88.—Hand-operated (rack and pinion) cutter.

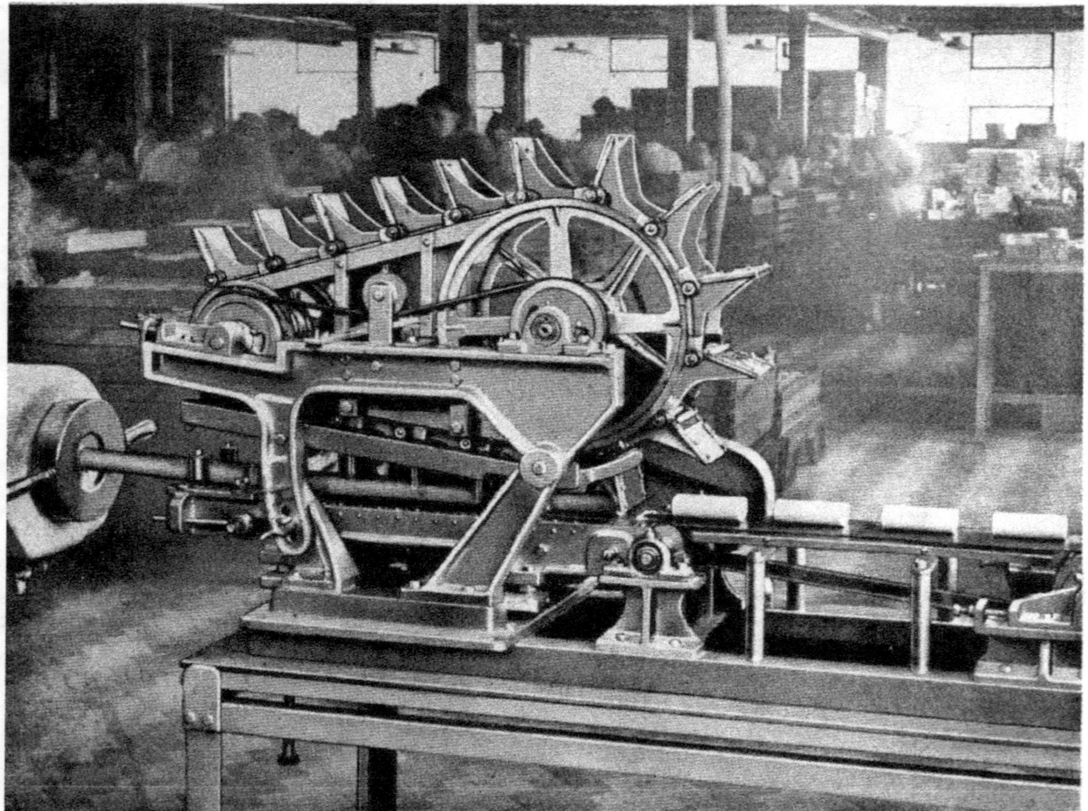

[*By courtesy of Henry Simon Ltd.*

Fig. 89.—Continuous cutting machine.

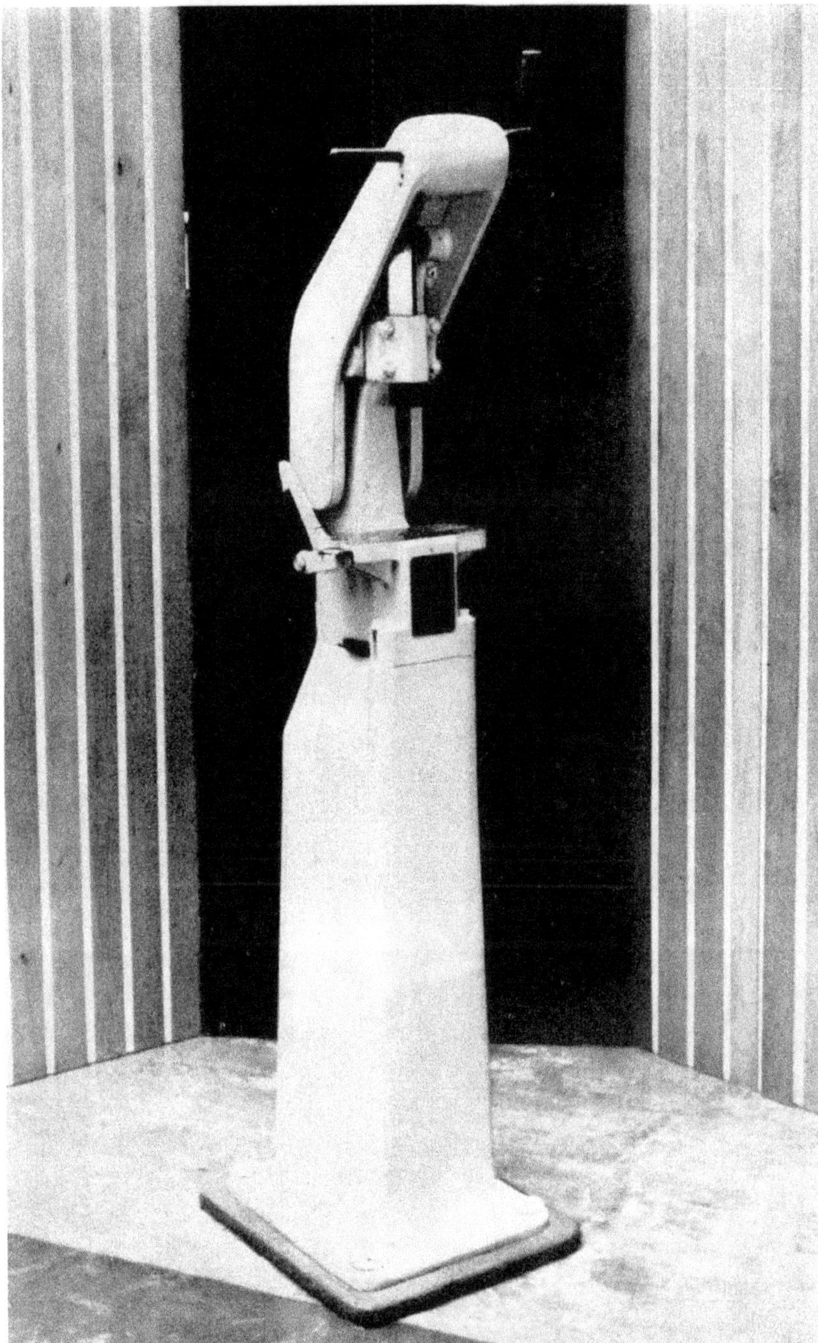

[*By courtesy of Vickers-Armstrongs Ltd.*

FIG. 90.—Hand-operated soap stamper (M.P. Mk. II).

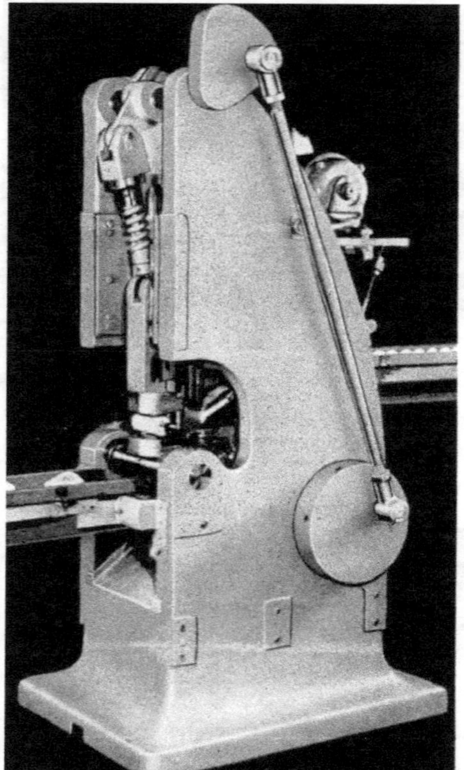

FIG. 91.—Jones type toggle R.

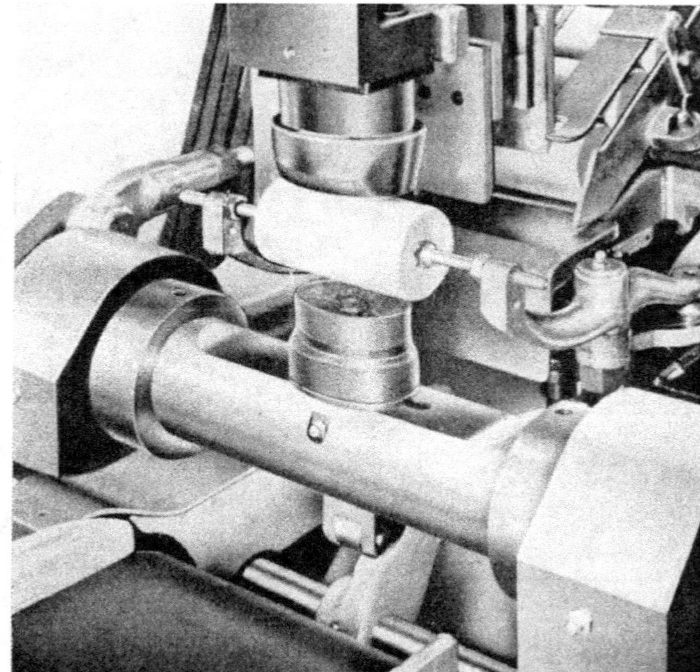

[*By courtesy of R. A. Jones & Co. Inc., Cincinnati, U.S.A.*

FIG. 92.—Jones type R toggle-operated pin tie press for toilet soap.

advantageous. (*See* " Additives in Shampoo Formulation ", Chapter 22.)

Apart from the dermatological angle, there are other technical factors involved in the addition of a certain amount of a superfatting material to soap, for example Glenn (*Soap, N.Y.*, 1939, **9**, 70) has enumerated the following :

(i) Reduced tendency of milled toilet soap to split or crack in use ;
(ii) Process of milling and plodding often made easier as the soap is rendered more plastic ;
(iii) The lather produced is usually smoother and closer in texture and the tablet in use has a velvety feel superior to that of ordinary soap.

As already mentioned such superfat may consist of white petroleum jelly, lanolin, cold cream, etc., added at the stage of amalgamating the soap chips with the opacifying agents, colour (if any), and perfume. Solutions, or dispersions of carboxymethylcellulose and allied derivatives, are sometimes included at this stage, with a view to improving the feel of the soap tablet and the quality of the lather in " washing down ".

Antiseptic Soaps

In recent years the development of antiseptics which are very effective in soap has enabled the manufacturers to market really effective products. One such substance is G-11 (Givaudan-Delawanna). Others are " Actamer " (Monsanto Chemicals) and " Anobial " (Firmenich & Co.). Claims have also been made for chlorinated xylenols in soap. These materials are discussed in some detail in Chapter 42. When incorporated in soap they are added dissolved in a suitable solvent, or dispersed in a dry state, during the process of amalgamation described earlier in this chapter.

CHAPTER 28

BATH PREPARATIONS

Bath Salts

These are used for the purpose of softening the water and at the same time providing it with a refreshing and attractive odour. There is no doubt that this latter function is of very great importance and that bath salts are often used in cases where the water requires no softening, solely on account of the psychological effect of adding coloured perfumed crystals to the water.

Three factors, therefore, appeal to the user: the colour, the general shape and size (i.e. appearance) of the crystals, and the fragrance of the perfume imparted.

In addition, of course, such preparations should leave the water soft and clear and not interfere with the lathering properties of the soap.

Requirements of a Bath Crystal

The requirements of such crystals are therefore:

(*a*) They should be readily soluble and effectively soften the water.

(*b*) Should possess an attractive appearance, be stable under ordinary climatic conditions, and should be easy to colour and perfume.

(*c*) should be reasonably inexpensive.

No one particular substance possesses all these desirable qualities and it is therefore necessary to compromise.

Substances Commonly Employed as Bath Salts

Sodium Carbonate. This is cheap, readily soluble in water and an effective water softener. Moreover, its crystals when tinted have an attractive appearance. Unfortunately it possesses a low melting point. At 33° C. a part of its water of crystallisation commences to dissociate, this acting as a solvent for the remainder, ultimately a sticky viscous mass results which is most unsightly. Such products must be protected therefore from direct sunlight. Even under ordinary conditions of storage, some efflorescence occurs, although this may be partially prevented by coating the crystals with a small proportion of a hygroscopic substance, e.g. glycerin, ethylene glycol, etc., dissolved previously in the dye solution.

Moreover, owing to its alkalinity, it is difficult to colour and perfume really well. These facts account for its diminishing popularity, particularly when better materials are now available.

Sodium Carbonate Monohydrate ($Na_2CO_3 . H_2O$). If the ordinary crystalline form of sodium carbonate is allowed to effloresce it ultimately reaches the composition $Na_2CO_3 . H_2O$ beyond which it does not lose further moisture. Conversely, if the anhydrous form of sodium carbonate is exposed to damp air it occludes water with the formation of the same monohydrate—which is therefore the most stable form of sodium carbonate under ordinary climatic conditions. A new process for the manufacture of this substance has been developed, and a product possessing an attractive physical form and of high chemical purity is now available in three different grades, viz. :

Large. (Passing a 3/16-in. sieve : retained on a 1/8-in.)
Medium. (Passing a 1/8-in sieve : retained on a 1/16-in.)
Small. (Passing a 1/16-in. sieve : retained on a 1/32-in.)

These grades consist of crystal agglomerates, and contain not less than 99·4 per cent. pure sodium carbonate monohydrate.

This retains its attractive appearance even in tropical heat, dissolves in water giving a clear colourless solution, and has a good solubility (26·5 per cent. at 20° C.). Its sole disadvantage appears to be its slower rate of dissolution, and to overcome this it should be added as soon as the bath water is turned on, in order to give it sufficient time to dissolve.

Sodium Sesquicarbonate ($Na_2CO_3NaHCO_3 . 2H_2O$). This is available in fine needle crystals of high purity. One of the best known supplies contains only 1 per cent. of normal sodium carbonate and 0·02 per cent. non-alkaline impurities. This salt is extraordinarily stable and does not require special precautions in packing ; it dissolves rapidly without residue in water, is easy to colour and perfume and has a bright, attractive appearance. It is the only product which can be marketed for this purpose, if desired, uncoloured, although its attractiveness is enhanced by dyeing it.

Trisodium Phosphate. This may be obtained in flake or globular form. It possesses the disadvantages of being difficult to tint, producing a milky appearance to the water when soap is used, and, further, the *p*H of its solution, in concentrations such as are normally used for bath salts, renders it unsuitable to be used alone.

Sodium Chloride. This occurs in colourless cubical crystals which are only slightly hygroscopic, and can be tinted and perfumed with the production of quite an attractive bath salt. It is said to refresh the skin. However, it is devoid of water-softening properties, and interferes with the production of a soapy lather. Although it may be utilised as a constituent of a foaming sea bath, in conjunction with soapless detergents, it is of no interest in the production of ordinary bath salts and needs no further consideration.

Borax. Borax does not affect the constituents of the perfumes normally used and is easy to tint. It possesses a mild detergent action and is obtainable in various grades of granulation. Its disadvantage appears to be its low solubility (8·7 per cent. at 40° C.).

Additives

The efficacy of the above bath salts may be increased by the use of one of the detergent builders and sequestrants such as sodium tripolyphosphate or sodium tetrapyrophosphate. (For further information on these substances, *see* Chapter 22.)

Having selected the substance it is desired to use, and/or any additives of suitable particle size, the next procedure is tinting and perfuming the mixture.

Method of Tinting

There are two methods of carrying out this operation:

(*a*) By spraying.
(*b*) By immersion.

The former is probably the easier for the smaller manufacturer, and it is also easier to judge the depth of colour which can be altered as desired by altering the density of spraying. The latter is better for tinting bath crystals on a large scale, although it has the disadvantage of slower drying unless a proportion of alcohol is included, or a centrifugal drier is utilised. The solvent, if aqueous, must be a saturated solution of the substance which is being dyed, otherwise solution will occur; alternatively, industrial methylated spirit may be employed. With spirit dyes a little ester gum or resin may be added to fix the colour.

Perfuming

These are best perfumed by spraying. The perfume used must be alkali stable, and may consist of essential oils (preferably terpeneless) mixed with a relatively large proportion of fixative, e.g. resinoid of benzoin, olibanum, etc. The most suitable perfumes for use are lavender, eau-de-Cologne, verbena and pine, although special bouquets may be purchased which are suitable for this purpose.

PACKING

In order to appeal to the fastidious woman, they should be packed in attractive wide-mouthed glass containers.

BATH CUBES

These consist usually of sodium carbonate, or sesquicarbonate and/or borax. The preliminary tinting of the material may be carried out by the processes described for bath crystals. Prior to compressing the tablets, particularly if sodium carbonate is used for this purpose—some disintegrating material such as sodium lauryl sulphate or starch should be included as failing this the sodium carbonate may set to a rock hard block which will be found very difficult to dissolve in the bath.

The following formulation for an effervescent tablet is from the *Drug Cosm. Ind.* ("Readers' Questions", Nov. 1950, p. 675) :

	per cent.
Sodium bicarbonate	55·0
Tartaric acid	20·0
Sodium sesquicarbonate	20·0
Perfume and colour	5·0

Procedure

Dry all the ingredients thoroughly. Mix, add perfume, compress and spray the colour in alcoholic solution on the tablets.

BATH OILS AND EMULSIONS

It is not proposed to discuss separate formulation of bath emulsions since emulsions for complexion or cleansing milks have already been given in Chapter 5. By including a fairly high proportion of perfume in place of some of the oil and by selecting perfume components that are stable at the *p*H of the "milk" to be used, such bath emulsions may readily be prepared. However, because of the relatively high concentration of perfume required, such "milks" are almost certain to discolour if made with one of the amino-fatty acid emulsifiers.

An alternative method is to emulsify the perfume in water by means of gums, acacia (or acacia mixed with tragacanth) utilising the pharmacopoeial methods of emulsifying essential oils. By this method concentrated dispersions of perfumes in water may be obtained, in the cold.

However, the main demand for liquid perfume preparations has been for bath oils. These are of two types. In the first type the perfume is dissolved in an oil, such as mineral oil, which is coloured and then encapsulated in a gelatin capsule. These *look* quite attractive but when dropped into the bath, take rather a while to dissolve, the perfumed oil floats on the surface of the water, and the gelatin capsule is left as a soggy mass near the plug hole which some people dislike. Alternatively, the same mixture may be put up in a bottle. The capsule idea, because of its small size, attractive appearance and " good price " appears to be more popular for this type than the bottle.

In the second type, the perfume is dispersed to form a transparent dispersion (*see* Chapter 41, Emulsions and Dispersions), which can be coloured, is water-soluble and can be added to the bath, sometimes producing a milky effect. Originally sulphonated oils were mixed with the perfume for this purpose but more recently the development of " tailored " emulsifiers, especially of the non-ionic type has provided an alternative, though rather more expensive medium.

Formerly such clear solutions of essential oils required a large proportion of alcohol to dissolve the perfume; non-ionic emulsifiers now permit a large reduction, or even replacement of the alcohol with water and emulsifier. Such " solubilised oils " (as discussed in Chapter 41) are transparent dispersions, or " transparent emulsions " (as may be shown by a cone of light impinged on the dispersion) and not true solutions.

The following formulations illustrate the use of such materials:

	Partial replacement of alcohol *per cent.*	*Complete replacement of alcohol* *per cent.*
Perfume compound	1·0	1·0
Alcohol	40·0	—
" Tween " 20 (Polyoxyalkylene sorbitan monolaurate)	3·0	6·0
Water	56·0	93·0

(*Courtesy, Atlas Powder Co.*)

Procedure

Dissolve perfume compound in " Tween " 20 and slowly add water at room temperature, with moderate agitation. [Similar results can be obtained by the use of Cithrol No. 6 (Croda Ltd.) 12 parts, perfume 1 part, water 93 parts.]

It will be noted that the concentration of perfume at 1 per cent. level is low and that hence a very concentrated perfume is required. Alternatively, the water may be omitted and solutions, or rather dispersions, of very much greater strength of perfume prepared which can be added to the bath. Unfortunately these are expensive because of the increased cost due both to the level of perfume and of non-ionic dispersing agent; moreover, since these are not anhydrous they are not suitable for packing in ordinary gelatin capsules (which would have allowed a " smaller dosage " at an enhanced price).

The following illustrate the use of higher levels of both perfumes and dispersant:

Solubilised essential oil	*per cent.*[1]	*Parts by weight*[2]
Essential oil	15·0	15·0
"Tween" 20 (Polyoxyalkylene sorbitan monolaurate)	85·0	—
"Cithrol" No. 6 (Croda)	—	170·0

Procedure

The oil is mixed with the solubiliser at room temperature and the mixture can then be diluted with any proportion of water without clouding.

[In the example quoted, *peppermint oil* is the essential oil used, nevertheless the same *principle* applies and by carefully studying which essential oils and synthetics are solubilised by the above process, a perfume compound may be built up.]

An example of the older type of formulation, utilising sulphonated castor oil is:

	per cent.
Perfume	5–10
Sulphonated castor oil	95–90

Whilst a cheap solubilised pine oil may be prepared thus:

	per cent.
Bornyl acetate	2·0
Sulphonated olive oil	98·0

For other methods of solubilising essential oils using high proportions of potassium oleate, potassium ricinoleate, triethanolamine linoleate, etc., reference may be made to the paper by Albert and Wyburn (*Soap Perfum. Cosm.*, June 1939, p. 498). Unfortunately the methods described in this paper are not suitable for dispersing delicate perfumes.

Foam Baths

Foam baths or "bubble baths" are a comparatively recent innovation and consist, as their name would suggest, of a bath full of light, dense, gleaming creamy lather.

In addition to their detergent action, they possess a definite psychological effect. The warmth, fragrance and softness of the foam induce a feeling of contentment at the end of a day's labour and act as a fitting sedative before a night's rest.

For the above reasons it is probable that their use will in the future become more general.

[1] Courtesy, Atlas Powder Co., Wilmington.
[2] Courtesy, Croda Ltd.

Factors Underlying Foam Production Stability

In formulating a successful foam bath it is necessary to consider the theoretical factors involved in the production of a stable foam.

The formulation of a bubble involves an increase in the surface area, which is opposed by the natural forces of surface tension. It is, therefore, obvious that the surface tension of the solution must first be lowered by the introduction of a suitable agent. Although thus diminished it will still be present and may tend to impair the permanence of the bubbles formed. For this reason the bubbles should be rendered more stable by the introduction of a substance capable of increasing the viscosity of the bubble wall, i.e. its rigidity.

This may be brought about without raising the viscosity of the solution as a whole, by including a surface-active agent capable of concentrating itself on the actual bubble surface, for example saponin.

Types of Foaming Agents

The use of soaps for such purposes is quite unsatisfactory. The lather obtained is wet and the bubbles large and unstable. Moreover, they are quite useless in waters containing appreciable quantities of dissolved lime or magnesium salts because a precipitation of calcium and magnesium soaps as a dirty hard scum will occur. Neither are the amino soaps suitable for this purpose.

Quite a number of journals, either in their " Enquiries " service to readers, or in definite articles, have suggested the use of effervescent powders for the production of foam baths, these usually being composed of sodium bicarbonate, tartaric acid and starch, etc. *These are of course quite useless.* The amount of carbon dioxide, or other gas, required to aerate a normal bath efficiently would require the use of several pounds of sodium bicarbonate—a demonstrable absurdity.

On the other hand, excellent foam baths can be prepared by the use of the foaming agents described below, in conjunction with cylinders of compressed air or carbon dioxide. Alternatively, special fittings for attachment to the water supply on the lines of a water pump can be used where the pressure of the supply is sufficiently high. The former equipment, although convenient for use in high-class beauty salons, is quite impracticable for home use. There is, however, no reason why cheap fittings of the latter type might not be put up for home use with the ordinary *foam bath* powder or liquid.

The mere beating up of the foam dispels some of the glamour with which such baths tend to be surrounded, and preferably such foam should be produced mechanically by the jet of water impinging under high pressure into the main solution.

One of the best surfactants for the production of a foam bath is triethanolamine lauryl sulphate, which will on agitation in water produce a fairly heavy layer of well-knit, small-sized bubbles. The amount and stability of these bubbles may be improved by the addition of saponin or other bubble stabilisers. Some of the mucilages and the cellulosic derivatives are helpful for this purpose. The following illustrates such a formulation :

	per cent.
Triethanolamine lauryl sulphate liquid	50·0
Foam builder and stabiliser	5·0
Water	45·0
Colour	*q.s.*
Perfume	*q.s.*

[Saponin, though it enhances and stabilises the foam, is not really very satisfactory as it darkens in alkaline solution on keeping.]

The various characteristics of the commonly available surfactants, builders, sequestrants, etc., are dealt with in detail in Chapter 22 and it is suggested that this chapter be consulted with a view to selecting materials for formulation and trial.

Many of the materials included in shampoos to increase their viscosity and efficacy can be included also in bubble, i.e. foam baths. Liquid foams or foam bath preparations give the best results, and offer the widest field for experiment.

There is one outstanding disadvantage of the present-day foam baths, they are not resistant to soap, and this must therefore be excluded for the toilet, when they are used.

Directions for use of Foam Bath Preparations

The usual direction given with such preparations is to remove all soap, by first rinsing the bath with hot water. The preparation is then placed under the direct stream of the tap and hot water run in to a depth of about four inches, this being then worked up to a high foam by means of the hands or a bath brush (possibly a specially shaped paddle could be supplied for such purposes, containing slots or holes to produce the greatest possible agitation).

The requisite amount of hot and cold water is then run in as usual. Massage the body with the foam, using no soap at all. To remove foam from bath wipe over with a soapy cloth.

PERFUMING AND TINTING OF SUCH PREPARATIONS

Pine oil perfumes are sometimes used for perfuming such preparations but to my mind these are improved by the use of a fragrant but fresh odour such as eau-de-Cologne, or one of the synthetic bouquets: lilac or lavender, etc.

The tinting is usually accomplished by the addition of a small quantity of a dye.

CHAPTER 29

SHAVING PREPARATIONS

Shaving Cream—Brushless Shaving Cream—The Pressurised-Dispensing of Shaving Creams—Electric Razors—Shaving and Skin Infections, Role of Antiseptics—Pre- and After-Shave Lotions—Powders.

AFTER many years in which development in shaving preparations has appeared dormant, the adaptation of the wartime insecticidal high-pressure spray (operating at greatly reduced pressures) to the dispensing of pressurised-shaving creams has, in the United States, led to a sudden demand for these products.

Although the solids content of such preparations is considerably lower than that of an ordinary shaving cream, the general principles of basic formulation and many of the same criteria apply. For this reason discussion is confined initially to the discussion of shaving creams in general after which some notes on the difficulties involved in the pressurised-dispensing of such (and other similar types of) products are included.

The absorption of water from a shaving soap or cream lowers the tensile strength of the hair, while the formation of lather supports the hair shaft in a convenient cutting position and at the same time acts as a protection against skin injury.

The use of shaving powders is now to all intents and purposes obsolete, except in barbers' shops; shaving soaps are, however, still popular since they are more economical than creams and are readily packed. However, there is a large and increasing market for modern soap creams which readily produce a soft lather, and which in some cases also contain substances to prevent or minimise skin injury.

CRITERIA OF A GOOD SHAVING-SOAP CREAM

(1) It must produce a rich, copious lather, composed of small bubbles, since large ones are watery and unsatisfactory.

(2) It must be non-irritant.

(3) It must have good wetting-out properties.

(4) It should be white, smooth, soft and entirely free from lumps.

(5) It must adhere readily to both face and brush and yet be readily removed on rinsing.

(6) It must retain a satisfactory consistency and texture over all temperature conditions likely to be encountered in use.

These qualities can be obtained only by a suitable choice of raw material. Stearic acid alone does not produce a sufficiently voluminous lather, and for this purpose some coconut oil is included. The ratio of stearic acid to coconut oil varies considerably with different products, but the inclusion of about 25 per cent. coconut oil with 75 per cent. stearic acid will usually be found satisfactory.

Saponification of the fat charge is usually accomplished with a mixture of potassium and sodium hydroxides. Carbonates are not recommended since they liberate carbon dioxide which is liable to become entrapped in the cream. Triethanolamine, isopropanolamine or other amino compounds such as 2-methyl-2-amino-1,3-propanediol ("Amino glycol") may be employed as alkali in conjunction with fatty acids, and a proportion of sodium hydroxide included to give the desired firmness.

The tendency of triethanolamine soaps under certain conditions to develop a yellow tinge may be overcome, according to Wolff (*Fette and Seifen*, March 1952, p. 142, through *Soap, N.Y.*, Dec. 1952, p. 97), by incorporating a small amount (1 to 2 per cent.; at most 5 per cent.) of sulphurous acid in the triethanolamine. It is stated that the triethanolamine appears quite normal except that it contains a small amount of sulphur dioxide and that its degree of whiteness cannot be matched by any process involving distillation.

In order to prevent too rapid drying out of the shaving cream, glycerin is included in the formulation. Opinions regarding its effect upon the lathering properties of the cream vary. A proportion of 10 to 15 per cent. will be found satisfactory. Part of the glycerin may be replaced by sorbitol syrup. (*See* Chapter 44.)

An emollient may be included with a view to the cream being "easier on the skin". Emollients which may be included for this purpose are, "free fat", lanolin, fatty alcohols such as cetyl alcohol, mineral oil or vaseline. The proportion of any such additive must be kept low (of the order of 1 per cent.) if the lathering properties of the cream are not to be impaired.

The total fatty acid in a cream varies between 35–50 per cent. and the final reaction of such creams is about pH 10·0. Attention has been drawn (*Mfg. Chemist*, Aug. 1933, **4**, 228) to the fact that the foaming power is not directly proportional to the fatty acid or glycerin content of a cream. The type of water with which the cream is to be used, if hard, will render the use of more soap necessary to obtain a good lather, and in very hard water areas it may be desirable to increase the proportion of coconut oil present in the fat charge.

Thomssen and Kemp (*Modern Soap Making*, New York, 1937) have correctly drawn attention to the fact that plasticity of a shaving cream is best obtained by a 5 : 1 ratio of potassium hydroxide to sodium hydroxide and the presence of 3-5 per cent. free fatty acid. For detailed information on soap shaving creams a monograph on soap manufacture should be consulted. The following, however, will serve as a guide for experiment, but it may be mentioned that the manufacture of a good shaving cream which will stand up to various climatic conditions, is like the making of a sponge-cake—a *fine* art. Much of our knowledge on these products is still empiric. (To appreciate the complex nature of such products, *see* Vanishing Creams, Chapter 9.)

	per cent.
Stearic acid	30·0
Coconut oil	10·0
Palm kernel oil	5·0
Potassium hydroxide	7·0
Sodium hydroxide	1·5
Glycerin	10·0
Water	36·5
Perfume	*q.s.*

Procedure

Mix one-half of the stearic acid with the oils, melt by steam heat, and bring to a temperature of 75°-80° C. Run in the alkali, water, and glycerin and stir well until saponification is complete. The remainder of the melted stearic acid is now added and any water which may be necessary to compensate for evaporation that may have occurred in the process of manufacture.

Ralph H. Auch (*Amer. Perfum.*, May 1937, p. 50) gives the following shaving-cream formulae :

	per cent.
Coconut oil	10·0
Stearic acid	35·0
Potassium hydroxide (100 per cent.)	6·8
Sodium hydroxide (100 per cent.)	1·5
Glycerin	15·0
Perfume	0·50–0·75
Water about	31·2

Procedure

The potash and soda are dissolved in about two-thirds of the cold water in an enamelled pot by the smaller cosmetic manufacturer. [The soap manufacturer or bigger cosmetic manufacturer has liquid soda and liquid potash available having bought them that way, or dissolved the solid drum caustic to a definite concentration, or Baumé, which he dilutes to the requisite strength.] The glycerin and coconut oil are heated to 165°–170° F. The caustic solution is run in, in a thin stream while agitating. When the saponification is complete and while the mass is still hot, the molten stearic acid is added followed by the balance of the water, while continuing the agitation.

Another procedure is to employ white soap (coconut oil soap) scrap as the source of both soda and coconut oil:

	per cent.
Stearic acid	37·0
Potassium hydroxide (100 per cent.)	7·0
Water (to dissolve lye)	12·0
Glycerin	15·0
White scrap soap	12·0
Water (to dissolve above)	16·5
Perfume	0·5

Procedure

Procedure is the same as with the previous formula if the scrap soap is superfatted, as is usually the case. If, however, it is neutral, it may be added last in chip form with agitation until a homogeneous mass is finally obtained.

An American formulation, containing sorbitol syrup ("Arlex"), olive oil, boric acid (rather a higher amount than usually included in British shaving creams), and menthol is given below:

	Parts
Stearic acid	25·0
Coconut oil	8·0
"Arlex" (sorbitol syrup)	3·5
Boric acid	1·5
Potassium hydroxide (42° Bé)	18·0
Sodium hydroxide (42° Bé)	2·5
Water	39·0
Olive oil	2·0
Cetyl alcohol	1·0
Menthol	0·22

(*Courtesy, Atlas Powder Co., Wilmington.*)

Procedure

The recommended procedure in preparing this cream is to heat the stearic acid and oils to 212° F. At this point the alkali, likewise heated to the same temperature, is slowly added with stirring. The mixture is then held at 210° F. for 16 hours and stirred every 3 or 4 hours. Next, the boric acid dissolved in half the water is added at 212° F. and mixed. Finally, the remaining constituents mixed with water at 212° F. are added and the composition is stirred slowly while cooling.

Doubleday (*Soap Perfum. Cosm.*, 1950, 7, 715) gives the following formulation for what he terms " a non-irritant " shave cream :

	Parts
Coconut oil	10·0
Castor oil	2·0
Fatty acid (myristic)	5·0
Stearic acid	25·0
Potassium hydroxide (89/90)	9·5
Borax	0·5
Diglycol stearate	2·0
Stearyl alcohol	1·0
Liquid paraffin	1·5
Sorbitol syrup	5·0
Water	45·0

Procedure

Fatty acids (without previously melting) are added to hot aqueous alkali (potassium hydroxide and borax solution). After saponification the remaining solid ingredients and liquid paraffin are added and stirred slowly. After being kept hot for an hour, the sorbitol syrup is added.

LIQUID SHAVING CREAM

According to *Amer. Perfum.* (" Questions and Answers ", Oct. 1949, p. 283) a liquid shaving cream may be made along the lines of the following formula adjusting the viscosity by alteration in the water content. [The author would suggest that the viscosity might be more readily controlled by the use of an aqueous dispersion of one of the cellulose derivatives such as sodium carboxymethylcellulose, or other water-soluble viscous material] :

	per cent.
Stearic acid XXX	8·4
Coconut oil	8·4
100 per cent. potassium hydroxide	2·5
Superfatting material	1·0
Glycerin	8·0
Alcohol	3·0
Water	68·7

U.S. Patents 2,435,828 and 2,435,829 describe a method for the preparation of soaps having the desirable characteristics of coconut oil soaps, but prepared synthetically from the higher saturated fatty acids produced in the United States from fats and oils of domestic origin. The most readily available is commercial stearic acid which is a mixture of palmitic and stearic acids, but lauric and myristic acids are also mentioned as raw materials. The fatty acid is first halogenated in the position *alpha* to the carboxyl group and the halogenated compound is then treated with the sodium or potassium derivative of a polyhydric alcohol such as ethylene glycol or glycerin. This reaction results in the formation of a soap having an alkanol group attached to the *alpha* carbon atom of the soap molecule through an ether linkage. If the starting materials were α-bromostearic acid and sodium ethylene glycollate, the product would be the sodium soap of α-ethylene glycol stearic acid. With the addition of an oxygenated side chain, the soaps of palmitic and stearic acid, it is stated, become very soluble in water and according to the patent, lather well even in hard water. In the example given below, the potassium soap is employed:

	per cent.
Potassium soap of α-glyceryl stearic acid . . .	30·0
Stearic acid	30·0
Potassium hydroxide solution (specific gravity 1·5) . .	12·0
Water	28·0

The substitution of up to 5 parts of an alkanolamine soap of α-glyceryl stearic acid to replace a corresponding amount of the potassium soap is said to improve the product.

The new soaps are claimed to hold water and not dry out so readily on the face in use, and to be free from the "harshness" of coconut soaps on the skin.

Alkali Free Fatty Acids and Total Fatty Matter

These are adjusted to the correct proportions by analytical determination. As has been stated under vanishing creams (Chapter 9) the neutralisation of even so simple a mixture as stearic acid with potassium hydroxide leads to the production of a number of complex soaps. Acid soaps can co-exist in the presence of alkali pockets. This condition is not brought out by ordinary laboratory examination since, when the cream is dissolved in alcohol and titrated against indicator, the analyst obtains a figure which is the sum of acid-soap and free alkali [which can react and "neutralise each other"] in alcoholic solution but which cannot indicate that no "free alkali" exists in pockets in the cream.

The Phenomenon of "Rotting"

There is evidence that shaving cream improves on storage. The period of storage may vary from a week to several weeks; some manufacturers give as long as three weeks for the cream to improve. The improvement can be traced to the formation of a smoother and softer cream. From microscopical studies which the author has conducted, it is evident that very complex changes occur in the structure of the cream and many changes in crystal formation can occur. This phenomenon is commonly known as " curing " or " rotting ".

Brushless or Non-Lathering Creams

More recently the brush type of cream has been challenged by the so-called brushless or latherless type. These are modifications of ordinary vanishing creams and are used, as their name implies, without the application of a brush, being merely applied to the face, which is then shaved with the razor in the usual manner. The cream is, however, not removed, but ultimately rubbed into the skin. Such creams bring the beard into position for cutting and also exert a softening effect upon the skin.

These creams are becoming increasingly popular, particularly in the United States, and there is no doubt that they are perfectly satisfactory, when properly prepared and used in conjunction with a keen blade.

A good blade actually cuts the hair close to its point of emergence, a poor one merely tears it from its follicle, bringing with it adhering portions of its sheath, and rendering the face blotchy. The major factor in any shaving preparation is still the cutting edge. Although the modern forms of such creams contain suitable wetting agents, their softening effect is, in general, not as rapid as that of the soaps. It is recommended by many text books to incorporate a little spermaceti to stop such creams vanishing too readily. Since the ultimate aim of an ideal cream would be to vanish after the shave was completed, we actually have two factors which are diametrically opposed, and the most we can do is to effect a compromise.

Desirable factors in a brushless cream are that it should :

(1) Spread evenly, be smooth and free from lumps.

(2) Possess a soothing, not an irritant action.

(3) Show no separation, but should maintain a satisfactory consistency and texture over all the temperature conditions likely to be encountered in use.

(4) Allow the beard to be readily cut without pain.

(5) Ultimately vanish, leaving the face with a matt appearance.

Although such creams might, theoretically, be compounded on the basis of some of the newer soapless detergents and wetting agents, in a mucilage adjusted to the requisite *p*H, in practice this does not appear to be satisfactory.

The following are examples of brushless creams:

	per cent.
Stearic acid	25·0
Cetyl alcohol	1·0
Isopropanolamine (or other equivalent alkali)	2·0
Glycerin	5·0
Water	67·0
Preservative	*q.s.*
Perfume	*q.s.*

A little mineral oil or vegetable oil may be included if desired. If the latter, one that does not readily become rancid should be employed. Additional wetting agents, provided they are compatible, may also be included.

The isopropanolamines may be substituted by triethanolamine if desired. The following brushless cream is quoted in the *Drug and Cosmetic Review*, 1946–47, p. 192:

	per cent.
Stearic acid	20·0
Mineral oil	2·0
Cetyl alcohol	0·5
Potassium hydroxide	1·0
Glycerin	7·0
Water	69·5

In general the method of manufacture follows that of a vanishing cream. The stearic acid and fat soluble constituents are melted at 70° C. and the aqueous solution of the alkali and glycerin added at the same temperature. (For details *see* Vanishing Creams, Chapter 9.)

The following formulation includes triethanolamine alginate and Turkey red oil:

	Parts
Triethanolamine alginate TS/RE	5·0
"Nipagin" M (preservative)	0·1
Stearic acid	20·0
Lanolin	5·0
Liquid paraffin	3·0
Borax	2·0
Menthol	0·12
Turkey red oil	1·0
Perfume	0·2
Water to	100·0

Procedure

The alginate, preservative and borax are dispersed in liquid paraffin and the water is stirred in. Then stir in the Turkey red oil and the lanolin. Heat the stearic acid separately to 70° C. then add the stearic acid to the solution and homogenise. When cool stir in the menthol dissolved in the perfume.

(*Courtesy, Alginate Industries Ltd.*)

The following formulation (Glyco Products Inc.) illustrates the use of polyethylene glycol 600 monostearate in a brushless shave :

	Parts
Stearic acid (Triple pressed)	16·0
White mineral oil	4·0
Lanolin (anhydrous)	3·5
Terpineol	0·1
Polyethylene Glycol 600 Monostearate	3·2
Potassium hydroxide	0·8
Propylene glycol	4·0
Water	68·2

Procedure

Manufacture follows the usual course. Fat-soluble substances dissolved in the mixed melted fats. Alkali in the water. Add the hot aqueous solution to the hot oil solution (temperatures of both about 60° C.). Stir, and when the temperature has fallen to about 45° C. add the terpineol dissolved in the propylene glycol.

Carbowax 1500 may be used to formulate so-called non-greasy brushless shave creams :

		Parts
(A)	" Carbowax " 1500	45·0
	Stearic acid	37·5
(B)	Triethanolamine	3·0
	Potassium hydroxide	1·6
	Water	2·0
	Sodium alginate	3·5
	Water	178·0
	Propylene glycol	12·0
	Carbitol	15·0
	Perfume	*q.s.*

(*Courtesy, Carbide and Carbon Chemical Corporation.*

Procedure

Heat (A) to 70° C., and add (B) with stirring. Add sodium alginate, then water at 70° C. Stir in remaining ingredients, adding the perfume dissolved in part of the Carbitol when the cream has cooled to 50° C. Pour at 45° C.

The following formulation is based upon the use of the non-ionic compounds, sorbitan monostearate and polyoxyalkylene sorbitan monostearate :

		per cent.
(A)	Stearic acid	12·5
	" Span " 60 (Sorbitan monostearate)	2·5
	" Tween " 60 (Polyoxyalkylene sorbitan monostearate)	1·0
	White petrolatum	10·0

		per cent.
(B)	Propylene glycol	5·0
	Water	67·0
	Preservative	*q.s.*
(C)	28 per cent. Ammonia water	2·0
	Perfume	*q.s.*

Procedure

Melt (A) and bring to 80° C., bring (B) to 82° C., add (C) to (B) and quickly add this mixture to (A), agitating moderately until the temperature drops to 55° C., perfume, stir slowly and pack at 45° C.

Brushless Shaving Stick

Thomas and Witham (British Patent 537,407) describe a brushless shaving stick which can be applied directly to the face and which leaves on the wetted skin a thin continuous smear, providing adequate lubrication, it is claimed, for the shaving operation. This stick is composed of fatty or waxy material to which hydrophilic properties have been imparted by suitable emulsifier, e.g. soap or partial fatty acid ester of polyhydric alcohol, so that the product is readily wettable by, but not more than very sparingly soluble in, water. Pigment, dyestuff or opacifier is incorporated to indicate presence of composition on face whereby application is facilitated.

The following example is quoted:

	per cent.
Sesame oil	35·35
Spermaceti	45·80
Stearin	7·60
Soap	5·00
Monoglycerides of C.N.O. fatty acids	3·00
Titanium dioxide	2·00
Perfume	1·25

Aerosols: The Pressurised-Dispensing of Cosmetics and Other Preparations

Aerosol Shaving Cream

Webster defines an aerosol as "a suspension of fine solid or liquid particles in air or gas". Today the term aerosol includes all those products which depend upon the power of a compressed liquefied gas to dispense them from their container.

There are three basic types:

(i) True aerosols, e.g. the insecticides and space deodorants.

(ii) So-called wet sprays for surface-coating work.

(iii) Foam products.

CROSS-SECTION OF TYPICAL AEROSOL PACKAGE FOR FOAM-TYPE PRODUCT.

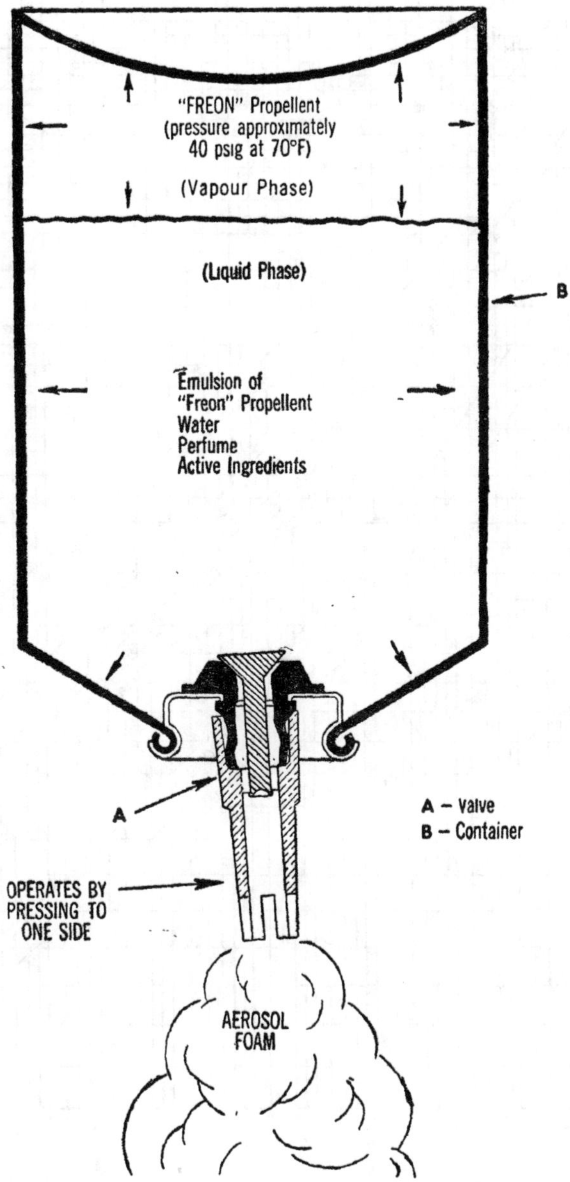

FIG. 93.

[*By courtesy of E. I. du Pont de Nemours & Co.*

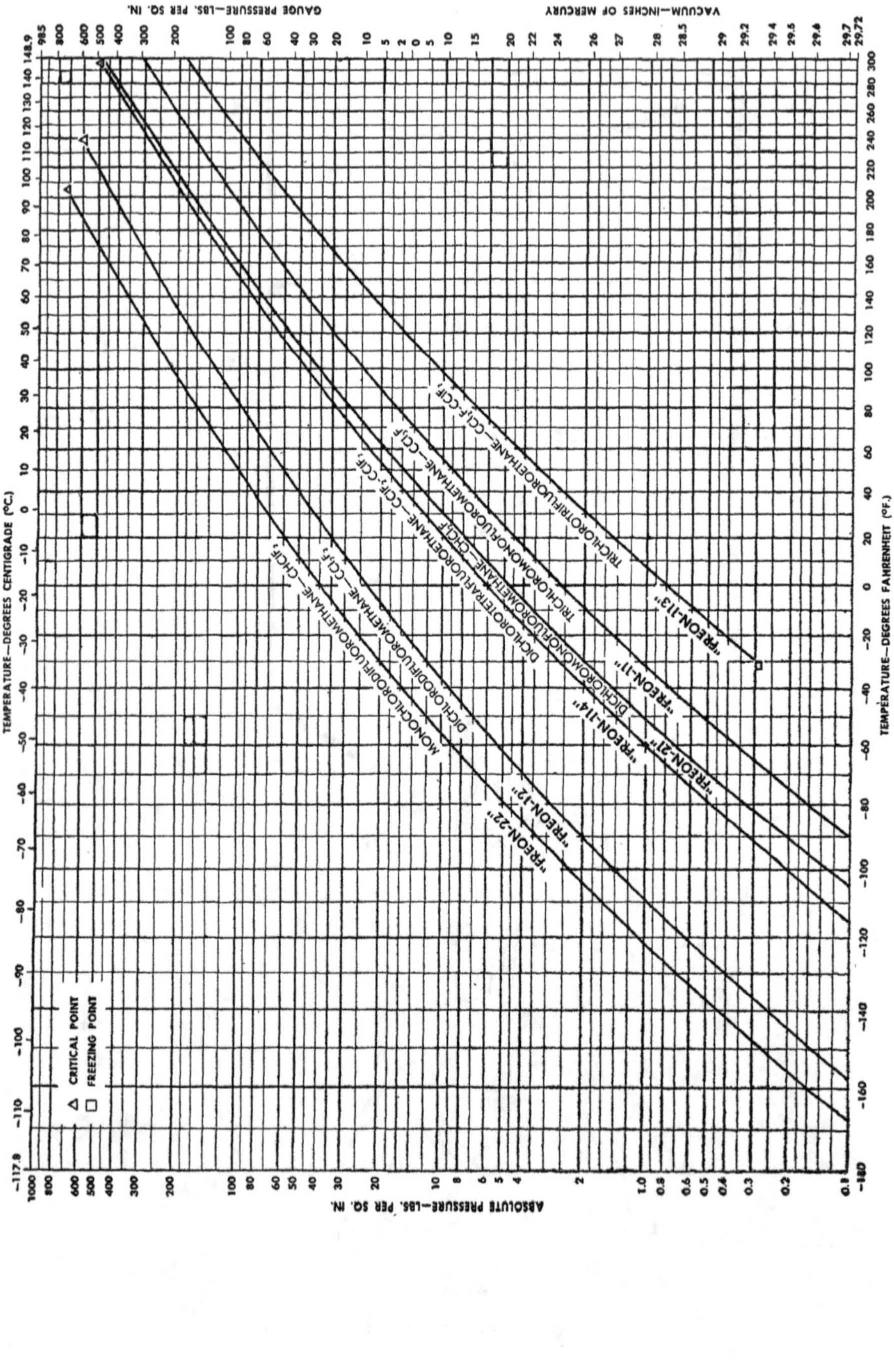

[*By courtesy of E. I. du Pont de Nemours & Co.*

FIG. 94.—Pressure-Temperature Relationship of "Freon" Propellents. ("Freon" is du Pont's registered trade-mark for its fluorinated hydrocarbon propellents.)

The patent basic to all such products is U.S. Patent 2,321,023, issued 8 July 1943, as a result of research by L. D. Goodhue and W. N. Sullivan and assigned to the U.S. Secretary of Agriculture.

Cosmetic aerosols are an adaptation of the wartime U.S. insecticidal high-pressure spray, but operate at very much lower pressures, less than 40 p.s.i. at 70° F. They consist of a mixture of the cosmetic product together with the propellent in a sealed container fitted with a specially designed dispensing valve Part of the propellent remains in solution as a liquid and part changes to a gas and fills the space above. The pressure exerted by this gaseous phase forces the solution out through the dispensing valve, when the valve is opened. On opening the valve, the propellent instantly changes into a gas and thereby disperses the product in the form of either a spray or as a foam. *Foam products are obtained by preparing a partial emulsion of the product and the propellent, using the appropriate propellent and correctly designed valve.* [The principle of foam aerosols is illustrated in the diagrammatic sketch, courtesy, E. I. du Pont de Nemours & Co.]

Propellents. In the United States, the propellents used are chiefly the *Freons* (" Kinetic Chemicals Division ", E. I. du Pont de Nemours & Co. (Inc.), which are chlorinated and fluorinated hydrocarbons ; and the *Genetrons* (General Chemical Division, Allied Chemical and Dye Corporation). Mixtures are frequently employed as some have high and others low vapour pressure. The amount of propellent used varies with the product, from 10 per cent. to 80 per cent.

In the United Kingdom, the " Freon " range of refrigerants were sold in this country, the General Chemicals Division of Imperial Chemical Industries marketing them and re-packing when necessary. With the production by Imperial Chemical Industries of dichlorodifluoromethane and monofluorotrichloromethane under the trade names of " Arcton " 6 and " Arcton " 9, connection with du Ponts on the " Freons " ceased. Dichlorodifluoromethane (" Arcton " 6) exerts at ordinary temperatures a vapour pressure of 57·7 lb. per sq. in., which is too high for use in relatively light walled containers. In order to reduce the pressure the refrigerant was mixed with a higher boiling member of the same family, monofluorotrichloromethane (" Arcton " 9) and by this means a propellent was obtained which exerted a pressure at ordinary temperatures approaching 30 lb. per sq. in. It is understood that this mixture has proved in practice to be suitable as a propellent in insecticidal aerosols or *where the ingredient is not in aqueous, or in some cases alcoholic solution.* Whereas monofluorotrichloromethane hydrolyses readily and hence is of no value for aqueous preparations, many of the other members of the family are more stable. Mixtures are frequently employed in the United

States, since some have high vapour pressure (Freon-12; dichlorodifluoromethane) and others low vapour pressures (Freon-114; dichlorotetrafluoromethane).

Whilst it is impossible to deal in so short a space with the many and varied problems involved in pressurising the dispensing of a cosmetic and toilet product, the following remarks may give some idea, particularly to British readers (since at the time of writing, these products are not on the British market), of the problems involved.

Special Problems Encountered in the Formulation of the Products to be Pressurised

(*a*) The product must be miscible with the propellent (or emulsified—in the case of foams—with it).

(*b*) It must be non-corrosive in respect of the valve and container.

(*c*) It must neither precipitate nor crystallise at the temperatures to which it is likely to be subjected.

(*d*) It must not deposit any gummy, resinous or other materials on the valve.

(*e*) The volume of the dispensed product must be adequate for the purpose.

(*f*) The product must be one that "justifies" pressurising.

A study of the above problems and of the optimum ratio of propellent and product, involves months of study using special pressure-resistant glass apparatus [so that problems of miscibility, precipitation, etc., can be observed] and the use by the scientific staff of protective eye screens, or goggles, etc.

Odour Problems in Aerosols

The evaporation of perfumed materials dispensed from a pressurised container differs from normal evaporation in that, instead of evaporating comparatively slowly, owing to the pressure in an aerosol, the dissemination of the perfume is claimed to be accomplished in an instant. It is stated that examination of perfumes by the usual blotting paper strip method gives little practical help in such cases.

Irritation Problems from Aerosols

Owing to the very fine particle size of the aerosol, perfumery materials which may be practically non-irritant under ordinary conditions of use, can become very irritant when sprayed in the form of an aerosol, an example of this quoted in the literature is that of benzyl benzoate.

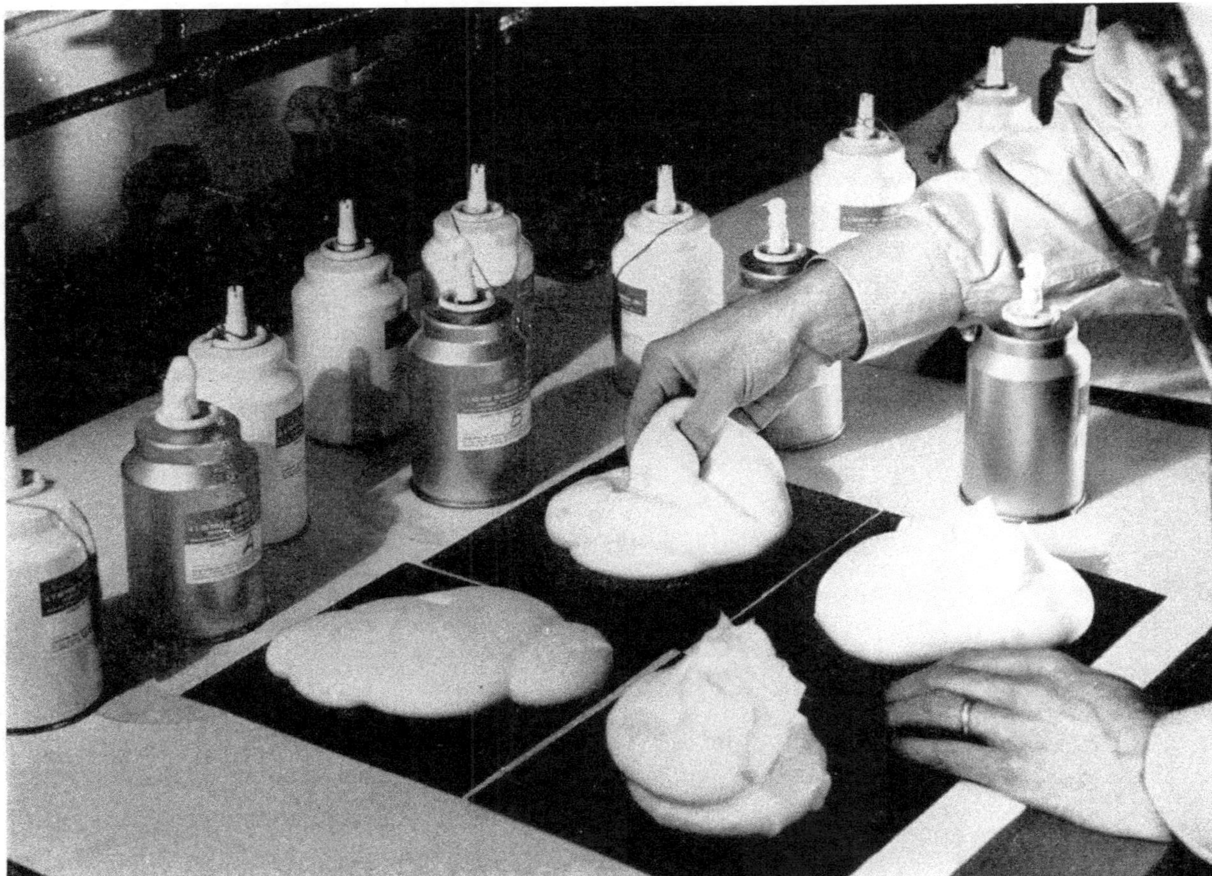

[By courtesy of E. I. du Pont de Nemours & Co.

Fig. 95.—Testing the efficacy of shaving cream " foam " formulations.

(*See* Victor DiGiacomo, " Perfumery Aerosols ", *Proc. Sci. Sect. T.G.A.*, May 1951.)

THE FILLING OF AEROSOLS

The filling of spray-type aerosols takes place in two stages, one in which the product to be pressurised is measured accurately into the container and the second in which the propellent is added to complete the contents. E. L. Rose (" Stability Testing of Low-Pressure Aerosols ", *J. Soc. cosmet. Chem.*, Dec. 1951, **5**, 315) has described the manner in which this is done and pointed out that " since the propellents are liquids boiling far below room temperature, it is important that the product be pre-cooled to temperatures that will permit accurate addition of the propellent with minimum loss. In order to accomplish this, extensive refrigeration equipment is required. Basically it consists of pumping the product through a cooler into a refrigerated filling tank. A constant head of material is maintained in the filling tank by a series of automatic valves. The filling nozzle on the tank is activated by a switch set off by the container as it passes the filling nozzle. This switch controls an electronic interval timer which holds the nozzle valve open for sufficient time to allow the required amount of product to flow into the container. The container with the cooled product passes now under the filling head of the propellent which operates in a similar manner. . . ."

Due to the very low temperatures encountered at the nozzles, condensation of moisture is, points out Rose, a serious problem since in the presence of water, many of the propellents hydrolyse and form corrosive acids. It is therefore necessary to use dry air or air-conditioning around the filling heads. At this point the contents are at a temperature usually below 0° F. and there is little evidence of gas loss.

The containers then pass through to the capper and are seamed. After seaming the cans are passed through a series of hot water baths, sufficient to raise the temperature of the contents of the can to about 130° F. ; in these baths leakers, overfilled cans, etc., can be detected and removed. The cans are then dried, labelled and cartoned.

FOAM-TYPE AEROSOLS

Fortunately for the cosmetic manufacturer these are filled in quite a different manner, since the amount of propellent used is small in comparison with that employed in the spray type of dispenser. In this case the product is introduced in liquid form at room temperature or above. The valve is attached, crimped into position and the propellent introduced through the valve as a liquid, using special type pressure piston filler. Check weighings after both filling procedures are necessary to

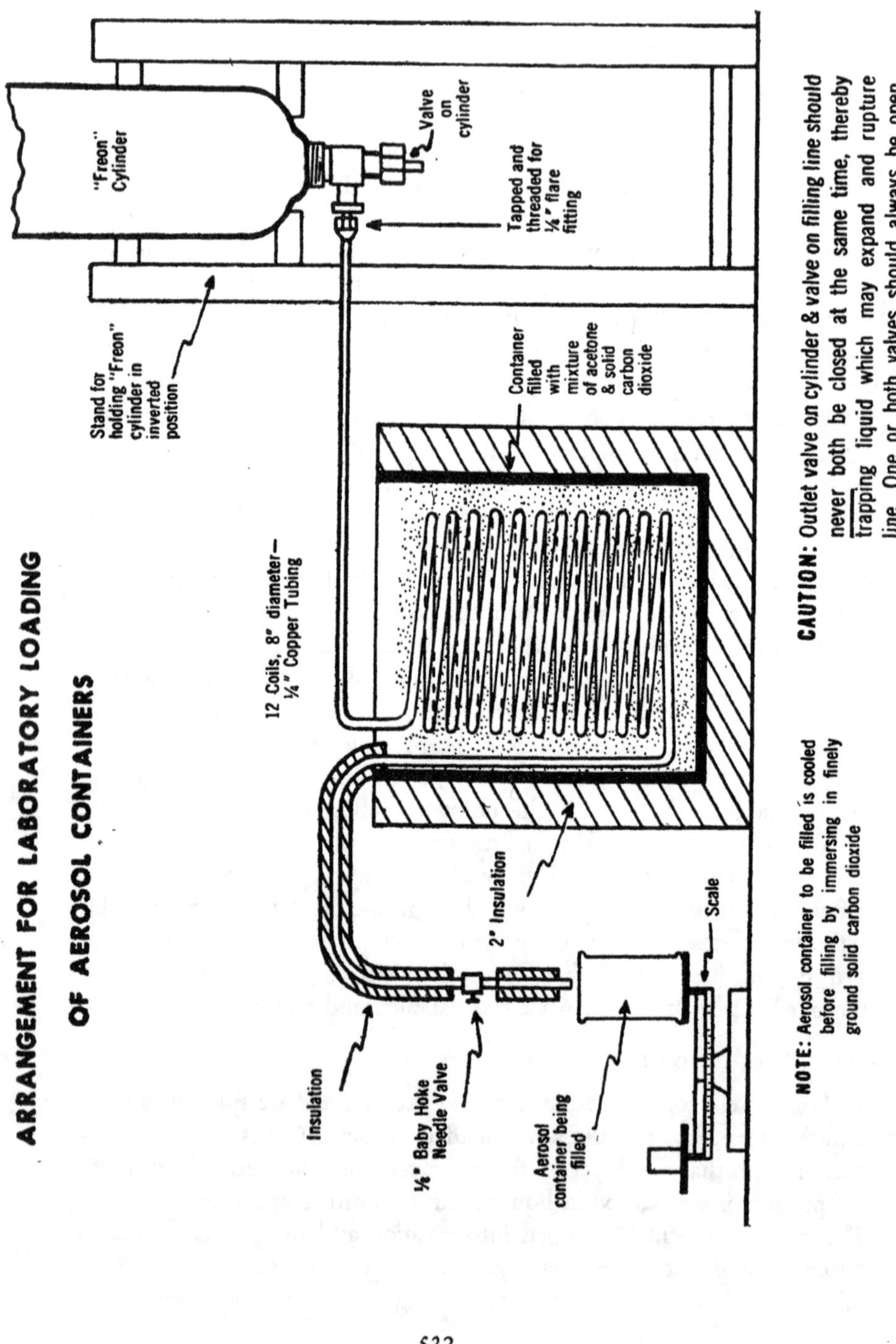

FIG. 96.—[*By courtesy of E. I. du Pont de Nemours & Co.*

ensure the accuracy of the fill, and the cans are sent through the water bath as above for testing.

For the manufacturer who wants to experimentally load a small number of containers in his own laboratory, a very simple set-up can be made. The sketch on facing page shows the details of such an arrangement. Messrs. du Pont point out that the cylinder of " Freon " must be inverted so that filling is done with liquid rather than gas, and that special attention must be given to obtaining adequate insulation around the copper tubing from the dry-ice containers to the outlet. If these precautions are observed, it is stated that satisfactory loading can be carried out without excessive " Freon " losses. In addition to the equipment shown, it is necessary to have a crimper for the can bottom or valve depending upon the container employed.

The following formulation for a Freon-Propelled Shaving Cream has appeared in the literature [*Schimmel Briefs*, July, No. 196] :

Freon-Propelled Shaving Cream

		per cent.
1 part " Freon " 12-" Freon " 114		
9 parts	Cetyl alcohol	2·40
	Hydrous lanolin	1·50
	Mineral oil, heavy	4·80
	" Avitex " C (E. I. du Pont)	16·20
	" Avitex " SF. (E. I. du Pont)	27·00
	" Triton " X-100 (Rohm and Haas)	3·00
	Stearic acid	1·00
	Perfume	0·20
	Water	43·90

Lesser (*Soap, N.Y.*, Nov. 1951) lists the following formula suggested to him by Beacher in a personal communication :

	per cent.
" Alrosol " S (Alrose Chemical Co.)	2·0
Stearic acid	9·0
Coconut oil	9·0
Potassium hydroxide	2·5
Glycerin	8·0
" Aeropon " 30 (Alrose Chemical Co.)	3·0
Water	66·5

The usual proportion of shaving cream to propellent is 90 per cent. of shaving cream and 10 per cent. of mixed propellent which may be a mixture of " Freon " 12 and " Freon " 114.

It is obvious from what has already been said, that the marketing of an Aerosol product involves a number of problems ; in most cases it will involve *not an alteration to the existing formula* but *a completely new formulation designed for the job in mind.*

In many cases considerable help will be obtained from contacting the leading manufacturers of propellents, containers and valves in the United States, where a number of firms specialise in pressurising and filling the customer's product. Some firms undertake both formulation and packing, since the setting up of a private filling line for cosmetic "aerosols" is a very expensive business only justifiable where a very large and regular sale of the product is envisaged.

Corrosion of Razor Blades

Kalish (*Drug Cosmet. Ind.*, 1937, p. 496) considers that since the reaction of shaving soaps is *p*H 8 (approximately) and upwards, and the brushless type of cream is nearly neutral, corrosion of the razor edge is more likely with the former.

This is contrary to many other opinions. Fash states that oxygen corrosion of steel occurs more rapidly at *p*H 7·2 than at *p*H 9·4, and that corrosion of the blade is more likely with the brushless type. This author cites interesting experiments which appear to show that the introduction of a small proportion of potassium chromate into creams having a *p*H of 7·2 decreases the rapidity of dulling and is non-irritant.[1] Apparently this effect is due to the formation of a thin invisible film of iron oxide which renders the edge passive. Sodium benzoate has been found to possess remarkable corrosion-resistive properties and may be of use in shaving preparations for this purpose.

Personally, I have not found undue corrosion with either type, in the case of ordinary safety razor blades, providing the blade is cleaned after use. The most important factor in the loss of edge in a blade is oxidation, and wiping immediately after use with a little mineral oil or grease increases the life of the blade.

The more rapid dulling of a razor blade when used with a brushless shaving cream is marked when compared with a blade used with a saponaceous cream. I find the life of the blade with a brushless cream to be approximately half of that when used with a saponaceous cream.

Electric Razors and Electric Razor Pre-Shave Lotions

Electric razors have become very popular in the United States and although they have not "caught on" to anything like the same extent in this country, their sales are increasing.

It is stated that ordinary methods of shaving result in the hair of the

[1] Covered by Patents. Flash, Brit. Patent 450,221; French Patent 788,572.

beard growing at an angle instead of at right angles to the skin surface, with the result that the user is often disgusted with his preliminary tests. After some two or three weeks, however, it is claimed that a good shave may be obtained. For use during this preliminary period, astringent lotions have been produced ; whether their local action assists in making the hair stand more upright or whether they merely cover up the minor trauma which the inexperienced user may inflict on his face does not appear to have been established.

Their use with such razors is, however, considered to be more conducive to a comfortable shave.

The basis of these preparations is almost invariably alcohol, together with either fatty matter or mild astringents, viz. :

	per cent.
Alcohol	45·0
Sorbitol	5·0
Lactic acid	1·0
Water	49·1

	per cent.
Zinc phenosulphonate	1·0
Distilled extract of Witch hazel	40·0
Alcohol	40·0
Water	19·0
Menthol	*q.s.* (trace only)

One theory has it that to cut the beard with an electric razor the hair should be stiff and dry, not soft and wet as in shaving with creams, and that the addition of alcoholic solutions of such a strength renders the beard dry and more readily cut. Whether the presence of oily or fatty matters interferes with such cutting action is not certain. The following illustrates such a product :

	per cent.
Isopropyl myristate	20·0
Alcohol	80·0
Perfume	*q.s.*
Antiseptic	*q.s.*

Whilst it may be quite true that after a short preliminary period, good shaves may be obtained, I, personally, find it quite impossible to get anything like so effective a shave as with the use of an ordinary razor and this is particularly evident on the neck and chin. Even dry-shaving with an electric razor may result in some trauma (*J. Amer. med. Assoc.*, **110**, 1748) and hence the potentialities of after-shave lotions and creams.

Shaving and Skin Antiseptics: The Role of Added Antiseptics

It is well known that the skin swarms with bacteria and other micro-organisms; that sebum is fungicidal to certain micro-organisms and that natural protective agencies: the drying (desiccation) of the skin surface—and possibly its *p*H reaction (which is about 5·5) all help to either inhibit or reduce the virulence of some of the pathogens present. How true this is, is well realised when the skin becomes chapped or fissured and infection sets in.

In the act of shaving, there is a certain amount of trauma and very often (particularly with a new razor blade) minor cuts occur; these, though small, are nevertheless breaks in the continuity of the skin; minor wounds from which major troubles can, and occasionally do, arise.

An American bacteriologist, A. H. Bryant, became interested in the effects of shaving and in 1951 published the results of his investigation, ("Hygienic Shaving Cuts Blemishes", *Amer. Perfum.*, Jan. 1951, p. 33).

Bryant's experiments were carried out on about 100 students and were designed to find the answers to the following questions:

(1) What effect the normal skin flora of bacteria may have in inciting skin infections following shaving.

(2) To what extent do unhygienic shaving practices affect casual causative agents in facial infections.

(3) What prophylactic measures might be resorted to in order to lower the incidence of such infections.

(4) The possible prophylactic action of antiseptic shaving creams and after-shave lotion.

(5) To what extent do old blades, razors and brushes harbour the skin flora of possible pathogenic bacteria.

(6) What mixed infection or secondary invaders are the probable aetiological factors in facial acnes, pustules, pimples and trichophytoses, etc.

As a result of his experiments, Bryant concluded that ". . . the use of antiseptics in shaving preparations is desirable because while adolescent acnes, folliculitis simplex, etc., may be the result of androgenic hormone disturbances, these infections seem to be made worse by local infections. The usual facial skin flora of possible pathogens, of staphylococcic and streptococcic groups were inhibited or killed by prophylactic measures including shaving creams containing penetrating non-irritant antiseptics. After-shave lotions containing alcohol and a bland antiseptic are valuable aids to shaving hygiene. . . ."

AFTER-SHAVE LOTIONS

These may be formulated along the lines of pre-shave lotions except that their alcohol content may be lower to avoid "smarting" on application; in point of fact some suggested formulations for after-shaves contain 40 per cent. and more alcohol. As antiseptic either a little G.11 "Actamer", or parachlormetacresol, may be added (*see* Chapter 42, Antiseptics and Preservatives), or a quaternary ammonium salt in low concentration included; for example:

Antiseptic After-Shave Lotion	*per cent.*
"Hyamine" 10-X (25 per cent.) (Rohm and Haas)	0·25
Alcohol	40·00
Menthol	0·005
Benzocaine	0·025
Water	59·72

(*Schimmel Briefs*, No. 190, Jan. 1951.)

It will be noted that the above preparation includes not only a cationic (Hyamine 10-X) but also a local anaesthetic (Benzocaine) and an anodyne (Menthol) which by its rubefacient action helps to allay any slight feeling of pain.

The following is by Kalish (*Drug Cosmet. Ind.*, 1937, **41**, 52):

	per cent.
Witch hazel	15·0
Alcohol	10·0
Alum	0·5
Menthol	0·05
Ethyl *p*-aminobenzoate	0·05
Boric acid	1·0
Glycerin	5·0
Water	68·4

AFTER-SHAVE CREAMS

These are applied after the usual *brush type*, i.e. soap cream and may be simple emollient creams tinted a flesh colour and suitably perfumed. Such perfume should be fresh rather than sophisticated, and eau-de-Cologne, lavender, lilac and certain bouquets are indicated.

Particular care should be taken in the perfuming of after-shave preparations since the skin is particularly tender after shaving. Substances which are irritant should be avoided. (*See* Vanishing Creams, Chapter 9, for basic formulations of creams which may be adopted as after-shave creams.)

Vanishing creams for men, for use after shaving, must not be associated with feminine articles if success is desired. Quite different sales psychology must be employed.

After-Shave Powders

For these to achieve popularity, they must be tinted so as not to be evident, and should be freshly and only lightly perfumed. Such powder must have high powers of adherence, otherwise it will dissipate itself over a suit on the slightest provocation and this may prove embarrassing.

	per cent.
Talc	85·0
Magnesium stearate	10·0
Boric acid	5·0
Colour	*q.s.*
Perfume	*q.s.*

For other formulations *see* Face Powders and Talcum Powders, Chapter 11, which by tinting to a flesh colour and incorporating suitable perfume may be adopted as after-shave powders.

CHAPTER 30

ANTIPERSPIRANTS AND DEODORANTS

ACCORDING to estimates by Krause (Wagner's *Handworterbuch der Physiologie*, 1884, Vol. 2, p. 131) and Taniguchi and Kamiyama (Y. Kuno, *The Physiology of Human Perspiration*, 1934, London : Churchill) about 2,380,000 sweat glands are present in the body surface.[1] There are two types of secretory glands, namely :

The Eccrine (or small coil glands). These are the true sweat glands, which occur all over the body. They secrete only water and water-soluble substances, no portion of the cell structure entering into their contents.

The Apocrine (or large coil glands). These are connected with a hair follicle, and are found in very few places on the skin. In general they are limited to the under-arm, breasts and genital regions. These secrete nitrogenous and fatty substances in addition to water and salt, and contain, in addition, portions of the inner cell layer.

The presence of iron in the secretion has been confirmed by Way and Mennesheimer (*Arch. Derm. Syph., Chicago*, 1938, **38**, 373) who used Mallory's potassium ferrocyanide test ; they found no iron in axillary tissue derived from five infants in which the eccrine type of gland alone was present.

The apocrine glands are actually secondary sexual characteristics and develop at puberty, being more developed in females than males, and probably undergo cyclical changes in activity coincident with menstruation. In earlier phases of the history of the human species they played an important part in sexual attraction, and even today it is not possible to say that they have ceased to have an influence, even if it be subconscious.

FUNCTIONS OF THE SWEAT GLANDS

The sweat glands are very largely concerned in the regulation of body temperature, evaporation of their contents leading to a loss of heat. In a normally healthy person this is automatic, unless the

[1] According to Montague (later in this chapter), negroes have three times as many sweat glands as white races.

surrounding air is hot or very moist, in which case evaporation is insufficient to prevent a sharp rise in body temperature and distress and even collapse may occur.

Their function is complementary to that of the kidneys, and they probably assist in maintaining the elasticity of the skin.

Kuno has shown (*The Physiology of Human Perspiration*) that sweat secretion differs in varying parts of the human body and that, contrary to feminine belief, the axillae (armpits) and internal femoral regions (thighs) sweat very little upon raising the temperature of the body; the head, neck, back and abdomen surfaces of the upper trunk sweating the most.

There are sexual differences in the response to sweating. In 1942 Kahn and Rothman demonstrated for the first time an interesting difference in the sweating response of men and women. Intracutaneous injections of acetylcholine produced medium to strong local sweating in 95 per cent. of the men tested, whereas only 10 per cent. of the women responded in this fashion. Kahn and Rothman considered there was no likely anatomic difference and suggested that possibly a hormonal background was responsible.

Lewis (*Clin. Sci.*, 1944, p. 5) reported that the introduction into the skin by iontophoresis of acetylcholine led to a definite whealing in female subjects whereas it did not lead to such whealing in male subjects.

In view of the lack of information on this subject Gibson and Sheeley (*J. invest. Derm.*, Aug. 1948, **2**, 137) carried out further studies in which they determined the local response to sweating of white and coloured subjects, males and females. Acetylcholine was introduced by iontophoresis and by injection both with and without prostigmine. Pilocarpine was introduced by intradermal injection. These investigators found that, in these tests, the sweat glands of both the white and coloured females proved to be much less responsive than those of the males, and that the sweat glands of the coloured races appeared to be slightly more responsive than those of the white race.

One of the strongest beliefs is that the negro possesses a unique and very objectional body odour. Montague (*Sci. Mon. Wash.*, 1944, **59**, 56) compared the physical characteristics of the American negro with those of the white race. It was found that negroes have three times as many sweat glands as whites (an adaptation for heat regulation in tropical climates). The limited experimental studies carried out suggested that the sweat of negroes differed only in quantity and not in nature from that of white persons. Perspiration was collected in test-tubes from white and coloured students after violent exercise in a gymnasium and these tubes then given to a number of white persons with instructions to place them in order of pleasantness. The results showed no consistent preference for the white samples; the samples considered most pleasant and that least pleasant were both taken from white students. [In assessing these results "body cleanliness" and diet must both be taken into account since sweat, when freshly secreted is not really unpleasant; it is only when mixed with skin debris and secretions from the apocrine glands, and when bacterial decomposition sets in, that the odour becomes obnoxious. So far as diet is concerned, it is well known that the odours of such things as garlic, spices, cheeses, tinned tongue, asparagus, etc., can be plainly detected both in the urine and in the perspiration.]

In general the palms of the hand and soles of the feet are unique in that though they constantly secrete some sweat this is not increased in proportion by a rise in temperature. Mental stress or fear, however, leads to an increase in such perspiration (Kuno, *The Physiology of Human Perspiration; see also* M. Kosaka, *J. Orient. Med.*, 1929, **10**, 75).

Kuno showed that the axillae, etc., became wet not because of excessive sweating but because sweat evaporates from these regions only with difficulty. These results are really in accord with our experience. We speak of "mopping the sweat from our forehead", whilst the novelist depicts the beads of perspiration on the hero's brow.

Even the commonly observed custom of spitting on the palms of the hands before heavy work can be regarded as a phenomenon transmitted from animal life. Mental stress (e.g. fear) produces palmar sweating, which confers a better grip for tree climbing to escape imminent danger, and in prehistoric time our forbears (when the odds were too great) probably spat on their hands and "legged it" to the nearest tree.

Sweat occurs as a colourless, opalescent fluid having a peculiar but not unpleasant odour. As secreted, it is slightly acid; rapidly, it becomes mixed with the fatty secretions of the sebaceous glands, and in some places of the apocrine glands. Bacterial decomposition starts under very favourable conditions of humidity and temperature. The decomposed fatty acids and the by-products of fermentation probably account for what we are told is "body odour".

The specific gravity is about 1·005 but may vary, being greater at the beginning of sweating. The acid reaction of sweat is due to the presence of fatty acids or acid phosphates of sodium and potassium which it contains. An adult secretes about 700 g. of sweat daily. Under the influence of heat, exercise, or disease this quantity may be vastly increased.

According to Way and Memmesheimer, sweat is made up mainly of a dilute solution of mineral salts, of which sodium chloride is the most important. Potassium chloride, alkaline salts, organic acids, some urea, a slight amount of fatty matter, odoriferous substances, volatile fatty acids, formic acid, acetic acid, propionic acid and butyric acid are also present. The volatile bases (trimethylamine and methylamine) and the fatty acids or their compounds (butyric acid, caproic ethers and valeric ethers) give to the sweat its foetid odour.

Favre (A. Favre cited by A. Gautier: *Leçons de chimie biologique normale et pathologique*, ed. 10, Paris: Masson & Cie, 1897, p. 446) gave the quantitative analysis of 1000 cc. of sweat as follows: sodium chloride, 2·230 g.; potassium chloride, 0·244 g.; alkaline sulphates, 0·012 g.; alkaline phosphates, traces; albuminates, 0·005 g; alkaline earth phosphates, traces; alkaline lactates, 0·317 g.; alkaline sudorates, 1·562 g.; urea, 0·043 g.; fatty matter, 0·014 g.; epithelium, 0·043 g.; and water, 995·573 cc. Substances similar to those found in the urine, such as urea, ammonia, uric acid, creatinine, chlorides, phosphates, sulphates and certain enzymes, also occur in the sweat.

B. A. McSwiney and G. C. N. Vass ("The Composition of Human Perspiration", *J. Soc. Dy. Col.*, June 1930) give the following average values calculated from the examination of specimens of sweat from 10 females and 14 males.

	pH	*NH_2-N mg./100 cc.*	*Urea-N mg./100 cc.*	*Amino-acid-N mg./100 cc.*	*Glucose mg./100 cc.*	*Chlorides g. NaCl 1000 cc.*
Average from 10 normal female subjects	6·57	6·0	19·23	6·5	20·0	3·00
Average from 14 normal male subjects	6·14	4·7	21·44	5·0	12·6	3·70

McSwiney and Vass found that in normal subjects the average glucose content was greater in female subjects than in males, and that obesity appeared to be associated with a higher glucose content than the normal, especially in the sweat of female subjects. They found that perspiration underwent considerable change on standing, and showed that these changes were due mainly if not entirely, to the bacteria normally present in freshly shed perspiration.

Klarmann ("The Cosmetic Aspects of Perspiration and its Control", *Amer. Perfum.*, July 1948) gives the following typical composition of perspiration:

Water	99·0200
Propionic acid	0·0062
Acetic acid	0·0096
Caprylic and caproic acids	0·0046
Sodium chloride	0·7000
Lactic acid	0·1000
Citric acid	0·0400
Ascorbic acid	0·0400
Urea	*Trace*
Uric acid	*Trace*

but points out that the quantitative composition of perspiration is subject to variation. Killian and Panzarella (*Proc. Sci. Sect. T.G.A.*, 1947, **7**, 3), in perspiration collected by "thermal sweating", found the sodium chloride content varying from 0·176 to 0·761 per cent. with a mean of 0·430 per cent.; the concentration of lactic acid ranged from 0·147 to 0·371 per cent. with a mean of 0·232 per cent. Prior to this Kuno (*The Physiology of Human Perspiration*) had reported extreme limits of 0·18 to 0·95 per cent. sodium chloride in perspiration on the basis of the findings of a number of investigators. Klarmann points out that the principal factors responsible for the divergence between the analytical figures reported by different investigators are:

(i) failure to take into account the degree of skin cleanliness at the time of collection;

(ii) differences in the conditions under which the sample is stored during the time interval between its collection and the beginning of the assay;

(iii) variations in the concentration of certain constituents of perspiration depending upon whether the body is in action or in repose; thus with respect to the last point it is known that during hard work the lactic acid content is increased since the sweat supplies the main avenue of excretion of this metabolic product.

As pointed out earlier in this chapter, diet may also affect the composition of perspiration.

Excretions of Vitamins in Sweat

Cornbleet, Kirch and Bergeim (*J. Amer. med. Ass.*, 12 June 1943, p. 426) found heat sweat to contain on the average about 150 micrograms of thiamine, 120 micrograms of riboflavin, 300 micrograms of pantothenic acid and 200 micrograms of nicotinic acid. These values per litre correspond for thiamine to about 5 per cent. of intake on a good diet, for riboflavin and pantothenic acid to about 3 per cent., and for nicotinic acid to about 0·5 per cent.

Mickelsen and Keys (*J. Biol. Chem.*, 1943, **149**, 479) reported their investigation into the composition of sweat with special reference to vitamins and some organic substances and to variations in composition of sweat collected from different parts of the body and at different times. For full details the original paper should be consulted, but the following is a summary of their general findings in respect of vitamin content:

Sweat was collected from various parts of the body of normal young men in rest and in moderate work. In most cases the temperature was 49° F., the humidity 25 per cent. relative saturation, but in some experiments humidities over 65 per cent. relative saturation were maintained at an air temperature of 37°-38° F. The following results were obtained:

Ascorbic acid. The concentration of ascorbic acid in sweat is generally less than 0·1 mg. per 10 cc., the true average being of the order of 0·03 mg. per 100 cc. The concentration is independent of the dietary intake of the vitamin.

Thiamine. The concentration of thiamine in sweat is of the order of 0·2γ or less per 100 cc.

Riboflavine. Riboflavine concentration is of the order of 0·5γ or less per 100 cc. sweat.

Nicotinic acid. The concentration of nicotinic acid or its biological equivalent in sweat is of the order of 0·1 mg. per 100 cc.

Sweat samples collected simultaneously from the hand, arm plus hand, face, torso and thigh, showed marked differences in total concentration and in concentration of individual constituents. Mickelsen and Keys concluded that under conditions of profuse sweating losses of ascorbic acid, thiamine and riboflavine are negligible from the standpoint of nutrition, but that the loss of nicotinic acid under these conditions could be significant.

Secretion of Sweat

The secretion of sweat is under control of the nervous system, the sweat glands being innervated by sympathetic fibres, and the nervous mechanism can be called into action by central stimuli, reflex action or peripheral stimuli. It would appear that the impulses are chemically transmitted by acetyl-choline liberated at the nerve endings and acting on the sweat glands.

Disorders of the Sweat Glands

Such disorders may take the form of hyperidrosis (excessive secretion of sweat) or anidrosis (diminution sometimes even cessation, of this secretion). The latter is of rare occurrence and necessitates medical treatment.

Hyperidrosis. This may be local or general. When general, it is denoted by the general colour or by the appearance of globules of moisture, and is usually the result of exposure to excessive heat, exertion, fever, or the action of certain drugs. Locally, it may occur (in particular under the arms and feet) without any visible outward sign.

Pathology of Hyperidrosis. The mental effect of this complaint may be out of all proportion to its severity. The sufferer may be acutely conscious, and the psychological effect may lead to a warped outlook in that individual's life. In addition, it may lead to actual physical harm. The skin exposed to the macerating effect of the secretions becomes irritated, inflamed, with the possibility of further secondary bacterial infection.

Although sage taken by the mouth diminishes sweating (and it has also been asserted that camphor gives good results) the usual methods employed in the treatment of this complaint are local. It is for such use that the cosmetician has formulated products which are not only harmless (when used with a little intelligence) but also efficacious.

It does not do any harm to use such preparations provided they have been carefully formulated. The diminution of the secretion over such a small area exerts not the slightest effect on the bodily health, if increased loss is desired the body will simply supply it at another (and probably less objectionable) spot.

Odour of Perspiration

As mentioned earlier in this chapter, the odour of freshly secreted perspiration is not unpleasant; the offensive odour develops as a result of bacterial action causing decomposition of the organic matter, both soluble and insoluble, carried by perspiration.

Killian and Panzarella (*Proc. Sci. Sect. T.G.A.*, 1947) have provided an elegant demonstration of the role played by bacteria in this scheme. These investigations showed that filtration of perspiration through a Berkefeld assembly (which removes any suspended bacteria) prevented any change of the original odour, and incidentally that of the original *p*H, during 24 hours. By contrast, an unfiltered sample developed a strong odour during the same period of time; its reaction changed from acid to alkaline (from *p*H 4·82 to *p*H 7·86) concomitant with a drop in urea nitrogen and an increase in ammonia nitrogen. The same authors proved also that the insoluble sediment of perspiration separated from the water-soluble phase does not give rise to perspiratory odour when inoculated with a culture of either *Staphylococcus albus* or the gram positive bacillus, previously found to be connected with the production of such odours. Only the coexistence of the insoluble and the liquid components of perspiration will give rise to odour development under the action of the typical bacterial flora.

MECHANISM OF ANTIPERSPIRANT (" ASTRINGENT ") ACTION

Because the substances found effective as antiperspirants were protein precipitants and on applying these to the skin, in a more diluted form in cases of so-called enlarged " pores " (in reality empty hair-follicles), such openings became less visible, it became generally accepted that these substances acted by precipitating protein and—by analogy with " astringent lotions "—in thus doing blocked the openings through which perspiration is excreted.

The plain, simple truth, however, is rarely plain and never simple and recent investigations into the mechanism of antiperspirant action indicate that the mode of action of such substances is nothing like so simple as was thought.

Sulzberger and co-workers (*Arch. Derm. Syph., Chicago*, 1949, **60**, 404) attempted to determine the exact mode of action of antiperspirants by histological examinations of the human skin after the application of such creams. By taking biopsy specimens from the axillary skin of healthy volunteers it was found that no narrowing of the ostiums could be observed microscopically; but a significant finding was that in all cases involving an effective reduction of sensible perspiration, a microscopically observable inflammatory reaction was present. It was pointed out, however, that this small inflammatory response is not necessarily harmful (the widespread use of antiperspirants disproves any such assumption) but it does help to explain the occasional clinical inflammatory case resulting from the application of such preparations. Although, at the time, no simple explanation of the action of antiperspirants could be given, it appeared probable that an inflammatory reaction with accompanying degenerative changes in the sweat glands was involved in the reduction of sensible perspiration by the application of astringent-containing preparations.

More recently Sulzberger, Herrmann, Keller and Pisha (*J. invest. Derm.*, Feb. 1950, " Studies of Sweating ", Part III) have carried out experiments in respect of experimental factors influencing the function of the sweat ducts. The important experiments of Shelley, Horvath,

Weidman and Pillsbury (*J. invest. Derm.*, 1948, **11**, 275) indicated that electrophoretic production of anidrosis was regularly successful only at the site of the anode, more or less regardless of what solutions of electrolytes were used. Sulzberger *et al.*, state that it was this finding of Shelley and co-workers which focused their attention upon the question of whether the electric charge, as such, influences the outpouring of sweat—and, if so, in what specific manner this influence is accomplished.

Various data suggested the presence of an electronegative charge somewhere at the border of the sweat ducts, which may be important for the regulation of normal outpouring and which might be diminished by the electrophoretic procedure of Shelley *et al.*, the anode being the active pole.

In order to investigate these questions, Sulzberger and co-workers decided to employ chemicals with a distinct and known polarity, applying these to the skin in place of the electric (galvanic) current previously used by Shelley. Should the hypothesis of Sulzberger *et al.* prove correct, it would be expected that *substances with a positive charge would tend to decrease or inhibit the outpouring of sweat; while substances with the opposite or negative charge would tend to increase the delivery of sweat.*

As a result of their preliminary investigations, these investigators believed they were justified in inferring that " . . . application of agents with biologically electropositive charges tend to reduce outpourings of sweat; and to produce miliaria rubra-like eruptions. . . ." Conversely, applications of biologically negative agents tended to increase outpouring of sweat.

The following statements are from their "summary of results and possible implications" of their work:

" . . . (1) External application of selected cationic wetting agents (quaternary ammonium bases), anionic wetting agents and of biologically electropositive and electronegative electrolytes in aqueous solution produced in most instances a local change in the delivery of thermal sweat in comparison to the appearance of sweat on the untreated control sites.

" (2) Biologically electropositive agents, for example, cationic wetting agents such as Roccal, and positive electrolytes like lithium thiocyanate, lithium iodide, lithium salicylate, sodium and potassium iodides, tended to reduce the outpouring of sweat. In a significant number of test subjects, this effect was associated with an eruptive response of the tested skin area, resembling miliaria rubra.

"(3) Biologically electronegative agents, such as anionic wetting agents like Aerosol O.T., or Duponol M.E., and 'negative' electrolytes like potassium sulphate tended to increase delivery of sweat to the surface.

"(4) These influences of both electropositive and electronegative agents were observed not only in skin areas with purely eccrine sweat secretion, but were at least as pronounced or still more conspicuous and uniform in the axillary vault, an area rich in apocrine glands.

"(5) Individual differences in the response of the test subjects were conspicuous regarding both degree and character of the changes in sweat delivery, and also regarding the tendency towards development of the eruptive response.

"(6) Special methods of vital staining produced selective staining at the spiral end-portion of the sweat duct. This selective staining is identical with the established selective attraction of the same dyes by other living structures which are characterised by physiologic electronegativity. . . . The findings suggest the presence of a negative electrical charge at the border of the terminal part of the sweat ducts.

"(7) The hypothesis is submitted that electronegativity of the distal end of the sweat duct maintains an electro-physiologic potential along the ducts which facilitates and expedites the movement of sweat towards the skin surface by electro-osmosis. This assumption is supported by the fact that vital staining at the spiral end of the ducts was distinctly weaker after application of electropositive forces which tend to inhibit the delivery of sweat to the skin's surface. . . ."

Formulation of Antiperspirants and Deodorants

There are two methods of approaching the problem of malodorous perspiration: the first is to attempt to *deodorise* the perspiration *without checking its flow* to any appreciable extent, the second method is to apply a substance which will *reduce the amount of perspiration* secreted. The first class of preparations are termed "deodorants", the second "antiperspirants". Actually the products sold as "deodorants" in many cases are antiperspirants rather than true deodorants.

Deodorisation of Perspiration

Chlorophyllins. Many claims have been made concerning the deodorant action of the sodium and potassium copper chlorophyllins (the so-called "water-soluble chlorophylls") and there is definite evidence to show that (i) where the chlorophyllins can actually come into contact with the malodorous material and (ii) an effective concentration of chlorophyll is present, deodorisation can, and often does, occur (for example, *see* J. A. Killian " Evaluation of In-vitro and In-vivo Methods of Testing Deodorants with Particular Reference to Chlorophyll and Its Derivatives ", *J. Soc. cosmet. Chem.*, March 1952, **1**, 30). Killian has pointed out that " . . . water-soluble chlorophyllins added to malodorous samples of perspiration effect prompt eradications of the perspiratory odours. At the same time these chlorophyll derivatives exhibit antibacterial actions.. . . In addition to their deodorising actions, the chlorophyllins, added to fresh samples of perspiration, inhibit the development of perspiratory odours under conditions of storage which are optimum for the production of obnoxious odours. . . ."

" . . . The results of the final series of experiments which are summarised . . . indicate definitely that the daily ingestion of water-soluble chlorophyllins . . . which in *in-vitro* tests had shown effective, failed to influence the capacities of samples of perspiration to develop offensive odours. . . ."

It would therefore appear that chlorophyll preparations to *ensure* deodorisation of perspiration should be applied locally. At the level at which such derivatives are really effective they also stain, temporarily, clothing and undergarments. For these reasons the local application of chlorophyllin preparations *as perspiration deodorants* is not considered further. So far as ingestion of chlorophyll is concerned, the evidence that this will banish the odour of perspiration which is undergoing decomposition is conflicting. (This is not to say that chlorophyllins may not have uses in other preparations ; the formula of chlorophyllins and the use of chlorophyllins in dentifrices is briefly discussed in Chapter 16.)

G-11 (*2,2′-methylenebis(3,4,6-trichlorophenol); 2,2′-dihydroxy-3,5,6,3′, 5′,6-hexachlorodiphenylmethane* (*Hexachlorophene*) (*Sindar Corporation*)

This substance was developed to fill the need for a truly antiseptic soap and quite a lot of clinical evidence is available to show its value. Apart from its use for antiseptic purposes, this substance has been incorporated in a number of soaps with claims for deodorant action on perspiration. Killian (*loc cit.*) has emphasised that all findings " . . . lead to the inescapable conclusion that control of bacterial populations on the surface of the skin is the *sine qua non* of the control of perspiratory odours. . . ." His experiments showed that a soap containing 2 per cent. G-11 was distinctly superior to ordinary plain soap in eliminating offensive body odours and inhibiting their re-development. Apart from its use in soap for this purpose G-11[1] (and G-4; 2,2′-dihydroxy-5,5′-dichlorodiphenylmethane) may be incorporated in deodorant creams and lotions. More recently another new antiseptic which is claimed to be effective in soap for reducing the bacterial flora of the skin—which are chiefly responsible for the decomposition of perspiration—has been developed. This substance "Actamer" (Monsanto Chemicals) is 2,2′-thiobis (4,6-dichlorophenol) on which preliminary reports in respect of efficacy and freedom from irritant and sensitising properties are very promising. "Actamer" is (like G-11) substantive to the skin. These antiseptics are discussed further in Chapter 42, meanwhile they offer relatively new materials for tackling the problem of "deodorisation". Other substances which can be employed for this purpose are quaternary ammonium compounds*, peroxides, chloramine compounds, formalin-containing compounds* such as hexamine, FS. 64 Hartke Co. K-G. (Hamburg), and various antiseptic substances used in cream, lotion or powder forms. More recently certain surfactants (*see* Chapter 22) have been found to possess deodorant properties, e.g. Nacconol NRSF.

Measurement of Odours; The "Osmometer"

In order to assess the deodorant action of various antiseptic substances upon perspiration, it is necessary to have some means of comparing the intensities of odours. Dr. Barail (U.S. Testing Co.) has devised an "Osmometer" for this purpose. Barail (*Soap, N.Y.*, June 1949; *J. Soc. cosmet. Chem.* 1950, **2**, 14) has pointed out that ". . . In order to obtain accurate results in the measurement of odours, it was necessary to build an apparatus of great reliability. As no way has yet been found to measure odours without using human olfactory nerves, such an apparatus should enable anyone to obtain reproducible results provided the following conditions be met:

(1) The amount of air to be smelled should be known.

(2) The air to be smelled should reach the nose of the technician under its own pressure. This pressure should be known.

(3) The air to be smelled should contain only the odour to be measured, and should have no odour of its own.

[1] ". . . A potential for controlling perspiration odour seems to be present in deodorant soaps containing G-11 to a degree beyond that of other types of soaps. Considerable evidence supports the conclusion that deodorant soaps containing G-11 are non-irritating for practical purposes and compare favourably with ordinary toilet soaps from the viewpoint of pharmaceutical elegance. . . ." (American Medical Association Committee on Cosmetics, Status Report on Deodorant Soaps, *J. Amer. med. Ass.*, 18 March 1950.)

* Caution should be employed in the use of these substances for such purposes!

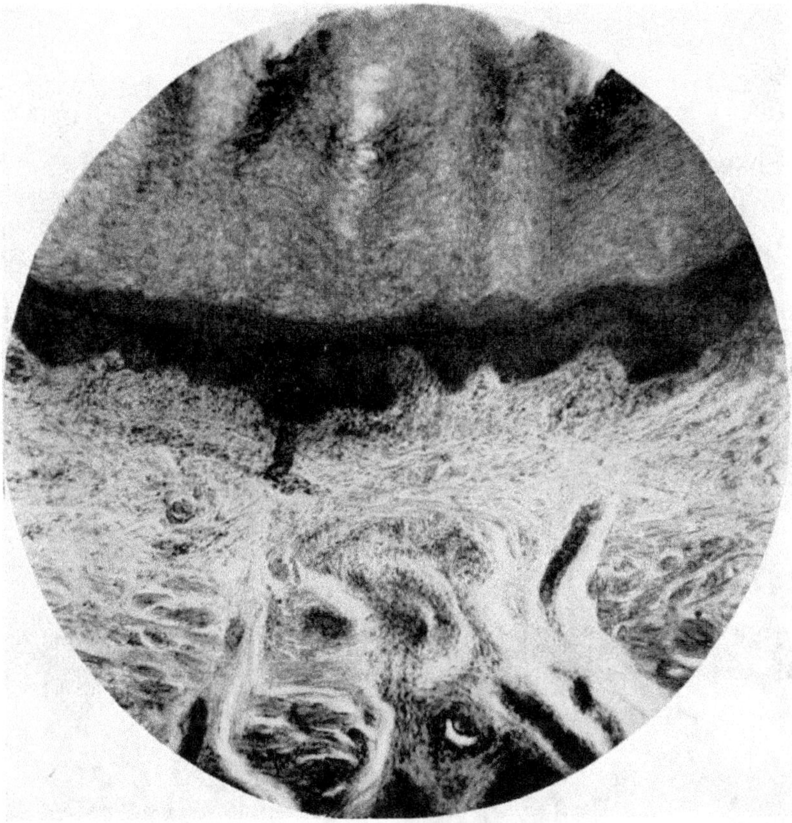

[*Illustration by the Author.*

FIG. 97.—Note sweat gland " corkscrewing " through the lower layers into the stratum corneum.

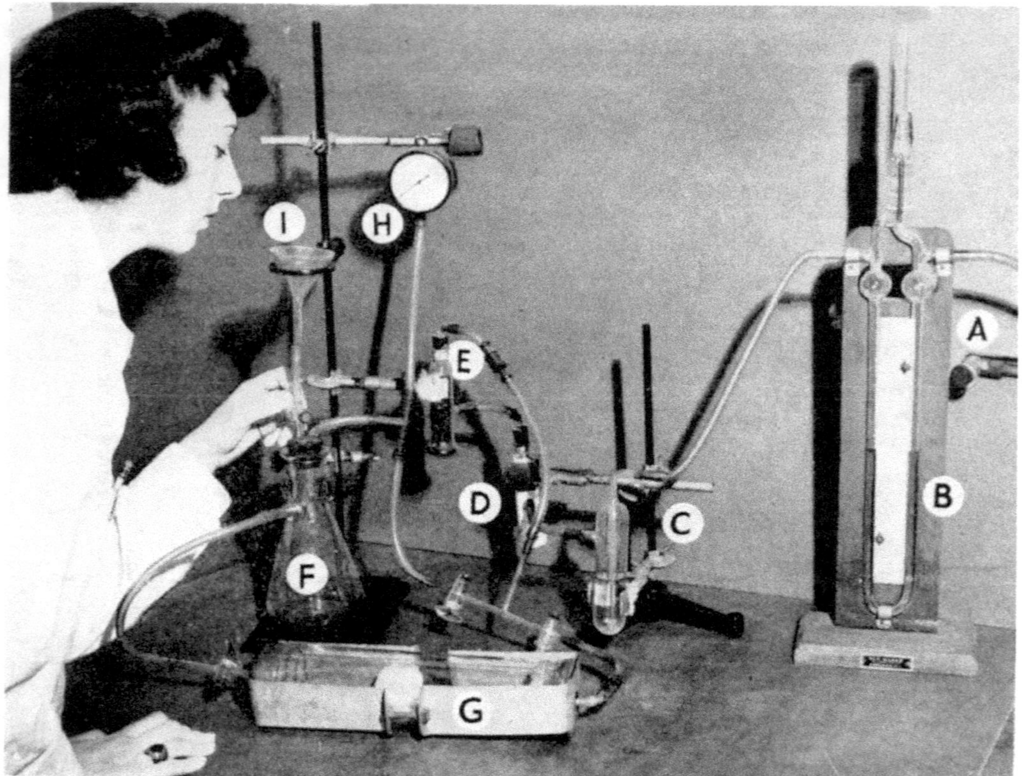

[By courtesy of Dr. Barail, U.S. Testing Co.

FIG. 98.—The Laboratory Osmometer (Single). (A) Source of compressed air. (B) Flow-meter. (C) Air-washer. (D) Dessicator. (E) Deodoriser. (F) Mixing Jar. (G) Sample-containing tube. (H) Pressure Gauge. (I) Outlet funnel.

(4) The air should be clean prior to its being contaminated with the odour to be tested. The moisture of the air to be tested should be known.

(5) All tests should be made under the same conditions.

DESCRIPTION OF THE OSMOMETER

" The osmometer is based on the air dilution principle, using quantities of odour-free and odorous air, which are diluted and mixed in various concentrations. The dilution is performed under moderate pressure, which can be made to vary from one to 300 mm. Hg. However, pressures higher than 150 mm. are seldom used.

" This pressure was found to be necessary for two reasons : First, a pressure difference was needed to move air from one container to another. Secondly, a stream of air which suddenly strikes the olfactory nerves will cause an immediate perception of odour if any may be present. The instrument is connected to a source of compressed air A. It consists of a flow-meter B, an air-washer C, a desiccator D, a deodoriser E, a mixing jar F, a sample-containing tube G, a pressure gauge H, and an outlet funnel I. The odorous material is placed in the sample tube, and a measured volume of washed, moisture-free and odour-free air is forced through the specimen and into the mixing jar. This, of course, increases the pressure in the mixing jar and also dilutes the odorous vapours in a known proportion, depending on the volume of air forced through the specimen and upon the volume of air in the mixing jar.

" Additional fresh air is then introduced into the mixing jar via a separate connection which by-passes the specimen tube in order to obtain a moderate pressure sufficient to cause a stream of air to pass through a narrow orifice upon the opening of a release valve. This final total pressure must be kept constant for all measurements.

" If no odour is detected when the air is suddenly released from the mixing flask, the experiment is repeated, this time with twice the volume of air forced through the specimen. The experiment is repeated until sufficient air has been pumped through the odorous object to produce the sensation of odour. The concentration at which the odour becomes just barely perceptible is called the ' threshold value '.

" This threshold value can be expressed numerically and this numerical expression is called the ' odour threshold number '. The ratio between the total final pressure and the pressure increment caused by the odorous air results in the odour threshold number :

$$\text{Odour Threshold Number} = \frac{\text{Total Pressure}}{\text{Odorous Increment}}.$$

"The odour threshold number gives the concentration of the odour in the air dilution which will just barely cause the sensation of odour. For strongly odorous substances, this concentration as reported in the odour threshold number will be low and the odour threshold number will be high. For weak odours it will be the opposite.

"The following classification of odour threshold numbers is used for the evaluation of the results of the tests. A threshold number in the range from 1·0 to 5·9 means a very slight odour; from 6·0 to 8·3, slight odour; from 8·4 to 13·0, definite or objectionable odour; from 13·1 to 26·0, strong odour; from 26·1 to 91·0, extremely strong odour."

ANTIPERSPIRANTS

The "active ingredients" of antiperspirants at present used, are certain metallic salts, such as aluminium, zinc, etc. Salts of other metals could be used were it not for certain disadvantages, for example, iron and silver salts discolour, lead, chromium, and mercury are toxic. The use of zirconium lactate has been patented (U.S. Patent 2,498,514).

Sulphates, chlorides, and phenolsulphonates of aluminium have been the most widely used salts for this purpose; the acetate and acetotartrate and others are also quoted in the literature.

More recently a basic salt of aluminium chloride, the so-called aluminium chlorohydrate, has been patented and is sold under the name "Chlorohydrol" (Reheis & Co. Inc.). Aqueous solutions of aluminium chlorohydrate are available in the United Kingdom. Aluminium Methionate (Aluminium Methane Disulphate) has been suggested for use as an antiperspirant. This material is claimed to be very soluble, non-toxic, more effective as a protein precipitant, and harmless to cloth whereas most astringents considerably weaken cloth ("Aluminium Methionate"; "Astringent", J. E. Christian and G. L. Jenkins, *Amer. Perfum.*, Feb. 1951, p. 107).

Other aluminium salts used are aluminium and zinc sulphamates (U.S. Patents 2,586,287–9) and aluminium dichloroaminoacetate (Grote, Holbert and Cross, *J. Amer. Pharm. Ass., Sci. Edn.*, 1949, **38**, 593).

The metallic salts vary in their "astringent" action depending upon the nature of both the cation and the anion.

EVALUATION OF ASTRINGENT EFFECT

Klarmann points out that a number of methods have been suggested for evaluation of the degree of astringent action. Govett and deNavarre (*Amer. Perfum.*, 1947, p. 365) suggested a method in which the capacity of precipitation of egg white is used as a criterion of astringent efficacy. In this method the metallic or other salt solution under test is added to a dilute solution of egg albumen producing a precipitate ; the amount, speed of formation, appearance and persistence over a given period of time are the determinative factors involved.

More elaborate tests for astringency depend upon the capacity of such substances to reduce the extensibility of frogs' lungs (Motolese, *Arch. Farmacol.*, 1940, p. 9), and to tan red blood corpuscles (T. Sollmann, *J. Pharmacol.*, 1920, **16**, 49 ; 1921, **17**, 63).

In view of the recent developments, reported earlier in this chapter, concerning the *mechanism of the action of antiperspirants* it may be that new methods of testing the efficacy of such products will have to be devised. Meanwhile, fortunately, there is always the final criterion—the user test.

FORMULATIONS

In considering the formulations given below, those preparations which are purely deodorant are given separately ; in the case of antiperspirants these sometimes contain, in addition to the active antiperspirant, a deodorant.

Antiperspirants and deodorants may be classified in four categories :

(i) Powder,
(ii) Stick,
(iii) Liquid,
(iv) Cream,

of which the last two types are by far the most important.

POWDERS

Klarmann quotes the following formulation for an antiperspirant and deodorant powder :

	per cent.
Talc	78·0
Corn starch	10·0
Sodium aluminium sulphate	2·0
Salicyclic acid	5·0
Boric acid	5·0

In general, powders " for deodorising only " are rarely satisfactory to the user. However, such preparations can be formulated by the use of an oxidising agent such as zinc peroxide in a powder base, which may consist of talc and chalk.

Alternatively, one of the antiseptic compounds (Chapter 42) may be dissolved, in alcohol or other solvent, and sprayed into part of the powder mass to make a concentrate, which, after sieving, can be blended off with untreated powder to the required dilution.

Similarly, by dissolving a little G-11 in an alcoholic lotion containing a little cologne perfume, a liquid deodorant may be prepared which is, I consider, a better proposition than the powder preparation. Alternatively cationics may be included.[1]

If a cream "deodorant" only is required, then an ordinary vanishing cream may be prepared by partially neutralising stearic acid and adding the sodium or potassium salt of G-11 which may be prepared in the laboratory by dissolving G-11 in the requisite amount of potassium or sodium hydroxides. [By dissolving the G-11 in the alkali hydroxide, prior to partially neutralising the stearic acid, the G-11 may be readily incorporated.]

In point of fact, unless the user is allergic to aluminium, the purchaser would probably prefer to use a cream that *checks*, not merely *deodorises*, the perspiration, although there is no objection to making a preparation that will achieve both objects.

For this reason, consideration in this chapter is given chiefly to "antiperspirants" rather than deodorants, particularly now that the development of substances such as G-11 allow deodorisation of the body to be achieved very largely in the normal process of "washing".

LIQUID ANTIPERSPIRANTS

Aluminium chloride and Aluminium sulphate. The earliest effective deodorants were those containing aluminium chloride or aluminium sulphate. The sulphate is sometimes preferred to the chloride on account of its greater stability to hydrolysis. Up to 25 per cent. of either of these makes an efficient product. The reaction of the solution of aluminium chloride is important. If too alkaline, precipitation of aluminium hydroxide or oxychloride will result, while if too acid, it will be irritant. It is desirable to add from ½ per cent. to 1 per cent. of borax, which will combine with any free hydrochloric acid (or sulphuric acid) with the production of sodium chloride and the comparatively mild boric acid. Aluminium chloride is obtainable in a crystalline form ($AlC_3 . 6H_2O$) and may be suitably diluted with water. Alternatively, of course, the sulphate may be used.

	per cent.
Aluminium chloride (salt)	25·0
Borax	0·8
Water	74·2

It is not easy to obtain transparent colourless solutions of aluminium chloride. A solution to the problem consists in adding about 0·25 per cent. of powdered aluminium (quoted in a letter from Ralph H. Auch by

[1] Such as the Quaternary Ammonium Compounds. These compounds, however, should be used with CAUTION for such purposes!

F. H. Overton, *Amer. Perfum.*), based on the weight of aluminium chloride used, to the warm solution (a little alcohol or acetone being used to wet the aluminium powder and render it miscible with the chloride), the solution is aged and then filtered. By this process any accompanying iron salts are reduced to the ferrous state.

Both aluminium chloride and aluminium sulphate suffer from the disadvantage that—as salts of a very weak base and a strong acid—they hydrolise in water with the liberation of the free mineral acid. This free acid is responsible for the skin irritation and the destructive effect on clothing which accompany their use. It was discovered that by the addition of chemical compounds characterised by the linkage

$$-\underset{\underset{\displaystyle O}{\|}}{C}-N<$$

which have feeble ionising properties, these disadvantages could be largely overcome. The compounds which contain this linkage include the amides, such as acetamide, butyramide, propionamide and the homologues including the higher molecular weight amides such as those of lauric, myristic, oleic and stearic acids. A similar effect is obtained with the addition of urea and this is utilised in several proprietary preparations. This forms a loose compound with the free mineral acid produced by hydrolysis and minimises its corrosive action on fabrics but still leaves sufficient acidity to prevent the precipitation of aluminium hydroxide. Wallace Laboratories (manufacturers of Arrid) brought a patent suit against F. W. Woolworth for selling Hinds Deodorant Cream, in which the Wallace Laboratories claimed infringement of U.S. Patent 2,236,387. The court, however, ruled that the expedient of introducing urea to promote the conservation of fabrics was well known prior to the application date of Wallace's patent. Whilst it was not shown that the part urea plays in arresting skin irritation was taught in any previous application, it was held that to devise such a new combination would not necessarily constitute a patentable invention.

Aluminium phenosulphonate. Weiss and Marcus (*Arch. Derm. Syph., Chicago*, 1941, **43**, 53) investigated the use of aluminium phenolsulphonate as a deodorant. Patch tests by them made on fifty subjects using solutions of 0·1 per cent. to 40 per cent. aluminium chloride and aluminium phenolsulphonate showed that at high concentrations aluminium chloride was the more irritant whilst at lower concentrations they were equal in respect of irritation.

Fifty-eight persons used a 20 per cent. solution and fifteen persons a greaseless cream containing 20 per cent. aluminium phenolsulphonate without any complaint in respect of effectiveness or irritation, and strips of linen, muslin and wool soaked in a 20 per cent. solution of this substance for one week showed no apparent damage.

Aluminium Chlorohydrate; Aluminium Chlorhydroxide Complex; "Chlorhydrol" (Reheis & Co. Inc.) $[Al_2(OH)_5Cl]_x$

This is a basic aluminium chloride complex in which the atomic ratio of Al : Cl is 2 : 1, as the above empirical formula shows, instead of 1 : 3 as in the normal aluminium chloride $AlCl_3$. Loosely associated with each molecular group there are, it is stated, two molecules of water.

The abnormal ratio of Al to Cl is reflected in the high *p*H value of "Chlorhydrol" solutions as shown in the following graph:

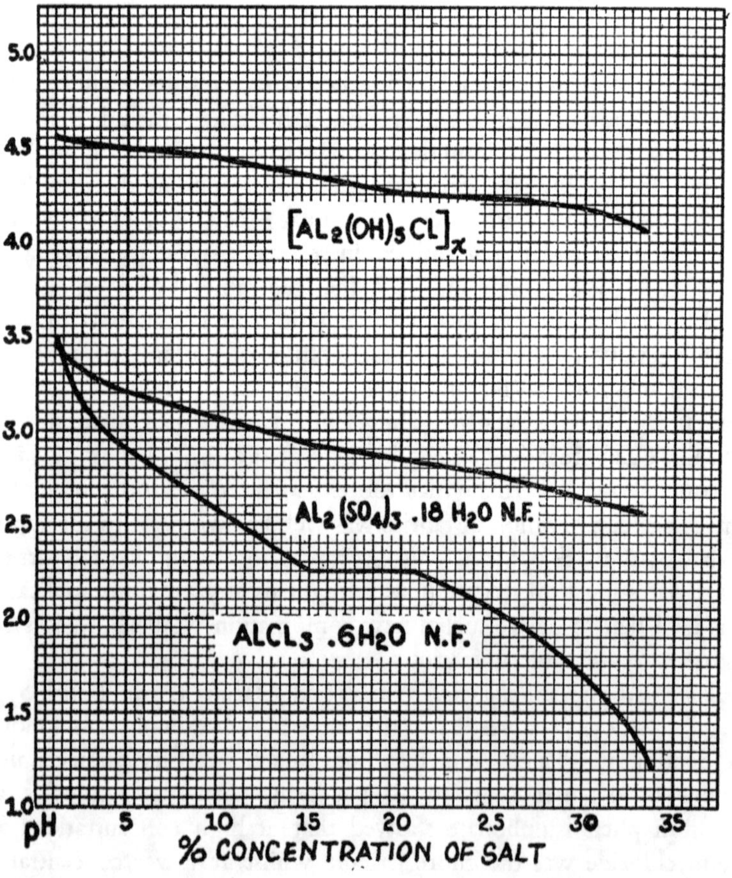

[*By courtesy of Reheis & Co. Inc.*

FIG. 99.—Comparison of *pH* values of Aluminium Chlorhydroxide complex (Chlorhydrol), Aluminium Sulphate, and Aluminium Chloride solutions.

Govett and deNavarre (*Amer. Perfum.*, 1947, **49**, 365), using a protein precipitation test in which preserved egg albumin was taken as being representative of undenatured protein, and in which the test solution was added to a solution of albumin in distilled water, obtained the following results:

	Precipitation	*pH*
Aluminium chloride	+ + + +	1·87
Aluminium Chlorhydrate Type E.1.	+ + + +	4·4
Aluminium sulphate	+ + + +	2·9
Aluminium citrate	+	2·4
Aluminium lactate	+	3·4
Aluminium sulphocarbolate	+ +	2·5

All the solutions were 10 per cent. w/v of the normal commercial salts. It is obvious that aluminium chlorhydrate is equal to aluminium chloride or sulphate, the best known astringents, and much superior to aluminium sulphocarbolate and the other aluminium salts.

This table shows very plainly the superiority of aluminium chlorhydrate (the high *p*H associated with lack of irritation and fabric destruction), together with the high protein precipitation value.

(In the test, egg albumin is diluted with equal parts of distilled water at room temperature. Five cc. of the solution is measured into a clean test tube. One cc. of the test solution is added.

Precipitation varies with the salt tested, as to quickness of formation, nature of precipitate and if it will remain insoluble over a 12-hour period. It is admitted that this test has its variables, but it is claimed that it does serve to determine relative values. Compounds known to be comparatively poor antiperspirants show little if any precipitate. On the other hand, formaldehyde, known to be a good antiperspirant, produces only a faint cloudiness.

Precipitation is denoted as +, + +, + + +, + + + +, increasing with the number of plus signs.)

"Chlorhydrol" is claimed to be absolutely stable in solution; test solutions showing no appreciable change in *p*H after being stored for 2 years. It is soluble in water in all proportions, though in amounts of 50 per cent. and over the solution becomes viscous and difficult to handle.

The following simple formulation exemplifies its use in a lotion:

	per cent.
"Chlorhydrol"[1]	20·0
Propylene glycol	5·0
Alcohol	10·0
Water	65·0
Perfume	*q.s.*

[1] A patent covers the use of this material in certain applications.

The viscosity of this solution may be increased if desired by the addition of a little colloidal magnesium aluminium silicate (R. T. Vanderbilt) "Veegum"; methyl cellulose, etc., and/or the alcohol level may be increased in order to simplify the perfuming of the preparation.

"Deodorant" antiseptic substances such as G-4 or G-11 may be added. (*See* Chapter 42, Antiseptics and Preservatives.)

Aluminium Methionate

It is claimed (Christian and Jenkins, *Amer. Perfum.*, Feb. 1951) that the utilisation of one of a series of aluminium alkyl disulphonates, viz. aluminium methionate (aluminium methane disulphonate), was superior to certain other aluminium salts. The pH of a 5 per cent. aqueous solution was about 3·5 and the substance was stated to be more effective as a protein precipitant and harmless to cloth.

Dichloro-aluminium amino-acetate, has, it is claimed, been successfully compounded with various cosmetic bases and has proved to be an effective underarm antiperspirant. ". . . Such preparations have been used by approximately 20 persons over a period of 3 years. There has been no evidence, so far, that such products tend to damage fabric or cause local skin irritation except in the case of one individual who appears to be sensitive to all aluminium-containing compounds. It is felt that the compound is worthy of further investigation. . . ." (Grote, Holbert, and Cross, *J. Amer. pharm. Ass., Sci. Edn.*, 1949, **38**, 593.)

Aluminium and Zinc Sulphamates

Three patents, U.S. Nos. 2,586,287-9, assigned to Colgate-Palmolive-Peet, claim that aluminium and zinc sulphamates are superior to aluminium sulphate as perspiration retardants and are practically non-tendering to clothing fabrics. In the case of aluminium sulphamate, however, some discoloration of cellulosic fibres was noted and Apperson and Richardson, the patentees, suggest four different groups of discoloration inhibitors as follows (*Drug. Cosmet. Ind.*, April 1952, p. 561):

Group 1. Amides which are neutral and contain the functional group:

$$-\underset{\underset{\displaystyle O}{\|}}{C}-NH_2$$

Group 2. Amino carboxylic acids $\equiv C-NH_2$.

Group 3. Compounds which are salts of non-hydroxy non-mercapto saturated carboxylic acids and ammonia bases.

Group 4. Compounds which contain the functional groups $\equiv C-S-H$.

Zinc sulphamate is said to be free of this discoloration factor.

Spray Antiperspirants

The newer types of antiperspirant liquids are packaged in polythene bottles, which, by means of a fine orifice, emit a spray when pressure is applied in quick jerks.

Liquid preparations utilising aluminium chloride, sulphate, or if the patent position permits, chlorhydrate may be used in the normal way for this purpose.

To such solutions, if desired, may be added antiseptics as "deodorants" (*See* Chapter 42.)

Aerosols ("Jet-Propelled Antiperspirants")

The development of the "aerosols" pressurised cosmetic preparations is briefly described in Chapter 29 (Shaving Preparations). As would be expected, corrosion problems in the use of aluminium solutions, of the type used as antiperspirants, are a serious hazard to the successful marketing of such preparations ; it is, however, said that aluminium sulphocarbolate has been successfully used for this purpose by using alcohol, up to 50 per cent., as cosolvent (Schimmel Briefs, No. 195, June 1951).

Antiperspirant Creams

Antiperspirant creams involve questions of compatibility of the antiperspirant with the emulsifier ; fortunately, owing to developments in the range of emulsifiers available to the cosmetic chemist, this is not an insoluble problem ; together with problems of hydrolysis and the possibility of the free acids formed by such hydrolysis reacting with other constituents of the cream.

Action of Cream Base *per se* on Perspiration

As pointed out earlier in this chapter, in discussing the mechanism of antiperspirant action, Sulzberger *et al.* have shown that anionic wetting agents such as "Aerosol OT", "Duponol" ME and negative electrolytes such as potassium sulphate, tend to increase delivery of sweat from the pores ; in these studies hexadienol, an oil-soluble, semi-solid alcohol was shown to act as a powerful stimulant to the sweat glands when applied to the skin. The experiments reported showed that apparently quite minor changes in the composition of the base may adversely affect the efficacy of the preparation. This is a comparatively new complication and whilst it is quite true that the concentration of antiperspirant is sufficient to exert a local antiperspirant action, it is obviously desirable to investigate this problem further with a view to producing an ideal antiperspirant which will have all the qualities desired, and which will produce this effect with the minimum concentration of materials foreign to the skin.

Action of Antiperspirant Creams on Fabrics

Klarmann (" The Cosmetic Aspects of Perspiration and its Control ", *Amer. Perfum.*, July 1948) in an excellent review of the subject draws attention to the fact that

" From extensive studies carried out with different antiperspirant products by R. R. Bien (*Proc. Sci. Sect. T.G.A.*, 1945, **4**, 8 ; *J. Soc. cosmet. Chem.* 1947, **1**, 2) it appears that whereas silk, wool and acetate rayon fabrics are resistant to such products, linen, cotton and viscose rayon are vulnerable ; a maximum amount of damage is produced by ironing directly, i.e. without a preceding laundering, for reasons discussed in connection with the need for buffering the astringent salts. The practical angle of these facts derives from the observation that garments and especially cotton and linen blouses or dresses often are subjected to pressing between launderings. Thus, if in the course of being worn, the garment picks up some of the antiperspirant cream from the axilla, and if it is then ironed without laundering the acidity of the cream will have been activated to such an extent than an irreparable damage to the garment will result.

" In order to obtain advance information as to the destructive effect on fabrics of antiperspirants and deodorants, a test procedure was evolved which provides for the exposure of a piece of cotton fabric to conditions approximately resembling those of actual wear, and for the determination of the loss of tensile strength which the fabric suffers as a result of such exposure. It was found that if this reduction is of the order of 20 per cent. or less, only a negligible damage would be caused by the antiperspirant cream to the fabric under the condition of use ; but if it was substantially more than 20 per cent., a serious damage could be anticipated as a result of ironing. While the original papers should be consulted for details of the testing procedure, it may be mentioned here that the several steps comprise application of the antiperspirant to the cotton fabric, maintenance in a humid atmosphere at 80° F. for 24 hours, pressing with an electric ironer (at 275° to 295° F.), conditioning in a humid atmosphere for 3 hours and testing in a motor-driven tensile strength apparatus. The comparison is made with an untreated control sample which, however, has undergone the same phases of exposure to humidity and ironing as the test sample. The percentage loss of tensile strength is calculated as an average of twenty-five individual ' breaks '.

" The acidity of the antiperspirant under test (as expressed by its pH) is an extremely important factor, which does not, however, of itself determine the product's safety to fabrics. Of two antiperspirant creams with the same *p*H at room temperature, one may affect the tensile strength at ironing temperatures to a much greater extent than another, depending upon the behaviour of the corrosion-inhibiting ingredient under those conditions, i.e. its capacity to neutralise the acidity to a point below the corrosive range. Incidentally, if the preparation shows a *p*H under 2·5, it is quite likely to cause fabric destruction regardless of the presence of any ingredient expected to act as a corrosion inhibitor. . . ."

The following formulations are illustrative of some antiperspirant creams :

Using acid-stable glyceryl monostearate

	per cent.
(*a*) "Tegacid" (Goldschmidt Co.)	20·00
(*b*) Glycerin	3·00
(*c*) Spermaceti	5·00
(*d*) "Chlorhydrol"	20·00
(*e*) Water	52·00

Procedure

(*a*), (*b*), (*c*) and (*e*) are mixed together and warmed under agitation close to the boiling-point. The emulsion thus formed is stirred until cooled to 30°-40° C., (*d*) is then added (dissolved in a little of the water kept back for this purpose) and stirred down to about 30° C.

(*Courtesy, Reheis & Co. Inc.*)

	per cent.
(*a*) "Tegacid"	15·00
(*b*) Glycerin	3·00
(*c*) Spermaceti	5·00
(*d*) "Tegosept" M	2·00
(*e*) Water	58·00
(*f*) Aluminium sulphate	15·00
(*g*) Titanium dioxide	2·00

Procedure

Similar to above adding (*f*) and (*g*) last. (*Note.*—This cream contains aluminium sulphate "straight" without an added buffer.)

(*Courtesy, Goldschmidt Chemical Corp.*)

Another formulation using aluminium sulphate and no buffer, and based on *non-ionic emulsifiers*, is :

	per cent.
(*a*) Stearic acid (triple pressed)	10·00
(*b*) Beeswax (white)	2·00
(*c*) Mineral oil (65/75)	1·00
(*d*) G-2152	5·00
(*e*) G-2160	5·00
(*f*) Water	62·00
(*g*) Aluminium sulphate (crystalline)	15·00

Procedure

Melt (*a*), (*b*), (*c*), (*d*) and (*e*) and bring to 80° C. Add (*f*) at 85° C., cool with agitation to 30° C. and work in (*g*) a little at a time. Make sure that each addition is thoroughly dissolved before adding more. Perfume and package immediately to obtain optimum consistency and stability.

(*Courtesy, Atlas Powder Co., Wilmington, U.S.A.*)

The following formulation (Reheis & Co. Inc.) illustrates an astringent liquid cream lotion:

		Parts
A	Cetyl alcohol	1·25
	Atlas G-2151	2·50
	Stearic acid	3·75
	Propylene glycol	1·00
B	Veegum HV (R. T. Vanderbilt & Co.)	0·75
	Water, distilled	20·00
	Chlorhydrol	20·00
C	Water, distilled	50·25
	Perfume	*q.s.*

Procedure

Heat A, B and C and mix at as low a temperature as possible.

CHAPTER 31

DEPILATORIES

THE value of preparations for the removal of unwanted hair was appreciated by the " dancing girls " of the East in ancient times, who apparently used " rhusma ", a mixture of one part of quicklime and two parts of arsenical pyrites, reduced to powder and mixed with aqueous alkali—possibly obtained from wood ashes—prior to use ; another preparation " orpiment " utilised for the same purpose consisted of arsenic trisulphide.

During intervening centuries there is little record of any development work having been carried out on so interesting a subject ; if " one used *anything*, one used *pumice stone* and didn't talk about such things ".

In the last twenty years there has, however, been an increasing interest in depilatories occasioned by an increasing scantiness in certain attire, " revealing " bathing dresses, the cult of sun bathing, evening dresses for which glabrous armpits are *de rigueur* and so on, including the introduction of nylon stockings.

The term " depilatory " is applied to preparations designed for the removal of bodily hair, in particular that occurring under the axilla and on the legs, without injury to the skin.

The advantage of such preparations as compared with the use of a razor is that, instead of merely cutting the hair at the skin surface, it removes them at the mouth of the hair follicle, with the result that a second treatment is necessary only after two or three weeks have elapsed, whereas if simple shaving is employed a dark growth will be visible once more after a few days.

Unfortunately, the hair shaft is of similar composition to that of the skin, and for this reason some small degree of local damage must necessarily occur as the result of applying such preparations. Providing the skin is reasonably healthy, that the time of application of the depilatory is not too long, and that this is correctly formulated, however, very little if any damage appears to be done.

Should a particular depilatory prove disappointing in action a second application (either of the same or any other similar preparation) should not be made for some days, and, preferably, a week or two should be allowed to elapse. On no account must depilatories be used on an inflamed surface, neither should they immediately follow, or be followed by, a deodorant.

With the above precautions in mind the requirements of a depilatory may be briefly discussed. These are that it should be:

(*a*) Non-irritant and innocuous.

(*b*) Efficient in action, removing hair in from 4-5 minutes.

(*c*) Preferably odourless.

After application for the above period, the hair should be observed to "corkscrew" and then may be wiped off with a damp cloth or sponge. Finally, the area denuded should be gently washed with soap and water, patted dry, and a little powdered talcum or calamine added.

If the skin shows any signs of roughness, a little calamine lotion or cold cream may be applied and left on overnight.

The depilatories most widely used today fall into two classes, namely:

(i) Those based on strontium sulphide; these are very effective and work in from 3-5 minutes after application. Whilst some people are sensitive to such preparations (as indeed are some people to shaving soaps), *if used according to the directions of the manufacturer,* they appear to be innocuous. Their main almost only disadvantage is the fact that they possess an odour of hydrogen sulphide. This odour is not very evident when the product is first applied to the skin and if the bulk is removed as advised with a wooden spatula (usually provided) before rinsing off the residue, the odour is comparatively slight and, in the author's opinion, not a lot worse than the odour which pervades the house when a cold wave is being carried out at home.

(ii) Types based upon the use of substituted mercaptans in the presence of alkaline reacting materials, for example, calcium thioglycollate. These preparations have the advantage of possessing less odour than the strontium sulphide type but have the very great disadvantage of taking over twice as long to do the trick. [If one has ever tried holding one's arm up for about 3 minutes and compares it with holding it up for 7-8 minutes the difference *will* be appreciated.] So far as skin irritation or toxicity is concerned, there is, in the author's opinion, little to choose between them.

The "ideal", odourless depilatory has not, as yet, been marketed; some of the stannite preparations showed promise but have not fulfilled that promise in practice. One keeps coming back to the fact that there are several ways to make a depilatory act more swiftly and to keep down its odour but, unfortunately, the method of so doing is the converse of that required to minimise skin irritation. That does not mean that the task is impossible but merely that it is a very difficult proposition.

Brief History of Depilatories

The use of sulphides has been known, as pointed out at the beginning of this chapter, for a very long time; however, it was not until 1885 that, in the United States, the first patent was taken out for the use of barium polysulphide for removing hair. In April 1891, the use of the monosulphide, polysulphide and sulphydrate of strontium for the same purpose was patented (U.S. Patent 450,032). These preparations were, however, mixtures rather than creams; the first depilatory in cream form being developed in 1921. Between 1930 and 1944 considerable attention was devoted to "soluble stannites" and to derivatives of thioglycollic acid, e.g. U.S. Patent 1,899,707 (1933) covers the use of sodium stannite as a preferred salt of tin, with Rochelle salts used as a stabiliser.

Stannites

U.S. Patent 2,123,214 (July 1938) draws attention to the fact that whilst the stannites have no appreciable odour, they suffer from instability, forming stannates in the presence of water. The Patent proposed the use, as stabilisers, of water-soluble organic compounds having three or more carbinol hydroxy groups, or three hydroxyl groups other than those in a carboxyl group and also soluble silicates; specific examples are triethanolamine, dextrine, sugars—and in the case of the silicate—potassium or sodium metasilicate. Brit. Patent 516,812 describes the addition of aqueous stannous chloride to aqueous sodium hydroxide containing sodium silicate to give a solution having a *p*H less than 12·6 (12·3). French Patent 840,552 also claims method for the preparation of a stable stannite.

Thioglycollates

Brit. Patent 484,467 (1938) granted to Karel Bohemen covered the use of calcium thioglycollate in a cream base. The base had the formula:

	per cent.
Stearyl alcohol	9·0
Sulphonated stearyl alcohol	1·0
Water	90·0

Sixty-six parts of the above base were mixed with 10 parts hydrated lime and 4 parts 90 per cent. thioglycollic acid, whereupon the cream liquefied and was stiffened by the addition of at least 20 parts of precipitated chalk.

U.S. Patent 2,352,524 issued June 1944 to Ralph L. Evans and E. G. McDonough, covered the use of two agents, substituted mercaptans (thioglycollic acid) and an alkaline-reacting material such as lime, a non-reacting paste-forming material and a perfume material. Substituted mercaptans, especially those having polar groupings, are preferred. The patentees claim that in order to obtain a desirable depilating action, the depilating agent must conform to certain general rules:

(i) *p*H value should be between *p*H 9·0 and *p*H 12·5.

(ii) Concentration of mercaptans should be between 0·1 and 1·5 mols. per litre.

(iii) The alkaline ingredient must have an ionisation constant greater than 2 times 10^{-5}.

(iv) In order to prevent skin damage, it is desirable that the concentration of the alkaline material in solution be not greater than twice the equivalent concentration of the mercaptans.

(v) Paste form is the most satisfactory.

(vi) Natural gums are used to give stable formulation.

Bohemen's discovery resulted in the issuance of patents in certain countries to him or his agent—Fletcher. In the United States, after litigation, a U.S. Patent was issued only to Evans and McDonough.

Because under the laws of certain countries, the Evans and McDonough patent conflicts with the Bohemen patent, the patents issued to Evans and McDonough cover the use of mercaptans other than mercapto-acetic acid in depilatories.[1] Intending manufacturers are advised to consult the *present* patent position in their country.

Guanidine Thioglycollate Depilatory, Brit. Patent 636,181 (1950) (R. L. Demuth), relates to depilatories in which the lower mercapto-carboxylic acid, e.g. thioglycollic, constitutes the active principle. The essential feature of this patent is the neutralisation of the mercapto-carboxylic acid with an alkaline earth compound, or with an organic base such as guanidine. The inclusion in the composition of hydrazine sulphate or like diamine derivatives is an important subsidiary feature in allowing the *p*H to be reduced whilst maintaining a rapid rate of depilation.

Strontium sulphide. Strontium sulphide prepared by the reduction of strontium sulphate by heating with carbon or carbonisable material, etc., is grey in colour. White or almost white grades for cosmetic purposes are prepared either by heating strontium hydroxide with sulphur or by purification of the grey material—unchanged carbon and coloured metallic sulphides being removed by leaching out with hot water, evaporation and re-firing. The grey commercial material normally contains 60–80 per cent. SrS, the white cosmetic grade

[1] E. G. McDonough, *Amer. Perfum.*, Nov. 1947.

contains up to 85 per cent. SrS—the balance being sulphate and carbonate.

A yellow form of strontium sulphide is sometimes used and prepared as described above by leaching and evaporation, but not re-firing; this is a mixture of hydrosulphide, polysulphide and hydroxide (Personal Communication; E. A. Roff, B.Sc., F.R.I.C.).

The *p*H of strontium sulphide depilatories is adjusted by the addition of strontium hydroxide or other alkali to the appropriate *p*H, since the depilating effect of the preparation is related to the alkalinity of the product.

Other Sulphides

Although from the theoretical aspect it might be considered that any of the water-soluble sulphides of the alkali metals could be used for such products, in point of fact only strontium sulphide is commercially valuable for this purpose. Lithium sulphide, although more expensive, possesses no advantage over sodium sulphide, whilst potassium sulphide as obtained commercially is a variable mixture of polysulphides. The toxicity of barium compounds in general, renders barium sulphide of little interest to the cosmetic manufacturer.

As Atkins ("Paper read before Section 14 of the 11th International Congress of Pure and Applied Chemistry", *Perfum. essent. Oil Rec.*, July 1947, p. 231) has pointed out, strontium sulphide is particularly suitable for depilatories of the sulphide type since discoloration is reduced to a minimum and the smell, whilst objectionable, can be controlled and masked. It has the minor disadvantage of limited solubility of strontium hydroxide with the result that strontium hydroxide tends to crystallise into hard particles. Whilst this difficulty can be overcome temporarily by milling the product, it may appear during storage under fluctuation in temperature.

So far as the odour of such preparations is concerned Atkins points out that ". . . In reality two problems are involved, the smell of sulphuretted hydrogen and the smell of by-products, such as mercaptans and other thio-substituted bodies, which may be formed in the perfume. So far as sulphuretted hydrogen is concerned, the conditions for its formation can be quite simply stated. Consider the hydrolysis of a typical sulphide, say sodium sulphide. This can take place in two stages:

$$(1)\ Na_2S + H_2O \rightleftharpoons NaHS + NaOH.$$

$$(2)\ NaHS + H_2O \rightleftharpoons NaOH + H_2S.$$

Thus primary hydrolysis produces an equilibrium of sulphydrate and hydroxide, which has a slight but not very objectionable smell of sulphuretted hydrogen, and is stable probably above *p*H 11. Below this, secondary hydrolysis takes place with a production of free sulphuretted hydrogen and a very marked offensive odour. This is the reason why many depilatories have comparatively little odour when applied to the skin, but fill the house with an intolerable smell of sulphuretted hydrogen when washed off. With proper manipulation this can be avoided. The procedure is to apply the depilatory in the ordinary way to the dry skin, leaving it on for the specified time, and scrape off with a dry wooden spatula or other convenient instrument. Do not wash this under the tap Wipe it on a dry piece of rag or newspaper, and burn it. Before washing the skin apply a small quantity of 5 per cent. zinc sulphate solution and then wash in the ordinary way. No sulphuretted hydrogen smell will develop because the small amount of sulphide remaining on the skin will be instantly converted into non-hydrolysable zinc sulphide, which of course, is not affected by water."

Thioglycerol

Brit. Patent 593,438 (1947), R. L. Evans and E. G. McDonough claims that " . . . whilst mercaptan substances generally were found to be chemically capable of depilating hair . . . nevertheless some of the mercaptans have certain drawbacks as compared with others of the mercaptans, when used in commercial depilatories. Thioglycollic acid is of such outstanding merit that it has, up to the present time, been generally accepted as the mercaptan suited for commercial depilatories. However, I (R. L. Evans, assignee of E. G. McDonough) have found that thioglycerol has remarkable advantages over the other mercaptans or any other substance used heretofore in depilatories and achieves new commercially significant and highly desirable results. It is so remarkably superior to other substances yet used for depilatories that it is a matter of contrast rather than of comparison. . . ."

Thioglycerol ($C_3H_8O_2S$), for which these advantages are claimed, generically describes dihydroxypropanthiol ($HSCH_2CHOH\ CH_2OH$) and dihydroxyisopropanthiol ($(HOCH_2)_2HCSH$. Advantages claimed are that this material and its alkali salts are hygroscopic and hence do not tend to dry out, are very stable, and do not form coloured substances when stored for long periods in collapsible tubes. It is also stated to be non-substantive to keratin so that residual skin odour is minimised.

The following examples are quoted in the patent :

Strontium hydrate	50·0 g.
Calcium oxide	12·0 g.
Colloidal clay	102·0 g.
Methyl cellulose	11·0 g.

Perfume	0·8 cc.
Water	300·0 cc.
Thioglycerol	12·0 cc.

and the following "general" formula:

	Parts by weight
Fatty alcohol	5–10
Sodium fatty alkyl sulphate	0·5–1·5
Alkaline earth hydroxide	5–20·0
Inorganic fillers	10–20·0
Thioglycerol	2–8·0
Perfume	0·3–1·0
Water (*q.s.* to form suitable consistency)	

"... Instead of using the fatty alcohol and the fatty alkyl sulphate, a mucilaginous material such as a 5 per cent. solution of polyvinyl alcohol or methyl cellulose, or mixtures of fatty alcohol and the fatty alkyl sulphate and mucilaginous solutions may be used. ..."

An example of the use of calcium thioglycollate (Evans and McDonough) is given, e.g.:

Calcium oxide	12·0 g.
Strontium hydroxide	50·0 g.
Colloidal clay	102·0 g.
Methyl cellulose	11·0 g.
Thioglycollic acid	12·0 cc.
Water	300·0 cc.
Perfume	0·8 cc.

The following formulation illustrates the use of calcium thioglycollate with guanidine and hydrazine sulphate (Brit. Patent 636,181):

	per cent.
Calcium thioglycollate	20·0
Guanidine	10·0
"Teepol"	30·0
Hydrazine sulphate *	5·0
Methyl cellulose (12 per cent.)	35·0

The following formulation includes both strontium and barium sulphides ("Readers' Questions", *Drug cosmet. Ind.*, Nov. 1952, p. 663):

	Parts
Strontium sulphide	15·0
Barium sulphide	10·0
Talc	10·0
Corn starch	20·0
Glycerin	18·0
Water	20·0
Perfume	2·0

(The author does not favour the use of barium sulphide.)

* Caution. *Toxic!*—Author.

It is the author's opinion that a better method of formulation for such a product lies along the use of non-ionic emulsifying agents, strontium sulphide as the depilating agent and adjustment of the pH to a sufficiently high figure by the addition of the requisite amount of a suitable alkali.

The formulation of depilatories depends upon very careful adherence to detail; slight departures from formulation in the process of manufacturing can produce remarkable differences between the efficacies of different batches of supposedly the same product. For this reason any formulation can be little more than a general guide.

Epilatory Preparations

These are really a sub-division of depilating preparations in that whilst "depilation" is the title for any process which removes the hair at the skin level, epilation describes any process of removing hair from beneath the skin, either by tweaking it out with a tweezers or by the application of sticky or waxy preparations to which the hairs adhere and may then be stripped off in a section.

From the author's experience of taking skin impressions by wax castings, the depilatory would win every time; the tweaking out of the hair is a most crude process which is bound to result in skin trauma and to a greater extent than with a well-formulated depilatory. However, such preparations apparently have their adherents.

Such preparations have been based, for very many years, on mixtures consisting essentially of rosin and beeswax, modified in some instances by the addition of mineral oil and/or waxes. The following examples are illustrative:

	per cent.
Rosin	75·0
Beeswax	25·0

(*The Chemistry and Manufacture of Cosmetics*, M. G. deNavarre, D. Van Nostrand.)

	per cent.
Light coloured rosin	52·0
Yellow beeswax	25·0
Paraffin wax	17·0
Petrolatum	5·0
Perfume	1·0

Procedure

Melt the rosin and waxes, mix and add the petrolatum, then, when the temperature drops to about 60° C., add the perfume and pour the melted mass into suitable moulds. When this wax is used it is melted and painted over the surface to be dehaired.

("Readers' Questions", *Drug Cosmet. Ind.*, Nov. 1949, p. 575.)

There have been no dramatic developments of a " painless " epilatory in the industry. Such developments as have taken place have been concerned with modifications in the method of application, such as the provision of a flexible backing strip, and also the provision of a preparation that does not require melting prior to use but can be applied cold, the preparation being based upon a mixture of glucose and zinc oxide (U.S. Patent 2,417,882). The use of a " rubber solution ", in which the solvent evaporates and the rubber film is stripped off is covered in U.S. Patent 2,067,909.

THE " IDEAL " DEPILATORY

The " ideal " depilatory, one which would have no odour, would remove hair in about 1 minute, could be used regularly without any complaints of irritation ; one that could replace the daily task of shaving, has yet to be devised. When such a product arrives it will certainly have a market.

Some interesting avenues of exploration have been opened up by recent researches into the depilating effect of certain unsaturated compounds.

Ritter and Carter (*J. indust. Hyg.*, May 1948, **30**, 192) reported that " . . . When commercial polymerisation of chlorobutadiene was undertaken in an aqueous emulsion some of the employees began to lose their hair after a few weeks or months. The loss of hair could be much reduced by frequent and complete change of the air in which they were working. The hair loss was predominantly on the scalp, and hair always grew again when the employees were transferred to other occupations. Microscopical examination of the hair showed that it came out at the root, a bulb being present at one end of each hair shaft, but there was no evidence of change in the shaft itself. A composite product containing various cyclic and short-chain polymers of chlorobutadiene was prepared : when two drops of this were placed on the back of a mouse or guinea pig, the area covered by the solution became completely denuded of hair in 4–10 days. In about 3 weeks hair was again visible over the denuded area and in 6 weeks it had completely regrown. . . ."

The interesting part of this observation is that, previous developments have been in connection with preparations which are intended to swell the hair near the mouth of the follicle and reduce its tensile strength to an extent that allows it to be " cork-screwed " away very readily. Since the hair and skin are both composed of keratin there is not a very wide *margin* between what will attack the one and irritate the other. The above observation shows the possibility of a *different method of attack ;* not damage to the hair (and skin) *per se*, but merely a *detachment of the hair bulb from the hair follicle*—such damage being, apparently, temporary since the hair grew again in from 3-6 weeks.

Obviously considerable research would be necessary to determine whether any commercial preparation could be developed along such lines and its toxicity and any effect of long-term usage would have to be fully investigated; moreover, the time lag between application and effect is too long. It may indeed be that such a time-lag could not safely be shortened. Nevertheless from a theoretical aspect, the above observations and those of Flesch and Goldstone discussed below are of interest.

Flesch (*J. Soc. cosmet. Chem.*, Aug. 1952, **3**, 2) found that squalene and a group of lipoid-soluble unsaturated compounds (with —C=C— groups) caused reversible complete baldness when applied to the skin of laboratory *animals*. These compounds include the synthetic dimers of chloroprene and certain esters of allyl alcohol, naturally occurring vitamin A, oleic and linoleic acids. Flesch postulated that the depilation is caused by the reaction between the —C=C— bonds and the sulphydryl group, of epidermal protein. Although Flesch has not, as yet, been able to depilate human beings with any of these unsaturated depilatory agents, these findings have suggested that human sebum may have an influence in hair growth. (This question is discussed more fully in Chapter 20, paragraph dealing with Sebum.)

Whether the above findings can be *safely* and *effectively* turned to a useful depilatory purpose is at present merely the object of speculation, but nevertheless an intriguing one!

Meanwhile, having regard to all the difficulties of this problem, it must be admitted that the leading makes of modern depilatories do a very good job, they are effective, reasonably innocuous when used correctly, and differ chiefly in respect of two characteristics only, odour and speed. If the odour is not objected to, the operation can be carried out effectively and safely in one-half to one-third of the time; if the odour is of paramount importance then one can obtain a product having less odour but it will take longer to perform its task. I would infinitely prefer either of these to "epilatory" preparations but that is only a personal opinion.

CHAPTER 32

COSMETIC STOCKINGS

LEG MAKE-UP

THE use of "Cosmetic Stockings" is not new. Elizabeth Arden introduced leg make-up in 1937 but some ten years prior to this the Doraldina Company had sold a similar preparation designated as such, in three or four different shades; even before Doraldina Leg Make-Up the Aubrey Sisters (in Chicago) had been marketing their "Beauty Secret" for some years. This product was used for covering up blemishes not only on the face, neck and arms but also on the legs (*Drug Cosmet. Ind.*, July 1942, 1, 53).

Although at least twenty years have therefore passed since the introduction of such preparations, they only jumped into prominence during the 1939-45 war, owing to the rationing of clothing and consequent loathness of women in Britain to part with the few clothing coupons they possessed for silk stockings which would ladder on but slight provocation.

The characteristics necessary to produce a satisfactory Cosmetic Stocking are:

(*a*) At a distance of a few yards the preparation should give the treated leg the appearance of being encased in a stocking, and hence should possess sufficient opacity to cover the nudeness of the leg and provide a *semblance of texture* yet it should possess sufficient transparency to obviate any suggestion that the leg has been completely encased in a heavy opaque paint; in addition, the shade of the preparation when dry should approximate to that in which silk, or nylon stockings are popularly marketed.

(*b*) The preparation must not wash away in rain, nor rub off on the clothing but should be capable of removal, when desired, by means of soap and water.

(*c*) The preparation should apply smoothly, yielding an even film and it should dry fairly rapidly.

(*d*) It is, of course, a *sine qua non* that the preparation should be neither a primary irritant, nor a sensitiser but should be dermatologically innocuous.

The development of the ideal preparation having all of the above characteristics is not at all easy and various types of preparations have been marketed in an endeavour to comply with the above conditions, e.g.:

(1) Liquid or solid suspensions of powder in an aqueous medium.

(2) Suspensions of powder in an oily or fatty base, such base being either in the free fatty state or emulsified.

(3) A compressed cake of powder.

LIQUID OR SOLID SUSPENSIONS OF POWDER IN AN AQUBOUS BASE

A " basic " formula upon which to elaborate a *liquid* type " Cosmetic Stocking " is:

	per cent.
Zinc oxide	6·0
Chalk (precipitated)	16·0
Methyl cellulose	0·5
Glycerin	16·0
Water	61·5
Additional	
Colouring matter	*q.s.*
Preservative	*q.s.*
Perfume	*q.s.*

More opacity in the finished make-up may be obtained by increasing the proportion of zinc oxide and/or including titanium dioxide, but an obviously artificial effect is undesirable. A little alcohol may be included in order to speed up the time of drying; the viscosity may be varied by the use of different viscosity grades of methyl cellulose or other cellulosic film-forming material, alternatively alginates or gum mucilages may be included but care must be taken that the finished preparation is not sticky.

To increase the time during which the pigmented powder remains in suspension (after shaking) whilst the preparation is being applied to the leg, a few per cent. of bentonite or other similar clays may be incorporated.

A certain amount of glycerin or similar non-evaporating and foundation-forming substance is desirable as this improves the adherence of the film of powder to the leg.

Colouring matters usually consist of mixtures of harmless yellow, red, and brown pigments, according to the shade desired, in addition some soluble dyes may be included to produce a slight staining effect on the leg and also minimise the appearance of separation between the aqueous and powder phase in the container.

Manufacture of such preparations is comparatively simple, the powder constituents being ground with the chosen colours, any water-soluble materials including preservative (and any additional water-soluble dye which it is desired to add) dissolved in the water and the two phases well mixed. Care should be taken in bottling to ensure that the powder does not separate from the aqueous phase as bottles showing—after standing on a display counter—an uneven deposit of pigmented powder are unsightly. Alternatively a measured amount of powder may be delivered to each container, followed by a measured volume of the aqueous phase and the containers then suitably agitated.

(Some information on water-resistant films may be obtained by consulting Chapter 39, Protective Creams and Industrial Cleansers.)

A formula utilising soluble-casein[1] was suggested by Kalish (*Drug Cosmet. Ind.*, Sept. 1941, **3**, 45):

	per cent.
Colloidal clay	10·0
Precipitated chalk	10·0
Talc	5·0
Alcohol	5·0
Sorbitol	5·0
Soluble casein [2]	3·0
Water	62·0
Dye and pigment	*q.s.*

The following formula appeared in the *Amer. Perfum.*, "Questions and Answers", June 1945, p. 37:

	per cent.
Zinc stearate	2·0
Titanium dioxide	3·5
Colloidal aluminium—	
Magnesium silicate gel [3]	20·0
Isopropyl alcohol	6·0
Umber	0·5
Yellow oxide	2·5
Red oxide	2·5
Propylene glycol	1·0
Methyl cellulose (1500 viscosity grade)	0·5
Water, perfume and preservative	to make 100·0

Cosmetic stockings in the form of a cream may be prepared by incorporating pigmented powder into a vanishing cream or other emulsified cream base which should be sufficiently low in viscosity to allow the preparation to be spread easily and which should also contain glycerin

[1] Casein preparations have a peculiar odour and require careful preservation.—Author.

[2] Prepared by dispensing 1 lb. of casein in 1 gallon of water with the help of 2 oz. of triethanolamine.

[3] Veegum, R. T. Vanderbilt & Co.

or other humectant, or in some cases oils may be included. (*See* Chapter 9.)

In answer to a reader's question, the following was stated to provide a good working formula for a liquid stocking:

	per cent.
Precipitated chalk	10·0
Talc	5·0
Titanium dioxide	3·0
Bentonite	2·0
Alcohol	8·0
Glycerin	3·0
Wetting agent	0·5
Methyl cellulose	0·5
Water	68·0
Dye and pigment	*q.s.*

It was pointed out that the colour of the preparation was important and the use of harmless earth colours and lakes made from certified dyes was suggested.

The following illustrates the use of glyceryl monostearate in a liquid stocking formulation:

	per cent.
Glyceryl monostearate S (Glyco Products)	0·4
Water	78·1
Glycerin	0·5
Titanium dioxide and earth pigments	20·0
Methyl cellulose	1·0

Procedure

Dissolve glycerin in the water and make a 5 per cent. dispersion of the glyceryl monostearate S in hot mixture, stirring until cool. Soak the methyl cellulose in the balance of the water (cold) until dissolved. Add this to the glyceryl monostearate dispersion and mill in the pigments.

(*Courtesy, Glyco Products Inc.*)

The use of "Veegum", essentially a hydrous magnesium aluminium silicate gel (R. T. Vanderbilt & Co.), in leg make-up is claimed to have the following advantages:

(i) reduces the tendency for the pigments to dust off;
(ii) keeps pigments in suspension longer;
(iii) a considerable reduction in the amount of glycerin or propylene glycol can be effected;
(iv) streaking is, to a large extent, overcome;
(v) Veegum is an excellent dispersing medium for pigments and fillers;
(vi) products made with Veegum feel creamy on application to the skin.

The following formulation illustrates the use of this material in a liquid leg make-up :

	Per cent. by weight
Veegum (5% dispersion in water)	25·00
Glyceryl monostearate	0·60
Methyl cellulose (4000 cps.)	0·80
Pigment 3122 (Kohnstamm)	8·00
Red oxide (Kohnstamm)	0·20
Titanium dioxide pure	1·00
Butyl *p*-hydroxy benzoate	0·02
Water [1]	64·28
Perfume	0·10

Procedure

Prepare the Veegum dispersion by adding Veegum to the water and stirring till smooth. Disperse the methyl cellulose in about one half of the water as follows: Heat the water to 80°-90° C., add the methyl cellulose, stir well and allow to stand over-night in the cold. A clear solution should result.

Disperse the glyceryl monostearate in the remainder of the water as follows : Heat the glyceryl monostearate to 65°-70° C., dissolve the butyl *p*-hydroxy benzoate and add to the water which has been previously heated to 65°-70° C. Stir with a mechanical mixer until cool.

Mix the above solutions, and add the colours, titanium dioxide, " Veegum " and perfume, mix well and pass through a colloid mill set at close clearance.

Note.—It is not important that the above colours be used unless a specific shade is to be matched. However, it is important that so called " Cosmetic Stocking Colours " be used. Several chemical houses supply these colours in a number of shades. Where possible it is preferable to use a " Cosmetic Stocking Colour " in preference to the red oxide used above as no bleeding of colour will then take place.

The viscosity of these preparations may be altered by increasing or decreasing the amount of " Veegum " at the expense of the water. This may be necessary as the viscosity of the methyl cellulose solution will vary from batch to batch. If pigments other than the above are used, the consistency should be adjusted accordingly.

(*Courtesy, R. T. Vanderbilt & Co., New York.*)

Cosmetic Stocking " Creams "

It is suggested that these may be based upon a foundation cream base, using the types of colours suggested in this chapter (cf. Chapter 9).

[1] Up to 10 per cent. additional water may be added after manufacture in case the above product is too thick.

CHAPTER 33

FOOT PREPARATIONS

ALTHOUGH some 60 to 70 per cent. of the adult population appear to suffer foot discomfort in one form or another, it is really amazing how little personal attention is lavished upon the much maligned human foot, although foot fatigue affects adversely both the physical and mental well-being of the sufferer, and leads to a sharp decline in the individual effort. Moreover, this effect is cumulative (tired and aching feet lead to ill humour, and meals eaten in a bad temper to indigestion) and ultimately often ends in various forms of stomach ailments plus the original foot discomfort.

This is not really surprising when we consider that the human foot has to maintain the whole weight of the body. In spite of the fact that it is equipped with a multitude of sweat glands, unequalled in any part of the skin surface, except the palmar surfaces of the hands, it is, under the dictates and necessities of modern civilisation, encased first in a woollen or cotton sock, and then in a leather shoe or boot. These leather encasements become saturated with nitrogenous organic substances derived from the sweat. The footwear is dried by evaporation and the process repeated. Bacterial infection occurs, as these organic salts act as nutrient media, and an optimum temperature (about 37° C.) is maintained in the boot or shoe in the presence of adequate moisture. The sock or stocking is washed from time to time, but no attempt is made to remove such accumulation in the footwear. It is no wonder that the shoe swarms with micro-organisms which very rapidly infect the new sock which may be put on.

In assessing the value which the cosmetician or manufacturing chemist can exert in the alleviation of foot ailments, the above facts should be remembered. First, it must be emphasised that *there is no substitute for a well-fitting shoe, and a foot that is automatically healthy.* The sufferer must select sensible and properly fitting footwear and, if suffering from what is commonly known as a *weak arch* (a common complaint in those persons whose work entails long hours of standing, e.g. shop assistants, policemen, plant operatives and laboratory technicians), an adequate foot support in the form of an *arch support* or *foot easer* should be fitted by an operator specialising in this branch of work. Given these conditions, and the absence of any organic disease, surgical defect, or bacterial or fungal infection, it is usually possible for the cosmetician or chemist to market certain products which will *temporarily* alleviate the foot discomfort. These products usually consist of foot lotions, foot bath preparations, creams, powders, and possibly an antiseptic *shoe* lotion.

Foot lotions need no special attention. For temporarily cooling the feet they may be formulated on the lines of a skin tonic or mild astringent lotion. For perspiration an astringent deodorant may be applied, full details of which will be found under their appropriate headings in this work. (*See* Chapter 30.)

Being an extremity of the body, and not having adequate exercise, the human foot, particularly when constricted in ill-fitting shoes, or by tight elastic or other suspenders around the leg, is prone to an inefficient circulation. Bathing the foot in hot water stimulates the blood circulation, eliminates stale sweat secretions, and bacterial infection is temporarily reduced. If the bath is alkaline it softens the hard keratinous layer of the skin and enables corns, callouses, etc., to be removed. Proprietary bath salts for the feet are put up for this purpose and consist essentially of alkali, often in conjunction with an oxygen-releasing substance such as sodium perbolate. Other types of powders are formulated so that the final bath solution approximates to sea water.

	per cent.
Sodium carbonate	20·0
Sodium bicarbonate	80·0
Perfume	*q.s.*

	per cent.
Sodium sesquicarbonate	100·0
Perfume (pine)	*q.s.*
Colour (Green)	*q.s.*

	per cent.
Sodium perborate	2·0
Sodium bicarbonate	45·0
Sodium carbonate	43·0
Borax	10·0
Perfume	*q.s.*

Fantus (" Technique of Medication ", 3rd edn., Chicago, *Amer. med. Ass.*, 1938, pp. 97, 94) has suggested the following composition to be used in the proportions of one or two teaspoonfuls to each quart of water :

	Parts
Menthol	5·0
Alum	10·0
Boric acid	20·0
Magnesium sulphate	30·0

Artificial sea-salt powders are sometimes used in foot baths, and relief sometimes attained by their use. Usually the main sea-water constituents of cheap commercial quality are purchased separately and mixed in an approximation of sea water, the powder being put up in packets. If the expense justifies it, they may be tinted green with an alcoholic solution of (1 per cent.) naphthol green and perfumed with cologne, or pine oil. The following are examples of such preparations:

	Parts
Potassium iodide	1
Potassium bromide	2
Magnesium chloride	250
Calcium chloride	125
Magnesium sulphate	250
Sodium sulphate	500
Sodium chloride	1500
Dye	*q.s.*
Perfume	*q.s.*

One part of this powder is sufficient for 20 parts water for a full strength product, i.e. about 1 lb for 2 gallons water.

	Parts
Potassium bromide	1
Potassium iodide	1
Potassium sulphate	25
Dry calcium chloride	100
Dry magnesium sulphate	1000
Crude dried salt	4000
Dye	*q.s.*
Perfume	*q.s.*

Very often the use of foot arch supports, in conjunction with perspiring feet, leads to the hardening of certain parts of the foot. By a thickening of the corneous layer, a type of pad is produced, especially near the heel of the foot. Soaking in an alkaline foot bath will soften the keratinous layer and it can then be removed by a little pumice stone, but this yields only a temporary relief. The new skin similarly thickens and the process is repeated. At the least, this is an unhealthy process, and may tend to produce proliferation of cells, and eventually, given suitable conditions, hardening and thickening of the corneous layer.

This may be obviated to a certain extent by frequent massage of the sole of the foot with a little bland vegetable or mixture of animal and vegetable oil, or by use of a lubricating cream.

Foot Creams

The following cream may be considered not only to assist in softening the skin due to the presence of fatty matter with sorbitol and glycerin (*see* Chapter 1, Hydration of the Skin) but to reduce bacterial decomposition of perspiration; thus reducing foot odour.

	per cent.
Glyceryl monostearate (self-emulsifying)	15·0
Lanolin	1·0
Sorbitol syrup	2·5
Glycerin	2·5
G-11 (Sodium salt)	0·25–0·50
Water to	100·0

Alternatively a preparation containing chlorophyllins may be formulated with a view to reducing foot odour. (For a discussion on the deodorising action of water-soluble chlorophyllins, *see* Chapter 16, The Tooth and Pathological Conditions.)

	per cent.
Lanette "Wax" SX	15·0
Petroleum jelly	3·0
Lanolin	1·0
Glycerin	3·0
Sodium copper chlorophyllin (80 per cent. or better)	0·1
Water	77·9
Preservative	*q.s.*

Procedure

The cream may be prepared in the normal manner by dissolving the lanolin, petroleum jelly and "Lanette Wax" SX at 75° C.; and the glycerin, preservative, water, and chlorophyllin at 75° C. and adding the aqueous solution to the fats. If a stock solution (5 per cent. or so) of chlorophyllin is made and stored, distilled or softened water should be employed to avoid any danger of precipitating calcium or magnesium salts.

Many of the formulations given under foundation creams may be adapted for foot creams. In general the amount of fatty materials is restricted. Some spermaceti or high-melting wax, or fatty acid such as stearic acid may be included to give a waxy film rather than a greasy layer on the foot. Camphor and methyl salicylate are commonly included to give a cooling sensation; a trace of menthol may be used for a similar purpose. The following formulation is in general along these lines:

	per cent.
"Tegin" (Goldschmidt)	12·0
Mineral oil	2·0
Glycerin	5·0
Spermaceti	5·0
Camphor	1·0
Methyl salicylate	1·0
Water	73·9
Preservative ("Tegosept" P)	0·1

(From *Emulsifiers*, Goldschmidt Chemical Corporation.)

FOOT POWDERS

Lehmann, in discussing dermatology in the U.S. Army, states that foot powders are recommended; they keep the feet dry and if they contain a fungicidal or fungistatic agent a better opportunity is presented for a more continuous application as perspiration dissolves the medicament. In the shoes they help to prevent reinfection. Lehmann (*J. Amer. med. Ass.*, through "Soap, Perfumery and Cosmetics", Aug. 1943, p. 435) quotes the following formulation as a serviceable one:

	per cent.
Thymol	1·0
Boric acid	10·0
Zinc oxide	20·0
Talc	69·0

It is pointed out that the use of foot powders containing as much as 3 per cent. salicylic acid is contra-indicated for soldiers because the salicylic acid adds to the macerating effect of the perspiration and causes a denudation of epithelium; thus it may defeat its purpose.

Another U.S. Army powder consists of (*Drug Cosmet. Ind.*, Sept. 1943):

	per cent.
Salicylic acid	2·0
Boric acid	6·0
Zinc stearate	3·0
Exsiccated alum	1·0
Starch	10·0
Powdered talc	78·0

Talc gives a product with adequate slip, starch is absorbent, and boric acid is often added as a mild antiseptic. Alum may be added for its astringent effect. Methylditannin, a compound of tannin with formaldehyde, may be used in dusting powders for the feet, or in ointments.

	per cent.
Methylditannin	5·0
Starch	95·0

For hyperidrosis and sore or tender feet

	per cent.
Boric acid	10·0
Starch	20·0
Oxyquinoline sulphate	1·0
Talc	69·0

	per cent.
Boric acid	10·0
Starch	45·0
Talc	45·0

The above may be mentholated by the addition of a small proportion of menthol, which may be dissolved in alcohol and the powders mixed and sprayed with this solution. Other antiseptic or deodorant substances may be incorporated in the above, e.g. hexamine, chloramine. In cases of excessive perspiration, astringent deodorants may be used as a foot preparation and this chapter should be read in conjunction with Chapter 30.

Corn Cures or Paints

Corn cures or paints contain salicylic acid in collodion either with or without extract of Indian hemp. Other preparations include lactic acid, trichloracetic acid, glacial acetic acid :

	per cent.
Salicylic acid	20·0
Flexible collodion	80·0

	per cent.
Salicylic acid	10·0
Indian hemp extract	10·0
Collodion	80·0

Five per cent. lactic acid, or 2½ per cent. acetic acid, may be included in the above if desired, and 5 per cent. castor oil may be added for its plasticising effect.

Skin-Softening Liquid for Hard Skin, Callous Softener, Etc.

	per cent.
Tribasic sodium phosphate	8·0
Triethanolamine	12·0
Water	80·0
Perfume (alkali stable)	*q.s.*

	per cent.
Potassium hydroxide	0·5
Glycerin	15·0
Water	84·5

This should be used with care and must not be left in contact with the skin as it is caustic.

Ten volume strength hydrogen peroxide applied on cotton wool for several minutes has mild but valuable skin-softening properties, and may be followed with advantage by a warm oil massage.

The cause of chilblains is still not satisfactorily explained. As Gourlay (*Brit. med. J.*, 21 Feb. 1948, p. 336) points out, the " first sign of a chilblain developing is a local redness and irritation which comes on whilst in bed or on sitting in front of a fire " ; subsequently the pain intensifies and "broken" chilblains may occur. Gourlay has drawn attention to the fact that whilst chilblains are a relatively common occurrence in Britain and Europe, they are rare in Canada and in the United States, and he has recorded the successful treatment of some cases with orally administered nicotinic acid (believed due to its vasodilator action).

Winner and Cooper-Willis (*Lancet*, 1946, **2**, 663) tested out an ointment having the following composition :

	Parts
Phenol	1·0
Camphor	6·0
Balsam of Peru	2·0
Soft paraffin	25·0
Hard paraffin	7·5
Anhydrous lanolin to	100·0

The instructions given were either (1) to immerse the affected part in hot water at bedtime, to dry it carefully and apply the ointment ; or (2) to rub in the ointment night and morning. Medical officers reported that the ointment eased the pain and caused rapid healing ; some describing it as the best remedy they had met. Winner and Cooper-Willis considered this ointment as an efficient palliative which probably acted by stimulating local circulation.

Although good results in the treatment of chilblains have been claimed by the administration of vitamin K (*Brit. med. J.*, 1 Nov. 1947, p. 689) it would appear that the best prophylactic measures to take, in our present state of knowledge, are, keeping the feet and hands warm with woollen gloves, socks, etc.

Athlete's Foot

Dermatophytosis of the foot, also called tinea pedis, trichophytosis pedis and ringworm of the feet is caused by the widely distributed fungi Trichophyton purpureum and Trichophyton gypseum. This is a very common complaint, particularly in certain parts of the United States, in camps and schools, etc. A considerable amount of literature has appeared on the treatment of this condition and a good review by M. A. Lesser appears in *Drug Cosmet. Ind.*, Oct. 1951, p. 468. Salts of certain fatty acids such as propionic and undecylenic, in conjunction often with the free acid, have been claimed to give good results in treatment and Keeney ("Medical Mycology", *Med. Clin. N. Amer.*, March 1945, p. 323) quoted the following formulations :

Propionate ointment	*Parts by weight*
Sodium propionate	16·4
Propionic acid	3·6

Propionate ointment	*Parts per weight*
Propylene glycol	5·0
n-Propyl alcohol	10·0
"Carbowax" 4000	35·0
Zinc stearate	5·0
Water to	100·0

Undecylenate ointment	*Parts by weight*
Undecylenic acid	10·0
Triethanolamine	6·0
Propylene glycol	14·0
Carbowax 1500	10·0
Carbowax 4000	40·0
Water to	100·0

Little difference in the clinical efficacy of these two ointments was found.

CHAPTER 34

INSECT-REPELLENT AND INSECT BITE PREPARATIONS

INSECT bite preparations are of two kinds, viz. those intended to prevent the insect biting, and those intended to alleviate the irritation produced by the bite itself. In connection with the latter it may be of interest to note that skin reactions to insect bites may be due to

(a) *Toxins* in which the effect is mainly due to the primarily toxic action of the insect secretion.

(b) *Allergy*, in which the sufferer is allergenically sensitive to the secretion, which in itself is not primarily toxic.

In general, the common reactions to insect bites are due not to a primarily toxic secretion, as is the general belief, but to a specific allergic sensitisation of the skin. This accounts for the extraordinary effect upon certain individuals of what must, after all, be an infinitely small dose of irritant. This sensitisation has usually been produced by a previous exposure to a minute dose of the same substance, possibly a previous bite, which, at the time caused no particularly ill effect, or by the exposure to a related agent. In this latter respect it must be remembered that in a modern civilisation we come into contact with an extraordinarily wide range of substances, dyes in furs, cosmetics, and in printing inks; proteins in foodstuffs; amino compounds and other nitrogenous substances in emulsified creams and glues, as well as in multifarious patent medicines and vitamin preparations, harmless in themselves but which may sensitise the human skin to a chemical substance akin to these substances but whose relationship would not be suspected even by a dermatologist. Apart from skin irritation and allergy, some of these biting insects carry disease (the rat flea carries bubonic plague; mosquitoes malaria and yellow fever; certain ticks may cause paralysis and spotted fever; lice may transmit typhus and trench fever).

The most important type of insect bite preparation, therefore, is preventive. The maintenance of armies in the tropics raised this question in acute form, since it was realised that prevention was better than cure.

The method by which insects are attracted to attack and bite human beings and animals is not known. Whether the insects are attracted to the organism by body warmth and "ride in along a beam of infra-red rays", or whether gases exhaled by the organism are chiefly responsible has still to be decided.

Darkness is certainly no deterrent since Anopheles mosquitoes generally bite during darkness.

Apart from these general observations (which apply to persons who have not used perfumed materials and to animals) there is little doubt in the author's mind but that insects—whilst they may also be influenced by the infra-red radiations of men and animals—are definitely influenced by perfumery materials and probably also by body odours due to constituents of the diet. Certain chemical substances are definitely attractants, others repellent. The power of insects to detect certain emanations such as odours has, it is understood, been shown in the case of the moth. In such experiments a female moth, shut in a gauze box was shown to attract male moths from many miles away, whereas if the moth was enclosed in a glass box, the males were no longer attracted.

It is also understood that the consumption of thiamine, leads to certain insects being repelled for a while, due it is believed to the odour of thiamine in the perspiration.

Prior to 1940, the commonly used insect-repellent substances were such odorous substances as citronella oil, clove oil, camphor, which, by modern standards, are relatively ineffective.

The outbreak of World War II and its development in the Eastern Theatre of Warfare led to an exhaustive investigation into the question of insect repellents.

Draize, Alvarez and Whitesell (*J. Pharmacol.*, 1948, **93**, 26) have pointed out that in the United States . . . "*approximately* 4000 *compounds, prepared by various universities and chemical concerns, were submitted during the war programme to the Food and Drug Administration for toxicological testing. Most of the compounds were organic chemicals; however, a few mixtures were also submitted. Ten thousand rabbits were used to determine the primary irritation and skin toxicity of these insect repellent candidates. . . . During the course of these studies many compounds did not survive the initial screening procedures because of excessive irritation, or because of systemic toxicity following initial exposure. Many of the compounds which passed the "screening for irritation" tests were eliminated in acute and* 3-*week subacute skin toxicity testing. In the final group surviving the initial tests there remained* 42 *compounds or mixtures which were studied intensively. . . .*"

Of these 42 potential repellent preparations, 18 were ultimately deemed safe for use by military personnel, whereas the other 24 did not pass the rigorous testing procedure and appraisal. It is pointed out (*J. Pharmacol.*) that the requirements and conditions of use for insect repellents by military personnel differ from those for use by the civilian population, since the military personnel is composed mainly of young adults under close medical supervision, whereas potential civilian users would include the very young, the aged and the infirm. On the other hand, amongst the numerous requirements for military personnel was the use of the preparation under tropical conditions, i.e. heavy perspiration and application to large areas of the body surface ; therefore the latter requirements are more rigorous than might be obtained in use in a temperate climate like the United States.

Among those considered safe for recommended use were :

Dimethyl phthalate.
2-ethyl hexane-diol 1,3 (*Rutgers* 612).
A mixture of the following composition :

Dimethyl phthalate	6 parts
2-ethyl hexane-diol, 1-3	2 parts
" Indalone "	2 parts

Di-isopropyl tartrate.
Cyclohexyl acetoacetate.
Hexahydrophthalic acid diethyl ester.
Piperonyl ether butoxide.

Amongst the better-known substances considered safe for *restricted use* was alpha, alpha, di-methyl alpha carbobutoxy-dihydro-gamma pyrone " Indalone ".

Travis and Jones (U.S. Patent 2,356,801) patented a mixture of 33·3 to 80 per cent. by volume of dimethyl phthalate and complementary equal parts of 2-ethyl-1,3-hexanediol and n-butyl mesityl oxide oxalate, for *free* use by the United States government. This mixture is effective against chiggers, fleas, flies and mosquitoes.

Dimethyl Phthalate

Dimethyl phthalate has been found to be an effective insect repellent and will prevent the bites of mosquitoes for 3-5 hours. (*Brit. med. J.*, 19 May 1945, p. 703.) When 50-100 cc. are applied to the clothing, protection was obtained for about a week. Since mosquitoes readily bite through clothing, this method is a valuable adjunct to skin application (Knipling and Dove, *J. econ. Ent.*, 1944, **37**, 477). It has also been used as a repellent against the vector of sandfly fever (Phlebotomus papatasi) and is effective against dog and cat fleas.

The author has used a 33 per cent. solution of D.M.P. in unperfumed alcohol extensively over some years and has found it effective against biting midges and no skin irritation has been experienced, either when applied to the skin or when used as a hair dressing to repel insects. Care should, however, be taken that this solution does not come into contact with plastics (such as are used in spectacle frames, etc.) as it possesses a solvent action. The application of dimethyl phthalate should be avoided in the region of the eyes or lips as it is likely to produce mild smarting.

2-ETHYLHEXANEDIOL-1, 3, ALSO KNOWN AS "RUTGERS" 612

(Proprietary designation of Carbide and Carbon Chemicals Corporation, U.S.A.; General Metallurgical and Chemical Ltd., London) was claimed by McClure (*Chem. Engng. News*, 1944, **22**, 416) to be among the best mosquito repellents found out of over 700 synthetic organic chemicals tested and can be used to repel biting flies, gnats, chiggers and fleas; approximately 4 to 8 hours' protection being obtained from one application. When incorporated in a cosmetic or toilet preparation, the protection afforded is usually reduced in about the direct relationship with the proportion of "612" present, e.g. if a neat fluid will repel gnats and midges for about 6 hours, a 33 per cent. lotion is effective for about 2 hours.

ALPHA, ALPHA-DIMETHYL-ALPHA'-CARBOBUTOXYDIHYDRO-GAMMA-PYRONE ("INDALONE", U.S. INDUSTRIAL CHEMICALS INC.)

"Indalone" is an effective insect repellent, the length of time during which it is effective depending (like other repellents) upon the kind of insect, climatic conditions, dilution, perspiration and other factors. The best results are said to be obtained from repellent lotions containing not less than 20 per cent. and up to 45 per cent. by weight of "Indalone"; such lotions are claimed to give protection for from 4 to 6 hours, although in some instances protection for as long as 19 hours has been reported. "Indalone" possesses anti-sunburn activity and it is claimed that a $\frac{1}{10}$ mm. film gives complete absorption of ultra-violet rays up to 3500 Å. Whilst "Indalone" can thus be used as a combined light filter in anti-sunburn preparations and also as an insect repellent, it is recommended by the manufacturers that when protection against sunburn also is desired, 0·25 per cent. of BK-5 (Butyl Cinnamoyl Pyruvate) be added since this greatly enhances the light-screening properties of "Indalone". (It should be noted that both "Indalone" and "BK-5" hydrolyse slowly on long standing in solutions or mixtures containing more than 10 per cent. water; when specially formulated to contain less than 10 per cent. water, excellent results are said to be obtained.)

OTHER REPELLENTS

Russian investigations into protective preparations against the bites of malarial mosquitoes have resulted in the discovery that anabasine sulphate solutions are extremely effective for this purpose according to a report of Nabokov (*Annual Review of Soviet Medicine*, 1945, **2**, 449 through *Drug Cosmet. Ind.*, Oct. 1945, **57**, 4). Anabasine sulphate, an alkaloid isolated from the plant Anabasis aphylla (Chenopodiaceae) has been used in Russia since 1931 against insects injurious to agriculture. In the present studies it was found that the application of a 5 per cent. aqueous solution of anabasine sulphate to the skin of a person exposed to mosquitoes affords a safe protection for 10 hours. Clinical and pharmacological investigations, it is stated, have shown that the external use of such a solution is harmless to the skin or health of the person treated. The mechanism of its action differs from that of other repellents in that it is not " repellent " but apparently *acts on the taste organs* [1] of the mosquito thereby discouraging it from biting. In the opinion of Nabakov, the ready solubility of anabasine sulphate, its lack of odour and its inexpensiveness make its large scale application possible and effective.

Ralston and Barrett (*Oil & Soap*, April 1941, p. 89) studying the activity of a number of fatty acid derivatives in repelling flies have shown that decyl, undecyl, undecenyl and dodecyl alcohols and aliphatic nitriles having 10–14 carbon atoms are highly repellent. Lauronitrile is stated to be non-toxic when applied externally or administered orally.

The following formulations illustrate various forms in which some of the more important of these insect repellents may be utilised :

LOTIONS

	per cent.
Dimethyl phthalate	33·0
Alcohol	67·0

Insect preparations applied to the skin in an irregular fashion are claimed to be ineffective in that they lead the insects to concentrate on the unprotected areas. A comparatively recent patent (U.S. Patent 2,496,270 ; through *Amer. Perfum.*, July 1950, p. 36) contains incorporated in the lotion a colouring material which vanishes shortly after application to the skin. Illustrating this principle is the following formulation which acts as repellent and, it is claimed, conditioner :

	Parts by volume
2-ethyl-1,3-hexanediol	10·0
Phenolphthalein (10 per cent. alcohol)	1·0
Glycerin	2·0
Alcohol	2·0

[1] I should have thought this effect too late, since presumably the mosquito must bite to taste it.—Author.

The above is blended with a little sodium carbonate and the excess removed by centrifuging. The resultant product is stated to be a somewhat viscous liquid with an intense red colour. All the colour disappears within a few moments of application to the skin.

Creams

The following formulation for a midge-repellent cream was issued by the Scottish Scientific Advisory Committee (*Mfg. Chemist*, Oct. 1950, p. 437):

	per cent.
Dimethyl phthalate	67·0
Magnesium stearate	10·0
Zinc stearate	23·0

Procedure

The mixture is gelled by means of heat. This preparation has the advantage of allowing the dimethyl phthalate to be applied to the skin in the form of a continuous and concentrated film and the mixed stearate film (in addition to its emollient properties) renders the applied film resistant to water and perspiration. The preparation is claimed to be harmless to the skin, but a warning is given not to let the cream come into contact with tortoiseshell or plastic spectacle frames.

The following two creams (Courtesy, *General Metallurgical and Chemical Ltd.*) illustrate creams containing "Rutgers" 612 (Ethyl hexane diol), zinc stearate and "Carbowaxes":

	per cent.	*per cent.*
2-Ethyl 1,3-hexanediol	30·0	30·0
Zinc stearate	20·0	20·0
Stearic acid	4·8	—
41 per cent. Potassium hydroxide (aqueous)	1·8	—
Water (distilled)	43·4	20·0
"Carbowax" 4000	—	30·0

The active ingredients of insect repellents are not easily emulsified by means of many of the ordinary cosmetic emulsifiers. The following formulation (*Drug and Cosmetic Emulsions*, Atlas Powder Co.) illustrates the use of "non-ionic" emulsifiers:

	per cent.
(*a*) Dimethyl phthalate	30·0
(*b*) "Span" 40 (sorbitan monopalmitate)	2·5
(*c*) "Tween" 60 (Polyoxyethylene sorbitan monostearate)	2·5
(*d*) Mineral oil 65/75	10·0
(*e*) Water	55·0
(*f*) Perfume	*q.s.*

Procedure

(1) Heat (*a*), (*b*), (*c*) and (*d*) to 55° C.

(2) Heat (*e*) to 60° C.

Add (2) to (1) with vigorous agitation at first, then with moderate agitation. Perfume at 55° C. and homogenise.

Note.—It has been my experience that perfumes, *if used at all*, need to be chosen with the greatest of care from materials which in themselves are not insect-attractant.

Gels

Dreyling (U.S. Patent 2,404,698) claims improvement of insect repellents by incorporation in a gel base, in that evaporation is retarded and packaging and handling are facilitated since there is no risk of spilling. The following is given as a typical formula :

	per cent.
Ethyl cellulose	2·7
Cellulose acetobutyrate	2·3
Propylene glycol monostearate	2·0
Dimethyl phthalate	55·8
2-Ethyl-hexane-1,3-diol (" Rutgers " 612)	18·6
" Indalone "	18·6

The product is claimed to be stable for long periods at extreme temperatures without liquefying or crystallising.

Insect-Repellent Sticks

A stick type of repellent as used by the American Army is as follows (*Drug Cosmet. Ind.*, June 1943) :

	per cent.
Hydrogenated castor oil	25·0
2-Ethyl-1,3-hexanediol	30·0
Colour mixture	38·0
Beeswax yellow	4·0
Lanolin anhydrous	3·0
Additional	
Phenyl mercuric benzoate	0·004

(The " colour mixture " was to provide the necessary camouflage of the features.)

Omohundro, Neumeier and Zeitlin (U.S. Patent 2,465,470) suggest methods for making insect-repellent sticks claimed to be transparent, stable at extremes of temperature normally encountered, non-friable, non-bleeding and easily applied to the skin. These sticks have a high proportion of active repellent and are made with a soap base, plasticised with glycerin to prevent brittleness :

	Parts
Dimethyl phthalate	18·2
2-Ethyl-1,3-hexanediol	18·0
Isopropyl alcohol (91 per cent.)	31·5
Sodium stearate (powdered)	20·3
Glycerin	12·1
Distilled water	3·5
Colour solution	1·2
Perfume	1·2

Procedure

The first three ingredients are mixed together, and to the mixture is added the soap, glycerin, water and colouring. The combination is heated at 81° to 82° C., with occasional stirring. When a clear solution is obtained (usually after 7-10 minutes), remove from heat and allow to cool to 60° C. Add the perfume and pour into moulds, cool to room temperature and remove.

In making such sticks, at least 30 per cent. or upwards of repellent should be present ; the gelling agent may consist of beeswax with the addition of other oils, fats and waxes to obtain the consistency desired.

In addition to the insect-repellent preparations mentioned, preparations for the relief of insect bites are marketed. With the exception of preparations intended for the treatment of wasp stings, most of the preparations are formulated with an alkaline reaction, containing, for example, ammonia, sodium bicarbonate, or lime water which usually give some relief. The addition of substances such as camphor, menthol, essential oils, or alcohol alleviates the skin irritation and itching which usually results. As stated in the beginning of this chapter, most of the inflammatory processes produced by insect bites are allergic in nature and hence local applications are not antidota. Attention has previously been drawn to the fact that painful swellings from insect bites may often be reduced by the immediate application of a strong (20-30 per cent.) aqueous solution of magnesium sulphate (R. G. Harry, *Mfg. Chemist*, May 1937, **8**, 160). If severe swelling follows a bite, or if systemic symptoms appear, a physician should be *immediately* consulted. Delay may prove dangerous.

Among innumerable formulae suggested in the literature is the following :

	per cent.
Menthol	1·8
Alcohol	75·0
Ammonia (28 per cent.)	23·2

A drop of the liquid applied to the bite is stated to exert an anodyne effect. The ammonia level is felt to be rather too high ; one-quarter of this amount should be sufficient, the balance being made up with alcohol.

Strauss (*J. Amer. med. Ass.*, 1949, **140**, 603) points out that the exact nature of bee venom is not known but that the active element is probably a basic alkaloid. Formic acid is present only in very small amounts and is not considered to be responsible for any of the phenomena of bee stings. There is some evidence that histamine, or a histamine-like substance, is responsible for many of the commoner symptoms, which may follow a sting. Strauss therefore employed an antihistaminic, " Thephorin ", in 5 per cent. concentration in an ointment base in 8 cases of bee and other stings. In every case the pain and stinging sensation were relieved within 1 or 2 minutes and no secondary effects observed. In the majority of cases there was no swelling.

Although not an insect repellent, " Circa 42 ", an itch remedy developed by Yeager and Wilson (*J. Lab. clin. Med.*, 1944, **29**, 177) in response to an acute wartime need for a means of alleviating skin irritation caused by attacks of insects such as chiggers, mosquitoes, yellow jacket stings and other miscellaneous conditions accompanied by extreme itching, is of interest. The composition of " Circa 42 " is as follows :

N-butyl-*p*-aminobenzoate	100·0 g.
Benzyl alcohol	170·0 cc.
Anhydrous lanolin melted	20·0 cc.
Corn starch	640·0 g.
Sodium lauryl sulphonate	64·0 g.

Procedure

This mixture is prepared by dissolving the N-butyl-*p*-aminobenzoate in the benzyl-alcohol, the melted lanolin is then added, keeping the mixture warm and stirring until as much of the lanolin as possible has gone into solution. The warm mixture is then added slowly, a little at a time, to a thorough mixture of the corn starch and sodium lauryl sulphonate and the mass carefully kneaded. Final preparation should be a doughy, non-greasy, cakelike material that can be packed in ointment jars (preferably non-metallic) or other suitable containers.

The preparation is rubbed on to the skin which has been previously moistened with water, until it forms a moderately thick layer over the affected region. No attempt should be made to rub the preparation into the skin. It will dry gradually to a powder which should be left on the skin undisturbed.

CHAPTER 35

BABY PREPARATIONS

INNOCUOUSNESS and emollient and soothing action must take precedence over mere odour or aesthetic appearance in preparations supplied to relieve the chafed or inflamed skin of babies, although, naturally, a combination of both factors is most likely to effect sales.

Babies frequently drool, and exposure of the wetted skin surface to varying weather conditions may result in painful sores. Remedial preparations may take the form of emollient creams in the early stages or, if the surface is broken and raw, a little 40 per cent. aqueous glycerin, or a light dusting of antiseptic powder or boric acid, until the surface is sufficiently healed to apply the usual emollient.

Babies suffer, in particular, from napkin eruptions and from chapped and roughened skin due to insufficient care in drying after washing. The former may be due to skin maceration brought on by decomposed urine, particularly if rubber pants are worn, to prolonged contact of the babies' skin with the stools, or possibly to the action of perspiration upon any residual soap left in the napkin after washing.

Abt, for example (*Pediatrics, Philadelphia*, 1926, **8**, 125), noted that such eruptions were definitely attributable to an excess of soap remaining in the napkins after laundering and sun-drying. In a series of cases observed at the Milwaukee Infants' Hospital, Crawford (*Penna. Med. J.*, 1922, **26**, 165) also stated that alkalis from the urine and from residual soap in the laundering were believed to be causative agents.

Biochemical agents also may take part in the production of such eruptions. Hart (*Canad. Med. J.*, 1921, **11**, 10) and Cooke (*Amer. J. Dis. Child.*, 1921, **22**, 5) have advanced biochemical explanations, the latter demonstrating a urea-splitting organism from the stools and urine of infants. The activity of this organism was said to be checked by antiseptics and acids.

McIlvenna (*Brit. med. J.*, 4 May 1940, p. 756) states that ammoniacal decomposition of urine will not occur, and consequently no associated dermatitis, if washed and dried napkins are steeped in saturated boric acid solution and hung out to dry without rinsing. I am not in favour of this procedure because of the insidious nature of boric acid as a poison, and the fact that the dry napkin in opening or shaking might distribute powdered boric acid over food in the vicinity.

Flett, Morgan and Hoyt (*Amer. Perfum.*, Sept. 1950, p. 231) state that clinical data obtained by pediatricians show that when diapers and infant garments generally are washed with a synthetic organic detergent such as " Nacconal NR ", either alone or in combination with soap, the dermatitis clears up in almost 100 per cent. of the cases. The irritation they believe is due to lime soaps. (It is of interest to note that the Nacconols have been found to possess antiseptic properties.) These investigators continue " . . . Pediatricians now instruct the mothers of young children to wash the infant garments with a synthetic detergent if moderately soiled. If the garments are heavily soiled, it is recommended that they be washed with a combination of $\frac{1}{4}$ to $\frac{1}{3}$ synthetic detergent and $\frac{2}{3}$ to $\frac{3}{4}$ soap, followed by 3 or more rinses, of which the second rinse can advantageously be made by adding a small amount, about 0·05 per cent., of synthetic detergent to facilitate removal of traces of lime soap. . . ."

Use of Hyamine 10-X to eliminate the cause of diaper rash was announced by Dr. Benson and Dr. Slobody, Professor of Pediatrics at the New York Medical College, Flower and Fifth Avenue Hospitals.

The Hyamine 10-X comes in tablet form under the name " Diaparene " and is dissolved in the final rinse water after washing. According to a medical report published in the October 1947 issue of the *Journal of Pediatrics*, a child may remain in a wet diaper, treated with " Diaparene " for as long as 15 hours without danger of diaper rash. (Information on this substance will be found in *Cosmetic Materials*, R. G. Harry, London, Leonard Hill Ltd., 1948, p. 115.)

Prevention of such rashes is best accomplished, therefore, by careful drying after washing, scrupulous cleanliness, frequent changing of the napkin, use of a mildly antiseptic powder, and in districts where the water contains excessive quantities of calcium and magnesium salts (i.e. where the water tends to be hard), the use of a diaper rinse after washing.

Baby Powder

The sale of baby powder is one of the largest individual items in the baby preparations market. Powders act on dry skin as a cooling application, radiation of skin heat probably taking place through their large surface area. They possess some absorbent properties and by absorbing surface moisture help to minimise maceration of the skin particularly in regions that are enclosed and subject to high humidity.

The raw materials, such as talc and other naturally mined minerals are liable to contamination by spore-forming organisms such as tetanus and such powders should be heat-sterilised by dry heat, at suitably high temperatures, prior to incorporating such materials as boric acid or perfume into the powder. In 1946 (*Sydney Sun*, 3 June 1946) deaths of five infants in New Zealand from tetanus following the use of baby powders (of more than one proprietary brand) were reported. The public were immediately advised not to use talcum powder, especially near broken skin, until Federal health authorities had investigated supplies.

It was reported that (*Mfg. Chemist*, Aug. 1946, p. 366) "... Sales of powder dropped considerably for some days but thorough investigations showed that the powder which caused the trouble was manufactured in Auckland from a consignment of Indian talc which, in its crude and finished state, contained tetanus spores. Several samples of powder were tested and a number of positive reactions were reported. At least one firm in New Zealand is having all its stocks sterilised and there is no doubt that this case will severely affect sales of talcum powder throughout New Zealand for some time to come. . . ."

I have consistently advised manufacturers to sterilise their supplies of talc before use and a number of leading British manufacturers are doing this as standard practice; in general, temperatures of 150°-160°C. for an hour are adequate and err if at all on the side of safety. It must, however, be remembered that this temperature for this time are the conditions which the *centre of the batch of powder must attain* and that to achieve this, a considerably longer time must be allowed (according to the size of batch) or alternatively suitable recording apparatus which reads the temperature *at the centre of* the batch should be employed.

The danger of any naturally mined material as a potential carrier of tetanus and other spore infections must be borne in mind in any preparation which may be used on an open wound or raw surface, baby powder or after-shave powder.

Zinc stearate possesses valuable adherent properties and is considered to give useful protection against voided urine. There have been criticisms of the use of this substance, for example, the "Special Committee of the Board of Trustees of the American Medical Association" (*J. Amer. med. Ass.*, 7 March 1925, p. 750) stated that details of 131 cases of poisoning had been received of which 28 had terminated fatally. They recommended that self-closing caps should be fitted to the tins and that the use of zinc stearate should not be encouraged for infants. On the other hand, the National Safety First Association approached Britich Chemical Manufacturers regarding possible health risks of zinc stearate. A summary of replies received with note on results of research of known literature of the subject appeared in Industrial Safety Bulletin for March 1936. Neither in the above Committee's report nor in available literature was there any real evidence of toxicity. It was pointed out that the main *industrial danger* was risk of dust explosion by a spark during sieving or milling (*Perfum. essent. Oil Rec.*, April 1937, p. 129).

However, there is no reason why *magnesium stearate* should not be used instead of zinc stearate for *baby powder* and in view of the habit that infants possess of sucking everything within reach, it is probably best (if a stearate is incorporated at all) to use the magnesium compound.

Lycopodium, the spores of the common club moss which contains about 50 per cent. of fixed oil consisting chiefly of lycopodium-oleic acid with some glyceryl myristate, resists moisture and is soothing but its expense and relative scarcity does not allow of its use in ordinary baby powders. Relatively pure powdered silica has been recommended for this purpose and it is claimed that 10 per cent. of this material added to an ordinary powder exerts a marked effect in increasing fluffiness. There is no clinical evidence to prove or disprove its value but the author would hesitate to recommend it for such a purpose until more is known of the causes of silicosis.

The following may be taken as straightforward baby powders with no special additives :

	per cent.
Sterilised talc	95·0
Boric acid	5·0
Perfume	*q.s.*

---

	per cent.
Sterilised talc	84·0
Starch	10·0
Boric acid	6·0

By grinding the talc with 2 per cent. of cetyl alcohol, or by the incorporation of 1-2 per cent. mineral oil, lanolin or vaseline, a product which is, theoretically, more emollient is obtained but it is doubtful whether the procedure is worth while, on the grounds of expense, since ordinary baby powders appear to fulfil their function admirably.

Baby Oil

Baby oils and lotions are widely used, particularly in the United States.

Hans Eisner (" A method for the study of the penetrability of liquid and semisolid films used in skin protection ", *J. invest. Derm.*, 1948, **10**, 273) has modified the method devised by Schwartz, Mason and Albritton (*Occupational Medicine*, April 1946, **1**, 376) for the evaluation of protective ointments and using his modified method, studied the penetrability of films formed by some samples of commercially promoted skin preparations for babies. The preparations selected were a baby oil and a baby lotion. As a result of his tests Eisner claimed that films of the baby oil, approximately $\frac{1}{5}$ mm. in thickness prevented for a period ot 2 hours or more, the penetration of aqueous solutions of *p*H values within and beyond the limits of those attained by normal and pathological body secretions. Moreover, urine and a suspension of faeces used as carriers for strong acid and alkali likewise failed to penetrate such oil layers. Films of oil-in-water emulsions of $\frac{1}{5}$ mm. thickness such as formed from commercially available hydrophilic ointments as well as from a baby lotion, established a continuous aqueous phase between their upper and lower boundary and thus permitted immediate and facile penetration of the aqueous electrolyte solutions tested.

The following examples of baby oils should provide a good basis upon to which to build any desired preparation :

	per cent.
White mineral oil	98·8
Lanolin	1·0
G-11 (Givaudan)	0·2

The G-11 may be added from a stock solution of this material in a fatty ester, such as isopropyl myristate, etc. The solution should be chilled and filtered. Perfuming should be the minimum necessary to cover any fatty odour. (A discussion of the various antiseptics such as G-11, G-4, "Actamer", D.C.M.X., etc., will be found in Chapter 42, Antiseptics and Preservatives.)

Oxyquinoline sulphate and benzoate have been employed as antiseptics in baby oils particularly in the United States. So far as the author is aware, although these salts are not absolutely free from complaints of skin irritation, the number of recorded complaints is believed to be very small.

The following formulation along these lines appeared in *Drug Cosmet. Ind.* (" Readers' Questions ", Dec. 1943, p. 697) :

	per cent.
White mineral oil (65-75)	45·0
Refined peanut oil	54·7
Oxyquinoline benzoate	0·2
Maleic anhydride	0·1

It is stated that " . . . the maleic anhydride and the oxyquinoline benzoate are dissolved in the peanut oil and the mineral oil is added. The preparation is then filtered. Whilst there is still some discussion as to the effectiveness of the test for oil-soluble antiseptics, it is stated that those who have worked with oxyquinoline benzoate have testified to its effectiveness. . . ." The following two formulations for "non-antiseptic" baby oils appeared in the same article :

	per cent.
Mineral oil	90·0
Lanolin	3·0
Ethyl stearate	7·0

---

	per cent.
Mineral oil	97·0
Cetyl alcohol	3·0

More recently the "Silicones" (organo-silicon oxide polymers), have been found effective as skin protectants and in the prevention and treatment of "nappy rash" (Talbot, MacGreggor & Crowe, *Jour. Invest. Dermatol.*, 1951, **17**, 125, see also Tajkowski and Reilly, *Proc. Scient. Section, T.G.A.*, Dec. 1953, **20**, 1).

Baby Lotions

These are usually emulsions of oil and water and may be formulated along the lines of complexion and cleansing milks, discussed in the appropriate chapter. Particular care should, however, be taken to use the minimum of perfume (the less the better) ; antiseptics known to be non-injurious to infant skin ; and if vegetable oils are employed, and an antioxidant is included, one considered to be dermatologically safe should be used at its lowest effective concentration.

K. E. Avis (*Amer. J. Pharm.*, 1947, **119**, 271) after a number of experiments with different surface-active agents, selected the following formulation as being the most satisfactory ; in his opinion the non-irritant character and the composition of the product would suggest it for use as a baby lotion :

	per cent.
Lanolin (anhydrous)	6·4
Liquid petrolatum heavy	8·8
Sesame oil N.F.	1·1
Corn oil	1·1
Emcol MS-16 [1]	2·0
Methyl cellulose (400 cp.) [2 per cent. mucilage] . .	20·0
Propylene glycol	20·0
Water	40·6

[1] A blend of glyceryl monostearate and a quaternary ammonium compound I, personally, would not recommend cationic preparations for infant skin without prolonged clinical trials.

The lotion was passed through a homogeniser after manufacture and was stated to produce a smooth emulsion of pH 3·6 which was stable after one year. In skin tests no indications of irritation were, it is claimed, obtained.

The following formulation (*Amer. Perfum.*, Feb. 1951, p. 105) illustrates the use of non-ionic emulsifiers :

		per cent.
(A)	Stearic acid XXX	4·0
	Lanolin (anhydrous)	2·0
	Sorbitan mono-oleate [1]	0·5
	Polyoxyethylene mono-stearate	2·0
	Isopropyl palmitate	2·0
(B)	Sorbitol syrup	2·5
	Propylene glycol NF	2·5
	Water	84·5
	Preservative	*q.s.*
	Perfume	*q.s.*

Procedure

(1) Melt (A) and bring to 90° C.
(2) Bring (B) to 95° C.
(3) Add (A) to (B) with rapid stirring at first, then stirring more slowly until the temperature has dropped to 55° C., add perfume and agitate slowly until cold.

Whilst Eisner, as reported earlier in this chapter, found baby oils more effective protectives than emulsified lotions, Perlstein, in an investigation into the evaluation of certain preparations for care of the skin of newborn infants (*Amer. J. Dis. Child.*, March 1948), took as his criteria the appearance of heat rash on the infant's skin. Perlstein concluded that anything that interferes with the evaporation of sweat such as oils or greasy ointments, generally predisposes to this condition. In the main Perlstein studied the action of three types of lotion in the case of 2,077 newborn infants and claimed that during the course of this study, the case incidence of miliaria was reduced from 55 per cent. in August 1942 to 3 per cent. in August 1945 and that this remarkable reduction appeared to be due to the use of an oil-in-water emulsion of the type described. In one part of the Report it states, however, that "... no cases of impetigo occurred during the two-year period in which the *water-in-oil* and one of the *oil-in-water* emulsions were used. These data corroborate the clinical impression that, in the prevention of impetigo, avoidance of miliaria is at least as important as antisepsis. *Work on the effect of the water-in-oil type of emulsion was dropped because it was said that the oil-in-water types appeared pharmaceutically superior, etc.*

[1] Atlas Powder Co., Wilmington.

It is the author's opinion that the inclusion of lanolin modifies fatty ointments and allows water to pass through the layer, slowly it is true but nevertheless it is considered to *reduce* the imperviousness of mineral greases. (*See* Hydration of the Skin, Chapter 1.) It is considered that baby oils and water-in-oil ointments are of definite value in protecting the skin. It would appear that apart from " pharmaceutical inelegance " the water-in-oil preparation was promising and with the newer emulsifiers becoming available the preparation of a stable w/o cream should be practicable. (Miliaria is discussed in Chapter 1.)

Baby Creams

The formulation already discussed for cold creams, for foundation creams and for " all purpose creams " may be modified to produce perfectly satisfactory baby creams. Special ingredients which may be added include lanolin, castor oil (many mothers have experienced the value of " zinc and castor oil ointment ", as advised by the various baby clinics), white mineral oil, white petroleum jelly, etc. The following provide a basis for experiment :

	per cent.
Lanette wax SX (Ronsheim and Moore)	15·0
Lanolin	2·0
Petroleum jelly	4·0
White mineral oil	4·0
Water	75·0
Preservative	*q.s.*

or using a non-ionic emulsifier :

	per cent.
Polawax (Croda)	14·0
Cetyl alcohol	1·0
Lanolin	1·0
Sorbitol	5·0
White mineral oil	7·0
Water	72·0
Preservative	*q.s.*

For formulations of the water-in-oil type, *see* All Purpose Creams.

Sun Screens

The action of sunlight on the skin and the dangers resulting from excessive exposure to ultra-violet light have been discussed in Chapter 13, which also includes details of formulations. Young children are often exposed to excessive sunlight with consequent ill effect. For very young babies, some *physical* form of screening (keeping the baby's face shaded) is suggested as far as possible, but where the child is active and the sunlight excessive, some form of sunscreen may be desirable, and reference concerning the general formulation of such preparations should be made to the appropriate chapter.

Shampoos

These do not differ from those described for adults in Chapter 22. Particular care should be taken to include in the formulation only those " surfactants " which come low on the list of corneal irritation and which have been found non-toxic. (The question of corneal irritation and toxicity of detergents is discussed in Chapter 22 to which reference may be made.)

Setting Lotions

Various setting lotions to " make baby's hair curl " are supplied under various proprietary names of which the following formulation is typical :

	per cent.
Gum tragacanth	1·0
Glycerin	14·0
Water	85·0
Preservative	*q.s.*
Perfume	*q.s.*

Such preparations are sometimes packaged in a tube with definite instructions about " diluting the product " in such a way as to render the hair curly. (For other possible lines of formulations, *see* Setting Lotions, Chapter 24.)

CHAPTER 36

THE NAILS

HISTORY OF THE NAIL

NAILS consist of protective translucent plates covering the top surfaces of the last bone joint of each finger and toe.

Like the hair, they are composed of horny epidermal cells which, instead of being shed separately in the form of flakes, as in the case of the skin, are first built up into a definite protective structure. Unlike the hair, however, this process of growth is not limited to the same extent, but is kept short only by the natural wearing away of its free edge, or by cutting, filing, or injury.

Anatomically the nail is composed of the nail plate and the nail bed upon which it rests. The nail grows towards its free edge and away from the matrix, or reproductive portion of the nail. This matrix is the most important part of the nail and is composed of polygonal cells similar to the Malpighian layer of the skin. These cells contain keratohylin which is considered to give them their peculiarly cloudy colour.

The most important constituent of the nails appears to be keratin, an amino acid containing a large proportion of sulphur, or some closely allied substance. Owing to the very compact nature of these keratinous cells, histologists have termed the material of which they are composed *onychin*, this being a substance very closely akin to keratin.

The nail bed plays a most important part in the nutrition of the nail itself, the latter becoming distorted or discoloured if separated through injury. Formerly it was believed that the nail in receiving fresh cells from the matrix was forced *over* the nail bed. This, as a matter of fact, is the usual statement appearing in text-books on nail histology. Krautz, however (*Dermat. Z.*, 1932, p. 239), *showed that the nail bed and plate grow outwards together* from the matrix and that should the nail bed be wounded after surgical removal of the nail plate this mark continues to grow *ahead* of the nail and is not covered by it. For this reason any injury to the matrix may affect both nail and bed. The lunula, or whitish half-moon, occurs at the base of the nail separating the nail bed and matrix, its colour being due, so it is believed, to the refraction of incident light at this separation. The fact that the nail rests directly

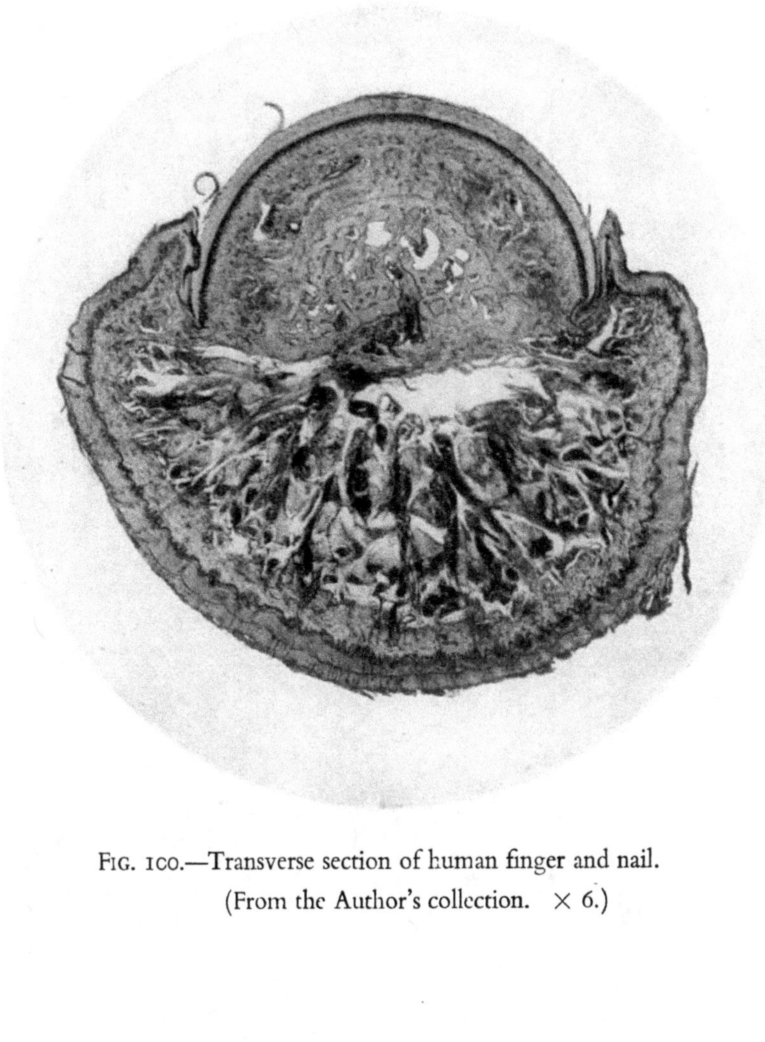

FIG. 100.—Transverse section of human finger and nail.
(From the Author's collection. × 6.)

upon a bed composed of prickly cells, overlying a papillary layer containing numerous sensitive nerves, accounts for the extreme sensitivity of the finger and toe nails to pressure or shock.

Rate of Nail Growth. Many of the older references to nail growth are inaccurate and contradictory. W. E. Le Gros Clark and L. H. Dudley Buxton, of the Department of Human Anatomy at the University of Oxford (*Brit. J. Derm.*, 1938, **50**, 221), measured nail growth in the case of undergraduates and school children by marking the nail with a notch at a distance of about 2 mm. from the margin of the lunula and recording the displacement each month by means of a Beck luminous magnifier. The margin of the lunula provides a fixed base line, for it marks the edge of the germinal matrix of the nail bed, which shows quite an abrupt structural transition into the sterile matrix. Their results showed that there is no variation in the rate of growth with age between 10 and 23 years old, that there is no conclusive evidence of sexual difference in nail growth, and only negligible difference between the rate of growth of the right and left hands. The rate of nail growth on the third digit was consistently greater than that of the others, while that of the little finger was consistently the least rapid in growth. The rate of growth so found averaged about 3 mm. per month, which is in good agreement with the statement by Goodman (*Cosmetic Dermatology*, New York, 1936, p. 412) that the average growth is about $\frac{1}{32}$ inch per week, i.e. an inch in 8 months. Goodman's statement that the nail grows at different rates according to the sex appears to require revision in the light of the above.

The Health of the Nail. R. W. McKenna (*Diseases of the Skin*, London, 1927, p. 430) has pointed out that transverse furrowing of the nails, a single furrow running across each nail, often marks the date of a severe illness, e.g. scarlet fever, typhus, while multiple furrowing, transverse or longitudinal, may be associated with rheumatism, gout, psoriasis, eczema, lichen planus, pemphigus. A pitted or worm-eaten appearance of the nails is very characteristic of psoriasis.

Many disorders of the nails have been attributed in the past to trophic changes, i.e. to influence of the nervous system, but G. Milian (" Maladies des Ongles ", *Nouvelle Pratique Dermatologique*, Paris, 1936, **7**, 275) points out that physiology has never proved such an influence unless exceptional cases such as Syringomyelia or Raynaud's disease are included. In actuality the trophic disturbances of the nail are due to insults to the matrix region. White spots in the nails (*Leukonychia puncta*) frequently occur and are not necessarily indicative of any disease. One opinion is that injury to the nail, with consequent production of an air bubble may be a factor, and cites the fact that the more frequent use of an orange stick by ladies coincides with its higher incidence in this sex. P. L. Singer (*Arch. Derm. Syph., Chicago*, 1931, **24**, 112) is, however, of the opinion that leukonychia is due not to the inclusion of air in the cells but to the presence of keratopyalin granules or enlarged acidophilic cells. These granules so diffuse light as to occlude the visibility of the pink vascular matrix below, causing the cells to appear white instead of pink.

H. Silver and B. Chiego (*J. invest. Derm.*, 1940, **3**, 133) gives the moisture content of the nail as varying between 7 and 12 per cent. with a fat content in finger nails of only 0·15–0·76 per cent., an exception being the nails of infants which, according to H. Langecher (*Hoppe-Seylers J.*, 1921, **115**, 38), contain 1·38 per cent. Wilkerson's (*J. Biol. Chem.*, 1934, **107**, 377) analysis of stratum corneum keratin showed a cystine content of 2·31 per cent. with 0·59 per cent. histidine ; 3·08 per cent. lysine and 10·01 per cent. arginine, the molecular ratios of the last three being in agreement with those obtained for the keratins of hair and finger nails.

Nail Brittleness, Nail Lacquers, and Dermatitis. Dermatitis from nail lacquers is comparatively rare but the number of reported cases appears to be increasing due, it is believed, to the plasticisers used (*see* Allergy and Dermatitis). H. Silver and B. Chiego (*J. invest. Derm.*, 1939, **2**, 6, 361) carried out over 5,000 patch tests on human subjects with nail lacquers and their ingredients, but failed to show sensitivity to the finished nail enamel. Their experiments further suggested that even in the case of certain dyes which give some reaction the enmeshing of such dye in the lacquer base renders it relatively innocuous. More recently cases of sensitivity to nail lacquer have been recorded and the sulphonamide-formaldehyde resins have come under suspicion. Silver and Chiego (*J. invest. Derm.*, 1939, **2**, 361) have also ascribed antiseptic qualities to liquid nail polishes when tested by the Reddish Cap method. Brittleness of the nail is relatively frequent. L. Hollander (*J. Amer. med. Ass.*, 1933, **101**, 259) stated that nail lacquers and manicuring aids produce scaling of the nail plates, while G. L. Woolcott (*Arch. Derm. Syph., Chicago*, 1940, **41**, 64) investigated the reactions of twenty-five business women using the same brand of nail lacquer, and found that nearly 50 per cent. showed brittleness and splitting of the nail but that the remaining 50 per cent. used the lacquer without any sign of irritation.

In view of the relatively low fat content of the human nail, Bernard and Chiego have drawn attention to the possible dehydrative action of solvents on the nail rather than their defatting effect. More recently (*J. invest. Derm.*, 1942, **5**, 95) these authors consider alkali degradation of keratin in the use of washing and cleansing preparations to be a primary factor in brittleness of the nails. Their experiments with N/10 caustic, however, represent conditions far removed, in respect of *p*H and titratable alkalinity, from those accompanying the use of ordinary soaps and cleansers in domestic practice. I consider it most probable that loss of moisture from the nail is an important factor in brittleness. (*See* Chapter 1, The Hydration of the Skin.)

The Effect of Vitamins on Nail Growth. This question has not yet been satisfactorily settled. That vitamins, particularly vitamin A, can effect the keratinisation of cells appears certain. How far this is true of the health of the human nail has not been accurately determined, although Schwemmer (*Münch. med. Wschr.*, 1939, **86,** 1226) reported that vitamin A increased nail growth. White (*J. Amer. med. Ass.*, 1934, p. 2178) observed that certain cases of ridged and furrowed nails were cleared up by administration of vitamin B and D after all other means had failed. The nails appear to improve during the summer months, but whether this can be ascribed to any direct vitamin D effect or merely to the general improvement in bodily health and diet remains to be proved.

Pardo-Costello (*Diseases of the Nail*, 1936, p. 159) has shown that occupation plays an important role in the causation of many nail infections. These appear to develop most readily in those who constantly immerse their hands in alkaline solutions, housewives, kitchen-maids, bar-tenders, etc. It is claimed that certain fatty substances, in particular cholesterin, appear to assist in maintaining the natural elasticity of the nail. In this latter connection, the water-in-oil emulsifying properties of cholesterol should not be forgotten as it may assist in maintaining the requisite degree of moisture in the keratin. Although much remains to be discovered it would appear that the use of a nail cream, containing oils in an emulsified form with water (and possibly incorporating a mild antiseptic), would be of value.

CHAPTER 37

MANICURE PREPARATIONS

Cuticle Remover—Nail Bleach—Nail White—Nail Polish and Nail Lacquer—Nail Enamel Removers—Brittle Nails.

Cuticle Remover

As already stated, the skin continually sheds its outer dead cells, which in the case of the nail collect around its grooves, and together with the natural fatty secretion form an irregular appendage, which detracts from the beauty of an otherwise well-kept nail. This is usually removed by the use of an aqueous alkaline solution, applied by means of an orange stick surmounted with a pledget of cotton wool. Potassium hydroxide being cheap and effective enters into the majority of such preparations, e.g.:

	per cent.
Potassium hydroxide	2·0
Glycerin	25·0
Water	73·0
Perfume	*q.s.*

Milky cuticle removers may be prepared by mixing about one part of mineral oil with one part of oleic acid and adding the desired proportion of this mixture to the alkaline solution of cuticle remover.

Trisodium phosphate may also be used for this purpose but appears to be less effective.

	per cent.
Trisodium phosphate	8·0
Glycerin	12·0
Water	80·0
Perfume	*q.s.*

More recently some success has been claimed with the use of some of the quaternary ammonium compounds which soften the nail at *p*Hs not far removed from neutrality but do not destroy it. Information on the efficacy of such preparations is lacking and at present there appears no real rival to potassium hydroxide for this purpose.

All of the above preparations should be packed in glass containers, fitted with rubber, bakelite or suitable alkali-resistant stoppers.

Attempts have been made to utilise potassium hydroxide and other alkali in cream form, on the grounds that such preparations are easier to transport and apply and are less of a potential risk to furniture, carpets, etc. One method of achieving this is to prepare a vanishing cream with potassium hydroxide, finishing this to be on the "alkaline" side of neutrality. Another method is to use one of the many non-ionic emulsifiers now available. The following was suggested as a basic formula for such a preparation ("Questions and Answers", *Amer. Perfum.*, Oct. 1949, p. 282):

	per cent.
Sorbitan monopalmitate	2·0
Polyoxyalkylene sorbitan monopalmitate	2·0
Mineral oil	15·0
Water	81·0
Cuticle remover	*q.s.*

Procedure

Heat the first three items above to 65° C. Add the requisite amount of water at the same temperature. Stir until cold. Dilute the cuticle remover with this emulsion.

(By reducing the water a firmer product may be attained; alternatively the mineral oil, in part at least, might be replaced by some mineral wax.)

NAIL BLEACHES

These are solutions or creams used for the removal of ink or tobacco stains, vegetable stains, etc., from the nails. Such stains may yield either to "oxidation" or "reduction" depending upon the type of stain. Oxidation may be achieved by the use of hydrogen peroxide *per se* diluted to about 1 : 4, or can be used neat; by chlorinous compounds such as the hypochlorites, by sodium perborate and zinc peroxide (the latter two substances decompose in aqueous solution). Sulphites with dilute acid are probably the easiest methods for achieving "reduction" in such preparations. These can be packed in two-solution form, one the stabilised "oxidising" or "reducing" agent, the second containing enough acid or alkali to shift the *p*H sufficiently (when the two solutions are mixed) to render the agent to be employed unstable and hence active.

(A 4 per cent. solution of concentrated hydrochloric acid in water and glycerin has also been recommended (*Amer. Perfum.*, 1938, 5, 32) for such purposes.)

The following formula for a nicotine stain remover has appeared in *Drug Cosmet. Ind.*:

	per cent.
Beeswax	10·0
Paraffin wax	5·0
Mineral oil	46·0
Pumice powder	8·0
Borax	0·5
Water	30·0
Perfume	0·5

Procedure

The heated aqueous solution of borax may be added to the melted oils and fats and the pumice incorporated when the mixture is commencing to thicken. Homogenisation or milling will improve the distribution of the pumice, but will cause wear on the homogeniser.

Nail White

In order to produce an even white edge to the nails, a paste or cream, incorporating an inert pigment is often applied, the pigment being chosen from zinc oxide, titanium dioxide, kaolin, talc or colloidal silica ; titanium and zinc oxides being the best.

For general purposes a fatty base is preferable. Titanium dioxide is incorporated in the following example :

	per cent.
Titanium dioxide	38·0
Petroleum jelly	62·0

This simple preparation is readily produced by milling the titanium dioxide into the melted petroleum jelly. Various mixtures of suitable fats and waxes may replace the petroleum jelly as desired.

Nail white pencils have largely replaced nail white creams, since they are easier to apply, are less messy in use, and simply require moistening with water before application to the under surface of the nail free edge, the pencil being recapped and then returned to the handbag.

A wax may be used as a base if desired :

	per cent.
Beeswax	55·0
Hydrogenated cotton-seed oil	9·0
Cocoa butter	9·0
Castor oil	8·0
Lanolin base	9·0
Titanium dioxide	10·0

Such base is ready for use and is not wetted before application. The usual type, which requires preliminary damping, is prepared by massing casein or gum arabic with the inert pigment, or by suspending it in a soap, e.g. sodium stearate base.

The making of white pencils is a job for firms specialising in the manufacture of ordinary pencils and not for the ordinary cosmetic manufacturer. Consistency of the base will have to be adjusted according to plant operating conditions and hence any formulations given here probably bear little resemblance to those actually operated by the pencil manufacturers.

Nail Polishes and Lacquers

A distinction is drawn between those polishes which by abrasive action bestow a gloss on the nail surface, and a nail varnish. The former, by reason of the friction set up in the buffing process draw the blood to the numerous capillaries of the nail bed and, by increasing the blood supply, may exert some slight stimulating effect upon the growth of the nail. The latter, which depend upon the deposition of a thin film of highly lustrous cellulose lacquer upon the nail plate, have increased enormously in popularity and have largely replaced the abrasive type, although the latter may also be used between two successive coats of varnish to enhance the lustre, in the manner of the French polisher.

Abrasive polishes consist of a suitably finely powdered abrasive which is applied to the nail and then polished with a shaped chamois leather pad. The principal constituents of such powders are stannic oxide, talc, silica, kaolin, precipitated chalk, etc., the first named being an excellent abrasive but rather more expensive than the others listed.

	per cent.
Stannic oxide	90·0
Powdered silica	8·0
Butyl stearate	2·0
Pigment	*q.s.*
Perfume	*q.s.*

Butyl stearate is included to render the product less gritty and may be replaced, if desired, by oleic acid. The method of preparation is by simple trituration in a mortar or revolving mill. By the addition of a suspending agent, methyl cellulose or tragacanth, together with glycerin or one of the glycol ethers, they may be prepared in liquid form, or compressed into a paste or pencil.

Wax polishing pencils embodying a large proportion of abrasive powder replaced the older powder and block type. They were effective and could be carried and used without the danger of spilt contents:

	per cent.
Hardened palm kernel oil	22·0
Synthetic wax (high melting point)	7·0
Stannic oxide	71·0

(A softer stick may be obtained by omitting the synthetic wax and making a simple mixture of abrasive powder with the hardened oil. Alternatively, a base of rosin, beeswax, ceresin and petroleum jelly, or other suitable combination of waxes, may be employed.)

Nail Lacquer (Nail Varnish)

Rosenbaum (*Drug cosmet. Ind.*, July 1948, 1, 36) pointed out that from all available figures the annual unit sales of nail enamel in the United States are *between* 100 *and* 115 *million bottles.*

The phenomenal rise of this industry consequent upon the evolution of the modern nitrocellulose lacquer is one of the most striking features in the study of cosmetic preparations. A preparation which before World War I would have been regarded as absolutely " brazen " has become a most essential part of modern beauty. This has been accomplished through the desire of obtaining an attractive lustre rapidly and with the minimum of trouble, combined with the impossibility of colouring the nail attractively by the use of ordinary polishing pastes.

Requirements of a Modern Lacquer

Morelle (*International Perfumer*, 1951, No. 4, p. 26) has suggested the following requirements for a nail lacquer :

(i) must be innocuous to the nail and cuticle ;

(ii) the dyestuff must be well distributed and should be as finely ground as possible in order to avoid premature settlement of the dye in use and also so as not to reduce the gloss ;

(iii) it should confer intense lustre on the nail which should not fade either on exposure to light or when the hand is immersed in alkaline detergent solutions, either hot or cold ;

(iv) apart from colour in such detergents, the adherence of the lacquer under all normal conditions of use must be good ;

(v) its hardness must be such that it does not wear unduly in working ;

(vi) its plasticity must be sufficient so that the film will retain its adherence without breaking ;

(vii) the lacquer must remain homogeneous and not separate into layers when bottled, nor must it expand excessively under the influence of atmospheric temperatures which might make the bottles burst ;

(viii) the colour must not alter on keeping due either to reaction with the other constituents of the preparation or to sedimentation ;

(ix) the varnish must not colour the nail by de-laking of the lake under the influence of solvents ;

(x) lacquer must dry evenly, 4 minutes at the most ;

(xi) varnish must not produce coloured marks on paper on which the nail is rubbed.

Morelle includes one extra qualification, " must not attack the nails or they may split". This would, however, appear to be covered by (i) above.

To the above criteria I would add just two more, namely :

(xii) it must not be too thin, otherwise accumulation will occur at the free edge of the nail, but must be thin enough to allow of ready and even application ;

(xiii) solvents should be chosen and adjusted so that blushing, i.e. deposition of a film of moisture resulting in cloudiness does not occur even under conditions of high humidity.

Consideration of the Raw Materials

In order to obtain good results a satisfactory grade of nitrocellulose, free from unconverted cellulose, must be obtained.

In many of the vast number of solvents which may be used for the base, the nitrocellulose appears to be in colloidal suspension rather than true solution.

Having selected the main solvents which it is desired to use, it is necessary to blend them carefully. This is a most important point. If the resultant mixture dries too quickly, the film may be streaky ; moreover, the latent heat of evaporation may, in its evaporation, lower the temperature of the film to an extent which will result in the deposition of moisture (blushing) from the atmosphere. To overcome these defects, a small proportion of solvents having a slower evaporating period is included.

Evaporating Period of the Solvent

The normal procedure in textbooks appears to be the listing of a number of solvents with their boiling points, from which the experimenter is expected, presumably, to select a judicious mixture of medium-, high-, and low-boiling solvents.

Unfortunately, what he is concerned with is not the boiling point, but the rate of evaporation which depends upon quite a number of complex factors such as vapour pressure, molecular weight, heat of evaporation, degree of association, to mention but a few.

In the case of cellulose lacquers, in which a mixed solvent is employed, the effect of the vapour pressure of the mixed solvents on each other, and that of any molecular attraction has to be considered. Even this by no means exhausts the variable complex factors involved. It suffices, however, to show the difficulties of any purely theoretical selection.

The cosmetician is concerned with the vapour pressure at that temperature at which the nail varnish is applied, whereas the boiling point only gives the temperature at which the vapour pressure of the substance is the same as that of the atmosphere—a very different thing.

In order to provide some simple approximate factors for evaporation rates of single solvents for the experimenter, 5 ml. each of the following were allowed to evaporate from dishes of standard diameter at a temperature of 60° F. and a humidity of 55 per cent. moisture by hygrometer. The times were recorded and compared with that of 0·720 methylated ether under the same conditions, and the resultant factor, i.e. the evaporation period compared with methyl ether, as follows :

Solvent	*Approx. evaporation period*	*Boiling range* ° C.
Ether, methyl (0·72)	1·0	34–35
Ether, petroleum (40°–60° C.)	1·3	40–60
Methyl acetate	2·0	56–59
Acetone	2·1	55–56
Ether, petroleum (60°–80° C.)	2·5	60–80
Cyclohexane	4·2	81
Ethyl acetate	4·8	74–79
Methyl ethyl ketone	5·0	79
Carbon tetrachloride	6·0	77
Ethyl alcohol	9·0	78
n-Butyl acetate	12·8	124–128
Amyl acetate	13·0	137–142
Xylol	13·4	138
Isopropyl alcohol	22·0	80
n-Butyl alcohol	34·0	115–118
Diethylene-glycol-mono-methyl ether	35·0	134
Diethylene-glycol-mono-ethyl ether	45·0	135
Ethyl lactate	90·0	150–160

The above list is by no means complete and a large number of ester and ketonic solvents, benzine hydrocarbons, alcohols and aromatic ring compounds are used for the same purpose. They do, however, include the majority of the commoner solvents in such mixtures. The above figures, on account of the factors already quoted, are approximate. Those interested in more exact figures should consult *Ind. Engng. Chem.*, 1932, **24**, 135, in which Hofman has critically examined the various methods of the determination of evaporating rates and by the use of the Poleich and Fritz apparatus has obtained consistent results.

Plasticizers

In order that the resultant film should adhere well, be flexible and not flake off, a plasticiser must be added.

Castor oil (about 5 per cent.) was one of the first substances utilised for this purpose, but more recent compounds include dibutyl phthalate, amyl stearate, triamyl citrate, butyl stearate, tributyl citrate, resorcinol diacetate, triphenyl phosphate, esters of organic compounds, chloro compounds, urea derivatives, etc.

A good plasticiser must :

(i) not cause the " finished product " to discolour ;

(ii) since it does not evaporate but remains in contact with the nail—be stable and odourless ;

(iii) have low volatility ;

(iv) be miscible in all proportions with the solvent, the nitrocellulose and the resins used ;

(v) be dermatologically innocuous and quite free from sensitising properties ;

(vi) must be compatible with any pigments incorporated ;

(vii) improve the plasticity and adherence of the lacquer.

Plasticisers which *could be used* for this purpose are too numerous to mention in so brief an article as this. Dibutyl phthalate still, in my opinion, remains one of the best, being fast to light and having a boiling range higher than many other materials ; others used are dioctyl phthalate, diethyl phthalate, etc.

RESINS

As H. J. Wing (*Proc. Sci. Sect. T.G.A.*, Dec. 1947, p. 9) has pointed out, plasticised nitrocellulose films do not possess a high lustre. Manufacturers of industrial enamels added resins such as damar, and later the alkyd resins ; unfortunately these were found unsuitable for nail lacquer since it made the lacquer films more susceptible to water. About 1938, resins of the sulphonamide-formaldehyde type were introduced which gave good lustre to nail varnish films and improved their resistance in detergent solutions and such resins have been used in many modern nail varnishes since that time. The number of persons who develop a sensitivity to the aryl sulphonamide-formaldehyde resin in nail varnish is quite large (though a small *percentage* of actual users). Such persons should use a varnish which does not include this resin.

PIGMENTS

In the majority of nail lacquers, insoluble lakes are incorporated together with about 5 per cent. of either lithopone or titanium dioxide in order to confer opacity and creaminess upon the lacquer. The colours used must be very carefully tested out in the finished formulation and in the United States only certified colours or inorganic colours of suitable purity may be used.

FORMULATIONS

The following formulation illustrates the basic principles of nail varnish production. *Because of the risks of grinding and dispersing nitrocellulose, this procedure is carried out by specialists in such work;* in addition, solvent hazards make the manufacture of nail varnish by individual cosmetic manufacturers an unattractive proposition. The majority of manufacturers have their nail varnish compounded for them by one of the outside lacquer firms specialising in such work.

Typical Modern Nail Lacquer Base

	per cent.
Nitrocellulose (about ½ second viscosity)	10·0
Resin	10·0
Plasticiser	5·0
Alcohol	5·0
Ethyl acetate	20·0
Butyl acetate	15·0
Toluene	35·0

(*After H. J. Wing* [*loc. cit.*].)

Comparatively recently, it has been claimed that the use of resins consisting of polymerisation products of acrylic acid and its derivatives, in nitrocellulose compositions, overcomes many of the disadvantages inherent in nail polishes (U.S. Patent 2,195,971 assigned to E. I. du Pont de Nemours and Co.).

Amongst the disadvantages said to be overcome are: shrinkage during drying, peeling at the edge of the nail, discoloration, thickening of the enamel by evaporation of volatile ingredients when stored in poorly stoppered containers and failure to achieve proper gloss and durability. A typical formula cited is the following:

	Parts
Cellulose nitrate	3·2
Denatured alcohol	1·4
Butyl acetate	19·3
Ethyl alcohol	19·3
Toluene	19·3
Propyl methacrylate resin	15·0
Plasticiser	3·2

Both high- and low-boiling solvents are said to be eliminated in the above formula and the enamel produced is said to afford excellent adhesion and to be remarkably resistant to soapy water, alkali, marring and scratching.

Enamel Removers

These consist of simple mixtures of solvents to which may be added a little oil or oily material; castor oil was originally used, today butyl stearate or other suitable ester may be used for the same purpose:

	per cent.
Butyl stearate	5·0
Diethylene-glycol-mono-ethyl ether	10·0
Acetone	85·0

Gamma-Valerolactone ($C_5H_8O_2$), a colourless and almost odourless solvent, has been suggested (Schimmel Briefs, Jan. 1947, No. 142) by the manufacturers as a nail-polish remover. Unlike the majority of organic liquids used for this purpose, GVL (as the compound is known) is completely miscible with water; a 50 per cent. solution in water is suggested for use as a nail-polish remover. It is stated to be non-irritating to the skin.

Cream Nail-Enamel Removers

More recently a number of creamy nail-enamel removers have been introduced, many of them patented. In general these consist of a fairly high-boiling lacquer-solvent introduced into a cream which may contain some lanolin or other emollient material, or alternatively they may be composed of a lacquer-solvent solidified by means of a suitable wax.

Dreyling (U.S. Patent 2,351,195) describes a creamy nail polish remover which contains about 70 per cent. by weight of a substantially anhydrous organic solvent capable of dissolving nitrocellulose, the remainder of the preparation comprising a mixture in the ratios, by weight, of 10 parts of a solid fatty acid such as stearic or palmitic, 2 to 4 parts of ethyl cellulose, 2–10 parts of a cosmetic aid (castor oil, olive oil and lanolin) and 2 to 4·6 parts of concentrated ammonia water; the following example is from the patent:

	Parts
Ethyl acetate	40·0
n-Butyl acetate	40·0
Castor oil	4·0
Perfume	0·1
Ethyl cellulose (60/80 Sec.)	2·8
Stearic acid	11·0
Ammonium hydroxide (Conc.)	3·8

The above ingredients (with the exception of the ammonium hydroxide) are mixed until complete solution is obtained (heating at 50°–60° C. will hasten rate of solution). When the composition forms a clear liquid, the ammonium hydroxide is slowly added and the mixture kept stirred.

An important and critical part of the above invention is stated to lie in the balance existing between the ratios of ethyl cellulose, stearic acid, ammonia, water. Attention is drawn to the fact that whilst ammonium stearate produced *in situ* is the emulsifying agent, it does not appear possible to produce a satisfactory preparation by the inclusion of a previously and separately prepared ammonium stearate.

Carter (U.S. Patent 2,268,642) describes a cream to remove nail polish consisting of an intimate mixture of water-soluble soap, free stearic acid (in greater proportion than the soap, the two together forming at least 15 per cent. of the cream) and a solvent for nitrocellulose. Ochs (Canadian Patent 412,396) describes a type of preparation comprising 4 per cent. lanolin, 11·5 per cent. wax, 2–6 per cent. alkali metal soap, 5 per cent. water and 70–80 per cent. of a solvent for cellulose nitrate (e.g. methyl ethyl ketone).

Carter (U.S. Patent 2,197,630) employed bentonite as an emulsifier in an earlier patent. This patent points out that in mixtures of oil and water bentonite collects at the interfacial boundary and acts as a protective colloid to stabilise the emulsion. A suggested composition, from this patent, is:

	per cent.
Sulphonated olive oil	10·0
10 per cent. Sodium hydroxide	1·0
Benzyl acetate	15·0
Acetone	15·0
Titanium dioxide	0·5
Bentonite	2·0
Water	56·5

The bentonite is mixed with 20 per cent. of the water and allowed to stand for about 12 hours. The pigment, oil, organic solvents, alkali and the remainder of the water are then added to the suspension in this order, with continuous agitation.

Vasic (*Soap Perfum. Cosmet.* 1952, **9**, 935) considers that because of their greater viscosity they are easier to apply than ordinary nail-enamel remover and more economical in use. Whilst they are slower in action than the clear liquid products they are less drying to the nails and, it is claimed, leave them shiny and less brittle. The following two formulations are from those suggested by Vasic:

	Parts
Stearic acid	9·0
Castor oil	2·0
Triethanolamine	3·5
Butyl acetate	70·0
Water	15·5

	Parts
Lanette Wax SX	16·3
Nonex 39	3·4
Castor oil	1·6
Butyl acetate	62·0
Water	16·5

It is remarked that the above two formulations, amongst others, when tested by a Beauty Editor were described as "... being effective, non-smearing and non-drying but much slower in action than the liquid type...."

BRITTLE NAILS

Nails are not porous in the normal sense of the word. They cannot "breathe" through any pores, so cannot be clogged by a "nail varnish", and, considered from this aspect, the latter exert no harmful effects.

Fragility of the nail may be influenced through the health of its nail bed, which in turn is dependent upon the blood supply. This accounts for the fact that such fragility is frequently, although not necessarily, associated with some derangement of the normal metabolic function (gout, rheumatism, and in the case of certain fevers).

The continual use of modern nail varnishes and varnish removers, without the occasional intermediate use of a suitable nail cream, may be conducive to the production of brittle nails, probably through removal of moisture. (*See* Histology of the Nail; *also* Hydration of the Skin, Chapter 4.)

The remedy lies in the application of a suitable humectant which can be included in an emollient cream. This should be applied after soaking the hands in warm soapy water, and thoroughly drying last thing before retiring for the night. Such procedure being carried out at least once, and preferably two to three times (i.e. on alternate nights) per week, depending upon the condition of the nail.

The following nail cream was suggested for use on nails made brittle by polishes and polish removers ("Selected Questions and Answers", *Amer. med. Ass.*, 1939, p. 316):

	Parts
Triethanolamine	10·0
White petrolatum	15·0
White wax	5·0
Anhydrous wool fat	5·0
Water	75·0

"... Application should be nightly and if possible during the day. Fingerstalls should be worn...."

The above formulation is a straightforward one and should be satisfactory. *In view of the important role of moisture in skin, and presumably nail dryness it should be helpful to replace a portion of the water in the above formulation by either sorbitol syrup or glycerin; between 5–10 per cent. is suggested, since lower amounts are likely to be ineffective in holding sufficient moisture whilst higher amounts are likely to prove too sticky.*

Alternatively any of the cold, vanishing, foundation or all-purpose cream formulae given in the various chapters in this book may be modified slightly—if necessary—for use as a cream for brittle nails, by the inclusion of a little lanolin or other emollient and an *adequate amount of humectant.*

CHAPTER 38

HAND CREAMS AND LOTIONS

THE skin secretes a natural lubricant termed sebum which serves to keep its surface soft, pliable and healthy.

On washing in soapy water some of this sebum is removed, partly by absorption, due to the colloidal state of the soap solution, and partly by the lowering of surface tension produced by the soap, which, with the agitation which occurs on washing, emulsifies such fats. That alkali produced by the hydrolysis of the soap is *not an essential feature* is demonstrated by the vigorous degreasing effect of certain soapless products which have an acid reaction.

The removal of this sebum more rapidly than it is normally produced, results in the skin becoming dry and scaly. Fissures appear in the skin surface (formerly unbroken) giving bacteria a chance of ingress, infection may result, the skin commencing ultimately to secrete a moist discharge and if neglected a condition of dermatitis may result. As discussed in Hydration of the Skin, Chapter 4, the moisture content of the skin is important ; sebum is believed to play a double role in providing a layer of emollient fatty substance and also in controlling the evaporation of moisture from the skin (Chapters 4 and 20, Sebum).

Because maintenance of the water content of the skin between—what is believed to be—fairly narrow limits is of importance, the condition of the skin is profoundly influenced by exposure to cold drying winds in winter and also to the drying atmosphere of heated rooms.

Whilst most skins will withstand the moderate use of soap and water for an indefinite period, providing no constitutional weakness is present, they will not stand up indefinitely to " drying " winds or indoor atmospheres, or the almost continuous use of soap and mixed patent cleaners (e.g. toilet soap, scrubbing soap, dry soap, washing and scouring powder, etc.) as used by the modern housewife unless they are protected in some way.

The function of a hand cream is simply to keep the outer corneous layer soft, supple and healthy, thus preventing cracking, which almost invariably leads to painful complications.

That such means are efficacious is proved by examining the hands of surgeons who continuously cleanse their hands with soap and water, spirit soap and antiseptics. In nearly every case it will be found that emollient creams or ointments are used as soon as the first signs of chapping occur.

On the other hand, housewives, housemaids, plumbers, washer-women, bartenders and fishermen suffer considerable inconvenience, and even pain, by not bothering to take suitable precautions. In the majority of cases it appears to be ignorance of the necessity for such precautions, although in others it is often sheer laziness. The public should and could, by judicious advertisement, be educated to take better care of their hands.

It should be clearly realised, however, that the market for such preparations is not confined to persons whose work necessitates the constant immersion of their hands in water, for by their use the incidence of chapped knees in children, and of chapped or roughened hands in workers of sedentary occupation may be diminished and the annoyance and pain associated with such conditions alleviated.

Hand preparations can be divided into four main groups :

(*a*) Gum mucilages and jellies containing no fatty matter.

(*b*) Mixtures of oils and waxes containing no water.

(*c*) Emulsified preparations of the oil-in-water type with or without the addition of gum mucilage.

(*d*) Emulsified preparations of the water-in-oil type.

Each of the above classes may be marketed in the liquid or solid form.

Greasy preparations containing a sufficiency of a humectant such as glycerin or sorbitol are probably the most efficacious except in chronic cases involving bacterial infection, when the application of fatty matter may be inadvisable. They are eminently suitable for use in those conditions in which the skin is becoming reddened and dry and they have a good protective effect. Their very greasiness, however, necessitates washing them off before ordinary duties can be carried out. When these creams are applied overnight, the hands are encased in thin gloves. This method, incidentally, is very effective.

Formulations

The role of lanolin and lanolin-derivatives; glycerin and sorbitol; of vitamins, and of hormones, has been discussed in detail in previous chapters (Skin Foods, Chapter 10; Skin Nutrition, Chapter 4, etc.). It is not proposed to duplicate this information unnecessarily. The problem of dry and chapped skin in the case of the hands is similar to that existent in dry skin on the face, except that it is likely to be presented in an aggravated form. Reference to the appropriate chapters should therefore be made. However, two additional materials, urea and camphor may briefly be mentioned here. *Urea*: Rattner (*Arch. Derm. Syph.*, 1943, **1**, 47) reported that a hand cream containing 3 per cent. urea was favoured in a proportion of 10 : 1 against a similar cream not containing urea. *Camphor* has been a favourite ingredient in preparations designed for chapped skin for many years, e.g. "Camphor Ice"; it may possess useful properties. "Aveeno" (Fougera & Co. Inc.), a concentrated, colloid-fraction of whole oatmeal which has been found a soothing demulcent and skin cleanser (Kierland and Ede, *Arch. Derm. Syph., Chicago*, April 1951; Raicus, *New York Physicn.*, May 1952), might also be of interest in such preparations.

The following formulae typify various types of hand preparations. Various oils, fats, and waxes may be included as replacement for similar fatty materials mentioned in these formulae.

Probably the simplest type of lotion is glycerin and rose water. Originally this was a mixture composed of equal parts of these substances, but today lower concentrations of glycerin are preferred, e.g.:

	per cent.
Glycerin	25·0
Rose water	74·9
Preservative	0·1

The inclusion of a preservative is a useful safeguard.

The following basic formulae are typical of preparations consisting essentially of gum mucilages and containing no fatty matter:

	per cent.
Gum tragacanth	2·0
Glycerin	10·0
Titanium dioxide	0·2
Water	87·6
Perfume	*q.s.*
Preservative	*q.s.*
Colour	*q.s.*

Soak tragacanth in glycerin and water overnight, heat to 70° C., allow to age for 48 hours. Stir in remaining ingredients. Homogenise if desired.

	per cent.
Irish moss	2·4
Glycerin	5·0
Alcohol	10·0
Water	82·6
Perfume	*q.s.*
Preservative	*q.s.*
Colour	*q.s.*

Soak Irish moss and glycerin in the water, overnight. Dissolve by heating to 60° C. the following day and proceed as above.

Colouring of gum mucilage preparations may be achieved either by the use of water-soluble chlorophyll or by the use of a mixture of F.D. and C. Yellow No. 5 and F.D. and C. Green No. 3 in cases where a green coloration or F.D. and C. Yellow No. 5 where a yellow coloration is desired. D. and C. Red 19 may be used for a strawberry tint. (M. G. deNavarre, *The Chemistry and Manufacture of Cosmetics*, New York: D. Van Nostrand, 1941.)

Mixtures of oils and waxes containing no water are represented by preparations with anhydrous lanolin and petroleum jelly. They are supplied in tubes or in hand blocks.

The following formulae are typical for fatty base hand block preparations:

	per cent.
Paraffin wax	26·0
Petroleum jelly	74·0

	per cent.
Lanolin	9·0
Ceresin	18·0
Amber resin	4·5
Paraffin wax	18·5
Petroleum jelly	50·0

To such mixtures may be added various herbal preparations such as chlorophyll, marshmallow leaves,[1] etc., essential oils, turpentine, eucalyptus, oils of cade, birch tar, etc., camphor, zinc oxide, monochlorthymol, etc., to build up a formula such as the following which is similar to a well-known British preparation:

	per cent.
Birch tar oil	0·06
Benzoin	0·05
Marshmallow leaves	0·15
Zinc oxide	0·10
Oil thymi	0·20
Oil citronella	0·10
Methyl salicylate	0·20
Camphor	0·10
Oil eucalyptus	2·00
Amber resin	8·00
Colour	0·05
Paraffin wax	24·00
Petroleum jelly to	100·00

[1] *See* Herbals, pp. 139–147. *Cosmetic Materials*, R. G. Harry, London, Leonard Hill, Ltd., 1948.

An old-fashioned and popular remedy is *Camphor Ice* which consists of 5-15 per cent. camphor incorporated in a mixture of white petroleum jelly and paraffin wax ; the hardness may be varied by altering the ratio of these two ingredients.

Emulsified preparations of the oil-in-water type often consist of a thin vanishing cream, with or without the addition of gum mucilage. Preparations containing a relatively small proportion of fatty matter emulsified in water and glycerin, with or without the addition of gums or cellulosic materials, are also popular. Goodman (*Cosmetic Dermatology*, New York : McGraw-Hill, 1936) gives the following example :

	Parts
Stearic acid	4·0
Potassium hydroxide	0·4
Glycerin	6·0
Water	32·0
Mixed with	
Quince seed	2·0
Water	64·0

A preservative should, of course, be included.

Musick (*J. Amer. pharm. Ass., Pract. Pharm. Edn.*, 1942, p. 264) found that a gum base was preferable to a water base for stearic acid hand lotions. Cetyl alcohol (0·5 per cent.) was found to improve the texture and smoothness of the product and to have a stabilising effect. It was found that products having the best sheen and stability contained 0·5 per cent. cetyl alcohol, 5 per cent. stearic acid and 0·5 per cent. triethanolamine or 0·5 per cent. cetyl alcohol, 4 per cent. stearic acid and 0·2 per cent. potassium hydroxide.

The development of pearliness in a lotion takes time. The use of about 5 per cent. alcohol and/or of stearic acid containing a small amount of oleic acid, the use of aminoglycol in place of potassium hydroxide and storage of the finished lotion in a warm place promote crystallisation (*Drug. Cosmet. Ind.*, July 1942).

	per cent.
Cetyl alcohol	0·5
Lanolin	1·0
Petroleum oil	14·0
Stearic acid	4·0
Isopropanolamines	0·8
Glycerin	5·0
Methyl *p*-hydroxybenzoate	0·2
Titanium dioxide	0·1
Distilled water	74·4

In preparing the above cream, the water containing the glycerin and alkali is heated to 70° C. and added to the mixture of the stearic acid, cetyl alcohol, lanolin, petroleum oil, methyl *p*-hydroxybenzoate, etc., warmed to the same temperature. The mixture is stirred until cooled down to room temperature.

The *Drug and Cosmetic Review*, 1940–41, p. 285, quotes the following example of an emulsified hand cream containing gum mucilage:

	per cent.
Stearic acid	1·5
Potassium hydroxide	0·2
Quince seed	1·0
Karaya gum	0·3
Glycerin	15·0
Cetyl alcohol	0·5
Lanolin	1·0
Perfume	0·5
Preservative	0·1
Water	79·9

In the case of formulae containing gum mucilage, the gum should be soaked separately in a portion of the water and stirred into the cream after the saponification.

The following hand cream is based upon "Manucol", glycerin and "calamine lotion". ("A Selection of Approved Formulae for Cosmetic and Toilet Goods", Alginate Industries Ltd.):

	parts
Manucol SS/LH	5·0
Glycerin B.P.	3·0
Calamine lotion	10·0
Nipagin M (preservative)	0·1
Rose perfume	0·2
Lanolin	0·5
Water	to 100·0

Procedure

All the components except the lanolin and the calamine are stirred into the water and, when they have dissolved, the lanolin is stirred in, followed by the calamine lotion.

[*Note.*—Water-soluble lanolin derivatives are now available (*see* Chapter 10). Alternatively the lanolin may be emulsified as an oil-in-water emulsion using a non-ionic emulsifier and a portion of this emulsion used to replace lanolin. Non-ionic is suggested because the hand lotion contains a zinc-compound.—Author.]

The following formulation utilises non-ionic emulsifiers of the "Span" and "Tween" types. It contains no special medicament but these can be included as desired:

		per cent.
(A)	Stearic Acid	10·0
	"Span" 60 Sorbitan monostearate	5·2
	"Span" 80 Sorbitan mono-oleate	1·0
	"Tween" 60 Polyoxyalkylene sorbitan monostearate	2·8
(B)	Water	81·0
	reservative	*q.s.*
	Perfume	*q.s.*

Procedure

Add (A) at 80° C. to (B) at 85° C., with rapid stirring. Perfume at 50° C. Pour at 45° C.

(*Drug and Cosmetic Emulsions*, Atlas Powder Co.)

As mentioned earlier in this chapter, humectants play a valuable role in keeping the skin soft and supple and may be included with advantage in the above formulation (*see* Chapter 44).

Non-ionic emulsifiers, available in the United Kingdom, include "Polawax" (Croda), a reaction product of ethylene oxide and stearyl alcohol; the "Collones" and "Texofors" in which the hydrophobic groups are combined with ethylene oxide [Glovers (Chemicals) Ltd., the "Spans" and "Tweens" (Atlas Powder Co.)] and the "Nonex" range of non-ionic compounds which comprise a series of fatty esters of polyethylene glycol (General Metallurgical and Chemical Ltd., London), etc. The following formulation illustrates the use of "Polawax" in a hand cream ("Polawax", Croda Ltd.):

	per cent.
"Polawax"	20·0
Beeswax	3·0
Lanolin	2·0
Water	75·0
Preservative	*q.s.*

Colloidal magnesium aluminium silicate gel ("Veegum") has been recommended for hand creams, since it is claimed it prevents sweating and separation, is non-sticky and non-greasy; the following formulation illustrates its use (courtesy, R. T. Vanderbilt, New York):

	per cent. by weight
Stearic acid (triple pressed)	22·00
Methyl *p*-hydroxy benzoate	0·05
Propyl *p*-hydroxy benzoate	0·05
Triethanolamine	1·80
Glycerin	7·50
Propylene glycol	7·50
Water (distilled)	40·60
"Veegum" (R. T. Vanderbilt), gel (5%)	20·00
Perfume to suit	0·50

Procedure

(1) Weigh the stearic acid into a suitable container. Heat to 75°–80° C., add the preservatives and Stir until dissolved.

(2) In a separate vessel measure out the water, "Veegum", and triethanolamine, and heat to 75°–80° C.

(3) Add the "Veegum" mixture to the stearic acid mixture with slow speed stirring and continue stirring until the temperature falls to 50°–55° C. and add the perfume. Stir very slowly till cold and either fill into jars cold or rewarm, stir and fill at about 35° C.

The following hand cream formulation illustrates the use of glyceryl monostearate:

	per cent.
(*a*) Glyceryl monostearate (self-emulsifying)	12·0
(*b*) Lanolin	3·0
(*c*) Mineral oil	3·0
(*d*) Spermaceti	3·0
(*e*) Sorbitol syrup	5·0
(*f*) Water	74·0
(*g*) Preservative	*q.s.*

Procedure

(1) Heat (*a*), (*b*), (*c*) and (*d*) to 70°–75° C.
(2) Heat (*e*), (*f*) and (*g*) to 70°–75° C.

Add (2) to (1). Stir down to 45° C. Perfume. Continue to stir down to 30° C.

Water-in-oil hand creams are less popular than the types mentioned above since they tend to be more greasy in use. However, if such a preparation *is* desired, details of formulations may be obtained by reference to water-in-oil All-Purpose Creams, in Chapter 9.

WATERLESS HAND CLEANSERS

Polyvinyl alcohol. Toxicological examination has shown this substance to be non-injurious to the skin and it has been suggested for use in various cosmetic preparations. If a simple aqueous solution of polyvinyl alcohol is well rubbed on the hands for a few seconds, it starts to peel off carrying all the dirt and grease with it. Before the war, collapsible tubes of this substance were sold in Germany for this purpose and proved very popular with motorists and mechanics (*British Plastics*, 16 March 1944, **178**, 127). [For a more detailed description of preparations for *protecting and cleansing* the hands, *see* Protective Creams and Hand Cleansers, Chapter 39.]

CHAPTER 39

PROTECTIVE CREAMS AND HAND CLEANSERS

THE term "protective cream" for preparations of the above type intended for feminine use is *psychologically* unsound, a preferable title for such preparations is the term "cream glove" or invisible glove. There is evidence to show that during the war it was the appeal to *fashion, hair styling, and skin beauty* which was the most efficacious in training women to utilise protective preparations and protective kit supplied.

The skin is exposed to all types of domestic and industrial hazards; in the home these are generally limited to dry dirt and dust—such as cleaning, sweeping, and fire-lighting—and to the use of aqueous detergents, such as dish-washing, paint-washing, clothes-washing, etc. In industry the potential hazard is very much greater. Schwartz (*Amer. Pract. Digest Treat.*, 1950, **1**, 1241) considers that occupational dermatoses constitute about two-thirds of all occupational disease reported by Compensation Boards. Schwartz has listed the chief predisposing causes of occupational dermatitis as:

(*a*) lack of personal and environmental cleanliness;

(*b*) excessive perspiration due to hot weather, personal idiosyncrasy, heavy work, and others;

(*c*) presence of other skin diseases or abnormalities which lower the natural defence mechanism of the skin, and

(*d*) allergy which accounts for not less than 20 per cent. of all dermatoses. (*See* Chapter 2.)

Race, sex, age and diet were considered to play only a minor role as predisposing causes.

In general, five types of industrial hazard are encountered:

(1) Dust and dry dirt.

(2) Aqueous solutions or suspensions.

(3) Organic solvents, including also oils and fats.

(4) Emulsified preparations.

(5) Physical hazards such as heat, cold, ultra-violet light and the action of sunlight, or ultra-violet light on photosensitising substances absorbed by the industrial worker.

No single preparation can give protection against all the above types of hazard, and protective creams are usually formulated with a view to their giving protection against one or other of them. Although such creams differ in composition according to the particular class of hazard against which protection is desired, the following features should be common to all of them:

(*a*) They must not be primarily irritant neither must they induce sensitisation.

(*b*) They should be capable of easy application, should form a continuous film over the skin surface, which must possess sufficient elasticity to stand up to the stresses involved under normal working conditions, and they should be capable of removal without the use of substances injurious to the skin.

(*c*) They should not be sticky or unaesthetic in use, as wartime experience has proved that, in general, workers will not apply an *unattractive* preparation no matter how *efficient* it may be.

Other authorities have advanced what they consider to be desirable attributes. Mumford ("Discussion on Industrial Dermatitis", *Brit. med. J.*, 21 Feb. 1942, p. 269) considers that the protective cream should be absorptive, should neutralise the irritant, should have a greater preferential solubility for the irritant than the skin and should lack penetrative power.

In my opinion, however, it is not desirable for the protective cream to possess the capacity of absorbing the irritant substance, since the irritant would then be *held* in a film close to the epidermal surface; moreover, owing to the thinness of the film of protective cream obtained under ordinary conditions, it is unlikely that the film could give adequate protection for more than a very short period of time as it would, in most cases, become saturated with the irritant substance.

So far as the power to chemically neutralise the irritant is concerned, a case may be made out for the use of an oxidising substance for use against Tetryl,[1] Lead styphnate, Mercury fulminate and Lead azide where—with care—the amount of contaminating dust may be relatively small and the risk of toxicity very high; but where protective creams are to be used in normal industrial operations involving in many cases the handling of a relatively large amount of the chemical irritant, it is not practicable to secure an adequate concentration of the neutralising agent in the film

[1] I am in agreement with the opinion expressed by Peters (Meeting of the Association of Industrial Medical Officers held at Manchester in 1942 to discuss "Industrial Dermatitis" reported in *Brit. med. J.*, 21 Feb. 1942, p. 269) to the effect that *ointments* should not be used in the case of workers who come into contact with Tetryl or T.N.T. In my opinion preparations for this purpose should contain no fatty matter at all.

applied. Moreover, even if a practicable concentration of the neutralising agent could be incorporated, the loading of the cream with this agent would, in many cases, itself lead to irritation of the skin.

(1) Protective Creams for use against Dry Dust

From a cosmetic standpoint such preparations are extremely useful in preventing the hands becoming ingrained with dirt in the case of women who have to carry out such domestic duties as fire lighting, handling coal, etc. Many of these preparations have a high degree of efficacy.

Such preparations contain essentially, a small amount of soap or soapless detergent to facilitate subsequent removal, a little fatty matter to prevent excessive dryness on the skin and to help to form a relatively flexible and resistant film, and in many cases a " filler " is included whose function it is to provide a mechanical barrier across the apertures of the hair follicles and sweat glands, this " filler " consisting, usually, of kaolin, talc, zinc oxide or mixtures of these, viz. :

	per cent.
(*a*) Stearic acid	6·00
(*b*) Cetyl alcohol	3·00
(*c*) Lanolin	3·00
(*d*) Petroleum jelly	2·00
(*e*) Sodium hydroxide	0·65
(*f*) Kaolin	18·00
(*g*) Water	67·35
(*h*) Preservative	*q.s.*

Procedure

(1) Heat (*a*), (*b*), (*c*) and (*d*) to 70°–75° C.
(2) Heat (*e*), (*g*) and (*h*) to 70°–75° C.

Add (2) to (1) with stirring then stir in (*f*), stir down to 45° C., add any perfume desired and continue to stir down to about 30° C. (The product may, with advantage, be homogenised at 33°–35° C.)

Downing, Ohmart and Stoklosa (*Arch. Derm. Syph., Chicago*, 1944, **49**, 436) developed the following protective cream based on similar principles :

	per cent.
Stearic acid	10·0
White wax	2·0
White petrolatum	4·5
Triethanolamine	1·5
Glycerin	8·0
Distilled water	54·0
Talc	20·0
Perfume	*q.s.*

Procedure

Melt wax, stearic acid and petrolatum, heat to 80° C. Mix triethanolamine, glycerin and water and bring to 80° C. Add the aqueous solution to the mixture of oils and fats, stir until congealed and mill in the talc and perfume.

[It is stated that this preparation was given several months trial in industries where workers were exposed to mechanical irritants and several types of grime and that this preparation was effective in reducing the incidence of dermatitis due to these causes.]

Cumming *et al.* (*Brit. J. industr. Med.*, 1947, **4**, 237) suggested the following cream based upon "Lanette wax SX" as a barrier cream for explosives workers (this may also be used against dry dust):

	parts
Paraffin wax	20·0
Petroleum jelly	40·0
Lanette wax SX	10·0
Filler	5–15·0
Water to	100·0

(The filler may consist of kaolin, fuller's earth, etc.).

The following formulation illustrates a modern cream formulated with non-ionic emulsifiers of the "Span" and "Tween" types:

	parts
Stearic acid	15·0
Span 60 (Sorbitan monostearate)	2·0
Tween (60 Polyoxyalkylene sorbitan monostearate)	1·5
Zinc stearate	5·0
Arlex (Sorbitol syrup)	5·0
4 per cent. Methyl cellulose (4000 cp.) mucilage	25·0
Water to make	100·0
Preservative	*q.s.*
Perfume	*q.s.*

Procedure

Melt all the fats including the zinc stearate and bring to 90° C. Dissolve the Arlex and preservative in the water and bring to 95° C. Add the water to the fats under rapid agitation. After the temperature has dropped to 55° C., work in the methyl cellulose mucilage under moderate agitation. Perfume at 40° C. and package while warm.

(*Drug and Cosmetic Emulsions*, Atlas Powder Co.)

(2) Protective Creams against Aqueous Solutions or Suspensions

Apart from water-insoluble plasticised films of nitrocellulose or plastics which require the use of organic solvents to remove them, and certain other substances which, though soluble or dispersible in water, dry to produce a film which is fairly water-resistant ; one of the simplest and most effective barriers against aqueous solutions is a layer of fatty matter, for example, petroleum jelly. By using a grade of low melting point excessive " drag " can be avoided and by including some 18 per cent. of zinc oxide or other inert filler excessive stickiness can be avoided. Such a preparation, suitably coloured with ferric oxide, etc., is in fact representative of certain types of cosmetic make-up bases employed by ladies (*see* Chapter 9). Though somewhat sticky when used on the hands, it is not unduly so and the film obtained appears to be tenacious, flexible and requires the use of soap and water, or soapless cleanser to remove it. A proportion of a " Silicone " may be added to still further increase its water-repellaney.

Where the industrial hazard encountered is really toxic, it may be necessary to apply a film of suitably plasticised nitrocellulose or other plastic, or of a gum resin (in spite of the fact that such preparations involve the use of powerful defatting solvents in order to remove them). Where the use of these preparations is imperative, the drying effect of the solvents can be minimised by the regular application of a suitable emollient hand cream, preferably overnight, the hands being encased in light gloves.

Schwartz (*The Medical Clinics of North America*, 1942) quotes the following formula for a preparation of this type containing gum benzoin :

	per cent.
Gum benzoin	5·0
Beeswax	2·0
Lanolin	5·0
Ethyl alcohol	88·0

(The method of manufacture given is to melt the beeswax with the lanolin, dissolve the gum benzoin in the alcohol and add the mixture of beeswax and lanolin.)

For less stringent purposes some success has been achieved by the incorporation of a relatively large proportion of petroleum jelly, and/or waxes or polymerised polyethylene derivatives into a cream using the minimum amount of emulsifier necessary to achieve stability. The addition of metallic soaps to increase the water resistancy, or in some cases to produce a reversed (i.e. water-in-oil) emulsion may also be helpful.

The introduction of a really effective protective cream against water, which would not be sticky or greasy, which would withstand warm soapy water and prevent water-logging of the hands and yet be easily removed would revolutionise domestic dish and other washing.

Unfortunately no such cream at present exists; moreover, the fact that detergent is present in such solutions, together with comparatively hot water, makes the successful formulation of such a product—with the materials at present available—doubtful. (In making this statement the properties of plastic and other water-resistant films dissolved in a solvent are not taken into account because of the necessity of using solvents for their removal.)

(3) Protective Preparations against Solvents, Oils and Fats

The materials used to form the barrier film for this class of preparation must be insoluble in the organic solvents and/or oils against which the protection is desired. Such preparations may be prepared from triethanolamine or sodium alginate, methyl cellulose and other synthetic cellulose derivatives, gum tragacanth, gum acacia, etc.; caseinates may also be included. These, when incorporated into an aqueous media, dry to produce an impervious film which is not readily removed by water but may be removed by soap or other dilute alkali. Polyvinyl alcohol is resistant to trichloroethylene and carbon tetrachloride but affected by water. Schwartz (*Industrial Medicine*, Feb. 1946, **15**, 175) gives:

	per cent.
Triethanolamine alginate	25·0
[Dry alginate content = 20 per cent.]	
Glycerin	2·0
Water	73·0
Preservative	*q.s.*
Colour	*q.s.*
Perfume	*q.s.*

A similar formulation (*A Selection of Approved Formulae for Cosmetic and Toilet Goods*, Alginate Industries Ltd.) is:

	parts
Triethanolamine alginate TS/RE	12·5
Nipagin M (preservative)	0·1
Kaolin	1·0
Glyceryl monostearate	1·0
Glycerin	3·0
Perfume	0·2
Colour (red)	*q.s.*
Water to	100·0

Procedure

Dry mix alginate TS/RE, kaolin and Nipagin M and dissolve in water plus glycerin. Heat to 70° C. Melt glycerin monostearate and add to alginate mix with stirring. When nearly cool, add colour and perfume.

(4) PROTECTIVE PREPARATIONS FOR USE AGAINST EMULSIFIED PRODUCTS

Such preparations contain an emulsifier (i.e. surface-active agent) and if this substance is present to any extent it raises special difficulties in that it may emulsify the layer of protective cream and cause it to " peel off" in the continuous phase of the emulsified product. If the emulsion is relatively dilute and contains a minimum of emulsifying agent, it may behave similarly to an aqueous *solution*, in which case the protective preparation effective against water *may* be employed with success. In general, where the emulsion is more concentrated or where the emulsifier is present to a greater extent, the problem becomes that of choosing a preparation such that the *dried out film* is resistant to both oil and water and is not emulsified by the emulsifier present. Here again casein in some cases has some useful applications.

Where the toxicity or irritation index of the substance is sufficiently high to warrant it, recourse may *have* to be made to plasticised films of nitrocellulose and other plastics in spite of the fact that their removal entails the use of organic solvents.

PROTECTIVE CREAMS FOR USE AGAINST PHYSICAL HAZARDS

Heat. The need for barrier creams effective against heat is—at the moment—slight. During the war, however, creams were developed to protect against flash burns and a cream of the following composition was developed to protect exposed skin surfaces against such burns and was adopted by the U.S. Army for issue to tank crews and flame throwers. Such a cream may have peace-time application in fire-fighting :

	per cent. by weight
Shellac	13·64
Isopropanol	29·90
Linseed oil	3·48
Stearic acid	0·14
Triethylene glycol di-2-ethyl butyrate	0·79
Diethylene glycol monoethyl ether	1·09
Menthyl salicylate	2·49
Titanium dioxide	36·82
Borax	2·24
Sulphated fatty alcohol	0·29
Mineral black	1·16
Magnesium oxide	0·40
Bentonite	4·87
Petrolatum	2·69

(From " Skin Protective Preparations Issued by the Quartermasters Corps ", R. Paul Schreiber, *Proc. Soc. Sect. T.G.A.*, Dec. 1945, p. 14.)

Protective Creams against Light

The formulation of protective preparations against ultra-violet rays, e.g. sunshine, is discussed in detail in Chapter 13, Sunburn and Sun-tan Preparations.

The Testing of Protective Preparations

Although laboratory sorting tests to determine the relative efficacy of protective creams have been described, none of them in their present form present a real criterion by which the behaviour of the protective cream in use can actually be predicted, though some of them give some useful indications, particularly in the negative aspect, in that they can help to "rule out" preparations which are *obviously* unsuitable, before the selected preparations are submitted to actual practical user trials.

Perhaps the simplest of the tests carried out, is that in which a film of the barrier or protective cream is applied to a series of clean glass microscope slides which, after allowing to dry for a prescribed period, are immersed in various solvents (such as water, alcohol, acetone, and various oils and other substances) against which the resistancy of the product is to be assessed. The slide may be subjected to standardised conditions of agitation, and the integrity of the barrier film after such treatment examined, preferably against a "control" preparation which has been found to be of promise.

In another test the preparation is applied to a porous supporting membrane (which can be filter or other paper, animal skin or other desired substance) and after drying, various solutions—the resistance of the barrier preparation to which it is desired to determine—are applied and the length of time which it takes the film test solution to penetrate the membrane containing the protective film is taken as a measure of the resistancy of the preparation to that preparation tested. Various modifications of this procedure, in which the pH of the test solution is made to change the colour of an indicator solution spotted on the reverse side of the membrane, in which the penetration of the aqueous phase renders a suitable indicator fluorescent under ultra-violet light, or in which the test solution merely contains a soluble dye which, on penetration, stains the far side of the membrane, have been employed but one of the main difficulties has been to obtain on the test membrane a layer of the protective substance of standardised thickness and area.

In order to overcome this difficulty, Schwartz, Mason and Albritton ("A Method for the Evaluation of Protective Ointments", *Occup. Med.*, April 1946, 1, 376) control the thickness of the film by placing it on the test paper by means of a specially shaped sheet of metal of standardised thickness which, after filling with the preparation to be tested, is subjected to a pressure of 5000 lb. by which the thickness of the film of protective cream becomes that of the standard metal shim. This "protective cream sandwich" is then transferred to a special optical viewing box. Resistancy of the film to 0·1 cc. of N/4 sodium hydroxide solution using neutralised phenolphthalein as indicator and to 0·1 cc. of N/4 hydrochloric acid using bromophenol blue as indicator is determined. All the materials and the equipment used in the test are maintained at 25° C. and 55 per cent. relative humidity.

Criticism may be made of the high pressure used by the above investigators to obtain their standardised film of the preparation as, at 5000 lb. pressure, there is a very real danger that the texture and behaviour of certain emulsified protective preparations would be profoundly modified. Moreover, it would be more in keeping with user conditions if the temperature in such tests, instead of being thermostatically controlled at 25° C. were controlled at 32° C. which is approximately that of the exposed skin surface with which we are concerned.

An apparatus for measuring the permeability of films of barrier cream was devised by Marriott and Sadler ("The Evaluation of Barrier Creams", *Brit. med. J.*, 23 Nov. 1946, p. 769) in which by reading the meniscus from time to time in a glass tube of fine bore, graduated in hundredths of a millilitre, the passage of the test solution through the barrier could be measured. In an endeavour to obtain an even film of the protective preparation, Marriott and Sadler stained the filter paper (used as membrane) with rhodamine and allowed it to dry, prior to applying the protective preparation. By this means it was possible to see more clearly where the film was thinnest so that in the second or third application these portions could receive a little more of the cream than the other portions. This led to a substantial improvement although perfection was not achieved. Experiments, it is stated, have since been carried out which suggest that satisfactory films can be spread on filter paper using a microtome, in which the filter paper is dropped into the hole of the microtome, to an adjusted depth, the space filled with cream and wiped off with a straight edge using the top surface of the microtome as a guide.

All the above tests, whilst they may have value as sorting tests, in that they serve to reject those creams which are unsatisfactory, omit to take into account the flexibility of the barrier film, and also its resistance under conditions of use where conditions of high humidity, or of electrolyte content, on one side of the film only, may be encountered. When it comes to finally choosing between a number of different experimental samples, all of which have shown promise in laboratory tests, then the final arbiter must be practical trials. At the same time, every effort should be made to reduce the number of samples sent for trial to a minimum, preferably not more than 2, or at the most 3 preparations, otherwise the trials may confuse rather than help.

It has been the author's experience that by applying the protective preparation to the hands, allowing to dry, flexing the fingers and then immersing the hands in various solutions (against which it is desired to determine the resistancy of the product, such solutions being highly coloured with an innocuous but soluble dye) a good idea of both the flexibility and general behaviour of the preparation in use may be obtained. It is of interest to note that in the experiments carried out by Schwartz, Mason and Albritton, mentioned above, anhydrous lanolin and petroleum jelly fell in the same class as the best commercial protectives, not only against alkali and acid, as might have been expected, but according to these investigators, against oil. It was also noteworthy that a far higher proportion of the preparations, stated by their manufacturers to be protective against oils or solvents, actually fell into this category under laboratory tests than those which claimed to be protective against water. It was concluded that, if anhydrous lanolin can be taken as a fair analogue of the human skin lubricant (sebum), then this natural lubricant is amongst the best general skin protectives. (Against this fact one must take into account, however, the aesthetic appeal and stickiness of the product. *See* condition " C " in the opening of this chapter.—Author.)

Industrial Cleansers

The requirements of a normal industrial cleanser are stated by Schwartz (*The Medical Clinics of North America*, July 1942) to be as follows :

(1) It should be freely soluble in hard, soft, cold, or hot, water.
(2) It should remove fats, oils and other soil without harming the skin.
(3) It should not extract from the skin its natural fats and oils.
(4) It should not contain harsh abrasives or irritant scrubbers.
(5) It should be handy to use, in cake form (or should flow easily through soap dispensers if in granulated or powder form).
(6) It should not deteriorate or become insect infested.

Schwartz considers that a normal industrial cleanser for general use should contain a wetting agent, a minimum of free alkali, and have a pH of 10·0 or less in a 1 per cent. solution, should not contain silica, quartz, feldspar, pumice, rosin fillers or organic solvents. The base for this preparation should be a superfatted neutral toilet soap, and he instances the following examples :

For General Use	*parts*
Neutral toilet soap (preferably sodium or potassium soaps of stearic, palmitic or oleic acids)	30·0
Colloidal clay (bentonite)	30·0
Synthetic detergent	10·0
Lanolin	5·0
Perfume	1·0

Manufacture

Mix the colloidal clay and detergent. Heat the soap and lanolin and mix with the clay and detergent. The product may be pressed into cake form or 27 parts of corn meal may be added to 75 parts of the mixture and the preparation mixed to form a powdered soap.

SOAPLESS CLEANSER

Schwartz considers that workers exposed to organic solvents, cutting and other petroleum oils which defat the skin, and also workers who have chronic eczema, dry fissured skin, or who are soap- or alkali-sensitive should be provided with a soapless cleanser on the following lines :

	per cent.
Detergent (Nacconol, Santomerse, Igepon or Duponol (Gardinol))	20·0
Lanolin	3·0
Colloidal clay	76·0
Perfume	1·0

Manufacture

Mix and press into cakes of suitable size.

Alternatively a liquid cleanser of the following general composition may be tried :

	per cent.
Neutral sulphonated castor oil	97·0
Pure castor oil	1·0
Detergent	2·0

In the course of investigations carried out by Morris and Tabershaw (*J. Amer. med. Ass.*, 1943, **121**, 192) on the removal of black chlorinated naphthalene ("Halowax") from the skin it was found that butyl stearate would remove the wax from the pores, this could then be washed off with soap and water leaving the skin clean. Subsequently the following one-solution cleansing agent was evolved which would appear to have applications as a cleanser:

	per cent.
Butyl stearate	22·5
Sulphonated castor oil (75 per cent.)	22·5
Oleic acid	5·0
White corn meal	50·0

Manufacture

The method of manufacture suggested is that of mixing the three first-named ingredients together, and then adding the corn meal or other filler.

(In view of the unlikelihood of obtaining corn meal in Britain for this purpose, this substance might be replaced by some other absorbent inorganic filler such as a cellulose derivative, care being taken to avoid any "wood flour" which comes from pine trees and other resinous products in case some persons are sensitive to such woods.)

The method of application is to rub the above mixture over the skin surface and then rinse off with water. It is considered important that the castor oil used should contain 75 per cent. of sulphonated oil and 25 per cent. of inert material, as oils with higher percentages of unsulphonated matter were found to be less effective.

CHAPTER 40

COSMETIC FACTS AND FALLACIES

Acid Skin (*see* Chapter 1)

The reaction of normal healthy skin is usually acid. Any preparation advertised to cure "acid skin" is based on ignorance and is not conducive to maintenance of skin health.

Alcohol and Skin Health (*see* Chapter 3)

In normal skin health the moderate consumption of alcoholic beverages is not deleterious to bodily health and natural beauty. Wines and spirits have a definite psychological and social value and are considered a token of hospitality. They repress psychological inhibitions: promote a general feeling of comfort and well-being, the value of which, in the strain and stress of modern life, should not be under-estimated. By stimulation of the gastric juices they improve the appetite and in moderation may thus improve the digestion. Spirits should be taken well diluted to avoid gastric irritation, preferably with four times their volume of water.

In skin diseases alcohol is better avoided as it produces dilation of the blood vessels. The red nose associated with chronic alcoholism can also be produced by the excessive drinking of strong tea or coffee.

Allergy (*see* Chapter 2)

There is no preparation which can truthfully be claimed to be non-allergenic.

Alopecia (Areata)

This form of hair fall is neither contagious nor infectious.

Bathing

There is no preparation which, added to a bath, will in itself cause any real loss of weight.

Birthmarks

No nervous connection exists between a mother and her unborn child and no shock to, or desire of, the mother can produce an impression of the cause of such shock (or desire) on the child. Birthmarks sometimes take the form of a strawberry, cherry, lobster, spider, etc.; these are due merely to the excessive dilation of the superficial blood capillaries and any resemblance to any particular object is incidental. Obviously every pattern can be likened to some object.

BLACKHEADS (*see* Chapter 14)

Blackheads are not caused by face powder or other cosmetics; neither do they consist of ingrained dirt. They are caused by an obstruction in the follicle which prevents the free excretion of the natural skin lubricant, sebum. This obstruction may be due to anatomical inheritance, e.g. not everybody possesses the same size follicles in relation to their rate of excretion of sebum. *The action of the endocrine glands is considered to be the initiating (and major) factor.*

CLEANSING CREAMS AND MILKS

Applied to the skin, already cleansed with soap and water, do remove further dirt as evidenced by wiping off the cream on a clean towel.

CLOGGING OF PORES

Neither face creams nor powders lead to "clogging of the pores". The openings referred to as pores are not even "pores" at all but are the openings of "hair follicles".

COLD SORES

Are produced by a virus infection.

CONSTIPATION AND SKIN HEALTH (*see* Chapter 3)

Role of constipation and skin health has been over-emphasised; even the term constipation is not easily defined. The assumption, however, that the bowels should be moved at least once every day to maintain normal skin health and beauty is an utter fallacy. The skin does not always mirror the health of the individual. One only has to study the milk and roses complexions of some consumptives, or the redness of the person with high blood pressure and compare these with the "blotchy", greasy face of the healthy adolescent boy to realise this.

COSMETICS (*see* "In Favour of Cosmetics")

Are not harmful to the skin. On the contrary, if correctly chosen in relation to the type of skin of the user, and used intelligently, they not only improve the appearance but are dermatologically and psychologically beneficial.

Crow's Feet

No externally applied preparation can eradicate crow's feet or crepey throat, once these are present, though the regular use of a suitable cream may, in some cases, *delay their premature onset* when this onset is not due to ill health or age.

Dandruff

Is a very common non-inflammatory disease of the scalp which does not, in itself, produce any true or permanent loss of hair. It does, however, appear to reduce the natural protection of the scalp so that other organisms are able to gain a footing.

Diet and Skin Health (Chapter 3)

The Hay Diet. The idea that carbohydrate and protein should not be eaten at the same time is a fallacy contradicted by experience and experiment.

Vegetarianism. Vegetable foods provide a valuable and comparatively inexpensive supply of carbohydrate, fat, protein, mineral salts and vitamins. Unfortunately a purely vegetarian diet is deficient in protein, (*a*) because such foods are less digestible, (*b*) owing to their cellulose content and bulk pass through the body at a more rapid rate without yielding all their protein. Moreover (*c*) vegetable protein may lack certain nutritive factors and not be as valuable for body building as animal protein. This lack of protein of high biological value may result in impaired development of growing children and in diminished powers of resistance to certain acute diseases especially in the convalescing stage. It has been noted that persons on a minimum protein diet make but slow recovery from such illness. This appears to be recognised by the so-called vegetarians themselves who eat also foods of animal origin such as eggs, butter, cheese, milk and even fish.

Dry Skin (*see* Chapter 10)

No externally applied preparation can *cure* dry skin but the regular use of a suitable cream can alleviate the symptoms of dry skin and keep the skin soft, hydrated, and oiled. (*See* Skin Foods—more correctly Lubricating Creams.)

ENLARGED PORES (*see* Chapter 1)

Are not " pores " at all but openings of the hair follicles. No preparation cures " enlarged pores ". Antiperspirants and astringents may correct the condition temporarily, or they may be disguised by the application of suitable " make-up ".

EYELASHES

No preparation can promote the growth of eyelashes nor make them longer or silkier.

FACE CREAMS CANNOT GROW HAIR (*see* Chapter 20)

There are no face creams nor any oil or fat which can possibly cause the growth of hair on the face or anywhere else! [An exception to this statement may be possible in cases of creams containing male sex hormones but even so the growth of hair is not due to the cream but to the male hormone itself.]

HAIR FACTS (*see* Chapter 20)

Baldness. The high brow (M type) baldness of males is not due to tight fitting hats, sedentary life, too frequent washing of the hair or working under electric light, but is believed to be a sexual inheritance characteristic of men only.

Cutting and Shaving Hair. Does not affect either its ultimate length, quantity or thickness.

Hair Food (*Hair Tonic*). The hair is nourished by the blood capillaries of the scalp and cannot be " fed " by external means. No hair tonic will eradicate any actual disease of the scalp or cause the growth of new hair. Friction used in conjunction with such lotions or " tonics " is of value in increasing the blood supply to the scalp ; moreover the incorporation of a mild antiseptic can temporarily reduce the incidence of bacterial infection. Alcohol lotions assist in removal of dandruff and the regular use of alcohol lotions can keep the hair free of dandruff scales—temporarily while the lotion is used. They cannot cure the condition nor remove the cause.

Grey Hair. Is not necessarily an indication of the state of health of the individual.

There is no evidence that any of the vitamins have any effect upon grey hair in human beings receiving a normal diet. Experiments on the anti-grey hair vitamins refer only to experiments on rats deprived of certain essentials in their diet. Evidence upon the sudden greying of hair is conflicting. While in the vast majority of cases greying of hair is a process involving months, there are some cases in the medical literature which suggest the possibility of the sudden appearance of gas bubbles in the hair shaft which gives the appearance of grey hair.

Necessity of Hair. Because we are accustomed to the "appearance" of hair, its presence is considered to be attractive, nevertheless from a scientific aspect there is no evidence to suggest the necessity of hair in modern life. In fact it would appear that the loss of hair may be a continued process of evolution, as witness the disappearance of the furry coats of our ancestors, until only occasional tufts remain on the body.

Permanent Waving. Properly carried out on normal healthy hair and scalp by an experienced operator and employing the technique of first making a "test curl" does not damage the hair. If any tendency to dryness becomes noticeable, it is counteracted by applying a hot oil shampoo and/or spraying the hair with a little light brilliantine. Iron waving carried out without proper heat control may be far more damaging to the hair than a permanent wave properly carried out.

Permanently waved hair should be regularly brushed to maintain the health of the scalp and also to distribute the sebum along the hair shaft, giving the hair a "sheen". The practice of sleeping in a hair net after the hair has been set, while unobjectionable when carried out for only a couple of nights, is reprehensible as a general practice.

Singeing of Hair. Is not beneficial. Split hairs should be cut and not singed.

NAILS (*see* Chapter 36)

Feeding of: No externally applied substance can feed the nail; neither can it encourage the growth of thicker or stronger nails.

Nails have no pores and therefore cannot breathe or become "clogged". There is no conclusive evidence that sexual variation occurs in the rate of nail growth and there is only negligible difference between the rate of growth of the nails of the right and left hand. Rate of nail growth is greatest on the third digit and least on the little finger.

PERSPIRATION (*see* Chapter 30)

No externally applied preparation will stop excessive perspiration other than temporarily. No harm is occasioned by checking perspiration in any local spot on the body providing the agent used is not in itself irritant. Deodorants should not be used on inflamed or suppurating skin.

POWDER PIMPLES

Are whiteheads not due to face powder at all.

Shampoos

Egg Shampoos. These have nothing to recommend them from a hygienic point of view. They are often recommended where it is desired to avoid soap or other cleansers having an alkaline reaction but this may be *equally well achieved with a soapless shampoo.* If soapless shampoos are too drying, use a reconditioning cream or apply a hot oil shampoo prior to the soapless shampoo or use a little light brilliantine in the form of a spray.

Superfatted Soaps. The statement that superfatted soap is better because it contains no free alkali is not true, though it may be easier on the skin (*see* Chapter 27).

Skin Foods (Lubricating Creams)

Designation " skin food " is a misnomer as the skin is fed through the blood capillaries, and so far as we know cannot be fed by external means.[1]

Such preparations, however, supply a valuable check to premature ageing of the skin through excessive dryness or climatic conditions, in that they keep the outer horny layer of the skin soft and supple and tend to prevent " chapping " with consequent risk of infection and " wind-burn ", both of which lead to earlier ageing of the skin. In delaying this they do delay the onset of wrinkles due to such causes.

They do not and cannot delay the ageing of skin due to the passage of years nor that due to disease. (*See* Chapter 4.)

Spots

A "spot" is not "better out than in". Many spots are due to staphylococcal infections and the particular health of the person and the appearance of the spot are not necessarily related.

A " spotted " face should not be massaged ; the application of greasy preparations to the spot is temporarily undesirable. Powder may, however, be used providing the spot is not an " open " one but merely a so-called pimple.

Sunbathing

It is difficult to overestimate the beneficial effects of sunlight in moderation but excessive exposure of the body to sunlight is dangerous and there is evidence to suggest that it may lead to increased susceptibility to cancer.

[1] It is not certain, however, that they cannot produce some local beneficial effect.

Sunbathing should be carried out gradually so that the body can form a "tan" and should not be indulged in between the hours of 11.00 a.m. and 2.00 p.m. The benefits of sunshine are due as much to the freely circulating air, to the change of scenery, to psychological effects, as they are to the actual ultra-violet rays. It is only necessary to compare the effect of a warm sunny day at the seaside at say 10.00 a.m. with that on a dull cloudy day at 12.00 a.m. when the quantity of ultra-violet light reaching the body may be the same—but what a different psychological effect! Or again compare sunshine and cold wind with sunshine and warm wind.

Sun-tan

Is not a sign of health but merely an attempt by the body to protect itself against the damaging effects which would be caused through the foolishness of man. (*See* Chapter 13.)

Teeth

A clean tooth is not necessarily a healthy tooth nor need dirty ones be unhealthy. (*See* Chapter 16.)

The claim of certain dentifrices to neutralise acid mouth is a fallacy. Normal saliva is acid when freshly excreted and no application of a dentifrice can effect more than a temporary diminution, if any, in the reaction of the mouth. Diet plays an important part in susceptibility to tooth infection and decay but *there is no convincing evidence to show that diet is the sole or major factor in the prevention of dental caries.*

Weight Reduction

No externally applied preparation can cause a genuine reduction in body weight nor affect the normal metabolism of fat in the body. No preparation added to a bath can effect, in itself, a genuine reduction in weight. On weighing after a hot bath there may be a slight loss in weight due to increased bodily metabolism and loss of water from the tissues but this is independent of any preparation that may be added. (*See* Chapter 3.)

Whiteheads

These can occur with or without the presence of acne. Whiteheads are small accumulations of sebaceous matter, more correctly termed milia or milium and can be removed in a similar manner to a comedone or blackhead. Milia should not be confused with miliaria which is an abnormal condition of the sweat glands (the commonest form being miliaria rubra or "prickly heat" due to exposure to excessive heat).

Wrinkles

Externally applied creams can delay the premature wrinkling of skin due to excessive dryness or to climatic conditions. No externally applied preparation can remove wrinkles nor prevent the ageing or wrinkling of skin due to advancing years or disease. (*See* Chapter 10.)

CHAPTER 41

EMULSIONS AND TRANSPARENT DISPERSIONS

Emulsions—Theories of Emulsification—Hydrophobic and Hydrophilic Balance —Classification of Surface-Active Agents by " HLB "—Emulsion Viscosity —Emulsion Creaming—Types of Emulsifying Agents and their Classification —" Tailored " Emulsifiers: The " Spans " and " Tweens "—Advantages of Non-ionic Emulsifiers—Determination of Emulsion Type—Dermatological considerations of Emulsion Type—Emulsification by means of Acoustic Waves—the " Pohlmann " Whistle—Rapisonic Emulsifier—Transparent Oil-in-Water Dispersions—Types of Micelli—Bimolecular Leaflets.

A VERY large proportion of cosmetical preparations (for example, cold and cleansing creams and lotions, vanishing and foundation creams, hair creams, etc., to name but a few) consist essentially of an emulsion of water and oil.

Certain transparent preparations, for example, bath oils and certain solubilised essential and other oils, may exist in the form of transparent dispersions, or bimolecular leaflets, and, with the increasing number of complex solubilising materials offered to the cosmetician, this type of preparation is likely to extend and replace certain cosmetical preparations at present sold in emulsified form.

Since the dispersion of water and oil to produce miscellaneous heterogeneous (though they may appear to the eye to be homogeneous) preparations enters so largely into the basic work of the cosmetician, a brief discussion of emulsions and dispersions is given in the present chapter subsequent to discussing the formulation of essential or cosmetical preparations under their appropriate chapter headings.

EMULSIONS

An emulsion is a system in which small droplets of one liquid (the dispersed phase) are suspended, in the form of globules, in a second liquid (the continuous phase). The two liquids most commonly employed in the formulation of cosmetic emulsions are oil and water respectively.

When oil and water are shaken together, one of them will disperse in the form of globules in the other to give, *temporarily*, an emulsion in which either the oil is dispersed in the water (i.e. an oil-in-water emulsion, sometimes known as an " obverse " emulsion) or an emulsion in which the water is dispersed in the oil (viz. a water-in-oil emulsion, also known as a "reverse" emulsion). If, however, either of these emulsions is allowed to stand undisturbed the dispersed globules will coalesce and the oil and the water separate as two distinct liquids. This is because in dispersing one of the above liquids in the other, we caused an enormous increase in the surface area of the phase dispersed. This increase in area is opposed by other natural forces acting in such a manner as to make its surface area a minimum. Though, by mechanical agitation, this force may be overcome sufficiently to yield a temporary emulsion, such a preparation will break under the influence of the force already mentioned. This force is known as the "surface tension".[1]

Ease of emulsification is almost entirely a function of the interfacial tension [1] existing between the two liquids; those having a low interfacial tension will emulsify very easily; those with a high interfacial tension with great difficulty, if at all, and then only with the application of considerable mechanical energy.

This interfacial tension may be altered by the introduction into either, or both, of the liquid phases of substances which are adsorbed at the interface. Such substances usually contain a polar group (e.g. NO_2, CN, COOH, COOR, NH_2, $NHCH_3$, CHO, OH, the halogens, or groups containing N . S . O, and double bonds), attached to a hydrocarbon chain, and thus exhibit hydrophobic and hydrophilic characteristics. Substances which have the property of reducing the interfacial tension and of producing mechanically stable interfacial films at the interface are often known as "emulsifiers".

Evidence has accumulated to show that, in an emulsion, a definite orientation occurs in which the polar groups mentioned above are turned towards the water, and the hydrocarbon portion towards the oil molecule, thus forming a film of the emulsifying agent around the dispersed globules. Donnan's work on interfacial tensions was extended by Bancroft (*J. Phys. Chem.*, 1913, **17**, 514) who showed that, since both oil and water wet the film of emulsifier, a difference of surface tension will exist on the two sides of the film, consequently the film bends, the side possessing the higher surface tension assuming a concave state. In order to prevent coalescence, the emulsifier should bend until it completely envelopes the globules of the dispersed phase. Moreover, the film should be tenacious and permanent. The electric charge on the surface of the dispersed droplets is important since in the presence of such a charge, the droplets will repel each other and tend to remain discrete rather than coalesce.

Schulman and Cockbain (*Trans. Faraday Soc.*, 1940, pp. 651, 661) advanced new and important considerations in respect of the stability and inversion of emulsions. For stable oil-in-water emulsions they found that

[1] The measurement of Surface and Interfacial Tension has been discussed in Chapter 22.

it is of great advantage to have present, in addition to a water-soluble emulsifying agent, a substance dissolved in the oil which will interact with the water-soluble emulsifying agent forming, at the interface, a complex film in which both these substances are closely associated. According to these investigators, the stability of mineral oil-in-water emulsions depends upon the following factors :[1]

(1) The interfacial film must be electrically charged.

(2) The interfacial film must be stable and in the condensed state, i.e. as many charged molecules as possible should be crowded into the interface.

(3) The above two conditions are satisfied when the interfacial film consists of a molecular complex of two suitable substances, one of which is an oil-soluble substance, and the other an ionisable water-soluble substance.

(4) The stability of the interfacial complex film is markedly increased by the presence of excess water-soluble molecules above that necessary for a monolayer around the droplets, whereas only a monolayer is necessary for the oil-soluble component.

The function of the charge is the same as in hydrophobic colloids, i.e. to produce repulsion between approaching droplets so that they do not collide and coalesce. In general, the same substances which form well-defined surface complexes at an air-water surface also stabilise emulsions the best, e.g. sodium cetyl sulphate in the water with cholesterol, or elaidyl alcohol in the oil, give stable complex films at an air-water surface and also produce stable emulsions whilst cholesteryl esters and the stereoisomeric oleyl alcohol produce neither. The proportion of water-soluble and oil-soluble substances should be that required to give a complete condensed interfacial film containing equal numbers of molecules of each substance, distributed over droplets not larger than 3 μ in diameter, preferably smaller. Excess of the ionised water-soluble material does not, however, impair the stability, on the contrary the stability is improved.

In the diagram on p. 652 is illustrated a representation of the conditions existing at the interface of a stabilised mineral oil droplet in water, with three different complexes which show marked differences in stabilising power. The three diagrams represent the three possible types of stereochemical packing at the interface. More molecules are crowded at the interface in diagram (1) than in (3) than (2). The emulsion stability actually decreases in this order.

Schulman and Cockbain, in discussing water-in-oil emulsions and the mechanism of phase inversion (a condition which cosmeticians sometimes

[1] Subsequently extended to cover non-ionic emulsifiers discussed later in this chapter.

encounter in the manufacture of cold creams made with beeswax-borax as the emulsifier), stress the necessity for an oil-in-water emulsion of the interfacial film being in the liquid condensed state and electrically charged and point out that if, however, the continuous phase of the emulsion were oil, the fact that the interfacial film consisted of charged molecules could not prevent the dispersed water droplets from coalescing because oil,

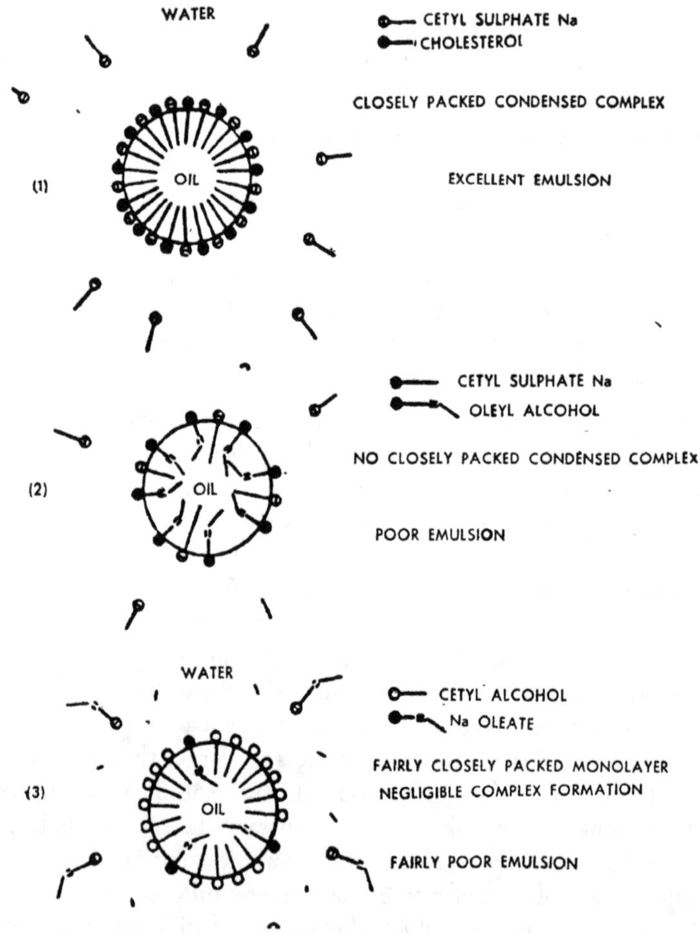

being a non-ionising medium, no electrical diffuse layer or ionic atmosphere could be built up around the dispersed droplets. If furthermore the charged interfacial film were an interlinked solid, no coalescence would be likely to occur for mechanical reasons. In the illustration opposite, Fig. (*a*) shows, diagrammatically, oil droplets dispersed in water and stabilised by a liquid condensed mixed film such as cholesterol + sodium cetyl sulphate. The adsorbed diffuse double layer of sodium cetyl sulphate is also represented and the oil droplets are given a negative charge because of the negatively charged cetyl sulphate ions.

In Fig. (*b*) is shown the state of affairs after the polyvalent kations (Ca^{++} or Ba^{++} for example) have been added to the oil-in-water emulsion. Adsorption of the kations has destroyed the negative charge

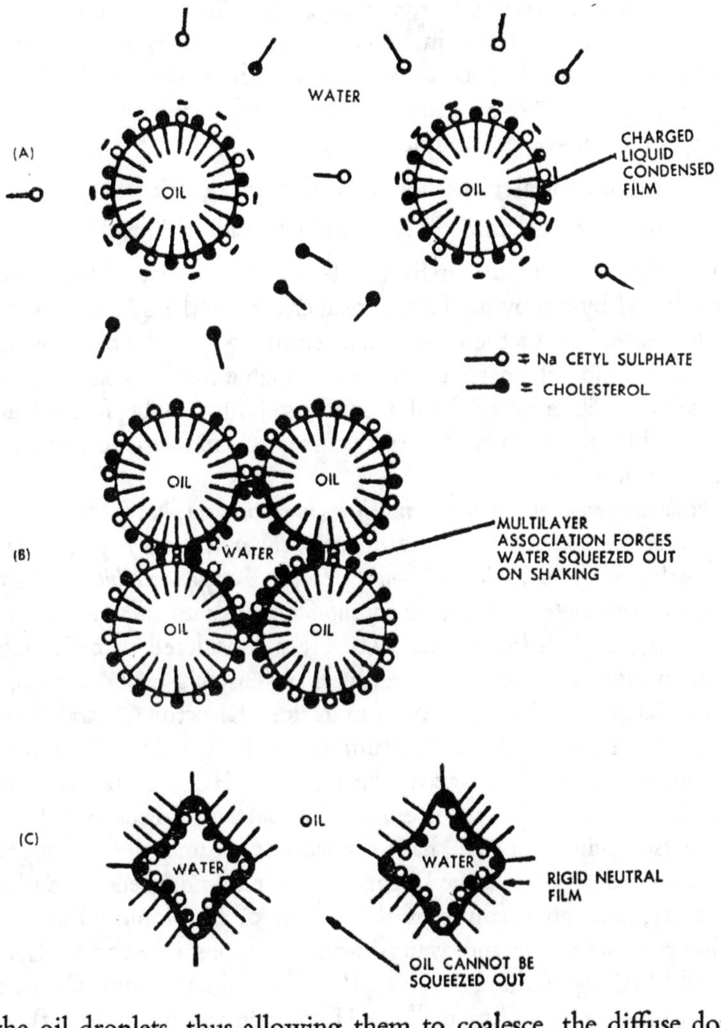

on the oil droplets, thus allowing them to coalesce, the diffuse double layer of sodium cetyl sulphate having been removed by kations in the process.

During the process of coalescence, water molecules can be squeezed out from between the oil droplets very readily because the interfacial film molecules have a strong tendency to align themselves with their polar heads together as in their normal crystal packing. Fig. (*b*) shows a number of oil droplets in the coalesced state after removal of the charge on the oil droplets. If, now, the interfacial film is rigid and especially if a cross-linkage of the film molecules has occurred to give the crystal packing arrangement already mentioned, the water "sacks" enclosed by the coalesced oil droplets will themselves be stabilised and will float away. This process is represented in Fig. (*c*). The emulsion is now of the water-in-oil type and the interfacial film molecules have their long hydrocarbon chains directed outwards from the water "sacks".

Schulman and Cockbain summarised the following conditions for the stability of oil-in-water emulsions:

(1) The interfacial film should possess an electric charge.

(2) The interfacial film should possess considerable rigidity.

Inversion of an emulsion from oil-in-water to water-in-oil may be accomplished by removing the electrical charge on the oil droplets, which leads to a breaking of the oil-in-water emulsion. If the composition of the aqueous and oil phases is such as to enable a solid condensed film, or better an "interlinked" solid condensed film to be formed at the interface, then an inversion process occurs with the formation of a water-in-oil emulsion.

The development of non-ionic emulsifiers in recent years has led to an extension of the above conception. Stable emulsions of the oil-in-water type, using non-ionic emulsifiers of the "Span" and "Tween" type, exhibit no charge as indicated by cataphoretic studies, are not substantive and are stable to the addition of various types of electrolytes and acids. It is considered that the stability of such emulsions is due to the emulsifier possessing a proper hydrophile-lipophile balance. (Private Communication, Director Central Research Laboratory, Atlas Powder Co., Wilmington, May 1950.) [The question of classification of surface-active agents by "HLB", viz. hydrophile-lipophile balance is reported in some detail later in this chapter.]

Professor Schulman *et al.*, have carried out a number of investigations on non-ionic detergents at the Department of Colloid Science, Cambridge University, and an account of the action of non-ionic emulsifiers in stabilising oil-in-water and water-in-oil emulsions is given in *Cytology and Cell Physiology* (edited by G. H. Bourne, 2nd edn., 1951, Chapter III, "The Monolayer Technique", J. H. Schulman, pp. 146-147). The emulsifying properties of the non-ionic detergents are considered to be straightforward. (Private Communication, Professor Schulman, Feb. 1953.)

The extension of the concept of emulsification is given in the following quotation (from Chapter III, "The Monolayer Technique," *loc. cit.*, pp. 146 *et seq.*) by Professor Schulman.

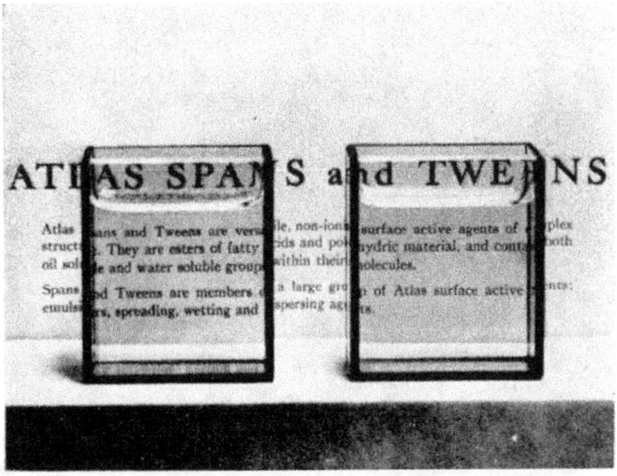

(*a*) A true solution (left) and a colloidal suspension (right). Both appear perfectly clear.

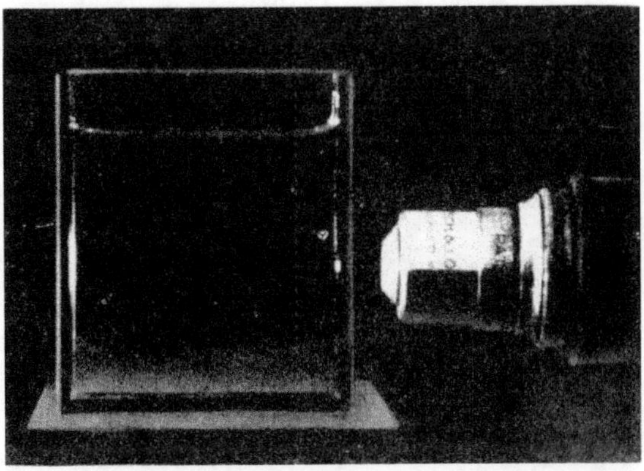

(*b*) A true solution does not reflect a beam of light directed through it.

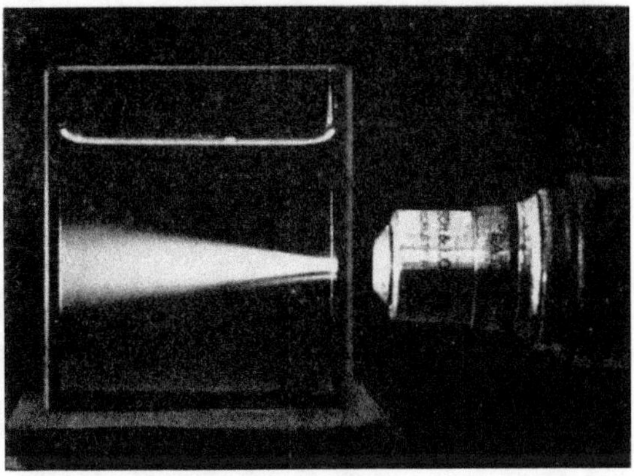

(*c*) Reflection of light beam reveals the presence of colloidal particles.

FIG. 101.

[*By courtesy of the Atlas Powder Co., U.S.A.*

Hydrophobic and Hydrophilic Balance of Interfacial Films in Relation to Phase Continuity in Emulsions.

" . . . There are three rules governing phase continuity in emulsions. These seem to hold for all systems of stabilising agents and for different oils. It must be remembered that the interfacial film counts as a phase, besides the oil and water phases.

" 1. If the interfacial film is charged by adsorption of positive or negative ions, or consists of anionic or cationic long-chain hydrocarbon stabilising agents present in dilute salt solution, then a diffuse ionic concentration gradient can be built up in the aqueous phase at the interface. This gives the droplet a zeta potential. Since the ionic gradient can only be held in high dielectrics, the charged droplets of the same sign will repel one another. Under these conditions it is necessary for the droplets to be oil and the continuous phase water. If this ionic concentration gradient be removed by addition of salts, or chemical means such as the tanning of cationic soaps with polyphenols, etc., one obtains an ion pair dipole or phenolic amine complex dipole, which answer to rule 2 or 3.

" 2. If the interfacial film of the stabilising agent, or agents, be more soluble in oil than in water, then oil will be the continuous phase. This is also the case if the contact angle with oil or water for a monolayer of the stabilising agents be greater with oil than with water at the oil/water interface.

" 3. If the reverse is the equilibrium condition, so that the interfacial film be more soluble in water, or the contact angle made by such a film with oil and water at an oil/water interface be greater with water than with oil, then water will be the continuous phase.

" If a single compound is used to stabilise an emulsion, then the oil or water solubility of that compound can give direct information as to which phase will be the continuous one.

" Interesting examples of this latter class are the non-ionogenic compounds, such as the condensation products of the long-chain alcohols with ethylene oxide.[1] In water-wetting power the oxygen atom equals three CH_2 groups in balancing out their oil-wetting power. One ethylene oxide group already containing two CH_2 groups equals one CH_2 group in the alcohol radical chain. Thus $CH_3(CH_2)_6O[(CH_2)_2O]_3H$ will give water/oil emulsions, and $CH_3(CH_2)_6O[(CH_2)_2O]_5H$ will give oil/water emulsions.

" If two stabilising agents are used, one of which is an oil-soluble agent, and the other a water-soluble agent, the phase continuity is governed

[1] Cohen (1948), *C. R. Acad. Sci.*, **226**, 1366.

by the nature of the monolayer formed at the interface. There are at least four possibilities. If no complex is formed between the two agents either the oil-soluble or water-soluble component will sit alone at the interface by displacing the other, according to the magnitude of the interfacial lowering properties of either agent. This is controlled by their mutual oil or water concentrations and their chemistry, which governs their mutual adhesion and cohesion to the oil or water phase.

"If there is complex formation between the two stabilising agents, it is usual for the equimolecular mixed monolayers resulting from the association to be more stable than the monolayer of either of the two components alone. This results in very low interfacial tensions, small droplet size, and spontaneous forming emulsions. The hydrophobic/hydrophilic balance of the mixed monolayer must now be considered, in order to establish which phase will be continuous.

Oleophobic Surfaces [1]

"A special case of interest is a surface that is not wettable by either oil or water. Such a surface is obtained by adsorbing long-chain polar compounds on to a base in which the polar group adheres strongly, or where the polar groups are bound together in double layers. This adlineates the CH_2 groups in the hydrocarbon chain in such a way that the end CH_3 group attached to each chain is tightly arranged in the form of a crystal monolayer lattice. The CH_3 surface cannot associate with the free CH_2 group or other hydrocarbon groups in any deposited oil. Contact angles of 42° with metals coated with long-chain amines having chain length of at least $(CH_2)_{14}$ have been obtained with hydrocarbon oils.[2] Any disorder brought into the CH_3 lattice array immediately permits the oil to spread, as on normal paraffin wax. . . ."

Emulsification by Means of Powders

". . . Pickering (*J. chem. Soc.*, 1907, p. 2001) was the first to show that solid powders could stabilise oil-in-water dispersions. Hildebrand (*J. Amer. chem. Soc.*, 1923, p. 2786) suggested that the reason why fine powders are emulsifying agents is that the powder particles are partially wettable by both oil and water. Oil would be the continuous phase of the emulsion if the powder was more wettable by oil, and vice versa.

"Recent investigations by J. H. Schulman and J. Leja ('Control of Contact Angles at the Oil/Water/Solid Interfaces in relation to emulsions stabilised by solid particles' ($BaSO_4$), Ernest Oppenheimer Laboratory, Department of Colloid Science, The University, Cambridge [in press])

[1] Schulman, 1948, *Discussion—Faraday Society*, "Interaction of Water and Porous Materials", **3**, 290.

[2] Bigelow, Pickett and Zisman, 1946, *J. Coll. Sci.*, **1**, 513.

give strong support to this theory. These workers investigated the relationship existing between the contact angle developed by a drop of oil deposited on a solid surface coated by an amphipathic agent and the stabilisation of oil-water emulsions by solid powders (of suitable size) similarly coated by the same agent. They found that :

(*a*) water-continuous emulsions, o/w, are stabilised by the solid powder when the contact angle at the oil/water/solid interface is slightly less than 90° (measured through the water phase) ;

(*b*) oil-continuous emulsions, w/o, are formed and stabilised by the solid powder when the contact angle is slightly more than 90° ;

and that the phase of the emulsion stabilised by the solid powder coated by the given amphipathic agent is usually opposite to that given by the system oil-water-amphipathic agent alone, without the solid powder.

" Solids capable of stabilising oil-water emulsions are either inherently wettable partly by oil and partly by water (only few solids possessing exceptionally low surface energies on their own, e.g. talc, molybdenite, graphite, diamond, sulphur) or are made partially wettable by coating them with a suitable agent. Such agent must be suitably chosen both as regards its polar group (giving anchorage to the solid surface) and its hydrocarbon chain. The contact angle developed at the oil/water/sensitised solid is the resultant effect of the density of coverage and the length of the hydrocarbon chain. The density of coverage by the amphipathic agent is regulated by the adsorption of the agent, and this depends on the state of the solid surface, the polar group of the agent, the nature and orientation of the hydrocarbon group, the concentration of the agent, *p*H, temperature and the inorganic ions present in solutions. In the investigations referred to, the variables studied by Schulman and Leja were limited to : the chain lengths of alkyl sulphates and carboxylic soaps, *p*H, and the concentration of the alkyl sulphates and soaps. It was shown that an inversion of the phase of a solid-stabilised emulsion, from an o/w into a w/o type, can be achieved by :

(*a*) a substitution of a short chain agent by a suitably longer chain of the same polar group agent at equimolar concentration ;

(*b*) a substitution of one type of an amphipathic agent (soap) by another (alkyl sulphate) possessing stronger adsorbing polar group and greater coverage power, at equimolar concentration and at equal chain length;

(*c*) suitable changes in the concentration of the agent employed and/or area of the solid surface available for covering ;

(*d*) an increase in *p*H from 7 to 12 when carboxylic soaps of $C > 12$ are employed.

"Production of too highly hydrophobic coatings on the surface of the solid particles leads to their dispersion within the oil phase (instead of their stabilisation of the oil-water interface) and results in unstable, poor oil-continuous dispersions. Penetration of a diffuse covered surface by long chain alcohol molecules takes place by molecular association."

Classification of Surface-Active Agents by "HLB"

The term "HLB" comes from the words hydrophile-lipophile balance. Surface-active agents have been classified in a variety of ways, including chemical groupings, etc. W. C. Griffin *et al.* ("Classification of Surface-Active Agents by "HLB", *J. Soc. cosmet. Chem.*, Dec. 1949, **5**, 311) have developed a classification which permits some prediction of behaviour, and reduces to some kind of rational order, the selection of an emulsifier, wetting agent or other type of agent. In this system, as applied to emulsifiers, Griffin *et al.* have assigned a low HLB number to an emulsifier that is lipophilic in character whilst to an emulsifier that is hydrophilic in character is assigned a high number. The midpoint is approximately 10 and the assigned values have ranged from 1 to 40. Griffin points out that, in this system, when two or more emulsifiers are combined, the HLB values are additive in behaviour. Attention is drawn to the fact that chemical type does not establish hydrophile-lipophile balance and thus soaps may range from strongly hydrophilic sodium laurate to strongly lipophilic aluminium oleate; esters may range from low to high HLBs, etc.

HLB is not the same as solubility, though there is, Griffin points out, an over-all relationship.

Thus materials which have a low value *tend* to be oil-soluble and materials having high values *tend* to be water-soluble. However, two emulsifiers may have the same HLB and exhibit different solubility characteristics.

The following discussion of the "HLB" is quoted, extensively, from the original paper by W. C. Griffin (by courtesy of this investigator; of the Atlas Powder Co., Wilmington, U.S.A.; and of the Society of Cosmetic Chemists). For full details, however, the original paper and the various publications on surface-active agents by the Atlas Powder Co., should be consulted.

Estimation of HLB Values for Emulsifiers and Oils

Griffin (*loc. cit.*) states ". . . In our proposed system, HLB values for new emulsifiers are estimated from a series of tests in which actual emulsification behaviour is compared. Comparison, by means of blends or mixtures, is made with agents of known HLB values, such as the series of Atlas emulsifiers. Emulsifiers, as used in industry, are almost always blends. The blend is usually most efficient if it combines lipophilic and hydrophilic emulsifiers. We usually recommend that 'Span'[1] and 'Tween'[1] emulsifiers be used blended. Glyceryl monostearate, self-emulsifying grade, is a blend. Even the monovalent soaps, generally used for o/w emulsification, are blends of soap and hydrolysed fatty acid.

"Variation of the proportions of the blended emulsifiers has been taught as preferred practice to obtain best results. When two emulsifiers of known HLB are thus blended for use with a given oil there is an optimum ratio that gives best emulsification and the HLB at this ratio is said to be the required 'HLB' for the oil (to give that type of emulsion, whether o/w, w/o solubilisation, etc.). This is expressed by the equation :

$$\frac{W_A \text{HLB}_A + W_B \text{HLB}_B (\text{optimum ratio})}{W_A + W_B} = \text{HLB oil}$$

wherein :

W_A = the amount (weight) of the first emulsifier (A) used, and

W_B = the amount (weight) of the second emulsifier (B) used at the 'optimum ratio', giving the best emulsion.

HLB_A, HLB_B = the assigned HLB values for emulsifiers A and B.

HLB oil = the 'required HLB' of the oil for the type of emulsion being studied.

"Since good emulsification may occur over a wide range of emulsifier ratios, or since emulsification in the entire series may be only mediocre, the optimum ratio may be obscured. By averaging results with several emulsifiers and several oils the estimation is made more precise. In conducting a number of these tests it will be apparent that the information will have relationship to many factors.

"To establish the necessary cross relationships, series of emulsions were prepared over a standard formula. The emulsions in these tests were prepared in a uniform manner in so far as possible.

". . . In Fig. 104, we show several series of samples in which heavy mineral oil is emulsified with several combinations or blends of emulsifiers. In each series, the only difference is the types of emulsifiers employed. Two emulsifiers are used in each row, one having a low and one a high HLB. The samples on the extreme left are emulsified with 100 per cent. of low HLB agents ; the samples on the extreme right are emulsified with 100 per cent. of high HLB agents. Blending permits coverage of the complete range of values between the two emulsifiers.

[1] Proprietary Range, Atlas Powder Co.

From top to bottom, the emulsifiers are blends of laurate, palmitate, stearate, and oleate ether-esters (the latter in addition being tri-esters). You will note that the weight percentages of the low and high HLB products required are not similar for best emulsification and that the gross efficiency of the systems are not identical. The important fact to us is that in each instance, the best emulsion is obtained at about an HLB of 10. This is one of the major points on which this system is based. *A given oil has an optimum HLB for a given type of emulsification.*

"Different oils require different values as may be seen in Fig. 103. In this figure, one of the pairs of non-ionic emulsifiers used in Fig. 104, 'Span' 40—'Tween' 40, is pictured with eight different oils or waxes; cotton-seed oil, lanolin, petrolatum, mineral oil, paraffin, cetyl alcohol, beeswax, and stearic acid. *It will be apparent that to choose an emulsifier for a formula we need to know the required HLB for the oil blend, as well as that of the proposed emulsifiers* . . . .

"Required HLB values for blends of oils may be calculated in a manner similar to that for blends of emulsifiers so long as the requirements for the components are known. . . .

"A natural question is the adherence of the HLB system to ionic or soap emulsions. Monovalent soaps, generally used for emulsification exhibit high HLB's, higher than required for optimum emulsification. However, soap alone is seldom, if ever, the sole emulsifier in a formula. We know that soaps hydrolyse, and the true emulsifier is a mixture, or blend, of soap and free fatty acid. This is illustrated in the accompanying figure where the samples with the arrows are the theoretically neutralised soaps, but in each instance, the samples to the left in which there is excess fatty acid are the better emulsions . . . .

"For a given oil and water there is one HLB for the total emulsifier that is best without regard to the concentrations of ingredients in the usual ranges . . . .

"In Table 5 we have listed several estimated 'HLB' values for emulsifiers. These were determined and correlated by preparing vast series of emulsifier-blend tests as in the illustration. Grouping in this table is according to composition as well as HLB since both are influential in choosing an emulsifier. We hope to extend this list, and expect to do so. The magnitude of this type of study is understood when you realise that each of these values was derived from approximately seventy-five emulsions. A more extensive tabulation of estimated HLB values for Atlas products is available in the Atlas Surface-Active Agents Booklet . . . .

"Chemical reactivity of an emulsifier can modify the behaviour of an emulsifier immensely. In the case of soaps, traces of multivalent ions completely change the HLB. Another instance that we have observed was with an amine-neutralised aryl sulphate, where the presence of acidic constituents lowered the HLB of the emulsifier markedly.

" Likewise, in Table 6 we have listed the estimated required ' HLB ' values for several of the more commonly used oils and waxes. These

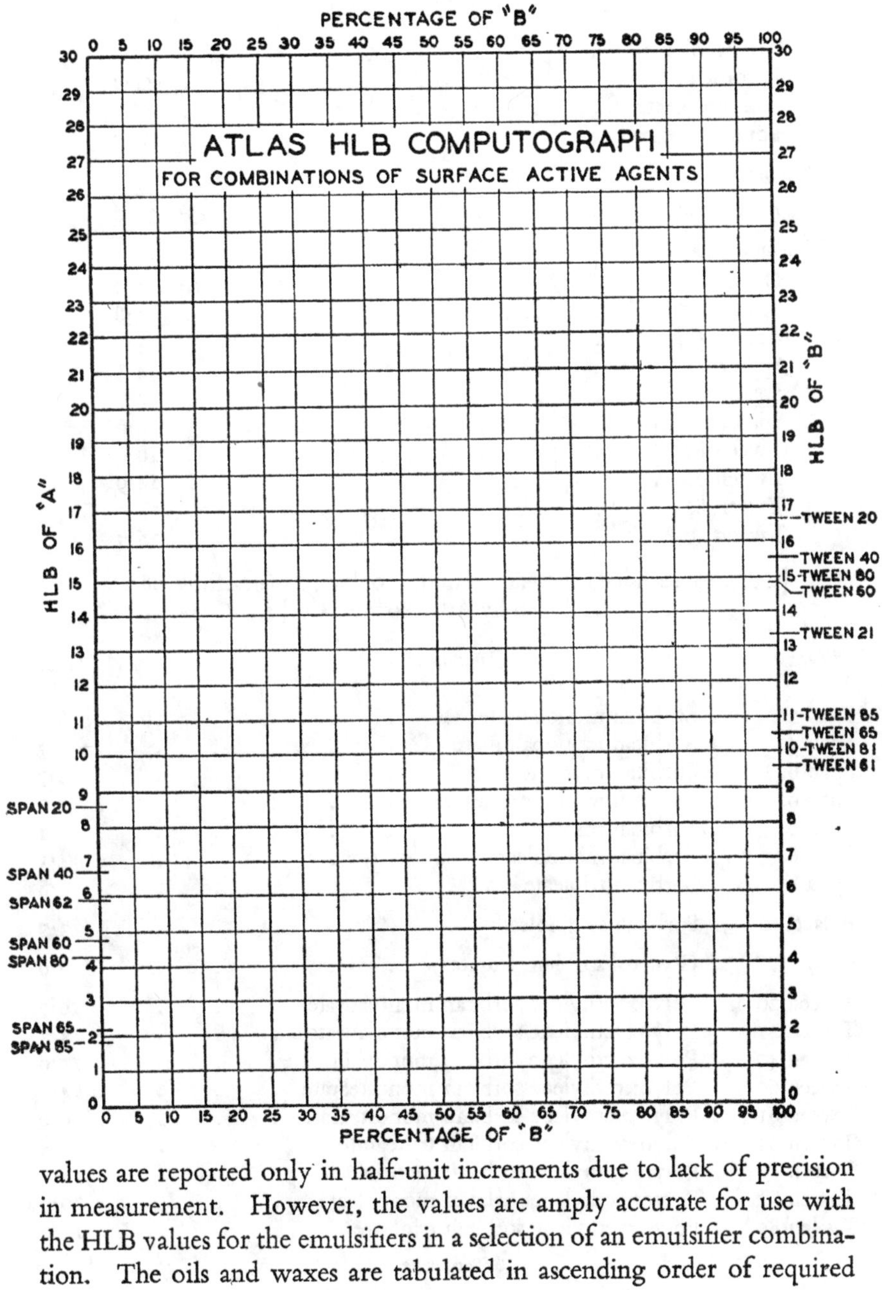

values are reported only in half-unit increments due to lack of precision in measurement. However, the values are amply accurate for use with the HLB values for the emulsifiers in a selection of an emulsifier combination. The oils and waxes are tabulated in ascending order of required

'HLBs'. As would be expected, similar values are noted for like chemical types.

TABLE 5

Emulsifier	*Estimated HLB*
Anionic	
T.E.A. oleate	12·0
Lecomene O	12·7*
Sodium oleate	18·0
Potassium oleate	20·0
Cationic	
Atlas G-251	25·0–35·0
Non-ionic	
Oleic acid	App. 1·0
Span 85	1·8
Arlacel C	3·7
Span 80	4·3
Span 60	4·7
Span 20	8·6
Tween 81	10·0
Tween 60	14·9
Tween 80	15·0
Tween 20	16·7

[Other values listed below are from the booklet, *Surface-Active Agents*, published by Atlas Powder Co.]

Name	*Compound*	*HLB*
Span 20	Sorbitan monolaurate	8·6
Span 40	Sorbitan monopalmitate	6·7
Span 60	Sorbitan monostearate	4·7
Span 62	Sorbitan monostearate	5·9
Span 65	Sorbitan tristearate	2·1
Span 80	Sorbitan monooleate	4·3
Span 85	Sorbitan trioleate	1·8
Arlacel C	Sorbitan sesquioleate	3·7
G-672	Glycerol sorbitan laurate	7·6
Tween 20	Polyoxyethylene sorbitan monolaurate	16·7
Tween 21	Polyoxyethylene sorbitan monolaurate	13·3
Tween 40	Polyoxyethylene sorbitan monopalmitate	15·6
Tween 60	Polyoxyethylene sorbitan monostearate	14·9
Tween 61	Polyoxyethylene sorbitan monostearate	9·6
Tween 65	Polyoxyethylene sorbitan tristearate	10·5
Tween 80	Polyoxyethylene sorbitan monooleate	15·0
Tween 81	Polyoxyethylene sorbitan monooleate	10·0
Tween 85	Polyoxyethylene sorbitan trioleate	11·0

* Tentative.

Name	*Compound*	*HLB*
G-7596-J	Polyoxyethylene sorbitan monolaurate	14·9
G-7596-P	Polyoxyethylene sorbitan monolaurate	16·3
G-7076-H	Polyoxyethylene sorbitan dilaurate	11·2
G-7426-N	Polyoxyethylene sorbitan monopalmitate	14·8
G-9446-N	Polyoxyethylene sorbitan monooleate	13·9
Myrj 45	Polyoxyethylene stearate	11·1
Myrj 49	Polyoxyethylene stearate	15·0
Myrj 51	Polyoxyethylene stearate	16·0
Myrj 52	Polyoxyethylene stearate	16·9
Myrj 53	Polyoxyethylene stearate	17·9
G-2162	Polyoxyethylene propyl glycol monostearate	15·7
G-1020	Polyoxyethylene sorbitol monolaurate	13·0
G-1061	Polyoxyethylene sorbitol pentalaurate	9·7
G-1050	Polyoxyethylene sorbitol hexastearate	2·6
G-2854	Polyoxyethylene sorbitol tetraoleate	3·4
G-2859	Polyoxyethylene sorbitol 4·5-oleate	3·7
G-2855	Polyoxyethylene sorbitol pentaoleate	3·6
G-1086	Polyoxyethylene sorbitol hexaoleate	10·2
G-931	Polyoxyethylene sorbitol cottonseed oil derivative	4·2
G-2800	Polyoxypropylene mannitol dioleate	—
Atlox 1045	Polyoxyethylene sorbitol laurate	11·5
Atlox 1045-A	Polyoxyethylene sorbitol oleate-laurate	13·2
NNO	Glycerol mannitan laurate	7·1
G-891	Sorbitan esters of mixed fatty and resin acids	6·4
G-8916-P	Polyoxyethylene sorbitan esters of mixed fatty and resin acids	14·6
G-8916-T	Polyoxyethylene sorbitan esters of mixed fatty and resin acids	15·4
G-1234	Polyoxyethylene sorbitol esters of mixed fatty and resin acids	8·6
G-1255	Polyoxyethylene sorbitol esters of mixed fatty and resin acids	10·7
G-1256	Polyoxyethylene sorbitol esters of mixed fatty and resin acids	9·7
G-1266	Polyoxyethylene sorbitol esters of mixed fatty and resin acids	10·6
Renex	Polyoxyethylene esters of mixed fatty and resin acids	13·5
G-1425	Polyoxyethylene sorbitol lanolin derivative	—
G-1431	Polyoxyethylene sorbitol lanolin derivative	—
G-1441	Polyoxyethylene sorbitol lanolin derivative	—
G-1702	Polyoxyethylene sorbitol beeswax derivative	—
G-1704	Polyoxyethylene sorbitol beeswax derivative	—
G-1706	Polyoxyethylene sorbitol beeswax derivative	—
G-1725	Polyoxyethylene sorbitol beeswax derivative	—
G-1726	Polyoxyethylene sorbitol beeswax derivative	—
G-1727	Polyoxyethylene sorbitol beeswax derivative	—
G-1734	Polyoxyethylene sorbitol beeswax derivative	—
Brij 30	Polyoxyethylene lauryl alcohol	9·5
Brij 35	Polyoxyethylene lauryl alcohol	16·9

TABLE 6

Oil or wax	Required HLB for o/w emulsion	Required HLB for w/o emulsion
Cottonseed oil	7·5	—
Carbon tetrachloride	9·0*	—
Paraffin (household)	9·0	4
Microcrystalline wax (Micropac Q, S-V)	9·5*	?
Mineral oil, white, light (Marcol GX)	10·0	4
Mineral oil, white, heavy (Nujol)	10·5	4
Mineral seal oil	10·5*	?
Petrolatum, white (white perfecta)	10·5	4
Silicone oil (G.E.)	10·5*	?
Kerosene	12·5*	?
Naphtha	13·0*	?
Cetyl alcohol	13·0	?
Orthodichlorobenzene †	13·0*	?
Beeswax, white	10·0–16·0	5
Carnauba wax	14·5*	?
Candelilla wax	14·5*	?
Lanolin, U.S.P. = United States Pharmacopoeia, anhyd	15·0	8
Dimethyl phthalate	15·0*	?
Orthophenylphenol	15·5*	?
Stearic acid	17·0	—

Method of Use of HLB Values

"We have developed a 'refined trial-and-error system' based on HLB values. In any emulsification problem one of two conditions can exist: (1) the problem can be to emulsify an oil phase of unknown composition, or (2) the approximate desired formula may be known including the composition of the oil phase.

"If the properties, particularly the required HLB, of the oil phase are unknown as in the first condition, a preliminary exploratory test is set up. This is usually done with a non-ionic emulsifier combination, such as 'Span' 60 and 'Tween' 60, of known HLB values.

"The first series of determinations are prepared with various ratios of these emulsifiers using a maximum amount of total emulsifier . . . A more accurate determination of the required HLB is next obtained by the preparation of a second series, using small increments of this same pair of emulsifiers. . . .

". . . After determination of the optimum point, the chemical classification for the emulsifier is studied by preparing a third test series . . . in which emulsifiers of selected different chemical types are tried, all of

* Tentative.

† Plus small amounts (3·5 per cent.) of pine oil and isopropyl alcohol.

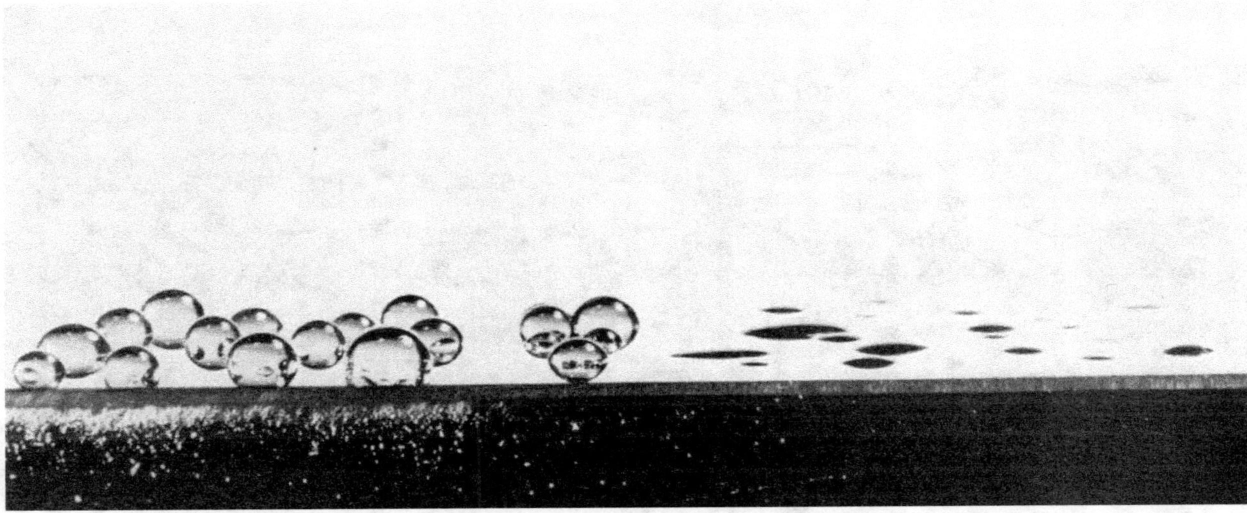

[*By courtesy of the Atlas Powder Co., U.S.A.*

FIG. 102.—Illustrating effect of a surface-active agent on the spreading properties of a liquid. At left are globules of water standing on a waxed surface of a pane of glass. (Parallel lines across bottom of photo are edge of pane.) At right are globules to which surface-active agent has been added, on same surface. Note how water spreads out in thin film.

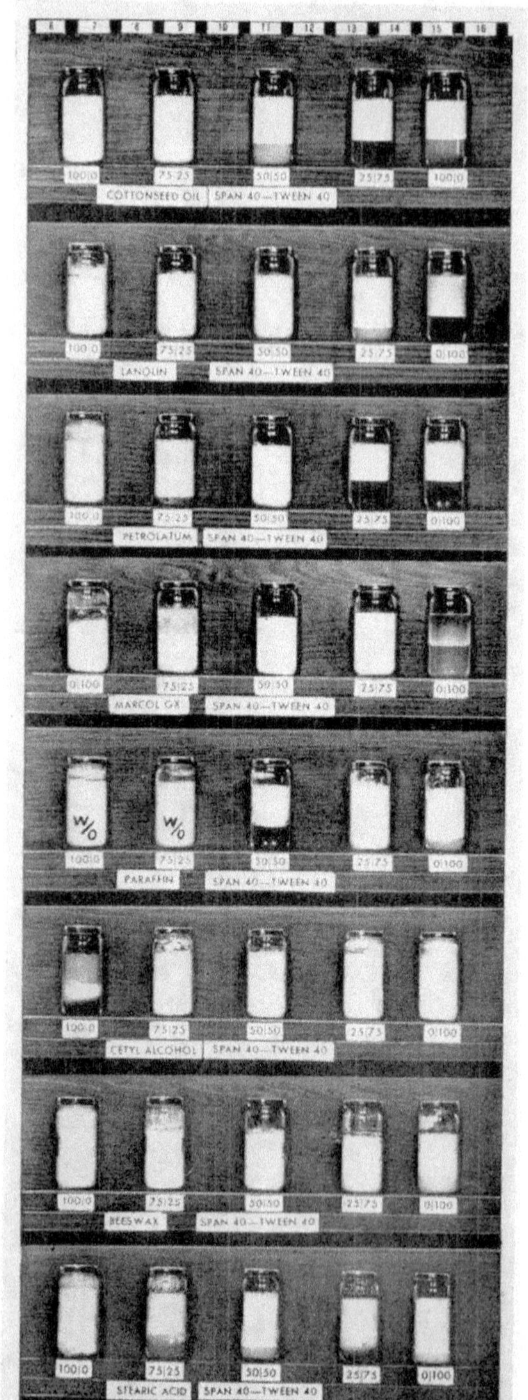

[*By courtesy of the Atlas Powder Co., and the Journal of the Society of Cosmetic Chemists.*

FIG. 103.—Behaviour of various oils with one pair of emulsifiers (different ratios best for different oils).

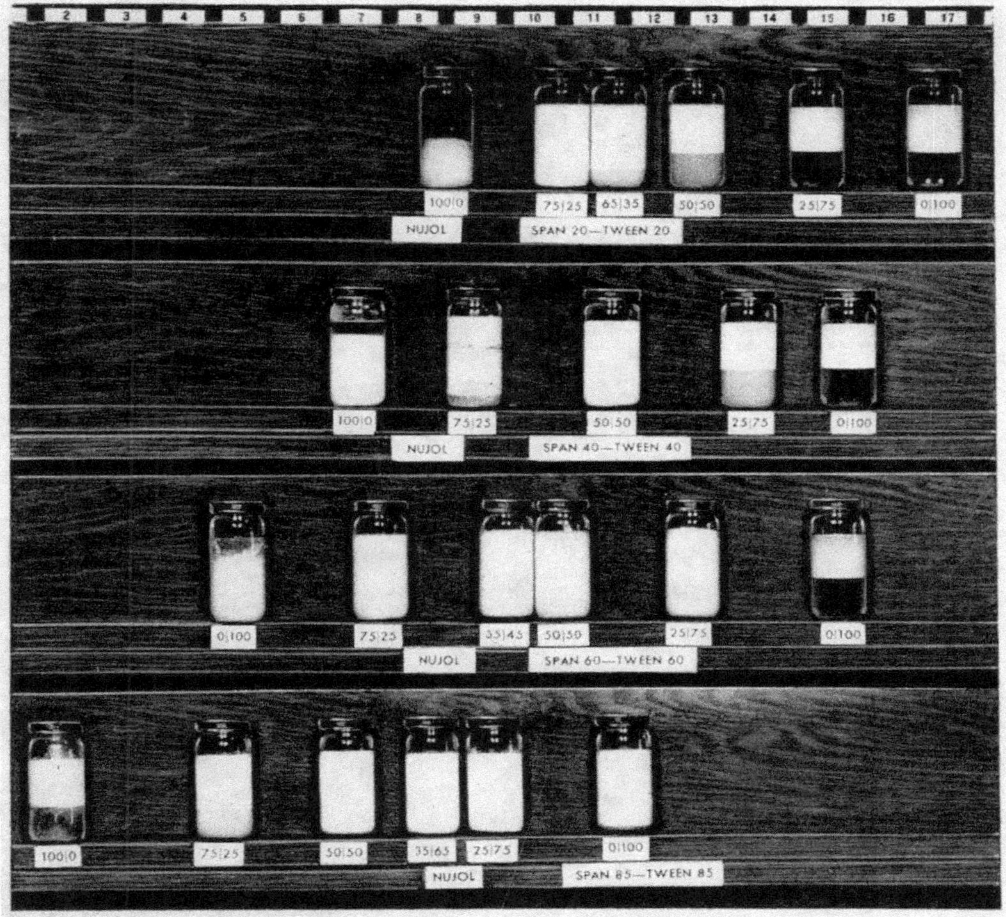

[*By courtesy of the Atlas Powder Co., and the Journal of the Society of Cosmetic Chemists.*

FIG. 104.—Effect of ratio of low and high HLB emulsifiers on emulsification (the same weight per cent. of emulsifier is not best).

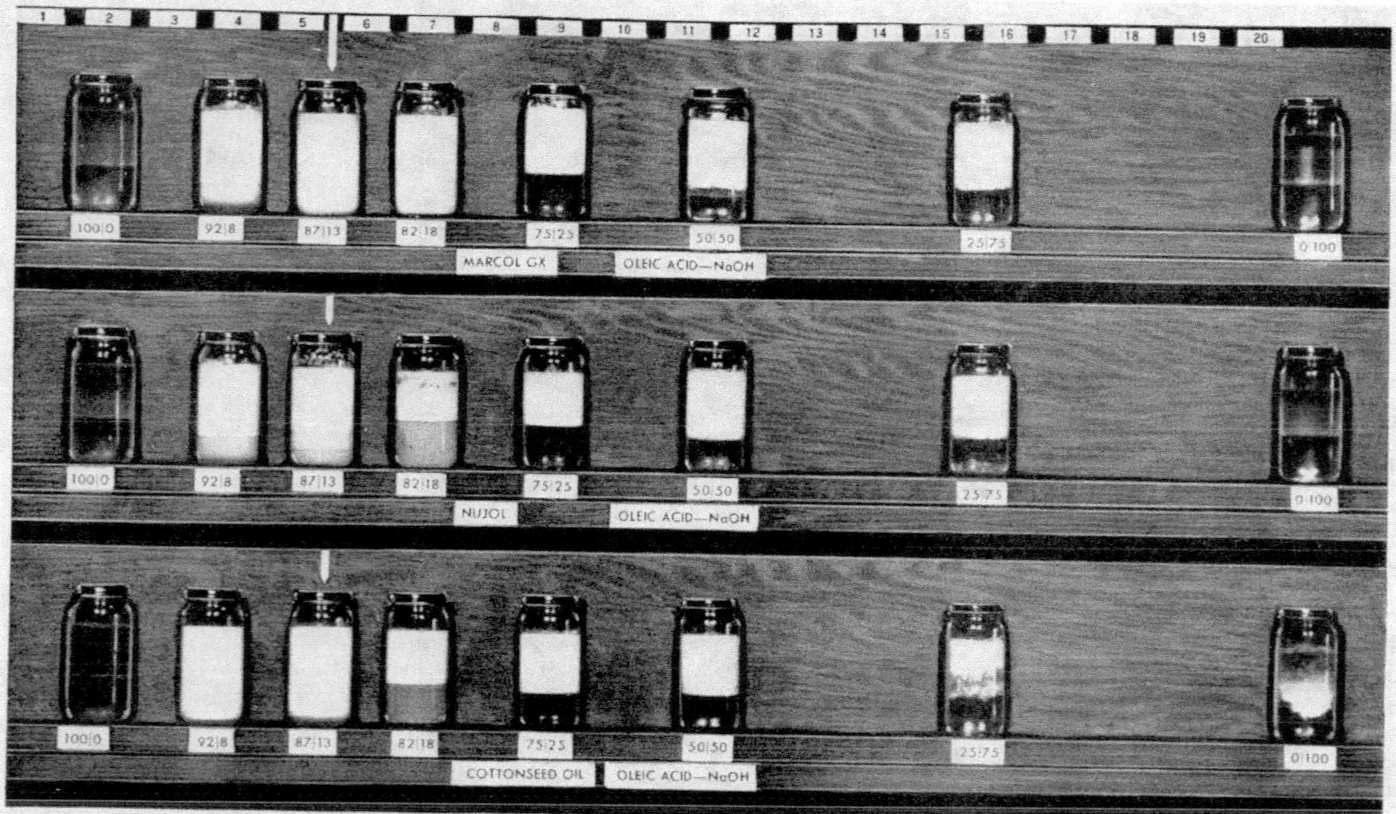

[*By courtesy of the Atlas Powder Co., and the Journal of the Society of Cosmetic Chemists.*

FIG. 105.—Behaviour of soaps—varying ratios of oleic acid and NaOH.

which have been previously blended to the required HLB. After choosing the chemical type, a final series usually suffices to provide a blend of emulsifiers of the chosen chemical type at the most favourable HLB and at the minimum required total concentration. This last series of samples is usually put through more extensive and more stringent stability tests.

" If the required HLB of the oil phase is known approximately, the first series of tests may be eliminated. If it is known with greater accuracy both the first and second series of tests may be omitted.

" For an example, an All-Purpose Cream has been chosen with a proposed formula of:

Beeswax	5
Mineral oil	26
Hydrogenated vegetable oil	18
Polyol	4
Emulsifier	5–10
Water	*q.s.* to make 100

" The oil phase, then consists of the following approximate percentages:

Oil or wax	*per cent.*	*Est. req. HLB*	
Beeswax	10	15	1·5
Mineral oil	53	10	5·3
Hydrogenated vegetable oil	37	9	3·3
Av. est. req. HLB			10·1

Calculation of an estimated required HLB gives a value slightly over 10. Therefore, the initial series with this oil phase can be prepared combining 'Span' 60 and 'Tween' 60 to give HLB values close to 10. . . .

'Span' 60	—	*'Tween'* 60	
50	—	50	9·8
45	—	55	10·3
40	—	60	10·8
35	—	65	11·3
25	—	75	12·4

The best ratio in this series is 45 per cent. 'Span' 60 and 55 per cent. 'Tween' 60 at a calculated HLB of 10·3.

" The evaluation of different chemical types of emulsifiers is then considered as previously mentioned. For this example, the stearate blend is the best chemical type . . . . It must be remembered that all blends must be at the correct HLB.

" It is interesting to note that the addition of polyol to the aqueous phase of an emulsion such as was just studied does not appear to alter the HLB appreciably. . . .

". . . Little difference is noted in the emulsification, regardless of the type of polyol used. This does not imply that the three polyols will produce similar cosmetic effects. These differences are well known and are due to the variations in hygroscopicities, co-solubilities, and other physical properties of the polyols themselves. The data indicate that at the proper balance of emulsifier, the emulsification will not be appreciably affected by the type and amount of polyol.

"The dividing line between ingredients and emulsifiers is often not clear. Stearic acid, lanolin, cholesterol, and beeswax are just a few examples of materials that may serve a dual role. An example of this is in soap-emulsified-facial-creams in which the stearic acid is partially neutralised. In this, the stearic acid forms a bulk of the oil phase, but portions of the stearic acid are present as emulsifier, both neutralised and as free acid. By examining a system, it is usually possible to evaluate each ingredient in the terms of its uses. . . ."

Solubilisation

". . . Solubilisation requires the highest HLB (for common uses) at 15–18. For this purpose, single high HLB agents are frequently used. Early work has indicated that the HLB can be too high for efficient solubilising. The effective range appears to be narrow even for different oils. No thorough study of solubilising *vs.* HLB has been undertaken. (*See* Transparent Dispersions later in this Chapter.)

"The HLB system, though it does not indicate the overall efficiency of the emulsifier, does tell 'what it will do', that is—what kind of an emulsion or product to expect. By so doing, it enables us to compare various chemical types of emulsifiers at their optimum balance. . . ."

It is claimed that the HLB system appears to be suitable for all types of problems employing surface-active agents.

Emulsion Viscosity

The role of viscosity has been much debated, and in a comprehensive series of articles Coutino (*Amer. Perfum.*, July 1938, p. 35; May 1940, p. 33) has emphasised, quite rightly, that the correct viscosity is of far greater importance than a merely high viscosity, since the latter will oppose not only coalescence but also globular diffusion. King and Mukherjee (*J. Soc. Chem. Ind.*, Sept. 1940), in an investigation of emulsions stabilised by hydrophilic colloids, demonstrated the importance of the "right" viscosity in the stability of their emulsions. High viscosity is a symptom, not a cause of stability. King (*Mfg. Chemist/Mfg. Perfum.*, Sept 1941, p. 213) has pointed out that the viscosity of an emulsion is a function of the concentration of the internal phase liquid—the greater the latter, the higher the viscosity. Emulsions containing 80 per cent. of one liquid dispersed in 20 per cent. of another are thick pastes. The same writer has also drawn attention to the fact that the nature of the emulsifying agent is also very important in determining the viscosity of the system.

Lawrence (*Chem. Ind.*, 1948, **39**, 615), who during the 1939-45 war was engaged on Admiralty work which necessitated a study of the breaking of emulsions of sea-water in fuel oil, has pointed out that all emulsion systems are theoretically dynamic and the reverse process of demulsification sets in as soon as the emulsion is made. He condemns as a fallacy the oft-repeated assertion that the stability of an emulsion is dependent upon the extent to which the interfacial tension between the dispersed and continuous phases is lowered by the introduction of an emulsifying agent. Surface activity is a necessary common property of emulsifying agents, necessary for the formation of an energy barrier at the interface, but not quantitatively related to the efficacy of the barrier so formed. Lawrence points out that the role of an emulsifying agent is mainly that of providing an energy barrier at the interface and thereby greatly reducing the ease of coalescence. Some emulsifying agents may, by increasing the viscosity of the continuous phase also limit the frequency of collision, but it is the energy barrier with its electrical and mechanical properties which is primarily responsible for emulsion stability. Where the barrier has a very high value, it may produce a system with a half-life period (i.e. 50 per cent. coalescence) of many years or even centuries. Lawrence adds that the increase in viscosity due to emulsification is caused by the resistance to flow from the " elastic bags " which encase each dispersed droplet. Consequently, for a given system, the measure of the viscosity is an indication of the efficiency of emulsification and also of homogenisation.

It is often assumed that globular size is of paramount importance in the formation of a stable emulsion, but this is incorrect.

Emulsion Creaming

It is necessary to distinguish between an emulsion break-down and the phenomenon of *creaming*. Creaming is the result of coarse droplets which rise under the influence of gravity as in the case of un-homogenised milk. This is inelegant and to prevent this, emulsions are usually homogenised with the production of fine particles of more or less equivalent size. These particles, if sufficiently small, are kept in motion by Brownian movement, but frequent collisions occur and as the globular size thereby increases we may get *creaming*. *This is not, however, a breakdown of the emulsion, and on shaking, such emulsions readily return to their former state, because there has been no separation of the internal liquid phase.*

Breakage of an emulsion, however, occurs when the dispersed liquid separates in its original form, as a distinct layer, and this may occur in an homogenised emulsion which shows no sign of *creaming*. This *cracking* of an emulsion occurs when the layer of emulsifier at the interface is too weak to prevent coalescence. Size frequency investigations have shown that some stable emulsions are actually of very coarse particle size.

The modern concept of emulsification therefore envisages three important phases, namely, the adsorption of the emulsifying agent at the interface, the building there of a stable interfacial film and the thermodynamical nature of the process which leads, eventually, to demulsification.

Many and varied have been the theories held in the past and it may be of interest to mention, very briefly, a few of the more important ones.

At one time the "orientated-wedge" theory was very generally accepted. Arising from the fact that the soaps of divalent metals usually formed water-in-oil emulsions, whilst those of the monovalent metals form oil-in-water emulsions, Harkins, Davies and Clark (*J. Amer. Chem. Soc.*, 1917, p. 595; *see also* Finkle, Draper and Hildebrand, 1923, p. 2780) suggested that, since in the divalent soaps there are two hydrocarbon chains attached to one metal atom, while in the monovalent there is only one chain, the molecules of these soaps were wedge-shaped, being wider at the water-soluble end in the case of the monovalent soaps and at the oil-soluble end with the di- and trivalent soaps. Thus a closely packed layer of these molecules would therefore curve with the concave side towards the oil in the case of monovalent soaps and with the convex side towards the oil in the case of the divalent soaps: thus the water phase would be the internal phase (as this has the convex curvature outwards) if divalent soaps are used as emulsifiers. For various technical reasons, this theory, in its original form at any rate, no longer seems tenable.

Two other theories are of interest, viz. the *solvation theory*, and the *cybotactic* one.

Solvation Theory

Fischer (*Fats and Fatty Degeneration*, N.Y., 1917, p. 5) postulated that emulsions can be produced only when the liquid which is to become the continuous phase is all used in the formation of the hydrated compound of the emulsifying agent employed; thus in an o/w emulsion stabilised with soap, the oil would not be considered a dispersion of *oil-in-water*, but as *oil-in-a (hydrated colloid of soap plus water)*. This theory has been strongly criticised in the past. However, King and Mukherjee in the investigation already mentioned, found support for the hypothesis that the efficacy of an emulsifying agent is due to its power of forming a solvated membrane of considerable strength at the oil-water interface, and found that agents which gel readily are capable of forming such membranes with production of stable emulsions. Further, it is a well-known fact that in attempts to crack the emulsions produced with organic protein material in chemical and toxicological analysis, particularly where chloroform has been used as a solvent, the addition of a few ml. of absolute alcohol (a dehydrating agent) is more effective than the addition of electrolytes. (It must be noted, however, that *large quantities* of electrolytes may also crack such emulsions, owing to their influence upon the relative degree of solvation.)

Cybotactic Theory

Speakman and Chamberlain (*Nature*, 1932, **130**, 274 ; *Trans. Faraday Soc.*, 1933, **29**, 359) considered this problem from the angle of X-ray investigation and showed that molecules within liquids undergo continuous association into groups or complexes of a transitory character. These cybotactic complexes break up after a brief period to re-form other complexes, and Speakman and Chamberlain suggested that the cybotactic state of the liquids employed is a determining factor in emulsion type. The tendency of paraffin to develop structure increases with length of the hydrocarbon chain, and it appears probable that paraffins of low density give o/w emulsions because little structure is present to resist dispersion ; whereas paraffins of high density possess sufficient structure to oppose dispersion, and water becomes the disperse phase. They concluded, therefore, that the formation of emulsions, especially in those cases of oils and related compounds of high molecular weight, is not determined simply by the magnitude of the interfacial tension and the formation of a stable adsorbed film at the interface, but that the cybotactic condition of the liquid which it is required to disperse was of equal import.

Chemical Constitution of the Oil and Emulsification

Some oils are more difficult to emulsify than others, and the difference is not merely that of specific gravity, viscosity or surface tension. Ordinary hydrocarbon oils are very easily emulsified, but if carefully purified, emulsification is exceedingly difficult. Strongly polar liquids are also difficult to emulsify. (*See* Classification by HLB.)

So far none of the theories of emulsification solves *every* problem. Perusal of the above will, however, explain many of the fundamental problems which arise in emulsion production ; for example, the necessity of small globular size to prevent creaming, achieved by the use of a colloid mill or homogeniser; the effect of temperature which controls both globular diffusion and collision in the mix; the variations attained with different types of emulsifiers according to their effect on the interfacial tension; and finally the differing effects obtained with the use of different oils in similar formulae. (In this latter connection, reference may be made to the following papers, viz.: Kernot and Knaggs, *J. Soc. chem. Ind. London*, 1928. **47**, 96T; Woodman and Taylor, 1929, **48**, 121T; Tartar and co-workers, *J. Phys. Chem.*, 1929, **33**, 446.)

Types of Emulsifying Agents

OIL-IN-WATER EMULSIFIERS

Carboxylic acids:

(*a*) Formation of insoluble salts, i.e. calcium alginate.

(*b*) Formation of soaps by the action of alkali, e.g. sodium and potassium hydroxides with stearic acid.

Amino derivatives: In conjunction with carboxylic acids (triethanolamine stearate, etc.).

Di-hydroxyl derivatives: Glycol monostearate.

Tri-hydroxyl derivatives, e.g. glyceryl monostearate.

Polyhydroxyl derivative, e.g. derivatives of sorbitol and mannitol. These can be tailored to give any desired HLB.[1]

Complex carbohydrates, e.g. the various natural gums.

Higher fatty acids: Condensed with amino derivatives, e.g. sapamines.

Sulphonated and Sulphated derivatives:

(*a*) O . SO_2 . OH group, e.g. sodium lauryl sulphate.

(*b*) O . SO_2 . OH + COOH groups, e.g. the sulphonated oils.

(*c*) SO_3H + NH_2 groups, e.g. the sulphonated amides.

Cellulose derivatives, e.g. methyl cellulose.

Phosphoric acid esters, e.g. lecithins, cephalines.

Glycol and glyceryl esters, e.g. glycol laurate; diethylene glycol monolaurate; glycol oleate; propylene glycol laurate; (oleate and stearate, glyceryl laurate; glyceryl monoricinoleate, etc.

Hydrophilic colloids (solid), e.g. bentonite, metallic oxides and hydroxides, particularly of aluminium.

WATER-IN-OIL EMULSIFIERS

Monohydroxyl alcohols, e.g. cetyl alcohol, stearyl alcohol, cholesterol.

Polyhydroxyl derivatives, e.g. mannitol mono-oleate; these can be tailored to give any desired HLB.[1]

[1] *See* Classification of Emulsifiers by the "HLB" System earlier in this Chapter.

Oxidised vegetable oils.

Salts of certain di- and tri- valent cations, e.g. Ca, Sr, Ba with fatty acids such as oleic acid.

Carboxylic acid, e.g. ursolic acid.

Surface-active agents differ markedly in respect of their relative emulsifying properties and their wetting, detergent and foaming characteristics, as the following table by Hollenberg (*Proc. Sci. Sect. T.G.A.*, 5 Dec. 1946, p. 15) clearly shows :

	Group	*Structure*	*Emul.*	*Wet.*	*Det.*	*Foam.*	*Disp.*	*Solu.*
Soaps	(*a*) Metallic	$C_{17}H_{35}COOK$	B*	C	B*	B*	C	D
	(*b*) Alkyl amine	$C_{17}H_{33}COON(CH_2.CH_2.OH)_3$	B*	C	B*	B*	B*	C
Sulphated or Sulphonated Compounds	(*a*) Vegetable oils	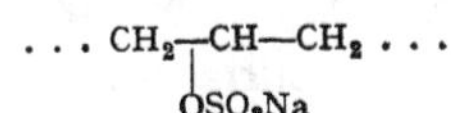	B	D	D	D	C	B
	(*b*) Alkyl naphthalenes	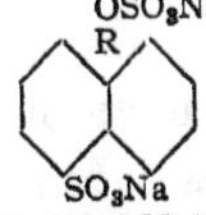	C	A	D	C	B	C
	(*c*) Fatty alcohols	$C_{11}H_{23}CH_2OSO_3Na$	B	C	B	A	B	B
	(*d*) Amides	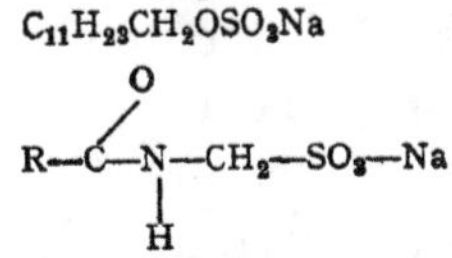	B	B	A	C	B	C
	(*e*) Dibasic acid esters	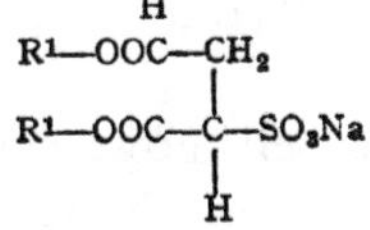	D	A	D	C	D	D
	(*f*) Petroleum derivatives	$R—AR—SO_3Na$	C	C	B	B	C	C
Mono-fatty acid esters	(*a*) Simple glycol or glycerol esters	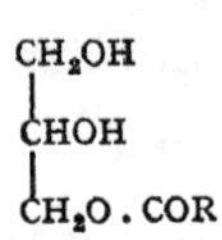	A	C	C	C	B	D
	(*b*) Modified sugar alcohol esters	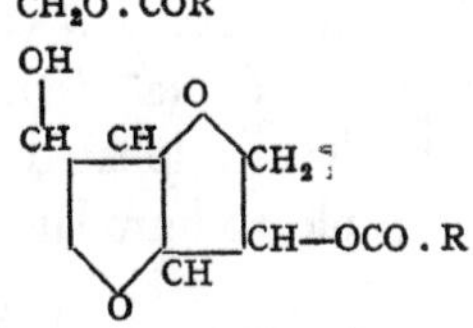	A	C	C	C	B	A
	(*c*) Polymerised poly-glycol esters	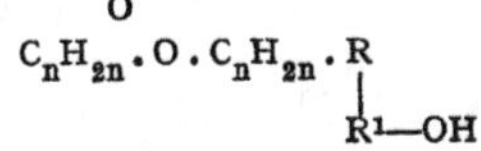	A	B	C	C	A	A
Nitrogen Compounds	(*a*) Fatty acid amide derivatives	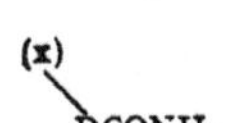	A	B	B	B	B	D
	(*b*) Quaternary ammonium salts	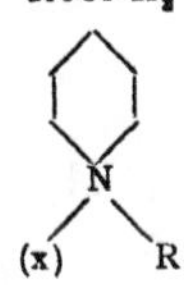	C	B	B	C	C	D

* In soft water A—Excellent B—Good C—Fair D—Poor

There are many different ways of classifying emulsifiers and other surface-active agents; for example, cosmeticians will frequently encounter references to *anionic*, *cationic*, and *non-ionic* agents. Whilst non-ionic emulsifiers may be used with anionic emulsifiers, anionic and cationic emulsifiers must not both be used in the same preparation since they are incompatible and the result of adding the anionic agent, if present in sufficient amount, will simply be to inhibit the action of the cationic agent.

Many well known emulsifiers are electrolytes and hence, like other salts, acids, and bases, dissociate in water, i.e. the molecule splits up or—more correctly—" ionises " to yield a positively charged portion and a negatively charged portion. If the active part of the emulsifying agent is contained in the negatively charged portion of the molecule, then the emulsifier is termed *anionic* (*anionic* because, in an electric field, the negatively charged portion of the surface-active molecule would be attracted to the positive electric pole, i.e. the anode). Conversely, if the active portion of the molecule is contained in the positively charged portion of the molecule then the emulsifier is termed *cationic* (*cationic* because, in an electric field, the positively charged portion of the molecule would be attracted to the negative pole, i.e. the cathode).

Some emulsifiers do not dissociate or " split up " into portions carrying an electric charge when dissolved in water and we term these *non-ionic* agents.

The following exemplify well known cosmetic examples of these three types of emulsifiers :

(*a*) *Anionic*

Soap is an excellent example of this class since it dissociates as follows :

$$R.COONa \longrightarrow R.COO^- + Na^+$$

where R represents a long hydrocarbon chain of more than 11 carbon atoms. [The positively charged Na^+ is not the active portion of the emulsifying agent.] The salts of sulphated and sulphonated fatty alcohols behave similarly ; for example, sodium lauryl sulphate ionises as follows :

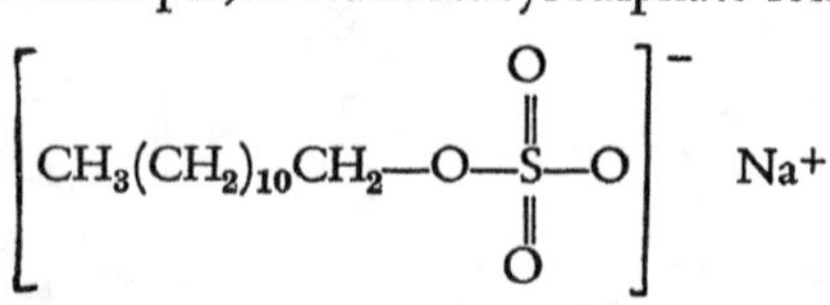

and sodium lauryl sulphonate :

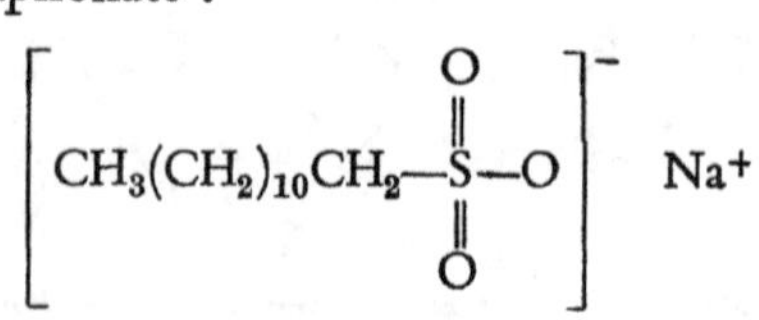

(b) Cationic

Cationic agents represent a more recent development in the field of surface-active chemistry. Such agents dissociate as follows :

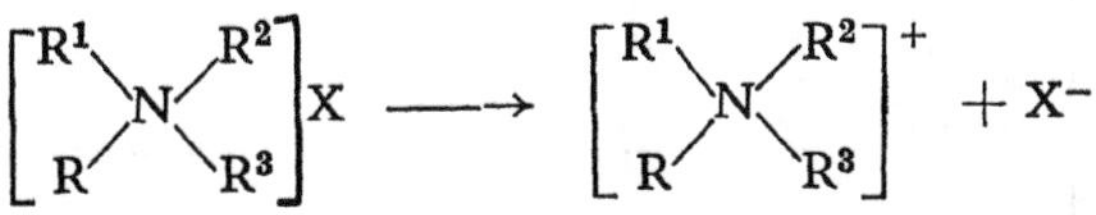

where R represents a long chain hydrocarbon, R^1, R^2, and R^3 represent quite short organic groups such as methyl, ethyl, benzyl, etc., and X represents any salt-forming acidic group, as, for example, the halogens, SO_4H, CH_3COO—, etc. The negatively charged portion X is, relatively, unimportant as the active emulsifying properties are contained in the positively charged, i.e. cationic, portion of the molecule.

A well known cationic active agent is, for example, cetyl trimethyl ammonium bromide which ionises thus :

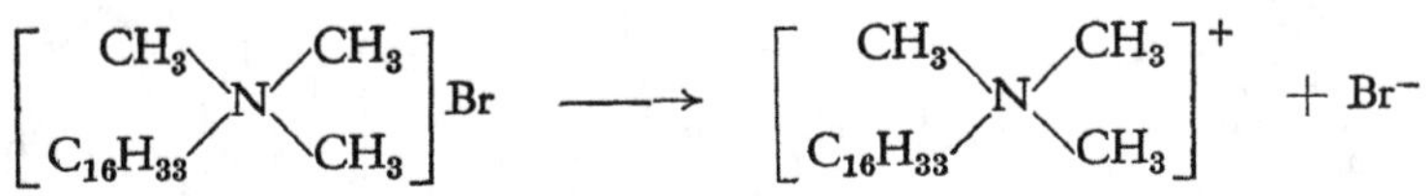

The sapamines (i.e. salts of diethylaminoethyloleylamide) are also well known agents of this class.

(c) Non-ionic agents

Some of the non-ionic agents are esters and can be represented by R . COOR′, where R represents a long hydrocarbon chain and R′ an alcohol or radicle containing a number of alcohol groupings.

Others are ethers of the type

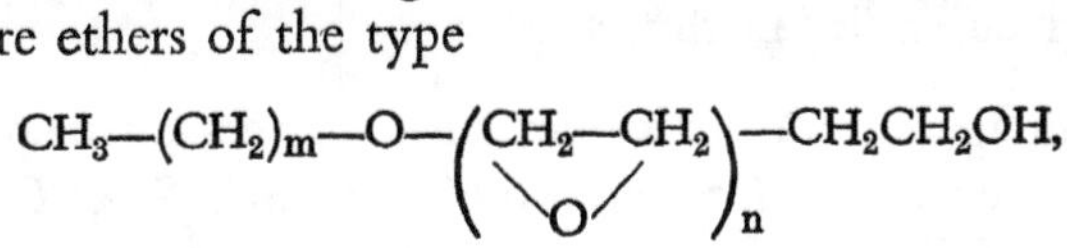

Well known cosmetic examples of non-ionic emulsifiers are the " Spans " and " Tweens ", " Carbowaxes ", " Polawax ", " Nonex " surface agents and certain of the " Collones " and " Texofors ". The number of proprietary names for such agents is constantly increasing.

" TAILORED " EMULSIFIERS

The " Spans " comprise a series of long chain fatty acid partial esters of hexitol anhydrides ; these hexitol anhydrides include sorbitans and sorbides, mannitans and mannides. The " Tweens " comprise a series of polyoxyalkylene derivatives of hexitol anhydride partial long chain fatty acid esters. (For HLB values of some of these emulsifiers refer to earlier discussion in this chapter.)

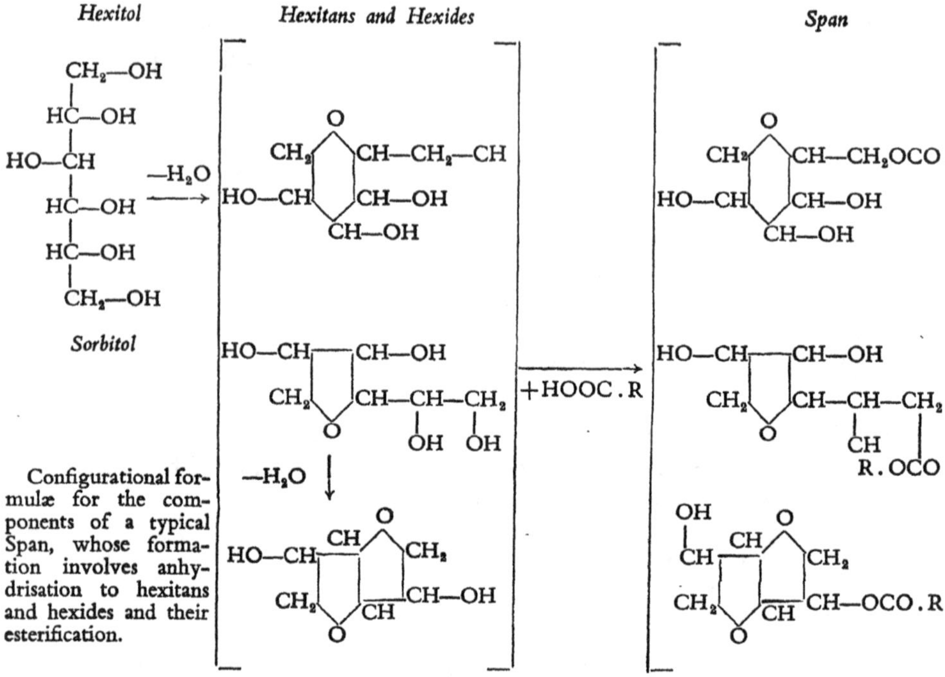

Configurational formulæ for the components of a typical Span, whose formation involves anhydrisation to hexitans and hexides and their esterification.

R = the residue of a long chain fatty acid.

(*Courtesy, Atlas Chemical Co.*

The chemical starting materials for these derivatives are the hexahydric alcohols, mannitol and sorbitol. Examples of some of the better known "Spans" and "Tweens" and their approximate constitution have been given earlier in this chapter.

The advantages of non-ionic over other surface-active emulsifiers have been summarised by Griffin and Rose (*Proc. Sci. Sect. T.G.A.*, 6 Dec. 1945, p. 17) as follows:

(1) They are neutral. As prepared and marketed, non-ionic agents may show a slightly acidic or basic reaction. This is usually due to a small amount of residual catalyst, the action of which is enhanced because there is only a small amount of water present. As employed in cosmetics they give neutral creams unless basic or acidic components are included for specific effects.

(2) They are versatile. By proper choice of emulsifier or emulsifier blend, wax combinations of widely differing character may be handled. (*See* Classification of Emulsifiers by HLB.)

(3) They are stable to freezing. Emulsions properly prepared using non-ionic emulsifiers are extremely resistant to freezing.

(4) They are stable to electrolytes. This characteristic has four aspects :

(*a*) Precautions need not be taken when hard water is to be used.

(*b*) Inorganic impurities in raw materials used in cosmetic formulations will have less harmful effects upon the emulsions.

(*c*) Antiperspirants and deodorants may be formed using aluminium salts, buffers, etc.

(*d*) Cosmetics having any desired *p*H may be prepared by using the proper additives.

(5) They are preformed. Many soaps are formed *in situ* and require skilful handling on the part of plant operators.

(6) They are compatible with many surface-active agents of the ionic type. Frequently they are valuable auxiliary emulsifiers for soap type cosmetics.

(7) They are generally non-toxic. During several years use in cosmetics of the hexitan fatty acid esters and their polyoxyethylene derivatives, there has been no evidence of toxicity.

Determination of Emulsion Type

Neither the dilution method, which depends upon the fact that an emulsion can be diluted only by the addition of the continuous phase, nor the indicator method, which depends upon the spreading of an oil-soluble dye (e.g. Sudan III) on the surface of an emulsion are to be recommended as they may lead to a reversal in type. Two suitable methods exist in (*a*) the electrical conductance method proposed by Clayton (*Brit. Ass. Colloid Repts.*, 1918, **2**, 114), and (*b*) that devised by Carriere (*Chem. Weekblad*, 1929, **26**, 413), based upon differences in refractivity, for full details of which the original paper should be consulted.

Clayton's method is based upon the insulating properties of oils as opposed to the conductance of water. If an emulsion is subjected to an electric current, then if oil be the continuous phase (i.e. if it is of the water-in-oil type), no current will flow, or at most only a fraction of a milliampere, whereas if water is the continuous phase (i.e. the emulsion is of the oil-in-water type) an appreciable current of 10-13 milliamperes may flow through the emulsion. As a simplification of this method, a lamp may be substituted for the milliampmeter, lighting of the lamp denoting an o/w emulsion, or at least the continuous phase is aqueous. The nature of the continuous phase is readily determined with a glass electrode *p*H meter, as a steady *p*H reading can only be obtained if the continuous phase is aqueous.

DERMATOLOGICAL CONSIDERATIONS OF EMULSION TYPE

Several theories regarding the relative efficacy and uses of oil-in-water and water-in-oil emulsions have appeared in the cosmetic literature.

Gattefosse (*Soap Perfum. Cosmet.*, 1939, p. 961) classified persons into those possessing one of four types of skin, viz. :

(*a*) greasy
(*b*) greaseless
(*c*) hydrated
(*d*) dehydrated

and suggested that the hydrated skins of the sub-Nordic type need fatty creams belonging to the w/o group, the o/w creams being used for persons resident in a warmer climate. Comparing the skin to a protein gel, e.g. he suggested that roughly similar effects may be obtained in the laboratory by demonstrating the physical reactions of such a sheet of gelatin.

Marriott (*Soap Perfum. Cosmet.*, 1940, p. 307) pointed out that dry proteins are preferentially wetted by oil rather than water so that application of greases produces an immediate water-resistant surface. He compared the problems of skin penetration with those governing the *currying* process of the leather industry where similar difficulties arise.

The assumption, however, that the human skin can be compared to either gelatin or leather with any accuracy in prediction is not correct in that the former is protected by an intact and normally impervious keratinous layer, kept flushed by secretions of the sebaceous and sweat glands, while in the filling of animal hides, the epidermis is previously *destroyed* by immersion in alkali. In the case of sheet gelatin the protective layer is absent.

Goodman (*J. Amer. med. Ass.*, 1940, p. 1005) also proposed a theory of skin irritation in which the skin was classified into two major groups (oil-in-water and water-in-oil). He claimed that the vehicle may be of greater importance than the active ingredient, recommending that applications to the skin be made by substances in the same phase. As an example he states that in cases of skin irritation in which the majority of practitioners stop further use of soap and water, they are, in reality, stopping the use of o/w emulsions, and to be consistent they should switch over to the use of a w/o type product of which lanolin bases are an example. Unfortunately, the example he gives can be more readily (and more satisfactorily) explained in other ways. Moreover, many skins intolerant of soap and water, are readily soothed by the use of an o/w emulsion containing an emollient oil, and of mild *p*H. In the case of an inflamed skin, however intolerant it may be to soap and water, it may be just as intolerant to w/o emulsions which inhibit the natural skin respiration and radiation and increase skin heat. Any irritation due to water or o/w emulsions, assuming perfumes and irritant substances absent, may be due to the *hypotonic* nature of such solutions, a point worthy of study. So far as lanolin is concerned, this has valuable emollient properties which are manifest not only in w/o but in o/w emulsions.

In dealing with *suppositions* such as the above, it would be as well to consider the *evidence* now available as to the efficacy of emollients in general and the effect, if any, of emulsification upon their penetrative properties. Clinical and pharmacological evidence regarding the former is conflicting, investigation of the latter—lacking.

Methods so far used to determine the efficacy of an emollient by the incorporation in it of a suitable drug which can be chemically determined in the urine are open to grave criticism.

All such experiments measure the absorption and excretion of the active drug and do not express the penetrating properties of the vehicle itself.

The writer has published (" Skin Penetration ", *Brit. J. Derm.*, March 1941) an extensive investigation into the above problems on post-mortem material of both sexes and varying ages, ranging from 18 months to 65 years of age, and on live guinea pigs, rabbits, and rats, some of the composite conclusions being checked in the case of a human amputation (*See* Chapter on Skin Nutrition).

The presence of polar groups, either with or without water present, was found to confer penetrant properties upon mineral oils and greases otherwise impermeable and to improve their adherence along the skin surface, but no evidence was obtained to confirm the theory that molecular chain length of the fat molecule was of major importance in skin penetration. In w/o emulsions the oil phase is partially absorbed (if of suitable constitution). In o/w emulsions, the effect is primarily cooling, due to evaporation of the aqueous phase, the film of residual oil containing a polar group is partially absorbed and the excess may either be spread over sufficient skin area *apparently* to disappear or it may be rinsed off with water.

There is naturally a *physical* difference between the characteristic feel of an o/w and w/o emulsion, the latter being greasy and the former non-greasy, due to the nature of the film surrounding the dispersed phase. The clinical effect, however, exhibits no appreciable difference, so far as *emollient* effect is concerned, though there may be dermatological reasons why one particular type of emulsion should be used (e.g. o/w for open, raw or inflamed surfaces, w/o for water-resisting properties, i.e. for protective creams for baby use as a protection against voided urine).

If two types of emulsion are prepared, one of the water-in-oil type and the other oil-in-water, each containing equal amounts of the oil and water, using closely related emulsifiers, and the products are homogenised, they will exert similar *oiling* effects on the skin surface. There is only one fundamental difference, i.e. the water resistancy of the w/o type.

For general pharmaceutical and dermatological formulation, the o/w type of emulsion is usually superior. Its non-greasy and aesthetic nature, non-interference with skin radiation, miscibility with serum and the fact that this type of emulsion does not inhibit bactericidal action, make it unique. Cosmetically, therefore, even lubricating creams, or so-called skin foods, need not necessarily be greasy (*see* Chapter 10).

Water-in-Oil Emulsions and Skin Infections

T. N. Rossides (*Arch. Path.* (*Lab. Med.*), 1927, **3**, 1008) has shown that non-virulent strains of staphylococci, which when injected alone produce no infection, do so in the presence of calcium salts, and R. R. Mellon (*J. Bact.*, 1928, **15**, 13) has observed that calcium salts enable bacteria to leave the aqueous phase of an oil-water mixture and enter the oily phase.

In view of the high degree of staphylococcal infections in wounds when treated with calcium compounds, K. K. Jones and M. Lorenz (*J. invest. Derm.*, 1941, **4**, 69) investigated this subject, and concluded that calcium ions in oil-water mixtures containing bacteria facilitate the passage of bacteria into the oil layer; moreover, the formation of insoluble calcium soaps, such as may occur in the presence of hard waters, may protect bacteria against disinfecting and bacteriostatic agents. Bacteria are viable for at least two weeks' time in calcium soap precipitates. Of importance to the cosmetician was the observation that the passage of bacteria into the oil phase by means of the calcium soap, enabled these organisms to enter follicles and sebaceous glands and produce infection.

It is likely that this action will be found to be shared by many water-in-oil emulsifying agents which are not in themselves bacteriostatic quite apart from calcium soaps, and that in view of the protective action of the outer oily phase, it may be desirable to include in such preparations an innocuous antiseptic in both the aqueous and oily phases, to keep such infections at a minimum. (*See* Chapter 42, Antiseptics and Preservatives.)

Emulsion Stability

Having discussed, very briefly, modern concepts of emulsification, types of cosmetic emulsifiers available and the inherent thermodynamical instability of emulsions in general, it is of interest for the cosmetician to consider those factors which, by greatly increasing instability, lead to a more or less rapid breakdown in emulsions.

Before so doing it is necessary to have some idea of what is known as a hydrated colloidal complex or "micelle".

Aqueous soap solutions, of suitable concentration, offer a good example of such a complex. Though of comparatively small size, the soap molecules are able to form, when dissolved in water, colloidal aggregates termed "micelles", in which the polar and non-polar portions of the soap molecule arrange themselves in such a manner that the hydrophobic (i.e. water-hating) portion of the molecule is orientated away from the water, whilst the polar heads of the molecule which are hydrophilic (i.e. water-loving) orientate themselves so that they are turned towards the water phase. Thus, if a soap molecule be represented graphically thus ●▭|, where ● represents the polar head of the molecule, and |▭| the long chain hydrocarbon portion, then we may consider a soap micelle as represented graphically by

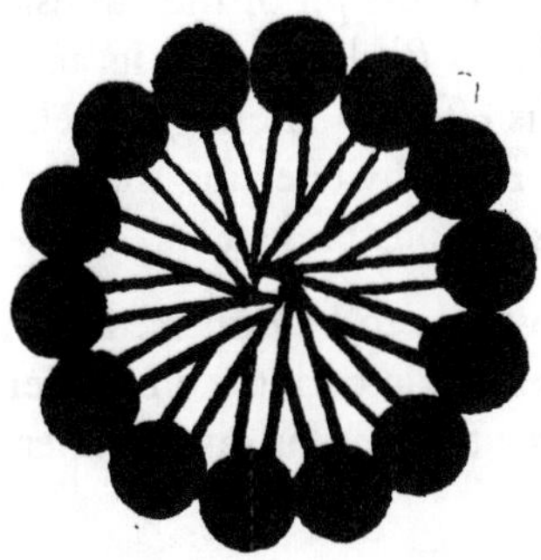

Such a micelle, by entraining and holding bound relatively large quantities of water, is capable of producing a hydrated complex which in turn considerably increases the viscosity of the aqueous soap dispersion. Such micelles are produced not only by soaps but by many of the emulsifying agents which ionise in solution. Because these micelles exhibit characteristics both of a colloid and of an electrolyte such micelles are often termed colloidal electrolytes.[1] (*See* Shampoos, Chapter 22.)

FACTORS LEADING TO INSTABILITY IN EMULSIONS

(1) The presence of electrolytes *may* produce instability, when present in an emulsion in sufficient amounts, in three different ways, viz.:

(*a*) If on ionisation their charge is opposite to the charge on the emulsified globules, they may neutralise this charge and coalescence of the globules may occur.

[1] This represents one type of micelle, some other representations are illustrated in Transparent Oil-in-Water Dispersions.

(*b*) Where the inclusion of an electrolyte introduces a different " ion ", ionic exchange may occur leading to inversion of the emulsion and/or precipitation of the emulsifying agent.

(*c*) Where the electrolyte is present in sufficient amount, it may—because of its affinity for water—withdraw water from any soap micelles or other hydrated colloids present.

(2) The presence of micro-organisms such as bacteria, yeasts or moulds, may, in the absence of adequate preservation, lead to emulsion breakdown in two different ways, i.e. :

(*a*) They may act directly upon, and alter, the emulsifying agent *per se*, e.g. protein emulsifiers, carbohydrates and other fermentable mucilages, or

(*b*) by fermenting or altering other constituents of the emulsion they may produce an alteration of the *p*H of the emulsion which can then lead to emulsion breakdown (i) directly by its action upon the emulsifier, e.g. soaps, (ii) by its effect in altering the electrical charge upon the dispersed globules or (iii) by effecting the size or degree of hydration of any colloidal dispersions present.

(3) A *p*H of the substance to be dispersed (or in which the substance is to be dispersed) incompatible with the emulsifier which rapidly leads to emulsion breakdown, for the reasons given under 2(*b*), (i), (ii) and (iii), respectively.

(4) The physical influences of heat or cold may lead to emulsion breakdown.

Heat because it may cause hydrated complexes to pass into solution and thus reduce the viscosity of the aqueous phase. Moreover, it increases the speed of reaction and may therefore increase the speed of demulsification.[1]

Cold may effect emulsions when the temperature is sufficiently low to produce freezing of the water in the emulsion. If this latter occurs, water is withdrawn from the hydrated complexes mentioned and may not be re-absorbed on thawing. Again the expansion of the water during the process of freezing may rupture the interfacial film of emulsifier.

[1] It must be remembered that the emulsifier itself is subject, particularly if a soap, to hydrolysis in which the reverse reaction, i.e. $R.COONa + H_2O \rightarrow R.COOH$ and $NaOH$ proceeds. Owing to the area of the dispersed phase, a large area of emulsifier is exposed to hydrolysis and there is a tendency for the products of hydrolysis to be continuously removed from the sphere of action ; the free fatty acid formed dissolving in the oil and the NaOH in the water.

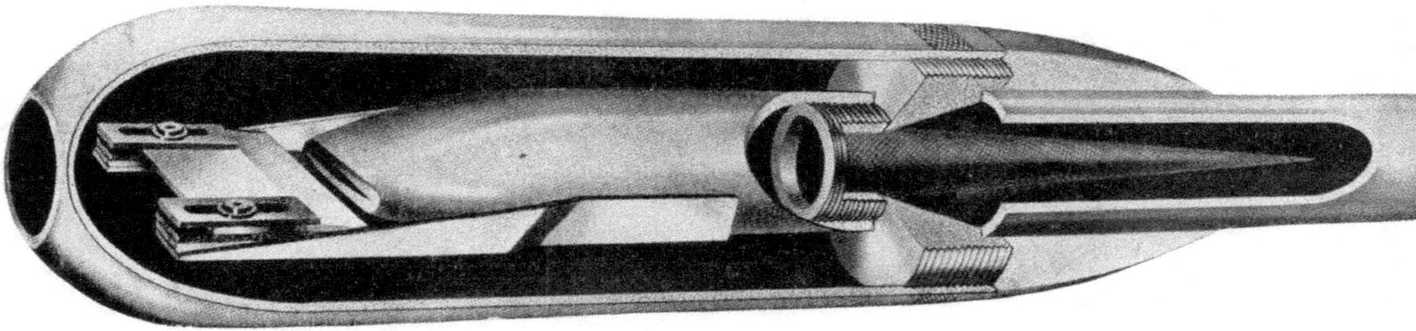

[*By courtesy of Ultrasonics Ltd.*

FIG. 106.—The " Rapisonic " emulsifier.

Determination of the Stability of Emulsions

In order that the manufacturer may determine the stability of his product prior to marketing, various rapid laboratory tests have been devised. For example, a particle size frequency analysis may be carried out at regular intervals to determine the rate of increase in the average particle size of the dispersed phase on storage.

Merrill (*Industr. Engng. Chem.*, Dec. 1943) described a rapid quantitative method of determining the mechanical stability of emulsions by measuring the rate of separation of the internal phase under a constant centrifugal force. The reciprocal of the initial rate of separation at a constant centrifuge speed was taken as a quantitative index of the mechanical stability of the emulsion. According to Merrill the method has been applied to both water-in-oil and oil-in-water emulsions stabilised by lecithin, soaps and vegetable gums and it is claimed that it yields in a few hours results apparently comparable to those obtained by other methods, involving a long-term study.

It is the writer's opinion, based upon many thousands of cosmetical emulsions formulated and examined, that whilst methods such as the above may be a useful guide, there is no satisfactory substitute for long-term storage tests under varying temperature conditions, as to the ultimate criterion. From an examination of the many complex factors at work to produce demulsification, described briefly above, this is to be expected !

To obtain emulsions of satisfactory stability the cosmetician should select an emulsifier suitable to the work in hand, avoid incompatibilities in the ingredient of his emulsion and in the *p*H of the finished preparation, include a suitable preservative (and, if necessary, antioxidant) to avoid decomposition of the constituents of the emulsion. Proper equipment and suitable temperatures should be employed in the process of emulsification and, in the majority of cases, the product should be homogenised to reduce the particle size.

Emulsification with Acoustic Waves

By reason of the very nature of his work the cosmetic chemist must perforce be acquainted with the practical problems of emulsification, some of which have already been discussed in this chapter. These invariably utilise an emulsifying agent, which is dissolved in the requisite phase, or phases of the preparation ; these phases are mixed by simple agitation and then, very often, are passed through an homogeniser. It is not proposed to enlarge further upon these well known operations. It is, however, considered of interest to dwell, very briefly indeed, upon newer commercial methods of emulsification by means of acoustic waves.

The terms "ultra" and "supersonic" have both been used to describe acoustic waves with frequencies beyond the audible human range. Alexander (*Mfg. Chemist*, Jan. 1951, p. 5)[1] has pointed out that since speed exceeding that of sound is invariably referred to as "supersonic", it is desirable (to avoid confusion) to confine this term to that purpose and to use the term "ultrasonics" exclusively when describing mechanical vibrations of high frequency.

Alexander points out that three levels of intensity of acoustic waves can be distinguished, viz. :

(i) those with an energy content of a small fraction of a watt per sq. cm., used for communication, submarine detection, echo depth sounding, etc. They produce no physical or chemical effects and cannot bring about emulsification ;

(ii) those in which the intensity is of the order of 0·5 to 3·0 watts/sq. cm. These waves can bring about cavitation and its accompanying effects such as emulsification ;

(iii) waves of very high intensity, up to and exceeding 10 watts/sq. cm. which have been used to produce a wide range of physical, biological and chemical effects.

Although there is no sharp division between the last two intensity ranges, it should be emphasised that it is not necessary to have the highest intensity sources for the production of emulsification ; in fact, this in many instances is undesirable since it may produce undesired side reactions such as degradation of polymers, denaturation of proteins and general oxidation. Whilst these side effects cannot be completely eliminated even when working at low orders of intensity such as about 1 watt/sq. cm., at such intensities, these side effects occur only to a very limited extent.

The primary effects, produced by acoustic waves in liquids are heat, radiation pressure, enormous acceleration of particles within the sound beam, and cavitation and one—or more—of these effects are responsible for the varied chemical and physico-chemical reactions which occur.

It is pointed out that when a vibrator is moving at high speeds the liquid surrounding it cannot, because of its own inertia, follow the movement and as a result there is a discontinuity between the liquid and the vibrator. This is known as a cavity, and the exact conditions of producing a cavity depend on the adhesive force between the liquid and the vibrator and hence will vary from system to system. Relatively stable emulsions can readily be formed under suitable conditions by the use of acoustic waves. It is even possible by the use of such waves to disperse mercury

[1] From which this discussion is extensively quoted.

in water ; in fact this is the only way of producing emulsions of this type. The outstanding merit of dispersion with acoustic waves, as Alexander points out, is that—in many instances—relatively stable emulsions can be formed without the use of emulsifying agents and this is probably the only practical way of producing such systems, which may have considerable practical advantages for some purposes.

There are four main methods of generating vibrations of high energy:

(*a*) *Piezo electric.* The principle of this method is that certain crystals contract when placed in an electric field. If an alternating field of the same frequency as the natural mode of vibration of the crystal is applied across the faces of a quartz crystal, oscillation of high amplitude will be induced.

(*b*) *Electro-magnetic.* High-intensity sound waves have been generated by exciting aluminium rods at their resonant frequency using the induction principle familiar in the moving-coil loud-speaker. This method has been used for the generation of waves in air but could doubtless be applied to liquids.

(*c*) *Magneto striction generators.* Joule discovered that certain ferro-magnetic materials, notably nickel, alter in length when placed in a magnetic field. The change in length is only very small (1–10 p.p.m.) and is independent of the direction of the field but varies with field strength up to a limiting value. By having an alternating magnetic field at the same frequency as that of the natural mode of vibration of a nickel rod, it is possible to obtain resonance and generate powerful waves in a way very similar to that of a piezo electric generator. There is, however, one distinct difference, in that magneto striction vibrator carries no current and can therefore be operated directly in water.

(*d*) *Mechanical generators.* Acoustic waves are, of course, generated by mechanical means in air by all the normal devices of making a noise (e.g. the whistle in an organ pipe). None of these methods can, however, be applied for the generation of powerful acoustic waves in liquids. *For the design of generators for use with liquids a new principle had to be found and this appears to have been done by Dr. R. Pohlmann.*

Alexander found details of the devices, which will be briefly described below, in the files of the Patent Section of the Research Department of Siemens-Schuckert in Berlin during a B.I.O.S. investigation in Germany.[1] No direct operating details nor the results of actual experimental runs

[1] Alexander, B.I.O.S. Report, 1504.

could be obtained. Preliminary experiments, however, carried out in the Research Department of Wolsey Ltd., confirmed in part at least the data found in Berlin. . . .

THE POHLMANN WHISTLE

Two modifications of the Pohlmann whistle appear to have been examined, although both work on the same principle of using a stream of liquid to produce vibrations. . . .

. . . (It is convenient, though not strictly accurate, to refer to the Pohlmann device as a whistle.) The basic design of the whistle is illustrated in the accompanying diagram :

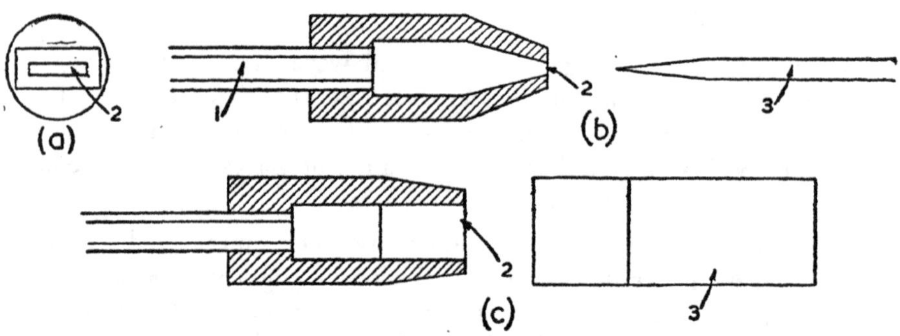

FIG. 107.—The Pohlmann Whistle.

In this figure 1*a*, 1*b* and 1*c* illustrate the construction of the simplest device and the one which has been tested by Alexander. Liquid is expelled through the pipe 1, through the adjustable slit 2 and against the firmly fixed blade 3. Figs. 1*a* and 1*b* show the cross-section and Fig. 1*c* the plan. For the blade an " Ever-ready " razor blade was employed, fixed about 1 cm. from the orifice, whose opening was adjusted so that the liquid was expelled at a pressure of 10-20 atmospheres. [The actual dimensions depend of course on the capacity of the pump used for driving the liquid. Under these conditions the frequency produced was approximately 15 kc.] . . .

. . . The basis of the generator is a jet of liquid which impinges on a blade and deflects it either up or down. The elasticity of the blade causes it to vibrate at its own natural frequency, which is governed solely by its physical properties and dimensions. As it vibrates it deflects the stream of liquid alternately up and down and in this way sets up powerful oscillations within the liquid. The waves are only intense near the actual edge of the blade, and it is in this zone that emulsification occurs. The actual intensity of the sound waves is not very great, but is just sufficient to produce a limited amount of cavitation and hence emulsification. Alexander *et al.*, were not able to detect in the Pohlmann whistle any of the chemical effects such as oxidation and depolymerisation associated with very high intensity sound waves. In Alexander's view a relatively low intensity is an advantage and not a disadvantage for emulsification, since the other effects would in almost every case bring about undesirable properties in the emulsions.

Alexander states "... There is no doubt, from my own experiments, that the Pohlmann whistle is capable of excellent emulsification of two liquids. . . ."

The illustration of the Rapisonic commercial ultrasonic emulsifier (Fig. 106), based upon the principles described, is by courtesy of Ultrasonics Ltd., Yorkshire, England.

The Rapisonic

This is the outcome of several years' research to find a method of producing effectively ultrasonic waves by *mechanical* means. It is the most economical system producing low frequency ultrasonics for emulsification and other dispersions.

Principle

Emulsification is effected by the blade which vibrates at its own frequency in the liquid stream. The vibration is inaudible to the human ear.

Cavitation is taking place continuously in the volume swept out by the vibrating blade. This causes violent molecular acceleration in the medium passing over the blade, and in effect minor local explosions are taking place continuously. Resultant pressures of the order of 30,000 lb. per sq. in. are released locally while the actual pressure at the pump is 150-250 lb. per sq. in.

The vibrating element and jet-form are all enclosed in a resonant bell which concentrates the vibrations and ensures that the velocity of the jet across the blade is maintained regardless of whether the vibrating element is submerged or above the level of the liquid.

Advantages claimed for the Rapisonic are:

(i) *Speed*. Faster and more effective than anything conceived hitherto. Output 300-420 gallons per hour.

(ii) *Efficacy*. Possible to produce particles of 1 μ.

(iii) *Economy*. Low h.p. of prime mover as compared with high output. For small batches necessary to run, for a few minutes only.

(iv) *Convenience*. Light and easily handled, yet robust. Clamping to the side of the mixing vessel is but a moment's work.

TRANSPARENT OIL-WATER DISPERSIONS

It has been known for some years that by the use of high concentrations of certain soluble soaps, for example, potassium oleate (20 per cent.), potassium ricinoleate (33 per cent.), triethanolamine linoleate solution containing free triethanolamine, or ammonium ricinolo-sulphate, it is possible to solubilise aromatic oils in water with the production of an apparently clear " solution ", or, more correctly, with the production of a transparent oil-in-water dispersion. The oil phase so dispersed is not visible under ordinary visual methods of examination. In recent years new surface active agents have become available by means of which stable mixtures of oil and water can be prepared which are transparent, the formula of such mixtures being described in U.S. Patent 2,402,373. The surface-active agents in question are the lauric acid monoesters of the sorbitol anhydrides (sorbitans) or mannitol anhydrides (mannitans) and condensation products of these esters with ethylene oxide.

X-ray diffraction bands of aqueous soap solutions of concentrations between 5 per cent. and 25 per cent. have been measured by a number of investigators (*see* Schulman and McRoberts, *Trans. Faraday Soc.*, 1946, 42B, 165). They considered that " the large dimensions given by the diffraction bands were those between the polar groups of layers of orientated soap molecules. These layers were close packed owing to the high concentration of orientated micelles consisting of approximately 80-180 vertically orientated soap molecules in the form of bimolecular leaflets with the polar groups pointing towards the water. The smaller X-ray spacings were considered to relate to the distance between the neighbouring molecules in the monolayers. It was thought significant by Schulman and McRoberts that these systems could absorb only a small quantity of a non-polar oil with a consequent small increase of the large X-ray dimensions and sharpening of the X-ray band, whereas by the addition of a polar oil (e.g. a long chain alcohol) together with a non-polar oil, to the aqueous soap solutions the o/w ratio could be varied within very wide limits and still give equilibrium conditions. These transparent o/w disperse systems of comparatively low viscosity could be either non-conducting or conducting depending on whether oil or water was the disperse phase. This was shown to be related to the constitution of the interfacial mixed monolayer and its wettability to either oil or water.

" These facts suggested that the systems were obtained by the combined action of the polar and non-polar oils. The swollen lamellar structure of the soap micelle is broken down by the penetration of the monolayer of soap molecules, by the polar oil, and by the swelling of the bimolecular leaflets by the absorption of the non-polar oil between the layers of the methyl groups. This results in a liquid or disordered system instead of an ordered system such as a swollen crystallite, thus enabling droplets of spherical shape to be formed, consisting of water dispersed in

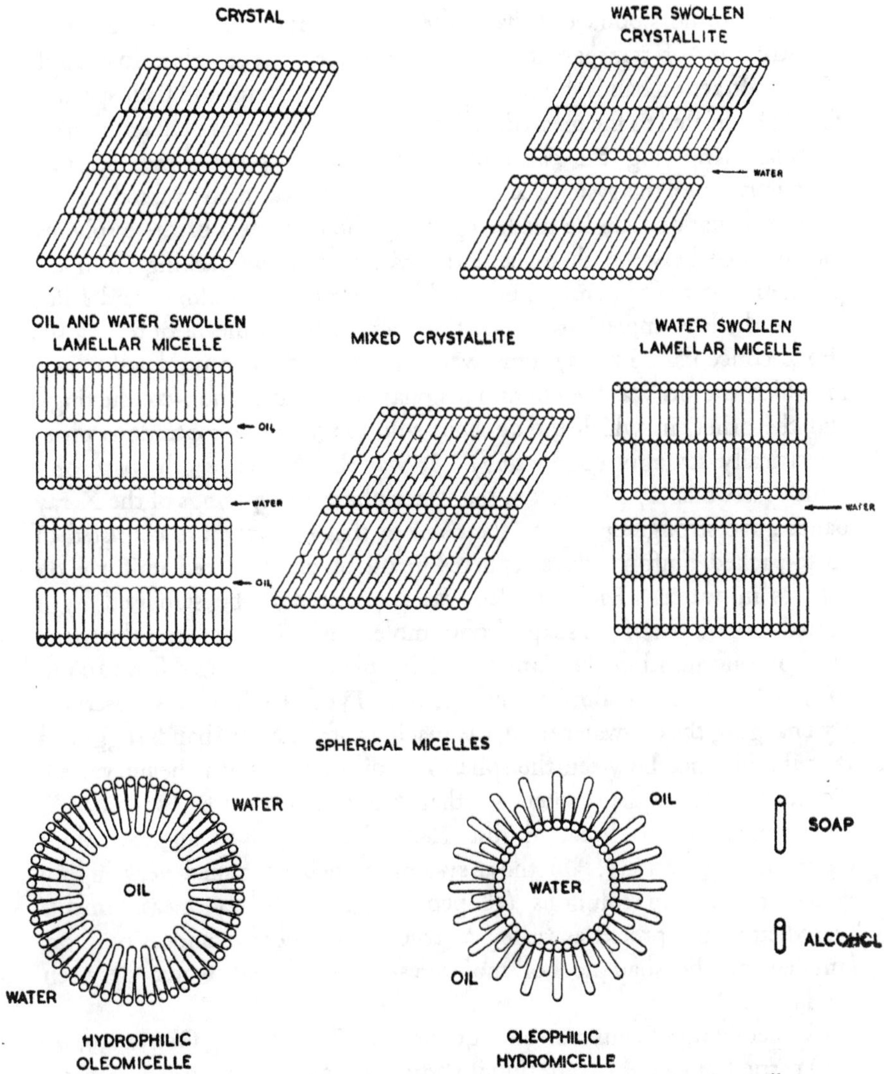

FIG. 108. Drawings illustrating formation of various types of micelle. [*Courtesy, Schulman and Riley.*

oil if non-conducting, or oil dispersed in water if conducting. These systems were then considered to consist of uniform spheres, in closest packing or nearly so, each droplet being covered by a mixed monolayer of the polar oil molecule and the soap molecule."

In Fig. 108 Schulman and Riley (*J. Colloid Sci.*, 3, No. 4, Aug. 1948) portray the various possible forms of associations of soap molecules in combination with non-polar oil, polar oil, and water, compatible with the physico-chemical and X-ray evidence.

These authors point out that if the concept given above be correct for the structure of transparent oil-water disperse systems, then low angle X-ray diffraction bands should be given by such systems, and their spacings should be related to the mean distance between the centres of neighbouring spheres. Knowing the ratio of oil and water phases, the electrical conductivity of the system, and the interfacial area of the mixed monolayer, calculations can be made regarding the diameters of these spheres, the distance between them, and the nature of their packing from the geometry of the system. The work reported by Schulman and Riley utilised the low-angle X-ray scattering technique as a means of testing the above concepts. Two systems were investigated in some detail ; one, in which the oil was the continuous phase (electrically non-conducting), and the other, in which the aqueous solution was the continuous phase (electrically strongly conducting). It was shown that, with soap solutions of less than 27 per cent. in the water phase, the spacings of the X-ray bands gave strong support to the concept that the structure consisted of close-packed uniform water spheres in oil or close-packed uniform oil spheres in water. Each droplet was considered to be stabilised by a mixed monolayer of the soap-alcohol molecules. By changing the soap-alcohol concentration, the diameters of the spheres were varied from 100 Å. to 550 Å., at which dimensions a strong Tyndall effect was observed. By changing the oil-water ratio, the spacings of the X-ray bands suggested that the distance between the spheres of oil or water was being varied. Conditions could be chosen so that the spheres were " squashed ", thus giving rise to broad diffuse X-ray bands and to an anomalous electrical conductivity. In those systems which contained very highly concentrated soap solutions (38 per cent.), the X-ray measurements were better interpreted as fitting a structure of short cylinders or short lamellae of the soap-alcohol molecules with oil and water between the layers.

Subsequently Schulman and Friend (*J. Colloid Sci.*, Oct. 1949, 4, 497) carried out a light-scattering investigation on such oil-water disperse systems in order to augment the information on their structure as found by X-ray and surface chemical methods. They found that the concept that the transparent non-birefringent oil-continuous oil-disperse system consisted of water droplets of uniform size and packing, surrounded by a mixed monolayer of soap and long chain alcohol molecules, was in agreement with the light-scattering results and that, by calculation, dimensions were obtained for the diameters of the droplets over the range 100–400 Å. agreeing with those calculated by surface chemical methods.

To summarise, it is now generally accepted that solutions of substances, relatively insoluble in water, only occur in water in the presence of micelle (i.e. aggregates of colloidal dimensions in which, in the case of ionic micelles, their polar heads are orientated towards the aqueous phase) and that the substances solubilised, if non-polar, are taken up into the interior of the micelle; substances which are water-soluble and oil-insoluble being taken up by the polar group of the micelle.

In addition to such cases as we have discussed above, in which we have considered the solution of substances (relatively insoluble in water), in water, there exists the converse of water being " taken up " in fatty materials. In connection with this phenomenon, the work of Schmitt and Palmer (*Cold Spring Harbor Symposium on Quantitative Biology*, Vol. VIII, 1940) is of interest. They studied the X-ray diffraction patterns of lipide and lipide-proteins and showed that bimolecular leaflets occur in emulsions of brain extracts.

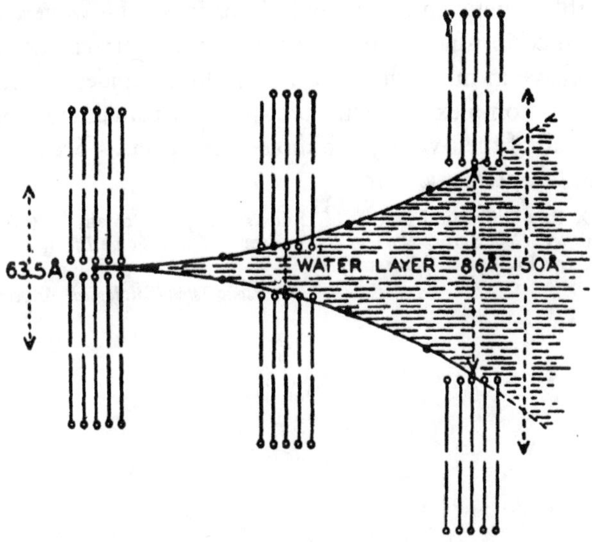

FIG. 109.—Schematic representation of the thickness of the water layers between bimolecular leaflets of mixed lipides as a function of the relative amount of water with which the lipides were emulsified. Points represent values obtained when the water content was 0 (dry), 25, 50, 67, and 75 per cent.

" The amount of water which occurs between the bimolecular leaflets in emulsions of brain extracts, these investigators state, is shown graphically in the above figure. In a 25 per cent. emulsion the spacing observed is 150 Å. of which not more than 65 Å. is due to the lipide double layers, leaving some 85 Å. for the thickness of the water layers. Stable emulsions are formed which give rise to the longest spacings when no electrolytes are present. Moreover, organic solvents may also penetrate the layers and cause considerable separation at the apolar interfaces.

" The presence of electrolytes has a striking effect on the interlayer water content of emulsions of mixed brain lipides. Univalent cations such as sodium or potassium reduce the spacing in amounts depending upon the concentration. In a 33 per cent. emulsion, approximately 0·6 M. potassium chloride was required to reduce the spacing to nearly that obtained from the longest lipides when dry. Calcium chloride was found to produce the same effect in a concentration of only 0·04 M. Schmitt and Palmer point out that the striking effect of calcium ion in expelling the water from between the layers may have considerable significance in physiological phenomena."[1]

At first sight, it might appear that the above work has little connection with cosmetic emulsions and dispersions. However, sterols and lecithin are used in toilet preparations, and in the presence of fatty acids probably behave in much the same way as brain lipides and it may well be that many complex cosmetic preparations containing lipoids, hold some, if not all of their water, as bimolecular leaflets. *See* discussion also on Lanolin, Chapters 4 and 10.

[1] From X-Ray Diffraction Studies of Lipide and Lipide-Protein " by F. O. Schmitt and K. J. Palmer, *Cold Spring Harbour Symposium on Quantitative Biology*, 1940. (With permission of the Biological Laboratory.)

Long Island Biological Association, U.S.A.

CHAPTER 42

ANTISEPTICS AND PRESERVATIVES

Before discussing the necessity of adding such substances to cosmetic and toilet preparations it is very necessary to understand clearly what is meant by the term " antiseptic " ; how it differs from the terms " bacteriostatic " and " germicide ", and also what is meant by the word " preservation ".

If the active agent incorporated *kills* the bacterial cell, so that under no method of treatment can it be rendered viable again, then that substance is a *germicide.*

An *antiseptic* has been defined as *a substance which will prevent growth either by killing or inhibiting the organism.* This definition of an antiseptic appears to me to be very loose, since if it kills the organism it is a germicide whilst if it only inhibits it, it does not differ from *a bacteriostat,* which is *a substance capable of inhibiting growth.*

If the active agent is incorporated merely to discourage the growth of bacteria, fungi or yeasts in the product itself, i.e. to preserve the colour, odour, and appearance of the preparation from deterioration due to by-products of bacterial and fungal metabolism, then the active substance is a *preservative.*

Whilst a preservative and an antiseptic can thus both possess the same property, namely, inhibition of growth, there is a well understood difference in that, when the term *antiseptic is used, it is understood that the concentration of active substance is sufficient to carry over to the skin or wound (which is being treated) sufficient of the agent to check the growth of organisms on that skin or wound (i.e. anti-sepsis—preventing sepsis), though—unless it is germicidal—it will not kill them.*

In general the cosmetic chemist is concerned with the aspect of " preservation " of cosmetic " make-up preparations ", etc., and with antiseptic action in the formulation of special soaps designed for surgical, deodorant, and other specialised purposes. In the case of shaving preparations the emphasis again is on *preservation* although in the case of after-shave lotions and other shaving specialities, antiseptic action may also be desired.

Necessity of Preserving Cosmetic and Toilet Preparations

The contamination of cosmetic preparations by micro-organisms may be (*a*) visible, (*b*) invisible.

Visible contamination. Probably the most obvious form of contamination is that of fungal growth either on the product itself, or on the wad or package. In general, bacterial growth is not so obvious though it may exhibit itself through degradation of one or more of the components of the cream. This may take the form of discoloration of the product, for example, liquefaction with coloured pools of liquid, or of decomposition of the perfume or other component of the cream usually with an accompanying disgusting odour.

Invisible contamination. This is almost invariably bacterial, the organisms being ones that have not affected any of the physical characteristics of the product though they may or may not be pathogenic.

Because of the obvious nature and frequency with which mould spoilage occurs, this aspect will be considered first.

Mould Growth

Even where conditions are entirely unfavourable for bacterial growth there will usually be found one or more species of mould capable of developing.

Mould spores are present in very large numbers in the air, and on growing and stored foodstuffs, timber, etc. It is therefore impracticable to attempt to market a product without adequate preservation since, however carefully the air may be conditioned in the factory and the container and wads sterilised, mould will develop when in use by the customer.

For growth, moulds require :

(i) *a high moisture content ;* present in most creams and lotions ;

(ii) *a source of carbon and nitrogen* as nutrients ; the commonest sources of carbon in cosmetic preparations are glycerin, sorbitol, etc. Ammonium salts, amino derivatives, protein and certain perfumery components may supply the nitrogen ;

(iii) *access of air.* As Galloway (*Perfum. essent. Oil Rec.*, 1952, **3**, 82) has pointed out, all moulds are anaerobic and the presence of air is essential ; thus mould growth should not be a problem in well-filled tubes but becomes one in jars and bottles ;

(iv) *suitable conditions of temperature.* Unfortunately as the optimum temperature range lies between 20°-40° (Galloway) this is usually provided in the ordinary shelf-life of the product.

The above reasons should make it evident that, in the majority of cosmetic preparations, conditions are very suitable indeed for mould growth and it is therefore necessary to add a fungicide.

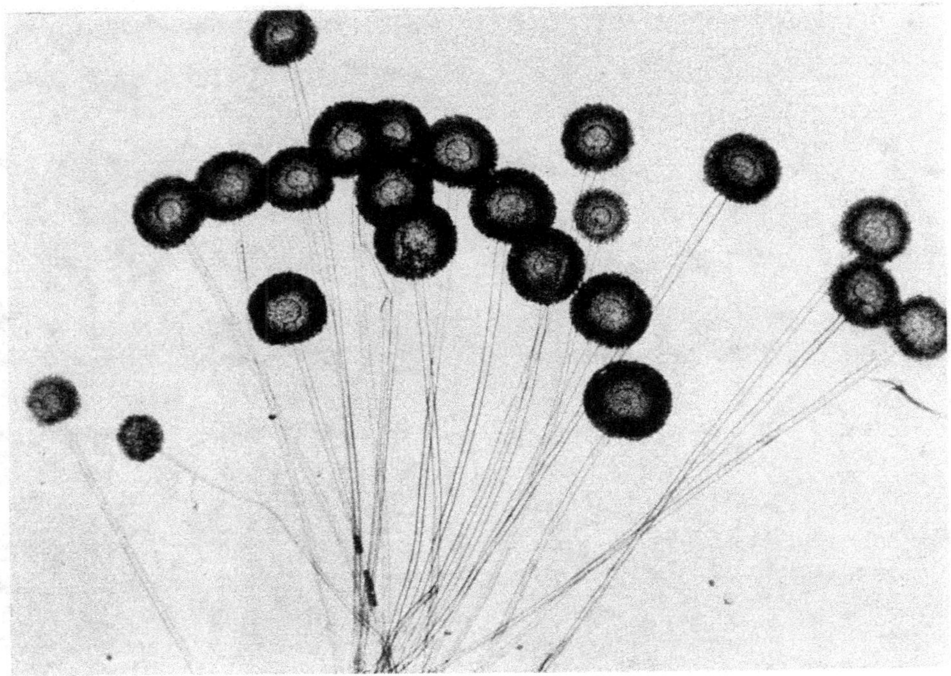

[*By courtesy of John & E. Sturge Ltd.*

FIG. 110.—Aspergillus Niger—culture from a single spore. (*a*) Spore-heads of Aspergillus Niger direct from a coffee bean.

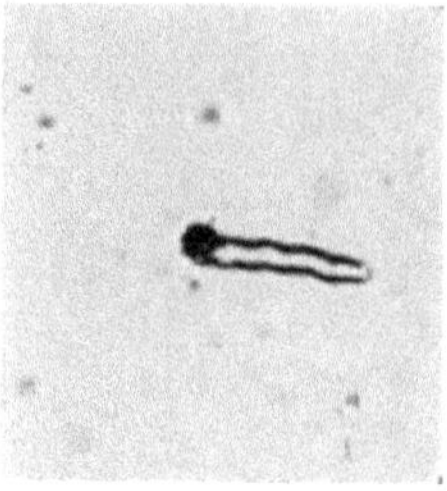

(*b*) single spore germinating.

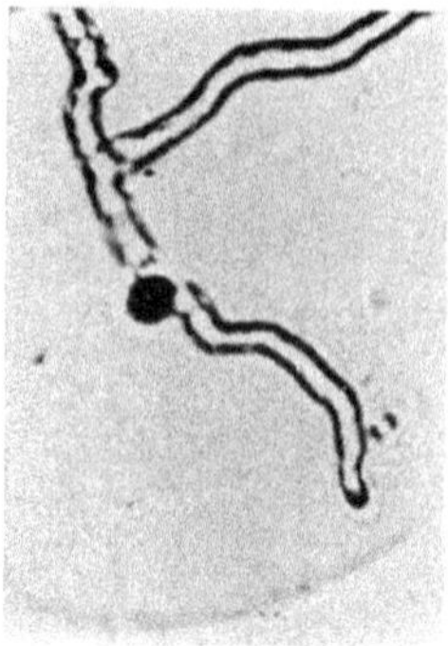

(*c*) 7 hours later.

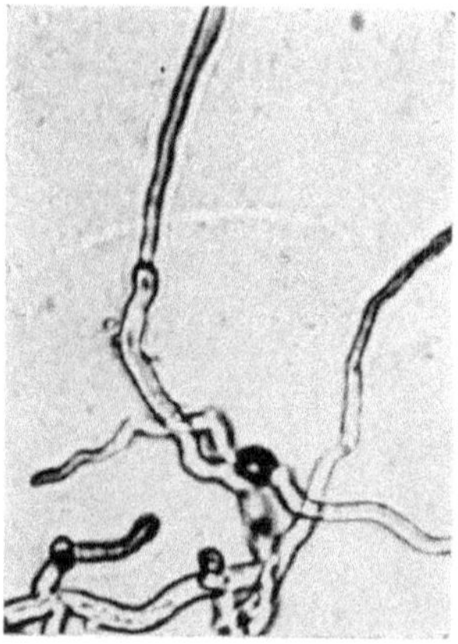

(*d*) after 24 hours.

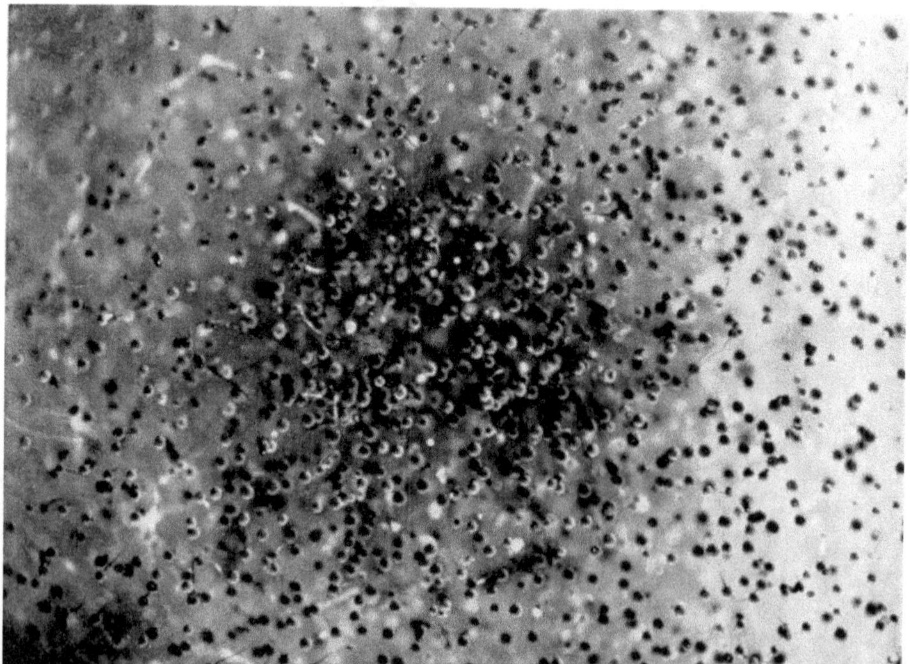

(*e*) and after 4 days, spore-heads fully formed.

[*By courtesy of John & E. Sturge Ltd.*

FIG. 111.—Aspergillus Niger—culture from a single spore.

Substances employed as fungicides (or fungistatics), i.e. killing (and/or inhibiting) the growth of fungi respectively, in cosmetics comprise esters of parahydroxybenzoic acid; chlorinated cresols and xylenols; salicylic acid, benzoic acid and benzoates (when the *p*H of the product is suitable), G-4, etc. These will be discussed more fully under their respective headings.

The rapid development of fungal growth under suitable conditions is well illustrated by Fig. 111, showing the development of Aspergillus Niger from a single spore ("Moulds in Industry", *Isolation and Selection of a Strain*, by courtesy John and E. Sturge Ltd.).

It is of interest to note that Agello, Grant and Dutzke (*Arch. Derm. Syph., Chicago*, 1951, **63**, 747) developed a method of maintaining viable cultures of pathogenic fungi by storing them in mineral oil. Similar results have been obtained in the case of bacterial spores as discussed later in this chapter. It would appear that the mineral oil merely acts as an inert atmosphere in which they can remain viable. The main interest of this work to the cosmetic chemist is to illustrate once again that it is not wise to assume the purity of any raw material purely on the basis of chemical analysis, and further, that the addition of a suitable antiseptic or preservative to any cosmetic preparation should be a *sine qua non*. In choosing such a preparation the relative solubility of the agent in the oil and water phases is important.

Bacteria

Whilst there can be no two opinions about the aspect of mould growth on products—the customer can obviously see it—the problem of bacterial growth from the aspect of the manufacturer is not quite so "clear cut". In general, apart from specialised products such as certain cheese, "mouldy" products are discarded and not eaten. The position with bacteria is quite different in that none of the food which we eat, unless it has previously been heat-sterilised, is free from bacterial infection. Further, the very process by which food is utilised in the human body, as well as the synthesis of certain vitamins of the B-complex (*see* Chapter 3) depends upon bacteria; in fact the suppression of such bacteria by means of some of the antibiotics now in use presents a serious therapeutic problem.

The skin swarms with various bacteria, although many of these are non-pathogenic and the dust in the house and the street is heavily contaminated with bacteria. It might be argued, why bother with cosmetics; bacteria do not reveal their presence, the user's hand will not be sterile anyway.

Whilst the above argument is true in some respects, there are exceptions in that many cosmetic preparations may be applied to *disguise* some scratch, some patch of erythema or even an infection of the skin, prior to going to a theatre or dance ; shaving creams, brushless and saponaceous, are applied prior to shaving in which operation the skin may receive a number of tiny cuts, whilst astringent lotions and after-shave lotions are applied, after shaving, to a face which may already have been abraded. In the latter instances, the excess brushless shave cream or after-shave lotion is often *rubbed into the skin*, and those preparations are likely to come into *contact with the blood prior to the formation of a protective clot*, whereas in the case of street dust the clot will already have been formed. Reference has been made in Chapter 29 to A. H. Bryant's investigation into the extent to which unhygienic shaving practices effect facial infections in men.)

On balance it would appear reasonable to conclude that whilst there is, at present at any rate, no case for insisting upon cosmetic and toilet preparations being *sterile*, pathogens should be absent and there is certainly a case for *condemning unhygienic preparations loaded with bacteria.*

Bacteria, unlike moulds, will not multiply except in the presence of sufficient moisture and in a medium of suitable *p*H, the optimum being about 7·0 ; on either side of which there are limits beyond which they fail to survive, for example :

	Acid limit *p*H	*Optimum* *p*H	*Alkaline limit* *p*H
B. coli communis	4·4	6·0–7·0	7·8
B. cholerae	5·6	6·2–8·0	9·6
B. paratyphosus	4·0	6·2–7·2	9·6
B. typhosus	4·0	6·2–7·2	8·7
Staphylococcus aureus	5·6	7·2–7·6	8·1

The majority of cosmetic preparations, brushless shave creams, foundation creams, etc., will be found to fall well within such limits.

According to Herbold (*Amer. Perfum.*, June 1938) the three bacterial organisms most commonly found in oily and cream preparations are staphylococcus aureus, Bacillus subtilus, and Escherichia Coli.

Bullock and Keepe (" Bacterial Survival in Systems of Low Moisture Content ", Part III ; " Bacteria in Fixed Oils and Fats ", *J. Pharm., London*, 1951, **3**, 717) have shown that spores of B. subtilis remain viable in oils, fats and liquid paraffin for over two years. This is true even when the spores are free from nutritive media and dried with acetone. S. faecalis has been shown to remain viable in oils, fats and liquid paraffin for over six months. These investigators point out that no indication was obtained of the multiplication of S. faecalis or the germination of spores of B. subtilis in oily media and no bactericide so far examined by them had exerted any marked action on the suspended organisms. Bullock and Keepe, however, add " . . . It should be clearly understood that the work described does not prove that bactericides in oily solution are useless. The organisms are viable in the sense that if the oily antiseptic is washed away *without the addition of moisture*, i.e. by a dry volatile solvent they are capable of multiplying to form a colony. If the oil is injected it is difficult to see how the oil could possibly be removed from the organism without the access of aqueous solutions, i.e. solutions of lipase. In these aqueous solutions the bactericide would presumably dissolve and might well kill the spore or bacterial cell."

Barail (*J. Soc. cosmet. Chem.*, 1948, 150), in discussing the bacteriological testing of cosmetic preparations, states : " . . . We have found amazingly high counts in cosmetics, so high that some of them almost defy comparison with any other polluted source of bacterial or fungal life. On the other hand, a great many cosmetic chemists have during the past years endeavoured to produce cosmetics that were of great bacteriological purity and sometimes even germ and fungus free. . . ."

What is the Most Suitable Germicide or Antiseptic for Cosmetic Purposes ?

Having agreed that it is desirable to include some kind of germicide, antiseptic, or bacteriostat, in a cosmetic preparation the difficulty is often to decide which of the many substances available is the best. In the first place, it is necessary to consider what criteria are available for such preparations and in what preparations is the use of certain substances contra-indicated.

Rideal-Walker Test. This test provides a " performance " test, in that it indicates the concentration of the test substance necessary, in distilled water, to ensure the death of Bacterium typhosum, in a specified time at 18°-20° C. As a reference standard phenol is used. Unfortunately the Rideal-Walker coefficient so obtained is not one which can safely be translated into any practical applicability.

In practice the organisms encountered on the skin are not Bacterium typhosum but organisms that behave very differently, moreover, practical usage conditions are quite different in so far as time and dilution are concerned ; the presence of certain salts may considerably affect the potency of the substances (salt in the case of phenolic compounds), the question of inactivators has to be considered (this is discussed later in this chapter) and such questions as the influence of emulsification and other changes in the physical state upon the efficacy of the substance being tested.

Mechanism of Neutralisation of Antiseptics

In 1948 Morton (through H. L. Davis, *J. Soc. cosmet. Chem.*, Dec. 1951, **5**, 295) showed that " . . . haemolytic streptococci treated with any of the three most popular mercurials showed *no growth in blood broth media* (lacking neutralisers) *but did kill many of the mice into whose abdominal cavities the organism-mercurial suspension was introduced.* In other words, these mercurials found—in animal tissues—chemicals capable of neutralising them and allowing bacterial growth to resume. . . ." At the same time Davis points out that it would not be fair to forget that complete bacteriostasis by an antiseptic which finds in tissues no neutralising mechanism is equivalent in effect to *sterility for that system.* This means that, in the last analysis, a clear demonstration by animals tests is the controlling criterion.

Davis has listed in tabular form the recognised mechanisms by which adsorbed antiseptics may be rendered innocuous, viz. :

Mechanisms of Neutralisation of Antiseptics

1. Insolubilisation—mercurials plus sulphides or thio compounds;
2. Complex formation—solubilisation—copper plus ammonia;
3. Desorption to another surface—phenol to charcoal, serum proteins;
4. Oxidation-reduction reactions—iodine plus thiosulphate;
5. Opposition of charge on colloidal particles and ions—anionics *v.* cationics;
6. Displacement from bacteria by strongly adsorbed innocuous substances;

and has emphasised that *in vitro* testing which relies only on dilution of the antiseptic-bacteria system is likely to give false indications of sterility. He suggests that sterility can be demonstrated by the application of a scheme, an outline of which is given, and which is reproduced on facing page. [With acknowledgment to H. L. Davis, " Introduction to Conference on Mechanism and Evaluation of Antiseptics ", *Ann. N.Y. Acad. Sci.*, 1950, **53**, 3-5, and to the Society of Cosmetic Chemists.]

Davis has suggested that when all other conditions are maintained constant, as the concentration of the antiseptic in a series of medication tubes is increased there is first an excitation of growth, then a gradual reduction in plate counts, and then plates showing no colonies. If one chooses the correct chemical, either as a separate intermediate neutralising bath or as a component of the culture medium, it will be found that organisms so treated can be " revived ". Finally, with increasing concentration of antiseptic, there will be found systems in which, even though one knows how to neutralise the antiseptic, one cannot get growth started again. Then, and only then, does it appear one is justified in applying the terms " sterile " and " bactericidal ". In 1948 H. L. Davis, A. Bloch, and A. A. Stonehill, " Criteria of Sterility ", *Bull. Nat.*

Formulary Comm., 1948, **41**, 69–76, outlined five steps by which any investigator can assure himself and his market as to just what his antiseptic

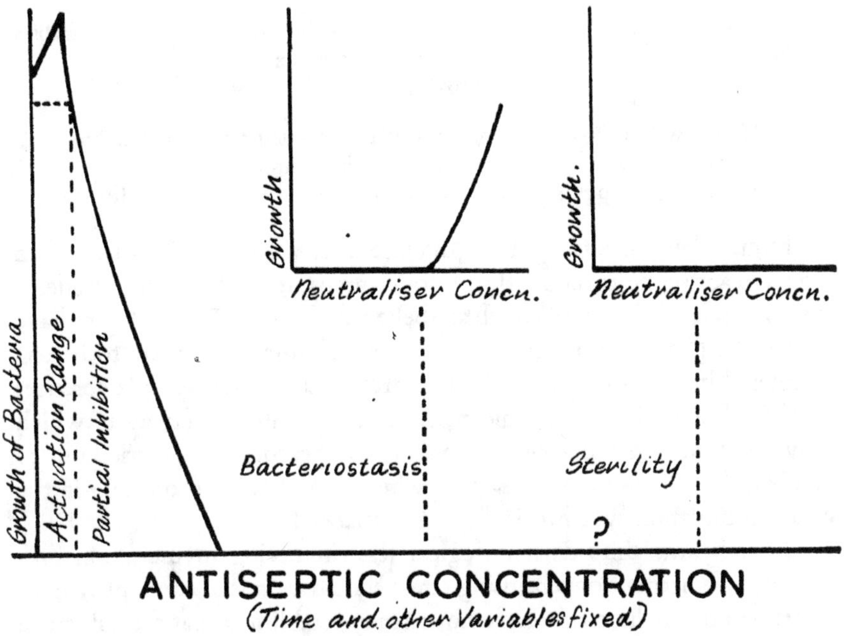

FIG. 112.—Relation between antiseptic concentrations and effects on bacterial growth. Criteria of sterility.

can do—the problem being one in which by successive approximation one fixes the concentration designated as the range between bacteriostasis and bactericidal effects.

EVALUATION OF ANTISEPTICS AND NEUTRALISERS

Step	*Procedure*	*Results*	*Interpretation*
1	Bacteria—medium	Growth	Viable culture, suitable medium
2	Bacteria—antiseptic	No growth	Inhibition *or* death ??
3	Bacteria—neutraliser	Growth	Neutraliser is not antiseptic
		No growth	Neutraliser is antiseptic—unsuitable
4	Bacteria—antiseptic, then neutraliser	Growth	Antiseptic bacteriostatic, neutralised
		No growth	*Antiseptic killed bacteria* or Neutraliser is not effective or Killed by antiseptic — neutraliser complex

Step	Procedure	Results	Interpretation
5	Bacteria—neutraliser, then antiseptic	Growth	Neutraliser effective against antiseptic *and* No killing by antiseptic—neutraliser complex
		No growth	Neutraliser is not effective

No growth in No. 4 and growth in No. 5—neutraliser is effective against *dissolved* but not against adsorbed antiseptic
Step No. 4 distinguishes between bactericidal and bacteriostatic effects

From what has already been discussed, it will be obvious that if an effective antiseptic is required in a toilet preparation, the first consideration is to select substances which are believed (from R.-W. values) to have germicidal properties against a wide range of organisms likely to be encountered in practice ; secondly, to search in the literature for references to the effect of blood organic matter, and possible inactivators which may be found in normal usage, and to have practical tests carried out to confirm the value of any antiseptics which appear to be promising in the exact formulation which it is desired to market.

At the same time dermatological tests involving investigation into any primary irritant or sensitising effect should be put in hand, providing references to the literature have not already established that the substance which it is desired to test has *been* indicated as a potential sensitiser. (There is no justification for skin tests involving the use of a known or suspected sensitiser on a human being, except possibly for the purpose of medical research carried out under medical supervision.)

It is naturally assumed that before lengthy investigations such as the above have been commenced, *the general compatibility of the active material* which it is desired to use *with the other ingredients of the preparation has been tested* and also any other relevant properties such as discoloration, odour, etc.

In the case of cosmetic and toilet preparations for which no antiseptic action is claimed, the position is rather simpler in that the tests required may be reduced to those required to establish that, in the final formulation, (*a*) the added preservative is non-toxic and is dermatologically innocuous, (*b*) that it prevents deterioration of the product due to the growth of micro-organisms and (*c*) that, in itself, it confers no undesirable physical property such as discoloration, odour or instability upon the preparation.

The various active substances which are added to toilet preparations in an endeavour to achieve these purposes are discussed below.

THE ESTERS OF PARA-HYDROXYBENZOIC ACID

Because of their low toxicity, lack of objectionable odour and compatibility with the majority of cosmetic lotions and creams, the various esters of para-hydroxybenzoic acid have been very extensively employed in all types of cosmetic and toilet preparations under various proprietary names. In the United Kingdom the "Nipa" series is probably the best known, though other brands are available.[1]

Methyl Para-Hydroxybenzoate	"Nipag*in*" M
Ethyl ,, ,,	"Nipag*in*" A
Propyl ,, ,,	"Nipas*ol*" M
Butyl ,, ,,	"Nipabutyl"
Benzyl ,, ,,	"Nipabenzyl"

The following table illustrates the different solubilities and melting points of these compounds:

Nipa esters	**Nipagin M*	**Nipagin A*	**Nipasol M*	*Nipa-butyl pure*	*Nipa-benzyl pure*	*Nipa-phenyl pure*
Molecular weight	152·14	166·17	180·2	194·22	228·24	214·21
Melting range ° C.	125-126	114-116	95-97	69-70	110-111	175-176
Solubility g. per 100 g. at 25° C.						
Acetone	64·0	84·0	105·0	240·0	45·0	34·0
Benzene	0·7	1·65	3·0	40·0	4·66	0·67
Carbon tetra-chloride	0·1	0·9	0·8	1·0	0·12	0·06
Ether	23·0	43·0	50·0	150·0	2·0	9·0
Ethyl alcohol	52·0	70·0	95·0	210·0	42·0	17·0
Methyl alcohol	59·0	115·0	124·0	220·0	41·0	15·0
Glycerol	4·5	1·5	1·0	1·4	1·5	0·3
Ground nut oil (Arachis)	0·5	1·0	1·4	5·0	4·5	1·5
Propylene glycol	22·0	25·0	26·0	110·0	12·0	23·0
Water at 25° C.	0·25	0·17	0·05	0·02	0·01	0·002
Water at 80° C.	2·0	0·86	0·11	0·15	0·05	0·01

* Registered Trade Marks in Great Britain and Abroad.

It is of interest to note that "Nipabutyl" is the only representative of the Nipa-Esters which is slightly soluble in hydrocarbons, e.g. it is soluble in paraffinum liquidum in a concentration of approximately

[1] For other brands *see* footnote on next page.

0·07 per cent. at a temperature of about 80° C. and remains in solution in this concentration at room temperature. In so-called micro-waxes Nipabutyl is soluble in concentrations up to 0·2 per cent. and may therefore be incorporated for the protection of the hydrocarbon phase in emulsions and for the treatment of paraffin waxed cork liners and adhesives.[1]

The following table gives the amounts recommended for various preparations.[2]

Material to be preserved	*Concentration of Preservatives* Nipagin M per cent.		Nipasol M per cent.		Nipasol M-Sodium per cent.
Agar emulsions	0·04–0·08	+	0·02		—
Alkaloid solutions	0·06	+	0·02		—
Almond lotions	0·15	+	0·05		—
Aluminium chloride solution	0·1 –0·15		—		—
Boric acid solutions	0·05	+	0·02		—
Carragheen (Irish Moss)	0·1 –0·2	+	0·04	or	0·25
Casein emulsions	0·2	+	0·1	or	0·25
Cod liver oil emulsions	0·1	+	0·02	or	0·1
CREAMS :					
Fat-free	0·05–0·15		—		—
5–10 per cent. fats	0·05	+	0·12		—
10–20 per cent. fats	—		0·15		—
Over 20 per cent. fats	—		0·2 –0·25		—
Creams with lecithin :					
Cholesterin and hormones	0·25	+	0·05		—
Drug infusions	0·15	+	0·05	or	0·25
Electuaries	0·1 –0·15		—		—
Emulsions	0·1	+	0·05		—
Eye drops or Washes	0·06	+	0·02	or	0·1
Flavour emulsions	0·15		—		—
Gelatin solutions ‡	0·1		—		—
Glucose solutions ‡	0·1 –0·2		—		—
Glycerin jelly or solution	0·15		—		—
Gums, solutions	0·12		—		—
Hair preparations	0·1 –0·2		—		—
Hydrogen peroxide	0·1 –0·15		—		—
Injection solutions	0·052	+	0·028	or	0·1
Lipsticks	—		0·2		—
Malt extract	0·1 –0·15		—	or	0·08
Milk preparations ‡	0·25–0·5	+	0·05	or	0·3

[1] Private Communication, Dr. Edrich Boehm.

[2] Other designations for these esters are " Baseptol ", " Paseptol ", " Maseptol " (benzyl, Propyl and Methyl esters) (A Boake Roberts & Co. Ltd., London), and the " Tegosepts " (Th. Goldschmidt, A. G. (Essen), Goldschmidt Chemical Corporation (New York), viz. " Tegosepts " E (ethyl), M (methyl), P (propyl), Tegosept Benzyl, and Tegosept Butyl.

Material to be preserved	*Concentration of Preservatives* Nipagin M per cent.		Nipasol M per cent.		Nipasol M-Sodium per cent.
Milk, skimmed, solution ‡	0·25	+	0·05	+	0·1
Mouth washes, antiseptic	0·26	+	0·14		—
Mucilages	0·1 -0·2		—	or	0·15
Oil solutions	0·15	+	0·15	or	—
Ointments, greaseless	0·1-0·15		—	or	0·2
Ointments, fatty	0·2	+	0·1		—
Pectin solutions	0·12		—		—
*Penicillin jelly bases	0·25		—		—
†Penicillin pastilles	0·26 g. for 200 pastilles				—
Pills	0·13	+	0·07		—
Prophylactic jellies	0·075	+	0·075		—
Soap bark	0·01	+	0·05		—
Soaps	0·1	+	0·1		—
Soaps, antiseptic	0·5	+	0·25		—
Sodium citrate solutions	0·06	+	0·02		—
Starch solutions	0·15	+	0·05	or	0·3
Sulpha drug solutions	0·06	+	0·02		—
Suppositories	0·15-0·5	+	0·1-0·25		—
Syrups, cough	0·06-0·15		—	or	0·15
Tannic acid solutions	0·08	+	0·02		—
Tea infusions ‡	0·1	+	0·05	or	0·2
Tooth pastes	0·1 -0·2	+	0·02	or	0·1
Yeast solutions	0·06	+	0·03	or	0·15
Zinc sulphate solutions	0·05	+	0·02		—

(*Courtesy, Nipa Laboratories, Ltd.*)

* See *Lancet*, 1946, 250, 127, no. 6387.

† *Brit. med. J.*, 2,686–689, 1944.

[‡ The use of *p*-hydroxybenzoic acid and its esters in food is not permissible in the United Kingdom. Article 4 of the Public Health (Preservatives, etc., in Food) Regulations prohibit the sale of any article of food whieh contains any preservative except those listed in Part I of the First Sehedule to the Regulations. Only sulphur dioxide and benzoic acid and benzoates are so listed and the amounts permitted, together with the article of food in which they are permitted, are specified. The term " food " is defined as food or drink intended for human consumption. *Author.*]

Eye Lotions

As pointed out in Chapter 19, although official bodies still recommend " Nipagin " M and " Nipasol " M as the most suitable preservatives for eye lotions in average concentrations of 0·04 per cent. " Nipagin " M plus 0·02 per cent. " Nipasol " M ; Nipa Laboratories have for some time developed a special preparation called " Nipasept " which consists of a combination of methyl, ethyl and propyl *p*-hydroxybenzoic acid esters. By using the " Nipasept " combinations, it is claimed that it is possible to produce a preparation which will function efficiently against all bacteria and fungi. The recommended concentration of "Nipasept" is 0·08 per cent. w/v.

A discussion and extensive bibliography of the advantage of the esters of *p*-hydroxybenzoic acid as preservatives was made by C. P. Neidig and H. Burrell (*Drug cosmet. Ind.*, 1944, **45**, 408).

They make the following points :

(1) Esters of benzoic acid and salicylic acid are less powerful than the free acids.
(2) Esters of *p*-hydroxybenzoic acid, however, are more powerful against micro-organisms than the free acid.
(3) The higher the alkyl group the more powerful is the preservative.
(4) *p*-Hydroxybenzoic acid esters are two to three times as effective as benzoic acid in preventing bacterial growth.

The methyl ester is, they state, generally more effective against moulds whereas the propyl ester is better against yeasts. The toxicity claimed to be low, especially that of the methyl ester. The esters are recommended for use in cosmetic preparations such as creams, hand lotions, gums, hair-waving fluids and soap, as well as for the preservation of pharmaceutical preparations.

A useful table of the amounts of each ester required to inhibit various micro-organisms is given.

Krajkeman (*Perfum. essent. Oil Rec.*, June 1952) points out that the use of the alkali-metal salts and especially of the sodium salt in place of the free esters has been suggested because of their much higher solubility in water, but that certain precautions must be observed in this practice (Heyden Chemical Co. Technical Data Sheet, No. 18-1 (1945). When aqueous solutions are prepared the temperature must not exceed 30° C since, being salts of a strong alkali and a weak acid the aqueous solutions of these compounds have an alkaline reaction and the ester may become hydrolysed. It is of interest to note that the zinc salts of these esters have been suggested as antiseptic dusting powders (U.S. Patent 2,089,197).

PHENYLMERCURIC NITRATE AND OTHER PHENYLMERCURIC SALTS

Weed and Ecker ("The Utility of Phenyl-Mercury Nitrate as a Disinfectant", *J. Infect. Dis.*, 1931, **49**, 440) published a report drawing attention to the bactericidal and fungicidal properties of phenylmercuric chloride and nitrate. Since that time this latter substance has been used in pharmacy and in cosmetic and toilet preparations as a preservative.

In 1943 deNavarre (*Amer. Perfum.* Aug. 1943, p. 29) drew attention to the value of the phenylmercuric compounds in cosmetics pointing out that his experience with these compounds began in 1934 and was applied to commercial practice in the cosmetic industry about 1936.

ACTION OF *p*-HYDROXYBENZOIC ACID ESTERS ON MICRO-ORGANISMS

Ester used	*Amount required per cent.*	*Organism*	*Nutrient*
Methyl	0·04	Aspergillus flavus and Penicillium glaucum	Syrup of senna
	0·07	Penicillium glaucum	
	0·1	Penicillium glaucum	
	0·125	Aspergillus flavus, Mucor mucedo and torula yeast	Liquorice juice
	0·04–0·05	Mucor mucedo	Syrup of cinnamon
	0·15	Bact. fluorescens, B. coli, B. prodigiosus, mucor and yeast	Ointment of glycerin
	0·05–0·15	Tubercle bacilli	
	0·1	Escherichia coli	
	0·125 0·1	B. coli, proteus vulgaris and mucor	Confection of senna, hard gelatin, soft gelatin, tamarind pulp
	0·075–0·1		Malt extract
Ethyl	0·15	Staphylococcus aureus, B. subtilis, proteus vulgaris, Penicillium glaucum	Acid or basic type gelatin
	0·03	Aspergillus flavus and Penicillium glaucum	Syrup of senna
	0·03–0·04	Mucor mucedo	Syrup of cinnamon
Propyl	0·08	Aspergillus flavus, mucor mucedo and torula yeast	Liquorice juice
	0·05–0·1	Bact. fluorescens, B. coli, B. prodigiosus, mucor and yeast	Ointment of glycerin
	0·15	Staphylococcus aureus, B. subtilis, proteus vulgaris, penicillium glaucum and dust	Acid type gelatin
	0·1	Escherichia coli	
	0·05	B. coli, proteus vulgaris and mucor	
Butyl	0·15	Staphylococcus aureus, B. subtilis, proteus vulgaris, Penicillium glaucum	Acid type gelatin
	0·02	B. coli, B. communis lactis aerogenes, aspergillus glaucum, P. terreste and mucor mucedo, Penicillium expansum	

In this time, it is pointed out, cosmetics containing these compounds were sold by the hundreds of thousands of units without one case of irritation or dermatitis being " reported ".

deNavarre states that in the case of karaya waving fluids, as little as 1 : 100,000 was found to prevent fermentation and the development of mould but considered that for general purposes this amount should be somewhat increased. The use of 1 : 25,000 of phenylmercuric borate for the preservation of cosmetic creams is suggested (*loc. cit.*) and evidence given to indicate that, at such dilutions, the use of such salts does not constitute a hazard.

Phenylmercuric nitrate has been used in this country for the preservation of several types of cosmetic products. It is therefore of interest to note that, in the Poisons List Order 1952 (S.I. 1952, No. 2085) and the Poisons Rules, 1952 (S.I. 1952, No. 2086), complete exemption from control is provided for by a Third Schedule entry which applies to " Toilet, cosmetic and therapeutic preparations containing not more than 0·01 per cent. of phenylmercuric salts as a preservative ". It will be noted that both the character of the preparation and the purpose of the mercury ingredient are taken into account in this classification.

Whilst phenylmercuric salts, *at the concentrations indicated, may be considered innocuous for cosmetic and toilet use*, it must be remembered *that phenylmercuric nitrate itself is a vesicant as well as being very toxic* and hence precautions must be taken (i) in supervising the addition of this materal (to ensure that plant operators do not have free access to such a material), and (ii) because of the vesicant nature of the concentrated material, to ensure that it is adequately and completely dispersed in the product in the course of manufacture.

It is known that even complex mercurials will react readily and stoichiometrically with certain thiol compounds, the resulting compound having no bacterial action (Professor H. Berry, " Disinfectants and Disinfection ", *Mfg. Chemist.*, October 1951, p. 395). This question of the neutralisation of antiseptic power has already been briefly discussed. In point of fact it reduces the phenylmercuric and other mercury salts from " germicides " to " bacteriostats ", though from the cosmetic aspect, as distinct from the antiseptic angle, this is not a grave disadvantage.

PARACHLORMETACRESOL [1] (" chlorocresol " B.P.), P.C.M.C. ; I-hydroxy, 3-methyl, 4-chlorobenzene

Parachlormetacresol occurs in the form of colourless crystals—with a

[1] Much of the information concerning P.C.M.C. and P.C.M.X. has been obtained through the courtesy of Monsanto Chemicals, St. Louis, U.S.A., and London, G-4 and G-11 through the courtesy of Givaudan-Delawanna, U.S.A.

characteristic phenolic odour—crystallising at 63°-64° C. It is soluble to the following extent:

	Per cent. w/w
In water at 20° C.	0·4
In water at 100° C.	2·0
In benzene at 30° C.	75·0
In toluene at 30° C.	62·0

It is freely soluble in alcohol, ether, fixed oils and in triethanolamine, caustic soda and in castor oil soap.

Parachlormetacresol was first suggested for use as a preservative for cosmetic and toilet preparations by the author in 1936 (R. G. Harry, *Mfg. Chemist*, 1936) this being found superior (for certain purposes) to the esters of parahydroxybenzoic acid. The efficacy of this substance has since been confirmed by Coulthard who investigated the destruction of bacterial spores by low temperature sterilisation and found that under ordinary conditions of pharmaceutical cleanliness, heating for 15 minutes at 100° C. in the presence of 0·25 per cent. parachlormetacresol was sufficient to *sterilise*. The main drawback of this substance from the toilet aspect is that its characteristic odour is somewhat persistent and requires careful perfuming to disguise.

Parachlormetacresol is highly toxic to a wide range of micro-organisms including common pathogenic and proteolytic bacteria, yeasts fungi and algae. The lethal concentration and the concentration required for inhibition depend upon the organism concerned and upon other factors.

Tested against B. Typhosus by the Standard Rideal-Walker method (B.S.S.-541), parachlormetacresol in castor-oil soap gives a phenol coefficient (Rideal-Walker) equivalent to approximately 25; in distilled water the corresponding R.-W. value of parachlormetacresol is only 13. (Communication, "Monsanto" Chemicals Ltd.) Such figures do not compare favourably with germicides such as Parachlormetaxylenol (P.C.M.X.).

Like the majority of other chemicals which are toxic to micro-organisms, parachlormetacresol is toxic to man; studies with experimental animals indicating a toxicity approximately that of pure phenol. Since parachlormetacresol is much more efficient as a bactericide than phenol, it may be employed as a preservative at very much lower concentrations; hence there is little or no toxic risk in the use of this material as a preservative other than in products intended for human consumption. Its use in food products is, however, forbidden. Under the terms of the current Poison Regulations operative in the United Kingdom, parachlormetacresol is not classified as a poison.

Cosmetic creams and lotions may be preserved by the addition of approximately 0·1 per cent. parachlormetacresol. At such low concentrations no ill effect on the skin is normally observed.

PARACHLORMETAXYLENOL (" Chloroxylenol " B.P.) P.C.M.X. ; 2 chloro-5 hydroxy-1,3 dimethyl benzene

Parachlormetaxylenol occurs as a white to creamy-white crystalline powder having a slightly phenolic odour. This material is soluble to the following extent :

In water at 15·5° C.	about 1 : 3000
In water at 100° C.	about 1 : 200

Parachlormetaxylenol is soluble in alcohol, ether, benzene, terpenes and fixed oils ; it is steam volatile. Melting point 114°–115·5° C.

Parachlormetaxylenol is very toxic to pathogenic bacteria particularly haemolytic Streptococci ; it is less effective against Staphylococci and Gram negative organisms such as Pyocyaneus.

Solutions and emulsions containing up to 5 per cent. parachlormetaxylenol are widely employed in surgical and obstetrical practice and as an antiseptic for cuts and wounds.

As parachlormetaxylenol may be considered to be virtually insoluble in water, it is necessary to use soaps, or other surface-active dispersants, in order to obtain antiseptic fluids of the requisite strength. Castor oil soap is the best dispersant to use for emulsification and with the correct proportion of this soap, parachlormetaxylenol has a higher activity than in the absence of soap. Its activity is, however, depressed in the presence of *excess* soap and a suitable ratio of these substances to employ is one part of part of P.C.M.X. to one part of anhydrous castor oil soap.

About 1 per cent. parachlormetaxylenol may be used in antiseptic creams. For cosmetic purposes 0·1 per cent. should be sufficient, especially in oil-in-water preparations.

DICHLORMETAXYLENOL ; 2 : 4 dichloro-sym-m-xylenol ; 2 : 4 dichloro-3,5 dimethyl phenol ; D.C.M.X.

Dichlormetaxylenol is a practically white and almost odourless powder, melting point 92° C. It is only slightly soluble in cold water. According to some authorities the solubility is about 1 : 9000 (Coalite and Chemical Products). Others consider it less than 1 : 30000 (Monsanto Chemicals Ltd.). It is soluble in alcohol, acetone, ether, etc., as well as in essential oils and certain synthetics [about 79 parts per 100 of industrial methylated spirit; 194 parts per 100 acetone, about 75 parts per 100 terpineol, etc.]. It is steam volatile and sublimes fairly readily.

Dichlormetaxylenol is claimed to have a relatively high R.-W. value against many common organisms such as staphylococci, streptococci, Ps. pyocyaneus, Streptococcus haemolyticus, etc.

It is not a scheduled poison in the United Kingdom and it is understood that no dermatological or toxic disturbances have as yet been reported.

The toxicity of dichlormetaxylenol is very low and of the same order as for parachlormetaxylenol. Tests have been carried out administering to mice both orally and intraperitoneally with the following results (*Courtesy, Coalite and Chemical Products, Ltd.*):

	Oral	*Intraperitoneal*
MLD 50 g. "D.C.M.X." per kilo body weight	4·0	1·0

(Identical figures were obtained on P.C.M.X under the same conditions of test.)

Because of its powerful germicidal activity and low cost, considerable interest has been aroused recently in this material (Gemmell, "A New British Base for Germicidal Soap", *Soap Perfum. Cosmet.*, Nov. 1952, p. 1160. Hexachlorophene *v.* D.C.M.X. in Soap, *ibid.* pp. 1158-59). A mild controversy has broken out over the relative germicidal properties of hexachlorphene (G-11) and D.C.M.X. D.C.M.X. on the evidence available appears somewhat more toxic to Gram-negative organisms whilst comparative skin de-germing tests indicate greater efficacy in this respect for G-11. [*Mfg. Chemist*, 1950, **21**, 237; *ibid.* 1952 (2), **63**; *ibid.* 1952, **25**, 836; *ibid.* 1952, **11**, 1158; *ibid.* 1953, p. 143.]

Dichlormetaxylenol appears to be an effective preservative for inclusion in cosmetic creams and lotions. Suggested concentrations are of the order of 0·05 per cent., subject to final experiments on the particular formulation in view in respect both of efficacy and dermatological innocuousness.

G-11 (Hexachlorophene is the generic name for G-11 approved by the Council on Pharmacy and Chemistry of the American Medical Association); 2,2'-methylenebis (3,4,6-trichlorophenol); bis (3,5,6-trichloro-2-hydroxyphenyl) methane; 2,2'-dihydroxy-3,5,6,3',5',6',-hexachloro-diphenylmethane)

G-11 is the bactericidally active ingredient in a large number of soaps and detergents used for medical, surgical and deodorant purposes. According to the system of nomenclature employed it may be designated chemically by any of the other names given above.

G-11 is a white, free-flowing powder practically insoluble in water.

	Solubility (g. in 100 ml. of solvent at 25° C.)
Ethyl alcohol	50·0
Acetone	191·0
Benzene	9·3
Toluene	5·6
Propylene glycol	24·5
Deltyl® (Isopropyl myristate-palmitate)	20·0

Soluble in vegetable oils and fatty acids with the aid of heat; practically insoluble in mineral oil, glycerin, petrolatum and paraffin.

G-11 was the first bactericide which, when added to soap, was consistently shown to produce a very considerably reduced bacterial skin flora, as shown by counts of the bacterial population of hand washings.

IN SOAP. Because there is a considerable volume of evidence regarding the efficiency of G-11 in soap, and because this subject is of interest in connection with toilet soap processing (Chapter 27) some of the more important findings will be briefly mentioned.

AS A DEODORANT. The American Medical Association, Committee on Cosmetics: Status report on deodorant soaps (*J. Amer. med. Ass.*, March 1950, **142,** 814) found that a potential for controlling perspiration odour seemed to be present in deodorant soaps containing G-11 to a degree beyond that of other types of soaps, and that consderable evidence supported the conclusion that deodorant soaps contiaining G-11 were non-irritating for practical purposes and compared favourably with ordinary toilet soaps from the viewpoint of pharmaceutical elegance.

In a recent study on deodorants Killian (*J. Soc. cosmet. Chem.*, March 1952, **3,** 30) emphasised that all findings "lead to the inescapable conclusion that control of bacterial population on the surface of the skin is the *sine qua non* of the control of perspiratory odour". His experiments showed that a soap containing 2 per cent. G-11 was distinctly superior to plain soap in eliminating offensive body odours and inhibiting their redevelopment.

AS A BACTERICIDE. Hexachlorophene and certain products containing this chemical, have been accepted by the Council on Pharmacy and Chemistry of the American Medical Association for admission to "New and Non-official Remedies". Tests and standards and dosage forms are given. Hexachlorophene is incorporated in soaps, detergents, etc., for topical application and the use of such products for pre-operative scrubbing, and pre-operative and post-operative preparation of the patient's skin is cited. "When used continually hexachlorophene is also an effective prophylactic agent in decreasing the incidence and severity of pyogenic skin infections including carbuncles, furuncles, miliaria, ammoniacal dermatitis, impetigo, etc. . . ." (*J. Amer. med. Ass.*, Feb. 1951, **145**, 563).

Studies by medical authorities have established the lowered incidence of skin blemishes produced by the use of soaps and detergents containing G-11. In one institution where the incidence of pyogenic skin infections was high, G-11 toilet soap was substituted for the normal toilet soap without the personnel involved being aware of the change. Detailed records over a period of one year showed a significant decrease in the number of skin infections. (J. R. Fuller *et al.*, *Amer. J. publ. Hlth.*, Sept. 1948, **38**, 9 ; E. F. Traub, *J. Soc. cosmet. Chem.*, June 1949, **1**, 251.)

According to the literature (Technical Bulletin H-6 Sindar Corporation) the United States Armed Forces have adopted the use of G-11 soaps and detergents for their medical personnel.

IN COSMETIC PREPARATIONS. A cursory examination of the literature might suggest that G-11 is effective only in alkaline media ; this is not the case. For example, when incorporated into a shaving soap containing a large excess of free fatty acids, it still retains its activity (Private Communication, Sindar Corporation). This is the basis of the U.S. patent to Gillette Company for the use of G-11 in shaving cream. Whilst the solubility of G-11 is low in water and the monosodium salt is not very much more soluble that G-11 itself (the disodium salt of G-11 cannot be prepared), none the less, it is understood that this concentration is in excess of the concentration at which G-11 effectively inhibits the growth of bacteria. Alcoholic lotions containing 0·25 per cent. G-11 have been shown to exhibit outstanding deodorant properties. G-11 has also been used in powders.

Spoor and Traub ("Efficacy of Hexachlorophene in Toilet Goods Preparations", *Proc. Sci. Sect. T.G.A.*, Dec. 1951, **16**, 16) found that under controlled usage conditions, certain mineral oil lotion preparations, fatty base, deodorants and both aqueous and alcoholic vegetable oil dressings containing G-11 were found to be effective against general skin and scalp organisms. However, G-11 was not as effective in these oil media as in soap solutions, even when its concentration present at the side of application was higher than that existing in the soap lather. Since G-11 is preferentially soluble in oils, the authors believe that it does not make as effective contact with the bacteria on the skin surfaces as when used in soap or other aqueous media.

G-4. (Sindar Corporation) ; "Dichlorophene" ; 2,2′-dihydroxy-5, 5′-dichloro-diphenylmethane ; 2, 2′-methylenebis-(4-chlorophenol- ; bis (5-chloro-2-hydroxy phenyl)methane).

G-4 is a potent fungicide and bactericide which is used in the United States to preserve cotton and woollen textiles and other materials. It has also been incorporated in hair lotions, and has been suggested for use in Athletes Foot preparations (Technical Bulletin 48-6, Nov. 1948, Sindar Corporation).

It is a white powder with a slightly phenolic odour having the following solubilities :

	g. of G-4 dissolved in 100 cc. of solvent at 25° C.
In water	0·003
In alcohol 10 per cent. by vol.	0·013
20 per cent. by vol.	0·022
50 per cent. by vol.	7·7
75 per cent. by vol.	35·500
95 per cent. by vol.	53·100
In isopropanol 99 per cent.	52·6
In propylene glycol	42·000
In acetone	76·500
In methyl ethyl ketone	67·200
In Deltyl Extra [1]	20·600
In corn oil	8·600

G-4 is also soluble to a limited extent in oils and fats ; however, it is recommended that the G-4 first be dissolved in a small amount of one of the solvents, and that this solution be added to the oil phase.

G-4, with one molecule of sodium or potassium hydroxide, forms mono-alkali-metal salts which are readily soluble in water. Powders containing G-4 have been found, it is stated (*loc. cit.*), to be beneficial, especially when excessive perspiration is present.

As pointed out G-4 is both bactericidal and fungicidal. The popularity of G-11 has tended to overshadow G-4 though this latter substance has virtues particularly where fungi are involved.

The acute oral toxicity of G-4 has been determined in guinea pigs and dogs : M.L.D. 1·00 g. kg. body-weight in guinea pigs, on the basis of a 60 per cent. rate of mortality (Applied Research Laboratories, Dayton, N.J.).

[1] Trademark Reg. U.S. Pat. Off. Deltyl Extra is a mixture of isopropyl myristate and palmitate.

M.L.D.$_{50}$ 3·00 g. per kg. in dogs (*North American Veterinarian*, Jan. 1946, **27**, 26). Skin irritation tests gave the following results :

Patch tests were made on 194 persons with an ointment containing 4 per cent. G-4 : 191 were negative, 3 positive.

Patch tests on 37 persons with a 12 per cent. G-4 ointment : 36 negative, 1 positive.

" ACTAMER " (Trademark Monsanto Chemical Co., St. Louis) ; 2,2′-Thiobis (4·6-dichlorophenol).

" Actamer " (2,2′-thiobis 4,6-dichlorophenol) has recently been found to possess exceptional bacteriostatic activity. Actamer is a colourless, tasteless, essentially odourless powder which has only a very low solubility in water, of the order of 0·0004 per cent. at 25° C. The addition of alkali such as sodium hydroxide to form the monosodium salt markedly increases the solubility, for example :

SOLUBILITY OF " ACTAMER " IN AQUEOUS SOLUTION

Aqueous solution	*Temperature*	*Solubility g./100 cc.*
Water	25° C.	0·0004
Water, 1 mol. NaOH	25° C.	0·29
0·2 per cent. NaOH	25° C.	0·7
0·4 per cent. NaOH	25° C.	1·3
2·0 per cent. NaOH	25° C.	8·2
4·0 per cent. NaOH	25° C.	16·2

Certain of the common organic solvents and fatty matters also act as solubilisers and hence should greatly assist the incorporation of this material into cosmetic and toilet preparations. The following brief list illustrates some of the more interesting examples :

SOLUBILITY OF " ACTAMER " IN ORGANIC SOLVENTS

Solvent	*Solubility (g./100 cc. at 25° C. except where indicated)*
Dimethyl acetamide	72·5
Polyoxyethylene sorbitan mono-oleate	19·0
Polyoxyethylene sorbitan monolaurate	19·0
Acetone	15·0
Lanolin	5·0 (42° C.)
Stearyl alcohol	5·0 (59° C.)
Ethyl alcohol	2·3
Stearic acid	1·5 (70° C.)
Olive oil	0·5
Propylene glycol	0·5
Glycerin	<0·2
Oleic acid	<0·2

The antimicrobial activity of 2,2[1]-thiobis (4,6-dichlorophenol) has been demonstrated by both *in vitro* and *in vivo* techniques. It is claimed to be particularly effective against the gram-positive cocci that make up a large proportion of the normal flora of the skin and which are believed to cause body odour and skin infections. *In vitro* tests have likewise shown this compound to have good activity against some pathogenic fungi. *In vivo*, " Actamer ", in bar soap at a concentration of 2·0 per cent., has been shown to reduce the number of resident bacteria on the skin by 97·4 per cent. after 12 days daily use. At 1·5 per cent. concentration approximately 94 per cent. reduction was effected. A concentration of 1·0 per cent. gave almost 92 per cent. reduction. " Actamer " is substantive to the skin and it is reported that no other compound has been found to have stronger skin substantive properties than " Actamer " without some undesirable effects. The acute oral toxicity, cumulative oral toxicity and cutaneous toxicity of this substance was found to be unexpectedly low for a compound of this type.

Irritation and sensitisation studies were carried out on 200 human subjects by patch tests according to the technique recommended by Schwartz and Peck (*U.S. Publ. Hlth. Repts.*, 1944, **59**, 17). In no instances were primary irritant or sensitisation reactions, which could be attributed to " Actamer ", obtained.

The close structural relationship existing between " G-11 " and " Actamer " is shown in the two formulae set out below :

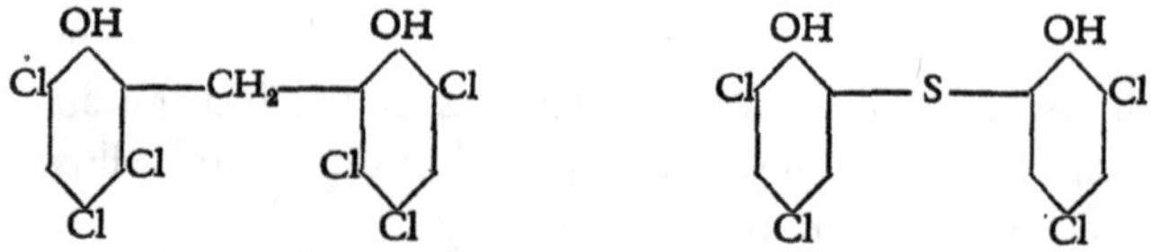

" G-11 " " ACTAMER "

Since soap containing " Hexachlorophene " (G-11) has been suggested (W. S. Gump and A. R. Cade, 1952, *Proc. 38th Mid-Year Meeting C.S.M.A.*, p. 81) as a standard for estimating the efficacy of antiseptic soaps, it is stated (Personal Communication from Monsanto Chemicals Ltd., St. Louis) that comparable washing tests have been carried out with " Actamer " and " Hexachlorophene " and are portrayed graphically at 2·0 per cent. levels in Graph 1, and at 1·0 per cent. levels in Graph 2. It is pointed out that the somewhat greater reduction of resident bacteria after 12 days and the slower return to a normal count can possibly be explained as due to a greater substantivity of " Actamer " to the skin, in as much as " Actamer " exhibits approximately the same degree of *in vitro* bacteriostatic activity as " Hexachlorophene ".

"*Anobial*" (the newest entry into the field of antiseptics active in soaps) is a chlorinated salicyl-anilide of the following structure:

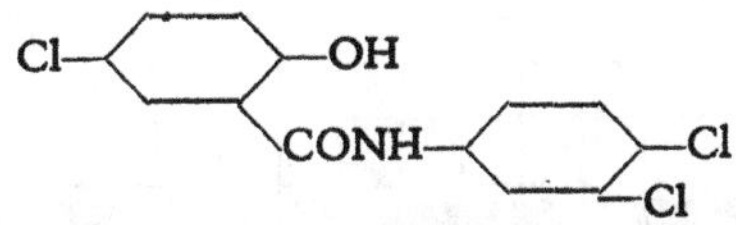

This substance, which is marketed by Firmenich & Cie. of Switzerland, is a powder of slightly yellowish-grey appearance having a very slightly phenolic odour, melting point 244°–246° C. It is claimed that "Anobial" keeps perfectly under normal storage conditions in the dry at a temperature not exceeding 40° C. but that under the action of light it discolours somewhat.

"Anobial" is only slightly soluble in the majority of solvents. Data on this point, according to Firmenich & Cie., are as follows:

	g./100 cc. at 25° C.
Amyl acetate	1·0
Acetone	0·58
Oleic acid	0·07
Ethyl alcohol 95 per cent.	0·25
Ethyl alcohol 70 per cent.	0·03
Isopropyl alcohol	0·25
Dimethyl formamide	23·0
Distilled water	0·0015
Glycerin	0·008
Olive oil	0·15
Castor oil	0·315
Methyl cellosolve	1·88
Propylene glycol	0·08

The sodium salt of "Anobial" is, however, more soluble. The bacteriological action is the same as that of free phenol. The salt solubilities are as follows:

	g./100 cc. at 25° C.
Acetone	4·9
Ethyl alcohol 95 per cent.	3·0
Distilled water	0·5

The bactericidal activities of "Anobial" *in vitro* have been determined by the method of successive dilution; the minimum concentrations obtained, it is claimed, were as follows:

	Mol.	*g./100 cc.*
Staphylococcus albus 1	$10 \cdot 10^{-6}$	0·00032
Staphylococcus albus 4	$5 \cdot 10^{-6}$	0·00016
Staphylococcus aureus (in soap solution)	$8 \cdot 10^{-6}$	0·00025
Proteus vulgaris (in soap solution)	$16 \cdot 10^{-6}$	0·00036

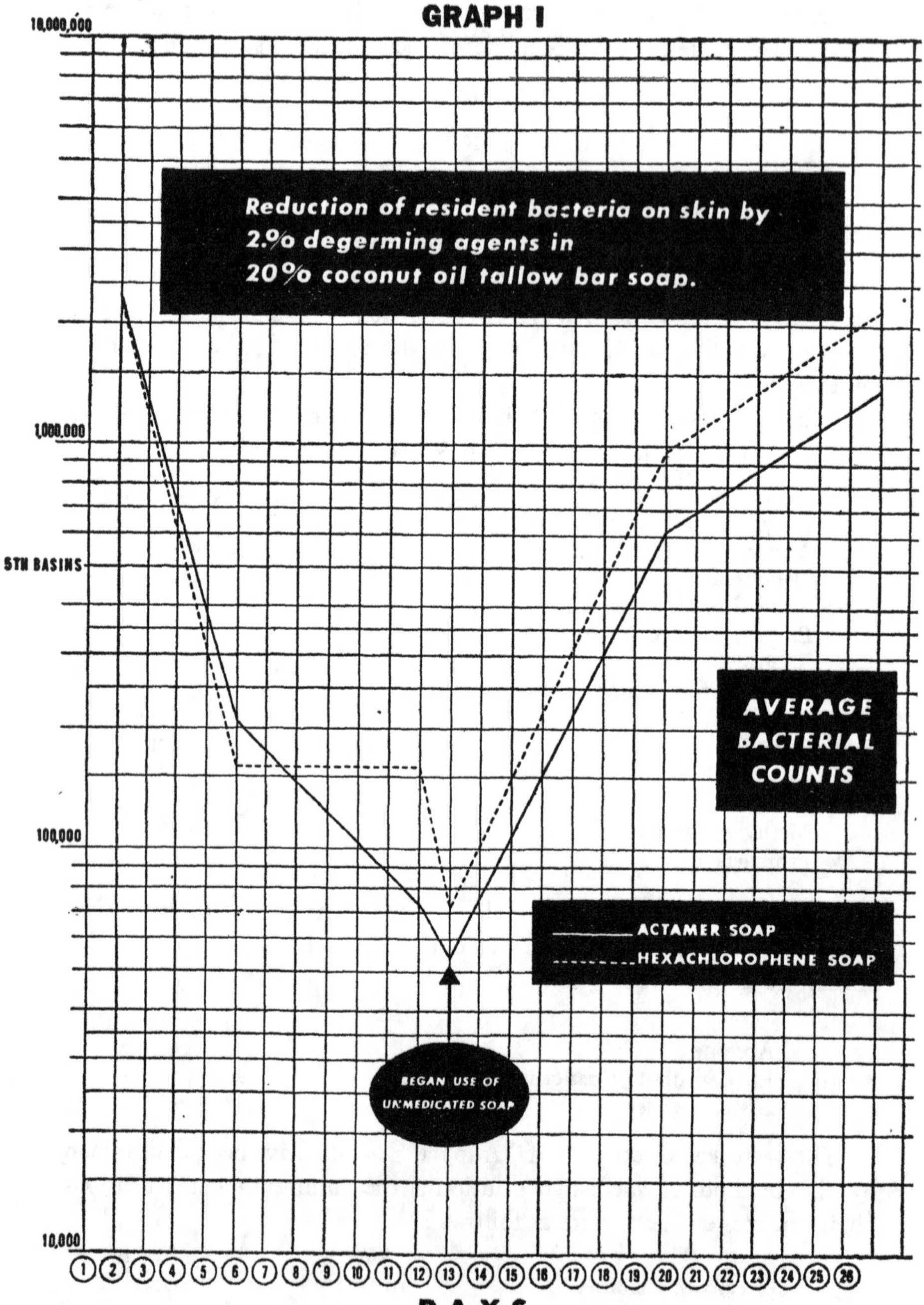

FIG. 113.

[By courtesy of Monsanto Chemical Co., U.S.A.

GRAPH II

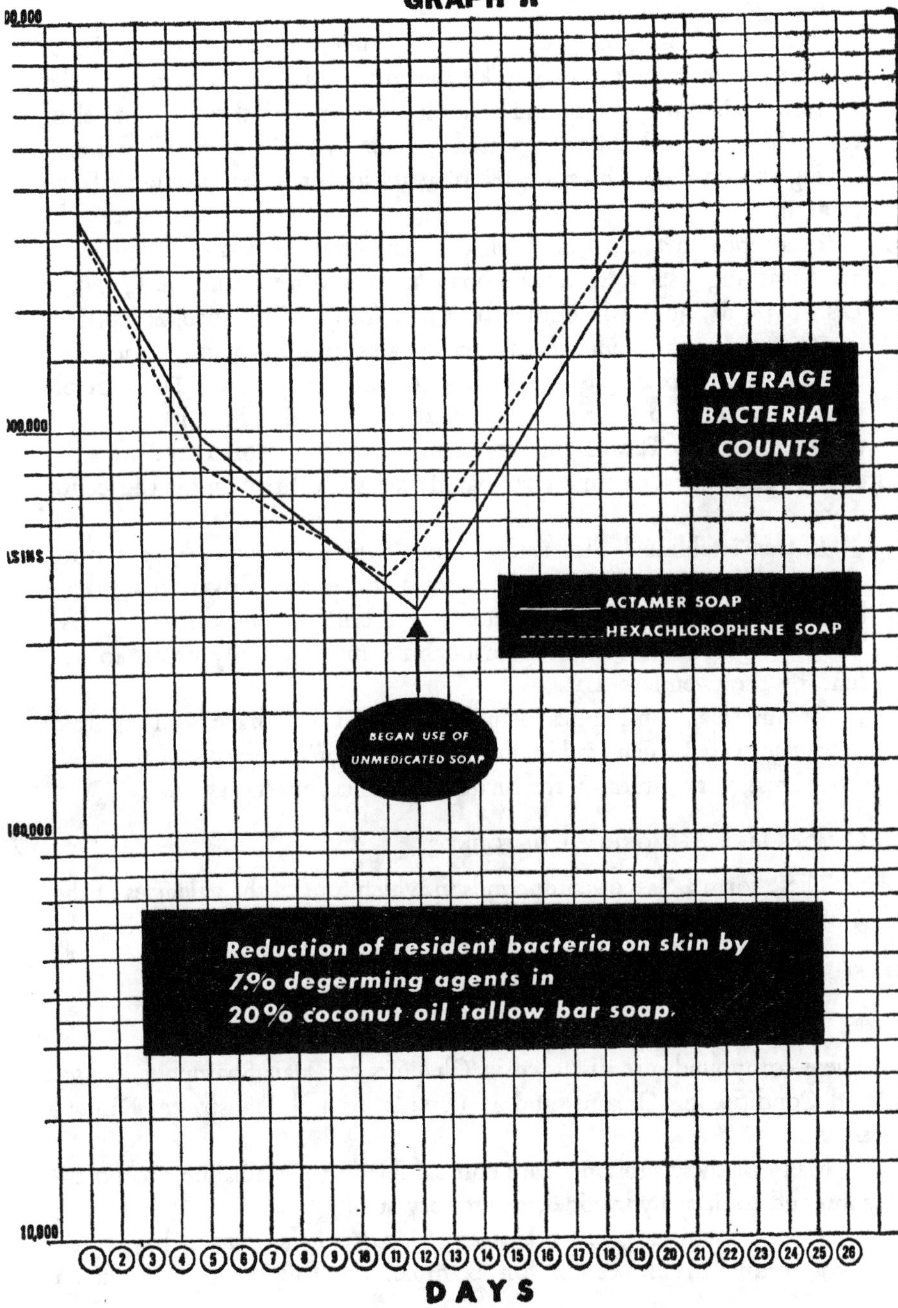

FIG. 114.

[*By courtesy of Monsanto Chemical Co., U.S.A.*

Like " Actamer " and G-11, " Anobial " has but little action on the gram-negative bacteria.

The lethal dose (LD_{50}) of " Anobial " determined on mice and rats is stated to be greater than 5 g./kg./weight and it is claimed that in the course of laboratory study and in preliminary practical tests, more than 100 persons have been in repeated contact with " Anobial " without having shown the slightest degree of irritation or of sensitisation of the epidermis.

It is reported that to establish the disinfectant action of " Anobial " hand-washing tests were carried out using the Price technique (*J. infect. Dis.*, 1938, **63,** 301) as modified by Cade (*Soap, N.Y.*, 1950, **26,** 35).

The study was made on thirteen groups of seven persons each and the tests took place each time over a period of twenty days. The controls were effected in principle on the first, fourth, eighth, thirteenth and twentieth days. The use of the disinfectant soap commenced after the control on the first day and terminated after the control on the thirteenth day.

It was established that using a soap which contains 1·5 per cent. " Anobial ", bacterial flora was destroyed at the rate of over 90 per cent. by the fourth day and more than 95 per cent. by the thirteenth day. The flora gradually formed again but in some cases only up to 40 per cent. by the twentieth day.

Because many antiseptics including G-4 and G-11 have been reported to be inactivated when used in non-ionic emulsions, users of such materials should test, very carefully, the finalised product for efficacy.

Quaternary Ammonium Compounds

These form a class of compounds in which four of the valencies of the ammonia nitrogen are substituted by organic radicles :[1]

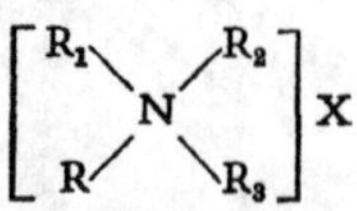

and dissociate this

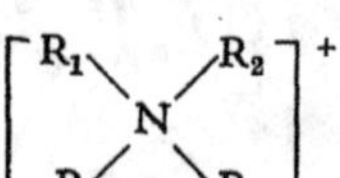

$+ X^-$

These compounds are discussed in Chapters 22 (Hair Shampoos, Rinses and Conditioning Creams) and 41 (Emulsions and Transparent Dispersions).

Many of these substances are comparable in their alkalinity to potassium and sodium hydroxides, being very strong bases.

These compounds, *in the absence of inactivating substances*, have very high germicidal properties, for example, the following table shows

[1] Where R represents a long chain hydrocarbon, R_1, R_2 and R_3 represent quite short organic groups such as methyl, ethyl, benzyl, etc., and X represents any salt-forming acidic group, as, for example, the halogens.

dilutions of " Hyamine 2389 " which proved bacteriostatic and bactericidal to certain bacteria :

HYAMINE 2389

Organism	*Highest dilutions which proved Bacteriostatic*	*Highest dilutions which proved Bactericidal*
S. pyogenes	1 : 4,000,000	1 : 1,000,000
S. aureus	1 : 1,000,000	1 : 512,000
S. fecalis	1 : 512,000	1 : 256,000
N. catarrhalis	1 : 16,000,000	1 : 512,000
B. suis	1 : 256,000	1 : 128,000
S. typhosa	1 : 32,000	1 : 32,000
P. vulgaris	1 : 4,000	1 : 2,000
Ps. aeruginosa	1 : 8,000	1 : 2,000

(By courtesy of Rohm & Haas Co., U.S.A.)

Berry (*Mfg. Chemist*, Oct. 1951, p. 395) has drawn attention to the fact that the first stage in the killing of bacteria is one of adsorption of the quaternary ammonium compound on to the bacterial surface. In this condition the organism, although still alive, cannot multiply even in a culture solution. This is a period of bacteriostasis and can be brought about, Berry points out, by quite low concentrations of bactericide. He adds that it has been shown that during this period the bacterial cells leak nitrogen and phosphorus compounds into the surrounding medium and unless the adsorbed layer is washed off or desorbed, the organism dies. Thus in ordinary circumstances the reaction is irreversible and leads to death. [The inactivation of antiseptics has been discussed earlier in this chapter.]

Quaternary compounds are not employed in ordinary cosmetic cream preparations since they are incompatible with anionic substances, as, for example, soaps, sodium lauryl sulphate and similar detergents and by " Calgon ", etc. However, they are sometimes incorporated in hair rinses to " condition " the hair, and in hair lotions, after-shave lotions—and " traces " have been suggested for use as preservatives in eye lotions [*see* Chapter 19, Eye Lotions. Great care must be taken in such usage to *ensure* that the concentration is insufficient to cause damage to the cornea (*see* also Chapter 22, paragraph dealing with Potential Hazards to the Eyes).]

So far as their action in " degerming " the skin surface is concerned, Blank and Coolidge (*J. invest. Derm.*, Sept. 1950, **3**, 249) point out that it has been shown that " . . . at a *p*H a little higher than the isoelectric point of keratin, the quaternary ammonium compounds change the charge on cutaneous surfaces from negative to positive. If the *p*H is then raised considerably higher than the isoelectric point the charge reverts to negative." It is pointed out (*loc. cit.*) that experiments with woollen cloth and skin have shown that *B. subtilus* spores are held on keratin surfaces when the electrical charge on the surface is changed to positive and released from these surfaces when the charge is negative. This mechanism explains the retention of bacteria on cutaneous surfaces treated with quaternary ammonium compounds, without the need of postulating the formation of a film of the agents under which the bacteria are retained.

It should be pointed out that the quaternary ammonium compounds are not very effective in killing " spores " and are also rather sensitive to low temperatures when they lose much of their activity.

CHAPTER 43

ANTIOXIDANTS

Physiologists have long recognised that rancid fats in the diet are harmful. According to Burr and Barnes (*Physiol. Rev.*, 1943, **23**, 256) such action is due to the fact that rancid fats destroy certain vitamins in the body and possibly other essential elements as well. In cosmetic preparations they not only spoil the odour—sometimes flavour, depending on the product—but may prove irritant. Dr. Dahle (*Proc. Sci. Sect. T.G.A.*, winter meeting 1943-44) pointed out that a rancid lipstick may cause an injury to the user's lips that cannot be explained away as allergy and moreover, that 601 (*b*) of the U.S. Food, Drug and Cosmetic Act holds that a cosmetic is deemed to be adulterated if it consists in whole or in part of a decomposed substance. Frank Atkins (*Perfum. essent. Oil Rec.*, 1935, **26**, 215) also drew attention to the fact that creams which have become rancid are notoriously irritating.

Investigations into the problem of the development of rancidity in certain oils on storage have shown that in such cases the unsaturated linkage of the fatty acids in the oil forms a centre of attack, oxygen attacking a double bond with the formation of a highly reactive and unstable peroxide (and possibly ring compounds or *moloxides*).

Oxidative Rancidity

Only in a few instances have such peroxides been actually isolated in a pure condition, and Staudinger (*Ber. Dtsh. Chem. Ges.*, 1925, **58B**, 1075) considered that " moloxides " are actually the first product of the reaction, e.g. :

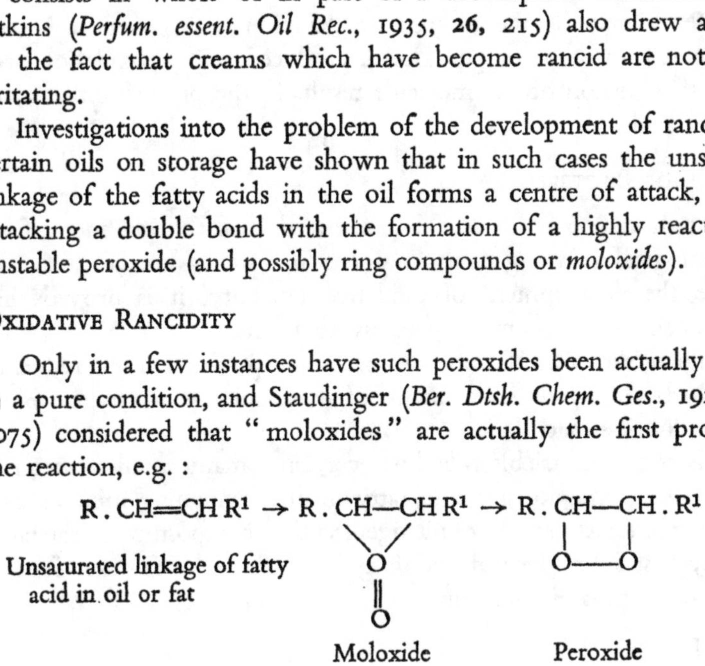

Farmer, *et al.* (*J. Chem. Soc.*, 1943, p. 541 ; 1943, p. 119 ; *Trans. Faraday Soc.*, 1942, **38**, 340), have postulated a hydroperoxide as the first compound formed in the autoxidation of olefinic type substrates (e.g. unsaturated fatty acids). This hydroperoxide is formed presumably by a free radical mechanism of olefinic peroxidation as follows :

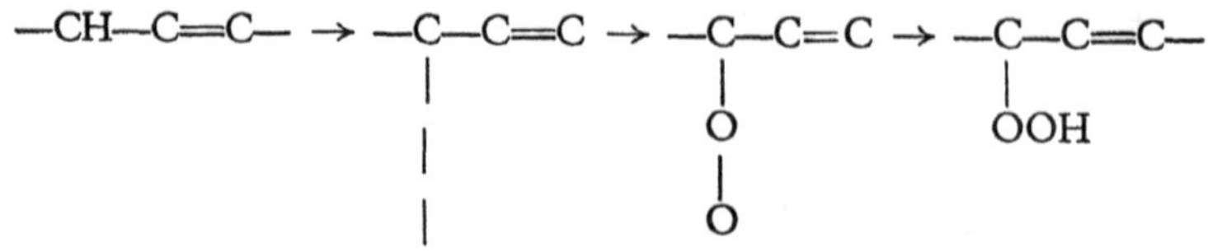

Evidence in support of this mechanism was obtained by the isolation of a rather pure hydroperoxide of cyclohexene and methyl oleate, and by the fact that the rate of loss of total unsaturation failed to parallel the rate of oxygen absorption by the substrate. These investigators indicated possible decomposition stages for the hydroperoxide as follows :

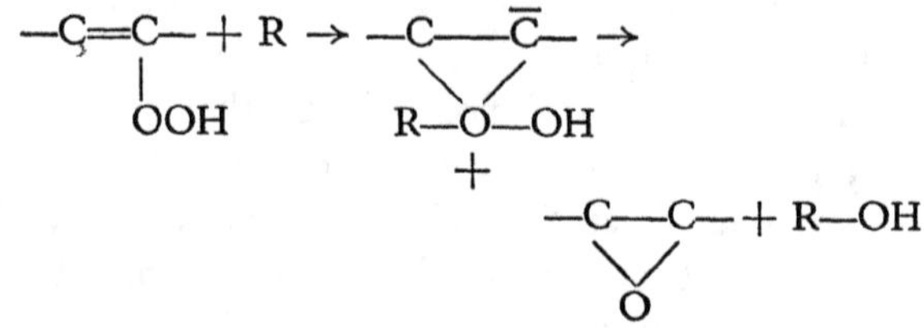

Whatever may be the ultimate explanation it is generally agreed that primarily an oxide or peroxide is produced, and as oxidation proceeds further, fission of the molecule results in the production of aldehydes and acids.

Influence of Bacteria

Although recent work has demonstrated that the presence of an active biological oxidising system, e.g. enzymes such as oxidase, etc., can accelerate the development of oxidative rancidity, it is proved that such a system is not in any way an essential factor.

In general, the metabolic effect of bacteria is production of a reducing system as denoted by the reduction of dyes, such as methylene blue, to their colourless leuco base.

This is not an invariable rule, however, since many moulds, bacteria, and yeasts can, and do, grow in fatty media, containing mineral salts or organic matter as a source of nitrogen, with decomposition of the fatty glyceride, first into glycerol and fatty acid, these being then further attacked and ultimately decomposed.

Ketone Rancidity

This form of rancidity is characterised by its perfume-like odour, produced by ketones, formed by the action of moulds, chiefly penicillium and aspergillus, on the fat, in presence of moisture and nitrogenous matter.

It appears that acids of relatively low molecular weight (i.e. containing less than 14 carbon atoms) are those chiefly attacked, e.g. butyric, valeric, caproic, capric, lauric acid, etc. Myristic acid (14 carbon atoms) is only slightly attacked under favourable conditions, and those of higher molecular weight (palmitic, stearic, oleic acid, etc.) do not undergo such ketonic rancidity.

The increasing use of amino compounds in cosmetics, which might act as a source of nitrogen for bacterial agencies, is countered by the adequate preservation which cosmetic and toilet preparations, unlike foodstuffs, receive.

Use of Antioxidants

It has been found that oxidative rancidity can be considerably delayed by the addition of traces of certain compounds, e.g. phenols, naphthols, etc., which act as negative catalysts or antioxidants. Their exact mode of action is still somewhat obscure. In one theory it is assumed that the antioxidant is oxidised by the active peroxide formed which is by this means reduced. Another suggestion is that the antioxidant is oxidised, and that the reaction product with the unstable peroxide involves a mutual reduction.

The above theories are not entirely satisfactory. Of interest is the activated chain theory of Christiansen, in which it is assumed that a molecule of oxygen combines with a molecule of the fatty substance, with the liberation of energy, which is passed on from molecule to molecule down the chain. The ultimate length of molecular chain effected will depend upon the efficiency of this transference and the absence of substances which might impede or inhibit it.

On colliding with an antioxidant, it is assumed that (though this latter is itself oxidised) it fails to pass on the energy and further fatty molecules are not activated.

Whatever the ultimate explanation, it is now a well-recognised fact of great importance that the addition of traces of such substances to an oil of vegetable or animal origin, inhibits rancidity, and increases its age resistance. For this reason such antioxidants are becoming increasingly used by the cosmetician.

Before discussing these products, it is necessary to mention briefly the chemical tests available for testing the relative value of such antioxidants, and the difficulties which arise in correlating the results with the observations of our physical senses. In general, chemical tests depend upon determination of aldehydes or peroxide. However, odour and taste are often due to a combination of factors, or secondary products, all of which are not measured by such chemical tests, though our nose or tongue may record this heterogeneous collection as an *entity*, and we call this *rancidity*. Moreover, the power of smell and taste differs widely from person to person, and it is astonishing how many mistakes a blindfolded person will make in judging types of flavour, particularly after the first few tests have been carried out and the sensitivity of the organ becomes deadened.

The difficulty is that an oil can absorb a relatively large amount of oxygen, and become technically rancid, while still organoleptically sound. Since in cosmetic and toilet preparations it is the organoleptic tests which the consumer applies, this must evidently be the final criterion, and the results of this, in conjunction with chemical tests, used wherever possible in assessment.

When it is desired to compare the efficiency of various antioxidants, the chemical tests are of special value, since an increase in aldehyde or peroxide content can be found much faster than by taste and smell. In this way some idea as to the *probable* value of a substance may be obtained. The result may then be checked up organoleptically.

Chemical Tests for Rancidity

The Kreis test, first described in 1902, is the one most frequently employed to determine oxidative rancidity. In this test 1 ml. of the oil (or melted fat) is shaken with 1 ml. concentrated hydrochloric acid for one minute ; then 1 ml. of a 0·1 per cent. solution of phloroglucinol in ether is added and shaking continued for a further minute. A pink or red coloration of the lower acid layer is considered to be indicative of rancidity, the amount of which is approximately (although not exactly) proportional to the intensity of the colour. A preferable modification of this method was suggested by the Committee of the American Oil Chemistry Society (*J. Oil Fat Ind.*, 1931, **8**, 269) in which the colour is measured by means of glass colour standards in a Lovibond tintometer.

This red coloration is produced by epihydrin aldehyde,

$$\underbrace{CH_2\text{—}O\text{—}HC}\text{—}CHO,$$

but it should be remembered that a fat, although it may respond to this test, is not necessarily rancid. Fresh, crude vegetable oils may give similar colours, although these usually disappear on refining. Essential oils and aldehydes which may be present in certain toilet articles and cosmetic products can give positive results ; hence such tests should be carried out on the unperfumed product.

A modified Kreis test applicable to cosmetic preparations in which aeration is employed together with a modified absorption reagent, has been described by J. H. Jones (*J. Amer. Oil Chem. Soc.*, 1944, **27**, 128). This test eliminates the interference of many other substances. Directions are given in the original article for testing various types of cosmetics.

The Schiff test for aldehydes appears to be slightly more sensitive, but the colorimetric evaluation is not so easy with this test and it offers no particular advantage. Since it may be readily found in any text-book, the exact procedure is not described.

Schibsted has developed this test (*Ind. Eng. Chem. Anal.*, 1932, **4**, 209) to be specified for aldehydes of a high molecular weight. However, the stipulated conditions must be carefully followed, and for these the original paper should be consulted.

C. H. Lea (*ibid.*, 1934, **6**, 241) has devised a method by which the relatively minute amounts of aldehydes in a rancid fat may be measured by a simple titration with sodium bisulphite. Some preliminary tests with cotton-seed oil appeared to indicate that this method correlated more closely with the organoleptic test than did the Kreis test.

Iodometric methods may be used for the determination of " peroxide oxygen ", and various methods are available. Wheeler's method is a rapid laboratory method suitable for a number of routine tests. In this 3 to 10 g. of the oil are dissolved in a mixture of 30 ml. glacial acetic acid and 20 ml. pure chloroform, and 1 ml. of a saturated solution of potassium iodide added. Exactly one minute after adding the potassium iodide, 100 ml. water are added and the liberated iodine titrated with a standard solution of sodium thiosulphate, using a little starch as indicator. Vigorous shaking is required for removal of the last tinge of iodine from the chloroform layer. Comparative results may be either recorded in mls. of standard thiosulphate used on a fixed weight of oil with varying antioxidants, or calculated and expressed by means of the following formula :

$$\text{Peroxide content (in millimoles per kilo)} = \frac{T \times N \times 500}{W}$$

where T = mls. of thiosulphate, N = its normality, and W = weight of oil taken.

Another test, which has been suggested for the determination of oxidative rancidity, is that employing a 0·025 per cent. solution of methylene blue in alcohol. About 2 ml. of this reagent are added to 20 ml. of the oil or fat, which is shaken and the amount of colour reduction taken as a measure of its rancidity. For a report on the determination of stability in an oil or fat, that of the American Oil Chemists' Society, 1935 (*Oil & Soap*, 1935, **12**, 187) should be consulted.

Lips, Chapman and McFarlane (*Oil & Soap*, 1943, **20**, 240) have applied the ferric thiocyanate method [previously described by Chapman and McFarlane (*Canad. J. Res.*, 1943, **B.21**, 133) for the determination of fat-peroxides in milk powder and modified for use with lard (Lips and McFarlane, *Oil & Soap*, 1943, **20**, 193] to the study of incipient rancidity in fats and oils. The oxygen absorbed by various oils and fats on storage, calculated from change in the peroxide value determined colorimetrically, was in good agreement with direct measurements in a Warburg-Barcroft manometric apparatus. It is stated that the proposed method is simpler and more sensitive than any previously described and is recommended particularly for the detection of incipient rancidity in vegetable oil products.

C. H. Lea ("Methods for Determining Peroxides in Lipids", *J. Sci. Food Agric.*, 3 Dec. 1952) states that the aerobic ferric thiocyanate method, although it gave high results in the presence of atmospheric oxygen and values too low in its absence, showed excellent reproducibility, required much less material than the iodometric method and under any one set of conditions gave results which appeared to be directly proportional to the iodometric values.

The following is a brief description of an apparatus which I used some years ago to investigate the effect of antioxidants in cosmetic emulsions. A current of air is blown continuously through the oil or fat containing the anti-oxidant, and kept in intimate contact with water by means of a high-speed stirrer, the whole apparatus being shielded from light and maintained at a constant temperature of 70° C. (in the case of solid fats; lower temperatures may be employed with oils) inside an incubator. In the case of oils and fats evolving volatile fatty acids on rancidity, such volatile fatty acids, if water-soluble, may be passed through a solution of a suitable indicator, the colour change produced operating a photo-electric cell which (at a definite colour change) switches off the whole apparatus and electric clock. In this way the relative time taken for a sample to reach a definite degree of rancidity may be measured and at the same time the oil or fat may be analysed by (1) the Schibsted modification of the Schiff test for aldehydes; (2) Lea's determination of aldehydes with sodium bisulphite; and (3) iodometric methods of determination of peroxide oxygen; (4) organoleptically.

The photo-electric attachment is an additional refinement and is optional. In its absence samples may be withdrawn from time to time and examined organoleptically and chemically. In oils or fats in which volatile fatty acids are either absent or are in too small a proportion to effect such a colour change, the photo-electric cell and relay is omitted and the method of withdrawing samples at fixed intervals and analysing

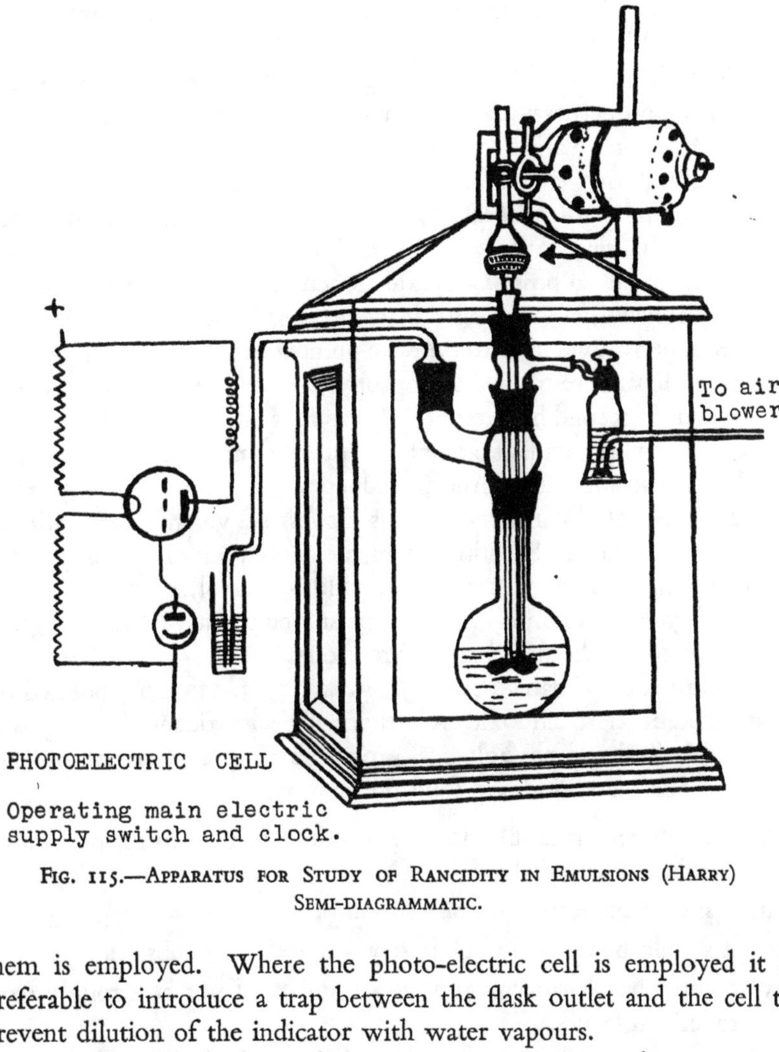

FIG. 115.—APPARATUS FOR STUDY OF RANCIDITY IN EMULSIONS (HARRY) SEMI-DIAGRAMMATIC.

them is employed. Where the photo-electric cell is employed it is preferable to introduce a trap between the flask outlet and the cell to prevent dilution of the indicator with water vapours.

By means of the high-speed mixer, intimate contact can be maintained between the oil and the water without the introduction of an emulsifier which might vitiate the results. Having thus investigated the action of water and air at 70° C. upon the oil or fat, varying emulsifiers *can* be included to study their effect, and, finally, the activity of antioxidants may be compared.

Choice of Antioxidants

Substances for the prevention of rancidity have been utilised since 1843, when Deschamps discovered that gum benzoin protected lard from oxidation and this fact has been utilised in pharmaceutical preparations (benzoinated lard).

Since then a number of investigators have attempted to correlate antioxidant properties with molecular structure (*see* Moureau and Dufraisse *C. R. Acad. Sci.*, Paris 1922, **174**, 258 ; 1922, **175**, 127 ; Tanaka and Nakamura, *J. Soc. Chem. Ind. Japan*, 1930, **33**, 129B ; 1933, **36**, 286B, 335B ; Mattill, *J. Biol. Chem.*, 1931, **90**, 141 ; and Greenbank and Holm, *Ind. Engng. Chem.*, 1934, **26**, 243), and a large number of compounds have been found to possess antioxidant activity. Though monohydroxy benzene (phenol) is practically inactive, substitution of certain groups in phenol derivatives leads to the development of activity. For example, ortho- and para-cresol, and 2-isopropyl-5-methyl-phenol (thymol) are active and if a second hydroxyl (OH) group is introduced in the ortho or para position antioxidant activity is greatly increased. This activity reaches a maximum with the introduction of a third hydroxy group (pyrogallol), tetrahydroxybenzene is far less active, and hexahydroxy-benzene is inactive. Substitution in the meta position yields products with but slight activity (resorcinol, phloroglucinol).

A very large number of complex substances have been suggested and patented for the retardation of rancidity.

Boehm and Williams (*Quart. J. Pharm.*, 1943, **232**, 292) pointed out that in addition to antioxidant activity, an antioxidant should possess certain physical and physiological properties if it is to be of practical value in pharmaceutical and food preparations :

(i) the antioxidant should not impart odour or taste to the preparation to which it is added ;

(ii) it should be nearly neutral in action ;

(iii) it should be easily and definitely soluble in the substrate ;

(iv) it must be pharmacologically safe and must not be strongly toxic to animal tissues.

Whilst the above criteria apply to food and pharmaceutical products they may equally well be applied to cosmetic preparations, with the addition that the antioxidant must also be *dermatologically innocuous* [i.e. free from primary irritating effects and from sensitising properties ; since the skin is often more sensitive to affront than is, for example, the stomach, and, in the case of lipsticks in particular, great care should be taken in choosing a suitable antioxidant material].

As an illustration of modern effective antioxidants permitted for use in foodstuffs in the United States in 1950, the following list (from C. H. Lea, "Problems Arising from the Use of Chemicals in Food-Antioxidants", *Chem. & Ind.*, 1952, p. 178) is of interest:

Antioxidants permitted in the U.S.A. (1950)	*Concentration not to exceed per cent.*
Guaiacum resin	0·10
* Nordihydroguaiaretic acid (NDGA)	0·01
Tocopherols	0·03
Lecithin	—
* Propyl gallate	0·01 (1948)
Thiodipropionic acid	0·01 (1949)
Dilauryl or distearyl thiodipropionate	0·09 (1949)
† Butylated hydroxyanisole	0·02 (1949)

The value of gum guaiacum as an antioxidant in certain cosmetic *emulsions* has been cited by the author (R. G. Harry, *Modern Cosmeticology*, London: Leonard Hill Ltd., 1944). The influence of water is of great importance to the cosmetic chemist. Lehmann and Watts (*J. Amer. Oil Chem. Soc.*, 1951, **28**, 477) found, after testing Nordihydroguaiaretic acid (NDGA), Butylated hydroxyanisole (BHA), Propyl gallate and alpha-tocopherol, that these antioxidants are effective in the order given, the first being the most effective in lard containing water. When water was added at a *p*H of 7·5, BHA was the best antioxidant used and NDGA was considered less effective. It was also found that ascorbic acid, generally considered to act with antioxidants as a synergist, in this case worked as an accelerator instead.

NORDIHYDROGUAIARETIC ACID (Lundberg, Halvorson and Burr, *Oil & Soap*, 1944, **21**, 33) is isolated from the common desert plant Larrea divaricata and frequently referred to as NDGA. This substance having the following structure

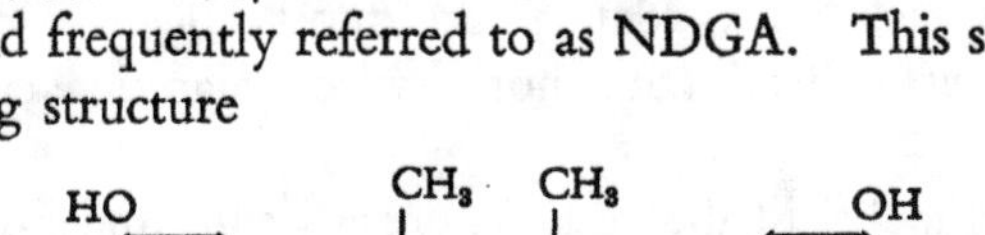

compares very favourably with other substances of the phenolic type in antioxygenic activity (Mattil, Filer and Longenecker, *Oil & Soap*, 1944, **21**, 160). It is only very slightly soluble in water; is appreciably soluble in hot fats and shows no tendency to crystallise out on cooling. Experiments show that at concentrations up to 0·1 per cent.

* May be used with 0·005 per cent. citric or phosphoric acid as synergist.

† May be used together with propyl gallate or NDGA, and with or without citric or phosphoric acid.

the acid has no deleterious effects on the other properties of lards and that its effectiveness in stabilising fats is carried over into baked products.

ETHYL AND PROPYL GALLATES

The valuable antioxidant properties of the esters of Gallic acid have been described by many investigators (*see* Boehm and Sabalitschka (Brit. Patent 542,833 ; U.S. Patent 2,255,191), Golumbic and Matill (*Oil & Soap*, 1942, **19,** 144), Boehm and Williams (*Pharm. J.*, 1943, **16,** 163), Hilditch (Paper read before a meeting of the Food Group of the Chemical Society on 13 Oct. 1943).)

Boehm and Williams found that from the practical and commercial standpoint, ease of solubility at low temperatures, acidity and colour, and from the point of general effectiveness, normal propyl gallate (i.e. normal propyl 3 : 4 : 5-trihydroxybenzoate) was the outstanding antioxidant amongst the gallic acid esters investigated. These investigators found that the protection afforded by 0·1 per cent. of the normal propyl gallate in lard, was equal to that obtained by ten times as much Siam benzoin and probably greater than that of thirty times as much Sumatra benzoin.

Further recommendation of the esters of gallic acid has been given by Stirton, Turer and Riemenschneider (*Oil & Soap*, 1945, **22,** 81). They compared the antioxygenic activities of nordihydroguaiaretic acid (NDGA), propyl gallate, benzyl hydroquinone, alpha-tocopherol and their synergistic combinations with citric acid, *d*-iso ascrobyl palmitate and lecithin in a number of fat substrates, viz. methyl oleate-methyl linoleate, methyl linolenate and the distilled methyl esters of lard. Nordihydroguaiaretic acid and propyl gallate surpassed the other substances in antioxidant activity. Citric acid showed marked synergism with each antioxidant ; the most effective combinations were those of citric acid with nordihydroguaiaretic acid and with propyl gallate.

Gallic acid is widely distributed in nature as a constituent of the tannins which are present in many vegetable foods and particularly in tea. About one-third of the aqueous extract of tea leaves consists of tannins, which are rich in gallic acid. Hilditch and Lea state in their publications (*Chemistry and Industry*, 1944, p. 70) that the possible toxicity of ethyl gallate has been thoroughly investigated by Professor J. A. Gunn, of Oxford, and Professor A. D. Macdonald, of Manchester, at the request of the Medical Research Council. From these investigations, they concluded that no symptoms of toxicity were observed in mice which had received, orally or subcutaneously, massive doses of ethyl gallate, in concentrations far greater than could ever be approached by human beings when receiving foods stabilised against oxidation by the ester.

Boehm and Williams (*loc cit.*) report that 0·5 g. of propyl gallate was administered orally to one of them on 6 consecutive days. An examination of the urine during this period, and for a further 6 days, showed that no albumen was present, abnormal sedimental contents were not observed, there being a complete absence of red blood corpuscles and casts of any kind. They also cite pharmacological tests received from the Pharmacological Laboratories of the College of the Pharmaceutical Society (University of London) which concludes as follows:

(1) Normal propyl trihydroxy-benzoate is less toxic than pyrogallol, when administered orally to mice (acute tests).

(2) There are no acute skin effects observable when a 10 per cent. solution of normal propyl gallate in propylene glycol is left in contact with shaven guinea pigs for 48 hours, or the human skin for 24 hours.

This contrasts favourably with the erythematous effect produced under similar conditions by a 10 per cent. solution of pyrogallol in propylene glycol.

PHYSICAL CHARACTERISTICS

	Progallin A	*Progallin P*
Theoretical Molecular weight	198	212
Melting point	150°–152° C.	146°–148° C.
Solubilities: w/w		
Acetone	40*	40*
Ethyl alcohol	35*	35*
Ether	40*	40*
Methyl alcohol	40*	40*
Propylene glycol	30*	30*
Arachis oil—at 25° C.	$<$0·005	0·05
at 37° C.	$<$0·01	0·2
at 60° C.	$<$1	1
(remaining in solution at room temperature)		
Water—shaking at 25° C.	0·25	0·2
after heating at 100° C. and cooling to room temperature	3·0*	0·5

* = Approximate Values.

*p*H VALUES OF AQUEOUS SOLUTIONS OF PROGALLIN A AND PROGALLIN P, AT VARIOUS CONCENTRATIONS

Concentration per cent.	*p*H *Values*	
	Progallin A	*Progallin P*
0·05	5·78	6·3
0·10	5·52	5·9
0·2	5·18	5·7
0·25	—	5·5
0·4	—	5·35
0·5	—	5·25
1	4·52	—
2	4·32	—
3	4·22	—

Progallin A was introduced as Nipa 48 and is the ethyl compound.
Progallin P was introduced as Nipa 49 and is the propyl compound.

(*Courtesy, Nipa Laboratories, Ltd.*)

BUTYLATED HYROXYANISOLE has been developed as a new and very effective antioxidant for animal fats. It is readily soluble in fats, practically insoluble in water and exhibits synergism with acids, hydroquinone, methionine, lecithin and thiodipropionic acid. Extensive toxicological tests in rats have failed to demonstrate any physiological effects when the antioxidant is used daily in food, even in amounts several hundred times larger than the maximum amount permitted in food (Kraybill, Dugan, Beadle, Vibrans, Swartz and Rezabek, *J. Amer. Oil Chem. Soc.*, Sept. 1949, p. 449).

NATURAL ANTIOXIDANTS—the "TOCOPHEROLS"

McConnell (*Amer. Perfum.*, Sept. 1947, p. 241) has pointed out that amongst pro-oxidant factors are *light* (which he says has perhaps greater influence on rancidity than any other single factor), *moisture* (the presence of even as little as 0·3 per cent. water in an oil will permit the growth of certain bacteria and moulds in fats, providing their nutritional requirements are met) and certain *metals*, which apparently act in the metallic form as surface catalysts without being attacked themselves (the concentration of metallic salts required for catalysis is very low, the effect of as little as 1 part copper per 100,000,000 being detectable).

It is typical of natural fresh oils and fats that they oxidise but slowly during the early part of their storage, then the rate of oxidation accelerates and is accompanied by the development of off-odours and flavours. This preliminary period of slow oxidation in which most oils and fats retain their fresh characteristics is termed the " induction " period.

This " induction " period has been shown to be due to the presence in the oils of natural antioxidants—usually the " tocopherols ". The tocopherols are now obtained in a highly concentrated form by molecular distillation ; the best known member of the family alpha-tocopherol, (5,7,8-trimethyltocol) ; (2,5,7,8-tetramethyl-2-(4′, 8′, 12′-trimethyl-decyl)-6-chromanol), being known as " Vitamin E ".

Associated, it is stated, with the tocopherols in vegetable oils is another inhibitor, chroman-5,6-quinone.

Alpha-tocopherol is a very suitable antioxidant for use in certain cosmetic and toilet preparations, only a very small amount is required.

Miscellaneous Antioxidants

DI-TERTIARY-BUTYL-PARA CRESOL, a trialkylated phenol has recently been shown to be an effective antioxidant for petroleum waxes. It is claimed (R. F. Scott and E. D. Andrews, *Modern Packaging*, Dec. 1952, p. 153) that " D.B.P.C." meets all the basic requirements of a good inhibitor and that its low order of toxicity suggests its application in all wax products including those destined for food packaging.

DIHYDROQUERCETIN, obtained from Douglas Fir heartwood, has been found to be an effective antioxidant for lard, cottonseed oil, etc. It is stated to impart no taste or colour to oils and fats and, like quercetin (3,3′,4′,5-7-Pentahydroxyflavone—widely distributed in the plant kingdom), appears to be non-toxic (E. F. Kurth and F. L. Chan, *J. Amer. Oil Chem. Soc.*, Oct. 1951, p. 433).

HYDROXY- AND AMINO- SUBSTITUTED DIPHENYLAMINES. Bickoff, Livingston, Guggolz and Thompson (*ibid.*, Nov. 1952, p. 445) have studied the possibilities of a number of compounds as antioxidants for carotene in mineral oil. The most effective antioxidants were found to be hydroxy- and amino- substituted diphenylamines, *p*-substituted phenylenediamines and derivatives of 2,2,4-trimethyl-1,2-dihydroquinoline.

Antioxidants for Soap

Antioxidants are added to soap in minute quantities with a view to restraining the oxidation of the soap and the rancidity and discoloration which would result from such rancidity.

One of the most widely used antioxidants for this purpose is ortho-Tolyl Biguanide " Sopanox " (Proprietary designation. Monsanto Chemical Co.)

"Sopanox" is a light grey to white powder, melting above 135° C. Its solubility in organic solvents is listed below.

A commonly used method of incorporating "Sopanox" in soap is to add "Sopanox" during milling. It can be added as a powder, as a water slurry, or in an alcoholic solution. As perfumes are sometimes dissolved in alcohol and added during the amalgamation operation, the "Sopanox" can also be dissolved in this alcoholic solution to ensure uniform distribution (*see* Chapter 27, The Processing of Toilet Soap).

The following will serve as indications for general soap practice :

In *medium and high titre soaps* and in those of greater stability, whether in the form of cakes, powder, chips, or flakes, "Sopanox" should be entirely effective when employed at a concentration of 0·04 per cent. to 0·05 per cent. on the basis of the soap weight.

In the case of *low titre soaps* and those having lesser stability, "Sopanox" may be required in greater concentration. However, 0·1 per cent. based on the soap weight, should give ample protection. The palm and coconut types of soap, though of low titre, exhibit good stability and are exceptions to the above recommendation. "Sopanox" at 0·05 per cent. concentration should protect these soap types from oxidation.

It must be emphasised that, to secure maximum effect from the small quantities employed, uniform distribution of "Sopanox" throughout the soaps is essential.

Solubility of Sopanox

Solvent	*g. per 100 g. solvent at 25° C.*	*at 75° C.*
Acetone	8	—
Alcohol	27	—
Ethylene glycol	15	120
"Carbitol"	70	175
Methyl "cellosolve"	85	240
"Cellosolve"	80	200
Water	1	5

(*Courtesy, Monsanto Chemical Co., St. Louis.*)

"SA-326". Ortho Biphenyl Biguanide (Monsanto Chemical Co.) is another antioxidant which is employed in soap manufacture and processing. Like "Sopanox" it is a light grey to white powder, melting point above 150° C.

It is employed in the same proportions and in the same manner as "Sopanox".

The solubility of "SA-326" in some organic solvents is listed below:

Solvent	g. per 100 g. solvent 25° C.	75° C.
Acetone	4	10
Alcohol	7	18
Carbitol	60	85
Cellosolve	40	65
Ethylene glycol	30	40
Methyl cellosolve	40	40

(*Courtesy, Monsanto Chemical Co., St. Louis.*)

Other new interesting synthetic antioxidants for soap are guanidine derivatives such as the para-tertiary amyl phenyl phosphoric acid salt and the mercaptobenzothiazole salt; polyamines, e.g. diethylene triamine, triethylene tetramine, and tetraethylene pentamine (U.S. Patent 2,409,056) and pyrene compounds (Brit. Patent. 572,458).

Sodium Dithionite (Brit. Patents 557,879 and 577,880) is claimed not only to improve the colour of soaps made from bleached fats but also to prevent the growth of fungi and bacteria (Paul D. Smith, *Amer. Perfum.*, Nov. 1951, p. 367).

CHAPTER 44

HUMECTANTS

HUMECTANTS are hygroscopic materials that possess the characteristic property of absorbing water from moist air until a certain degree of dilution is obtained; this dilution depends upon the character of the humectant and the moisture of the surrounding atmosphere.

Humectants are added to cosmetic creams, particularly of the oil-in-water type, with a view to reducing the *drying out* of such creams on exposure to the air. Such *drying-out* is judged by the consistency of the cream, any shrinkage from the walls of the container and—in particular—any evidence of the formation of a *crust* on the surface of the product. In addition, the hygroscopic properties of the film of humectant which remains on the skin may be an important factor in influencing the *feel* and *condition* of the skin after application. (*See* Chapters 4 and 10, The Hydration of the Skin.) It is also believed to minimise *balling up* when a cosmetic cream of the oil-in-water type is "rubbed-out" on the skin.

Evidence recently provided indicates that the rate of loss of water from an oil-in-water cream is not directly related to the amount of *crust formation* on a cream, neither is this *crust formation* a function of the humectant added (W. C. Griffin, R. W. Behrens and S. T. Cross, "Hygroscopic Agents and Their Use in Cosmetics", *J. Soc. Cosmet. Chem.*, March 1952, **3**, 5).

Hygroscopicity data are usually published in the form of equilibrium moisture contents at various humidities; such information is not really significant in cosmetic formulation, since very rarely, if ever, is sufficient humectant (to maintain the original moisture level of the preparation) added; such a product would feel sticky on the skin. In investigating *comparative hygroscopicity data* a number of complicating factors arise which make evaluation a difficult task. This information has, however, been badly needed by the cosmetic industry. The recent data published by Griffin, Behrens and Cross (*loc. cit.*) fulfil a long-felt want and, because of their importance, are extensively quoted in this chapter (with acknowledgment to these investigators, the Atlas Powder Co., Wilmington, and to the Society of Cosmetic Chemists):

"... Two conditions may exist when a humectant is being used. First, while the humidity is changing, or has just been changed, the humectant or product in which the humectant is used will *gain* or *lose* water, at which time the *rate* of change is of importance. Second, if conditions are constant for a suitable time, *equilibrium* is finally attained, at which time the *amount* of water held is important. Unfortunately, many of the published data represent a combination of these conditions, at times further complicated by loss of the humectant itself. This promotes confusion in the interpretation of hygroscopicity data and the choice of humectants.

"The three properties of major importance are defined as follows :

"*Equilibrium hygroscopicity* is the state or condition that exists when an aqueous solution will neither gain nor lose water at a given relative humidity. In our work this is usually expressed as the weight percentage of water in the solution in equilibrium with the given relative humidity. A single value does not characterise the behaviour of a compound ; rather the values must be expressed as a curve of solids content *vs.* relative humidity.

"*Dynamic Hygroscopicity* is the speed with which a compound or its aqueous solution will gain or lose moisture while approaching equilibrium. Since the rate depends on both the initial and final conditions as well as the exposed area-to-volume ratio, absolute units are usually not assigned and the dynamic hygroscopicity is expressed in comparison with another material.

"*Volatility* is the tendency of the product to evaporate and may be expressed as weight loss per unit area at a given temperature. Volatility is usually of importance under practical conditions of use, usually room temperature, and is proportional to the vapour pressure at room temperature.

"It will be seen that these three properties are directly related to the determination of water retention of humectants either when tested as such or when added to a cosmetic, etc., and evaluation methods must take these factors into account.

"*The properties of an ideal humectant are briefly summarised below* :

"1. High hygroscopicity—The product should hold an appreciable amount of water.

"2. Narrow humectant range—For a given change of relative humidity there should be a minimum change in water content.

"3. Desired viscosity—The lower the viscosity of the humectant the more easily it may be mixed with the materials to be conditioned. (Mixing is usually done in aqueous solution so that the actual viscosity of the humectant may be of secondary importance.) For some applications high viscosity is desirable.

"4. Low viscosity index—The usual terminology for viscosity index refers to change of viscosity with temperature. In this case a low viscosity change with both temperature and water content is desirable.

"5. Good compatibility—The product must be compatible with a wide variety of materials.

"6. Low volatility—complete lack of volatility is desirable.

"7. Low cost.

"8. Lack of toxicity.

"9. Good colour, odour, and taste.

"10. Lack of corrosive action.

"11. Low freezing point.

"In general humectants are divided into three classes: inorganic, organic, and metal-organic. The inorganic type, of which calcium chloride is an example, finds only limited use because of their corrosive nature and lack of compatibility. Organic humectants, the most widely used type, are usually polyhydric alcohols and their ethers or esters. The metal-organic type, such as sodium lactate, is not too generally employed.

"Considering inorganic humectants in view of the above list of qualities, we find that their hygroscopicity and viscosity characteristics are favourable, since they hold large quantities of water and the viscosities of the aqueous solutions change little with wide changes in water content (until a solid state is attained). Salts and their hydrates generally have hygroscopicity curves that progress in a stepwise fashion until complete solution is attained. For the most part they are highly corrosive and they exert a 'salting out' effect on organic colloids. They are non-volatile and—the major reason for their use—they are low in costs. . .

"Polyhydric alcohols comprise the most important subclass of organic humectants. Ethylene glycol is the simplest polyhydric alcohol and we may progress from it in several ways. Considering the family of *polyhydric* alcohols strictly the progression is: ethylene glycol, glycerin, to the hexitols, etc. A second progression for ethylene glycol is by the addition of ethylene oxide. This group of compounds actually comes under the classification of dihydric rather than polyhydric alcohols and the progression is ethylene glycol, diethylene glycol, tri, tetra, etc. A second class of dihydric alcohols may be based on propylene glycol and propylene oxide. Combinations of any base polyols with various alkylene oxides is possible to give a vast number of products. . . ."

After pointing out that care must be exercised in the determination of hygroscopicity in order to differentiate between equilibrium hygroscopicity, dynamic hygroscopicity and volatility, Griffin, Behrens and Cross outline the method they used in their investigations, and continue.

EQUILIBRIUM HYGROSCOPICITY DATA

"... These data were determined as previously described, the found values expressed as per cent. solids in equilibrium with the chosen relative humidity, and the successive values plotted. From the resulting curves, values of per cent. solids were read off at 30 per cent., 50 per cent., 70 per cent., and 85 per cent. relative humidities. These data are presented in Table 1.

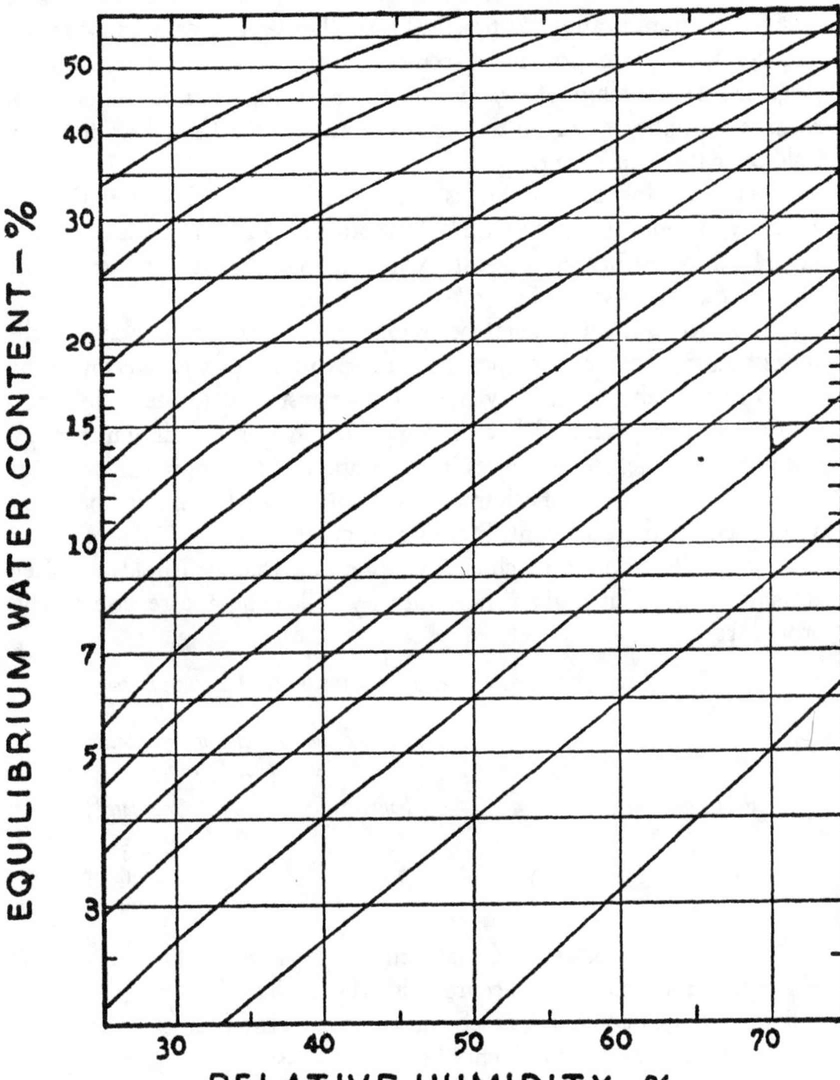

FIG 116.—Humectants Estimation of Equilibrium Moisture contents from 50 % R.H. value.

[*By courtesy of the Atlas Powder Co., and the Journal of the Society of Cosmetic Chemists.*

"In addition, Table 1 lists available physical data on these humectant compounds including viscosity and specific gravity *vs.* temperature and concentration, vapour pressure *vs.* temperature, boiling point, freezing point *vs.* concentration, water solubility and other information. A graphical method of choosing humectants for a desired equilibrium hygroscopicity and for calculating the effect of combinations of humectants has been proposed by Livengood.[21] This method represents a desirable simplification for practical use. However, the hygroscopicity data presented are not in agreement with published data, and his proposed relationship of water content as a logarithmic function of relative humidity from 20 to 100 per cent. relative humidity does not hold over this humidity range.

"The semilog relationship is true over a limited range within an accuracy of about $\pm$ 5 per cent. H_2O for most organic humectants. A revised form of the Livengood graph with a corrected family of curves on a limited scale is shown in Fig. 116.

"To ascertain the general behaviour of an organic humectant, the water holding power at 50 per cent. relative humidity is determined by reference to Table 1. This value is then transferred to the 50 per cent. relative humidity vertical line on Fig. 116. A curve is drawn through this point, parallel to the curves in the graph and the approximate water retention properties of the humectant at any desired humidity between 25 per cent. and 75 per cent. is then read off the curve. The graph and table may also be used to choose a humectant that will hold a desired amount of water at a given humidity by following the reverse of this procedure.

TABLE 2. HYGROSCOPICITIES OF BLENDS OF HUMECTANTS

	Per cent. water held at equilibrium 50/50 Arlex–Glycerol	
R.H., per cent.	*Found**	*Calculated†*
30	8·7	8·3
50	17·6	16·6
70	32·0	30·9

"Blends or mixtures of humectants apparently do not exhibit hygroscopicities exactly in accord with the arithmetic average of their individual hygroscopicities, as seen in Table 2. However, since moisture control by humectants is influenced more by the surrounding atmosphere than by the overall choice of humectant, an arithmetic average will

* Points from curve plotted from actual data.

† Arithmetic average of points taken from curves plotted from actual data.

Name	Ref. index 25° C.	Sp. heat	Flash point °F. (†)	Specific g vs. Concentration 100%	75 %
Ethylene glycol	1·4274[23]	0·575[19]	240[7]	1·116[19]	1·095[19]
Diethylene glycol	1·4311[24]	0·551[10]	275[7]	1·118[27]	1·104[27]
Triethylene glycol	1·4578[13]	0·54[7]	310[7]	1·125[27]	1·110[27]
Polyglycol 400	—	—	435[27]	1·130[27]	—
Polyglycol 600	—	—	475[27]	1·130[27]	—
" Carbowax " 1000	—	—	>450[27]	—	—
" Carbowax " 4000	—	—	>475[27]	—	—
Propylene glycol	1·4293[10]	0·590[10]	210[7]	1·038[9]	1·048[9]
Dipropylene glycol	1·439[7]	0·55[7]	244[7]	1·025[27]	—
Glycerin	1·4729[14]	0·591[19]	345[19]	1·262[19]	1·195[19]
Polyoxyethylene glycerin	—	—	—	—	—
Alpha methyl glycerin	—	—	—	1·24	—
Xylitol	—	—	—	—	—
Sorbitol (Arlex)*** (85% soln.)	1·488	—	—	—	1·310
Sorbitol (Sorbo)*** (70% soln.)	1·459	—	—	—	—
Mannitol	10% 1·345	0·321	—	1·51	—
Sorbitan (A-810)	—	—	—	—	—
Sorbide (A-815)	—	—	—	—	—
Polyoxyethylene Sorbitol (G-2240)	—	—	—	—	—
Polyoxyethylene sorbitol (G-2320)	—	—	—	—	—
Glucose	—	—	—	—	—
" Nulomoline "	—	—	—	—	—
" Mordex "	—	—	—	—	—
Propylene glycol glucoside (A-850)	—	—	—	—	—
Triethanolamine	1·4852[14]	0·64[1]	380[1]	1·124[14]	—
Sodium lactate	—	—	—	—	—
Triethanolamine lactate	—	—	—	—	—
Urea	1·484[14] 1·602	—	—	1·335[14]	—

*** Reg. U.S. Pat. Off. † Cle

TABLE 1.—PHYSICAL PROP

…gravity …n ** (20/20)		Freezing point °C. vs. Concentration**				Viscosity, cp. vs. Concentration**		
50%	25%	100%	75%	50%	25%	100%	85%	70%
1·065[19]	1·032[19]	−11·5[23]	−65[9]	−37[9]	−11[9]	19[9]	12[9]	7[9]
1·074[27]	1·037[27]	−10·45[14]	—	−28[9]	−8[9]	38[9]	17[9]	9·5[9]
1·080[27]	1·037[27]	−5[14]	—	−24[9]	−6[9]	45[9]	—	20[9]
—	—	4 to 10[27]	—	—	—	—	—	(75%) 43[5]
—	—	20–25[27]	—	—	—	—	—	—
—	—	35–40[27]	—	—	—	solid[5]	—	—
—	—	50–55[27]	—	—	—	solid[5]	—	solid[5]
1·040[9]	1·022[9]	—	—	−33[9]	−10[9]	55[9]	21[9]	11·2[9]
—	—	—	—	—	—	—	—	—
1·128[19]	1·061[19]	17·0[19]	−29·8[19]	−23·0[19]	−7·0[19]	1499[25]	112·9[25]	22·94[25]
—	—	—	—	—	—	—	—	—
—	—	—	—	—	—	viscous liquid[16]		—
—	—	—	—	—	—	—	—	—
1·195	1·075[3]	—	—	—	—	—	3500‡	110‡
1·193[3]	1·090[3]	—	—	—	—	—	—	110‡
—	—	166	—	—	—	—	—	—
—	—	—	—	—	—	—	1000‡	—
—	—	—	—	—	—	—	200‡	—
—	—	—	—	—	—	(95) 975	250‡	53‡
—	—	—	—	—	—	—	—	—
—	(24·03)† 1·096[28]	—	—	—	—	—	—	—
—	—	—	—	—	—	—	—	—
—	—	—	—	—	—	—	—	—
—	—	—	—	—	—	—	—	—
—	—	21·2[1]	−40	−14[1]	−2[1]	1013[1]	135[1]	45[1]
—	—	—	—	—	—	—	—	—
—	—	—	—	—	—	—	—	—
—	—	132·7	—	—	—	—	—	—

…eveland Open Cup. ** Weight per cent. solids. †† 25/4.

Properties of Humectants

, cp. ...** (20° C.)		*Viscosity, cp. vs. Temperature °C. (100%)*					*Vapour pres. vs. Tempera*
50%	25%	0	25	50	75	100	*mm. at temp.*
4[9]	1·8[9]	50[9]	17[9]	6[9]	2·0[9]	(120) 0·35[2]	30 at 110[19]
4·6[9]	2·0[9]	100[9]	28[9]	8[9]	5[9]	—	8 at 130[19]
6·8[9]	2·3[9]	—	35[9]	14[9]	7[9]	—	0·42 at 100[9]
14[5]	1·5[5]	solid[5]	—	—	—	—	—
14[5]	1·5[5]	solid[5]	—	—	—	—	—
21[5]	1·5[5]	solid[5]	solid[5]	—	—	—	—
—	17[5]	solid[5]	solid[5]	solid[5]	—	—	—
5·2[9]	2·0[9]	—	40[9]	12·5[9]	5[9]	—	0·2 at 20[9]
—	—	—	—	—	—	—	0·03 at 20[9]
6·050[25]	2·095[25]	solid[19]	945[19]	—	—	—	—
—	—	—	—	—	—	—	—
—	—	—	—	—	—	—	5 at 134[16]
—	—	—	—	—	—	—	—
9‡	2‡	—	—	—	—	—	—
9‡	2‡	—	—	—	—	—	—
—	—	—	—	—	—	—	—
—	—	—	—	—	—	—	—
—	—	—	—	—	—	—	—
12‡	—	—	—	—	—	—	—
—	—	—	—	—	—	—	—
—	—	—	—	—	—	—	—
—	—	—	—	—	—	—	—
—	—	—	—	—	—	—	—
—	—	—	—	—	—	—	—
10[1]	4[1]	—	(35° C.) 280[1]	115[1]	32[1]	17[1]	—
—	—	—	—	—	—	—	—
—	—	—	—	—	—	—	—
—	—	—	—	—	—	—	—

— Data not available. ‡ 25° C. || Solid when dry and does

ressure, mm. erature (°C.) mm. at temp.	*Boiling point* (760 *mm.*) °C.	*Equilibrium hygroscopicity* % *Solids vs. R.H.* % 30	50	70	*Name*
369 at 175[19]	197·2[9]	88	75+	56—	Ethylene glycol
195 at 200[19]	244·5[24]	90	82	60[7]	Diethylene glycol
60 at 200[9]	287·4[27]	91+	84	63[7]	Triethylene glycol
—	—	95—	89	79+	Polyglycol 400
—	—	96—	90	80—	Polyglycol 600
—	—	98—	92	—	"Carbowax" 1000
—	—	99+	99—	96	"Carbowax" 4000
40 at 110[9]	188·2[27]	91	82	68	Propylene glycol
20 at 130[9]	231·8[27]	96[7]	89[7]	77[7]	Dipropylene glycol
0·23 at 118	290[3]	89+	80	65+	Glycerin
—	—	94	87+	76+	Polyoxyethylene glycerin
25 at 171[16]	—	—	—	—	Alpha methyl glycerin
—	—	92	84—	71—	Xylitol
—	118‖	96+	87+	75+	Sorbitol (ARLEX)*** (85% soln.)
—	105‖	X	X	75—	Sorbitol (SORBO)*** (70% soln.)
—	decomposes	X	X	X	Mannitol
—	—	95	87—	75+	Sorbitan (A-810)
—	—	97	91+	80	Sorbide (A-815)
—	decomposes	—	88—	—	Polyoxyethylene sorbitol (G-2240)
—	decomposes	91—	90+	—	Polyoxyethylene sorbitol (G-2320)
—	decomposes	94	88+	79	Glucose
—	decomposes	93	86+	76+	"Nulomoline"
—	—	93+	88—	78	"Mordex"
—	—	89—	84+	77—	Propylene glycol glucoside (A-850)
—	150 mm. 277-9	92[21]	80[21]	52	Triethanolamine
—	—	84—	68—	50—	Sodium lactate
—	—	—	81—	—	Triethanolamine lactate
—	decomposes	X	X	(80%) 51	Urea

es not exhibit a boiling point. X Crystalline.

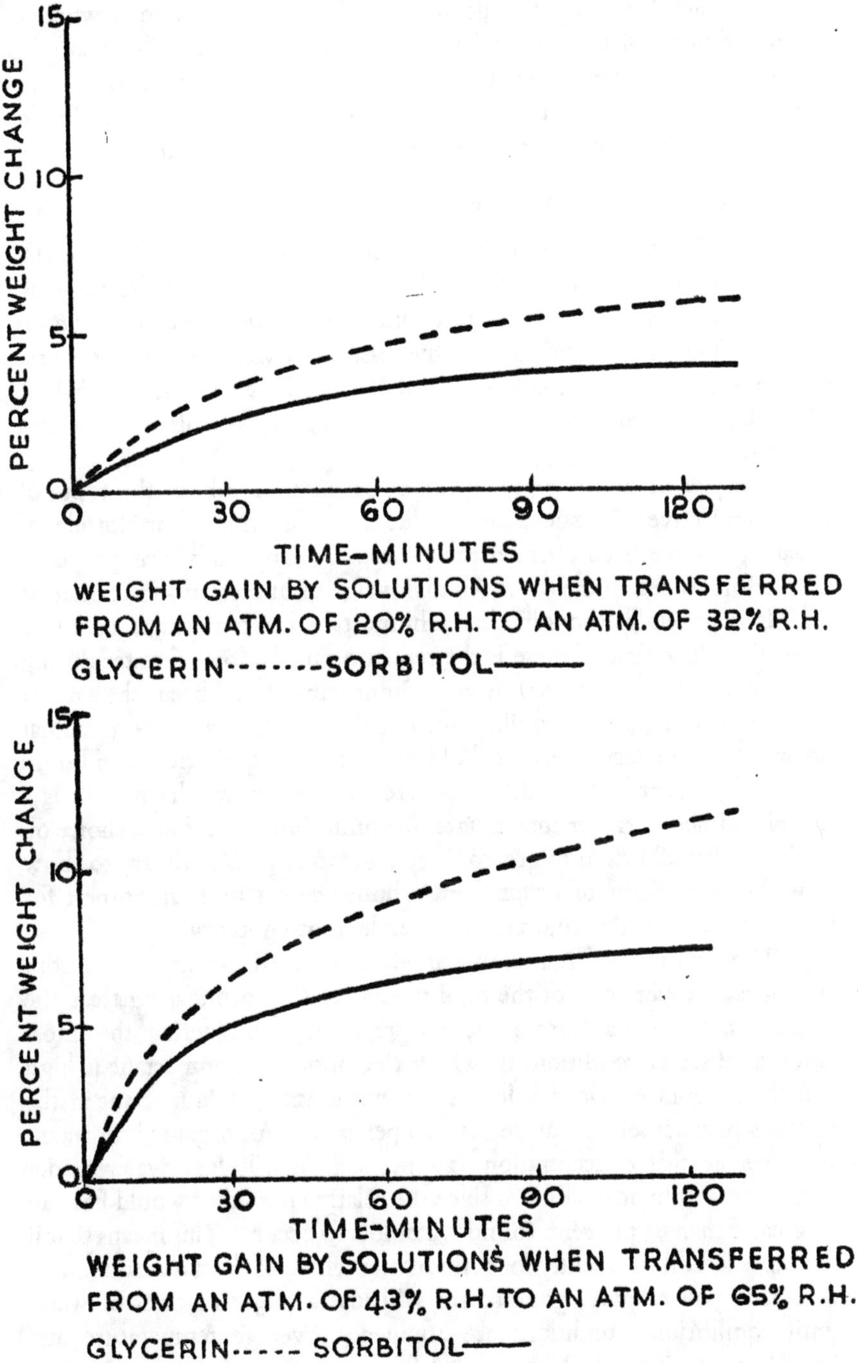

FIG. 117.

[*By courtesy of the Atlas Powder Co., and the Journal of the Society of Cosmetic Chemists.*

usually suffice for estimate calculations. There are occasions wherein blends of non-volatile and volatile humectants are used, for example, sorbitol and propylene glycol. Here, when a large surface to volume is exposed, the over-all hygroscopicity will change due to the change in composition and net remaining weight of the humectant. . . .

HYGROSCOPIC AGENTS IN COSMETICS—O/W EMULSIONS

" . . . The three humectants most used in cosmetic manufacture are, in increasing order of molecular weight and viscosity, propylene glycol, glycerin and sorbitol. Under equilibrium conditions, glycerin is the most hygroscopic and sorbitol the least ; in dynamic hygroscopicity, sorbitol exhibits by far the lowest rate of change of weight. Propylene glycol has the highest volatility, glycerin is slightly volatile, and sorbitol is non-volatile.

" The use of hygroscopic agents in cosmetics has been the topic of many subjective discussions in the literature in which a multitude of advantages have been claimed for their use. Our study was proposed as an effort to determine the *hygroscopic* value of humectants in cosmetics.

" It is generally thought that a humectant has two major uses in a cosmetic. The first of these is the reduction in the loss of water during times when the cap is removed. Humectants have been chosen for this use on the basis of equilibrium hygroscopicities with the idea that because these materials tend to hold water under equilibrium conditions they will prevent ' drying out ' of a cream. However, drying out is a rate phenomenon rather than a state of equilibrium, therefore a choice on the basis of equilibrium hygroscopicity is incorrect. We will try to show how the rate of loss of water from a humectant is more important for this purpose than the amount of water held at equilibrium.

" The amount of humectant used in cosmetic creams is seldom as much as 10 per cent. of the total weight of the formula, whereas the water content varies from 40 to 80 per cent. Considering the most favourable set of conditions in which the amount of humectant is high and the amount of water is low, the concentration of humectant in the aqueous phase is seldom more than 20 per cent. All organic humectant solutions at this concentration (20 per cent.) will lose water under normal atmospheric conditions since the relative humidity would have to be greater than 95 per cent. for no water loss to occur. This means that if the cap is left off sufficiently long, no matter which of the standard humectants that you employ, your cream will lose a major amount of water until equilibrium conditions are attained. Average temperature and humidity conditions in New York[2] for example, during June and July are 74° F. and 70 per cent. R.H. while during December and January the average conditions are 33° F. and 70 per cent. R.H. The important difference in summer and winter seasons is that in the summer indoor and

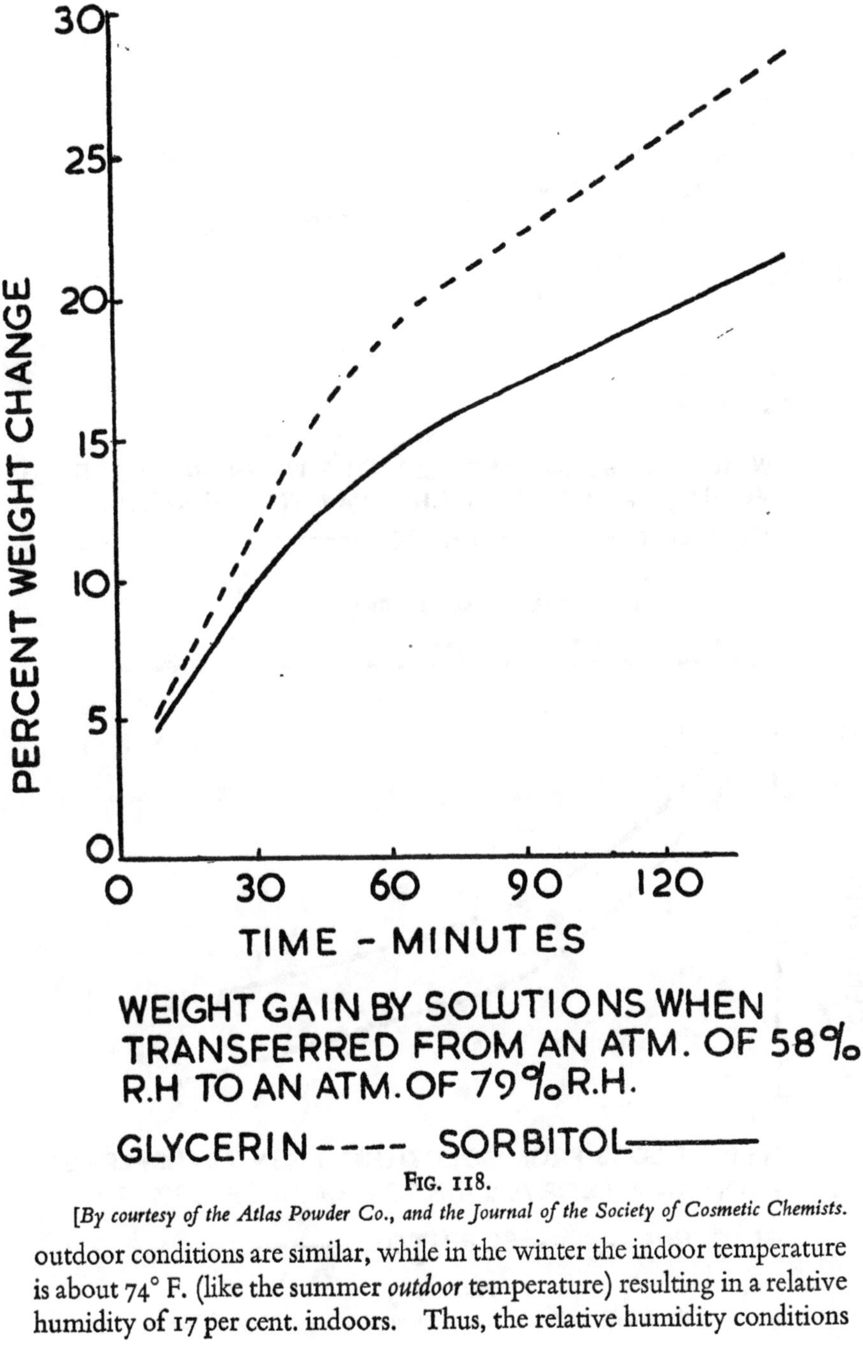

FIG. 118.

[*By courtesy of the Atlas Powder Co., and the Journal of the Society of Cosmetic Chemists.*

outdoor conditions are similar, while in the winter the indoor temperature is about 74° F. (like the summer *outdoor* temperature) resulting in a relative humidity of 17 per cent. indoors. Thus, the relative humidity conditions

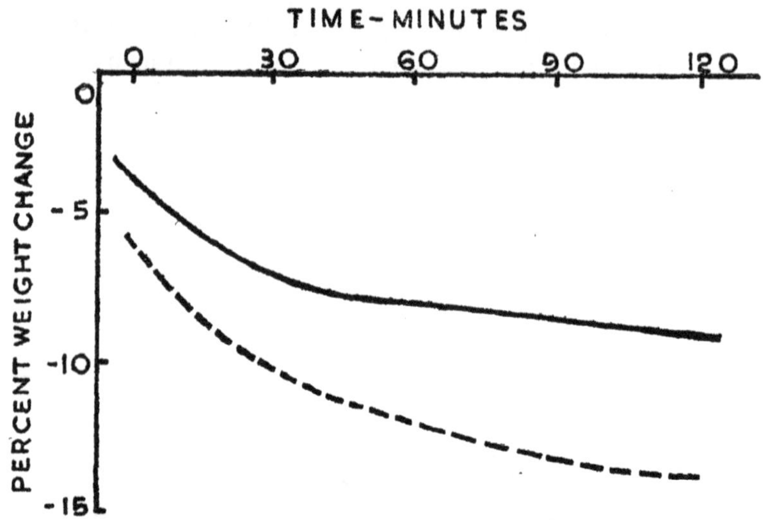

WEIGHT LOSS FROM SOLUTIONS WHEN TRANSFERRED FROM AN ATM. OF 58% R.H. TO AN ATM. OF 32% R.H.

GLYCERIN ----- SORBITOL ———

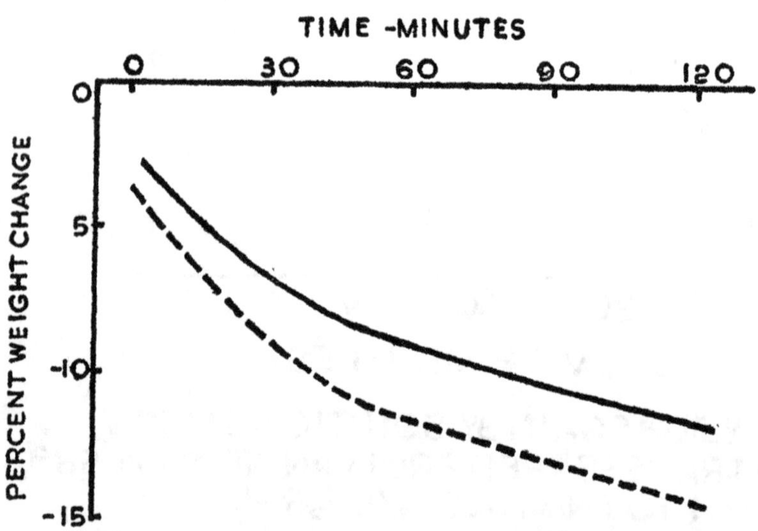

WEIGHT LOSS FROM SOLUTIONS WHEN TRANSFERRED FROM AN ATM. OF 79% R.H. TO AN ATM. OF 65% R.H.

GLYCERIN ------ SORBITOL ———

FIG. 119.

[*By courtesy of the Atlas Powder Co., and the Journal of the Society of Cosmetic Chemists.*

to which cosmetics are exposed are seldom greater than 70 per cent. R.H. and average a great deal less for most of the year. Similar conditions exist throughout most of the East. Even under the most favourable high humidity conditions, for the aqueous phase to be in equilibrium with the atmosphere it would of necessity contain almost three parts of humectant to every part of water. It is doubtful if products made with such high concentrations of polyhydric alcohols or other humectants would be satisfactory from a cosmetic standpoint regardless of the increased cost. From these considerations you will see that it is not practical to prepare cosmetics that are *in equilibrium* with the surrounding atmosphere. Also, it is apparent that existing creams will lose water and that the amounts of humectant that are added do not alter the *equilibrium* hygroscopicity of the creams appreciably. However, it is desirable to retard the loss of water and this immediately becomes a study of rate rather than of equilibrium. It is most interesting that *dynamic hygroscopicity is apparently not a function of equilibrium moisture holding power of humectants.*

" This effect has been illustrated in our recent study of the hygroscopic properties of cosmetic creams. The purpose in these studies was not to determine the equilibrium hygroscopicity of the cream as a whole but to note the rate of loss of water under standard conditions. Loss in weight was determined on a large number of samples at one time. In our equipment, as many as 77 separate samples could be observed at one time. The samples were placed on a screen tray in a cabinet in which the relative humidity and temperature were controlled. Loose fitting covers were removed simultaneously by a multiple magnet arrangement. By this arrangement creams having various formulae were exposed for lengths of time varying from 5 minutes to 48 hours under chosen conditions.

" Cessna *et al.*[6] found that aqueous solutions of humectants lost weight at a more or less constant rate until the concentration of the solutions approached that of the equilibrium values. Earlier work that we had done indicated that a similar behaviour could be expected from o/w cosmetic creams. From these data it was estimated that several days would be required to lose an amount of water sufficient to allow the humectant to exert an influence based on its *equilibrium* moisture holding power. In addition, it was believed that cosmetic creams would be unacceptable from a cosmetic standpoint long before this amount of water had been lost. Therefore, for our tests the maximum exposure of a cream was chosen as 48 hours and the rate of loss in this time was compared. Forty-eight hours is probably the longest time that a cream would be accidentally exposed without a cap (unless it was forgotten and allowed to dry out completely). In 48 hours the weight loss is about 10 per cent. of the total weight of the cream which is from 15 to 25 per cent of the net water content and represents an adequate loss from which to estimate rates. The formulas used in our study are shown in Table 3. Two series of o/w creams were used, both containing approximately 15 per cent. stearic acid and varying from 0 to 20 per cent. humectant, and differing in that one series was emulsified with soap and the other with a blend of non-ionic emulsifiers.

"Weight losses of these creams prepared with 0, 2, 5, 10, and 20 per cent. of either propylene glycol, glycerin, or sorbitol were observed at 30, 50, and 70 per cent. relative humidities at 80° F.

Table 3—Test Cream Formulas

Number→	1	2	3
Type→	*o/w Stearic acid*	*o/w Stearic acid*	*w/o emollient*
Emulsifier→	*Soap*	*Non-ionic*	*Non-ionic*
Stearic acid	15·0	15·0	—
Isopropyl palmitate	2·0	1·0	—
Paraffin	—	—	12·0
Petrolatum	—	—	40·0
Mineral oil	—	—	5·0
Lanolin	—	—	4·0
Arlacel 60	—	2·0	—
Tween 60	—	1·5	—
G-1500	—	—	4·0
Potassium hydroxide	1·0	—	—
Magnesium sulphate	—	—	0·2
Humectant	20·0– 0·0	20·0– 0·0	—0·0
Water	62·0–82·0	60·5–80·5	—34·8

"The two base formulas, with soap and non-ionic emulsifiers and with no added humectants, were found to have almost the same rate of weight loss, the non-ionic emulsified cream losing weight slightly faster. It was apparent that the soap-emulsified cream formed a crust on its exposed surface which retarded water loss slightly, but at the same time it made the cream unfit for use as a cosmetic. In 48 hours, the maximum exposure time, the weight loss observed for the creams was 10–20 per cent. of the total weight of the composition. Since the soap type and non-ionic type formulas behaved differently, they will be discussed separately.

Rate of Weight Loss from Soap-Type Creams

"On examination of the data obtained for weight loss *vs.* time for exposed soap-type creams to which concentrations of up to 20 per cent. sorbitol, glycerin and propylene glycol have been added as humectants, marked differences are evident between sorbitol, glycerin, and propylene glycol in inhibiting loss of water. Where creams have been exposed for periods up to 48 hours at 30 per cent. R.H., concentrations of sorbitol as low as 2 per cent. provide protection against drying out of the cream whereas the addition of glycerin does not offer any protection until concentrations of greater than 5 per cent. are added. At glycerin concentrations of 5 per cent. and less, the creams actually show a greater loss of water with increasing time than those with no humectant present. Propylene glycol does not begin to offer any appreciable advantages until concentrations of 10 per cent. and greater have been added. At low concentrations, as in the case of glycerin, the creams actually lose more water than those with no humectant present. . . .

"Where the creams were exposed at 50 per cent. R.H., those containing propylene glycol lost more water at all concentrations than the cream with no humectant present. Glycerin was also ineffective at this humidity even at concentrations of 20 per cent. As in the case of 30 per cent. R.H. storage, creams containing small concentrations of glycerin and propylene glycol lost considerably more weight than in similar cream containing no humectant. Sorbitol additions reduced the rate of weight loss at all concentrations. The reference formula (no humectant) at 50 per cent. R.H. showed more of a loss in weight than would be expected when comparing the values at 30 per cent., 50 per cent., and 70 per cent. R.H. The 50 per cent. reference cream value is representative of nine separate tests with later triplicate checks. Apparently this anomaly is related to uncontrolled factors such as rate of crust formation, etc.

"Where the soap-type creams were exposed at 70 per cent. R.H., data similar to that obtained for 30 per cent. and 50 per cent. R.H. storage were obtained with propylene glycol being ineffective at concentrations of 5 per cent. and less and with glycerin being ineffective at concentrations below 10 per cent. Sorbitol inhibited water loss at all concentrations.

Rate of Weight Loss from Non-Ionic Type Creams

"In the case of weight losses for the non-ionic type creams, the data were much more erratic than those obtained for the soap-type creams. The actual per cent. losses for the creams containing no humectant were approximately the same as the soap-type creams at 30 and 70 per cent. R.H., however at 50 per cent. R.H. the value for the soap-type cream was considerably lower than that obtained for the non-ionic cream. On storage at 30 per cent. R.H., all of the humectants were effective in inhibiting weight loss. At 2 per cent. humectant, propylene glycol was the most effective with sorbitol next and glycerin last. This was also true at 5 per cent. glycerin and 10 per cent. humectant ; however, as the concentration of humectant is increased the difference in effectiveness becomes negligible. At 50 per cent. R.H. storage all of the humectants provided protection with no appreciable differences apparent. This was also true at 70 per cent. R.H."

"Crust Formation"

Griffin, Behrens and Cross go on to state that it is their belief that some of the differences in the rate of moisture loss between the various samples are related to the formation of a crust on the exposed surface. On the soap-type creams the crust formed was sufficiently thick and dense so that it could be felt and measured.

It was pointed out that texture and consistency could not be correlated with loss of water alone and that, in fact, texture and the formation of a hard crust on loss of water are a function of the type of emulsifier used. Soap-emulsified creams developed a crust in less than 24 hours exposure but no measurable or apparent crust was formed in 48 hours when non-ionic emulsifiers were employed. An apparatus for the measurement of this crust is described (*loc. cit.*).

Water-in-Oil Creams

Based upon their experience with a test w/o formulation using Arlacel C as the emulsifier and upon earlier experiences Griffin, Behrens and Cross consider that additions of humectants to w/o creams should be based on desired cosmetical properties rather than on the reduction of moisture loss, since this is adequately controlled if the product is an efficient w/o emulsion. The following table illustrates the order of losses obtained in these experiments :

Weight Loss from w/o Emulsions

Test No.	*per cent. Polyol*	*per cent. Arlacel C®*	*Type Emulsion*	*per cent. wt. lost from 4-oz. sample*	
				15 days	*12 days*
1	None	1	Dual ?	0·8	1·1
2	Sorbitol, 10 per cent.	1	Dual ?	0·4	1·5
3	Glycerin, 10 per cent	1	Dual ?	1·6	2·3
4	Propylene glycol, 10 per cent.	1	Dual ?	1·2	3·2
5	None	5	w/o	0·6	0·9
6	Sorbitol, 10 per cent.	5	w/o	0·5	1·5
7	Glycerin, 10 per cent.	5	w/o	1·3	1·9
8	Propylene glycol, 10 per cent.	5	w/o	0·5	1·9

BEHAVIOUR OF HUMECTANTS IN EMULSIONS

Experiments carried out by deNavarre (*Proc. Sci. Sect. T.G.A.*, 1945, 4, 22) indicated that the polyols, glycerin, sorbitol and propylene glycol were not interchangeable in that in a w/o cream the sample containing propylene glycol and the control sample had the greatest stability whilst that containing glycerin showed the most oil separation. Conversely in an o/w emulsion, the sample containing glycerin and the control remained fluid whilst those containing propylene glycol and sorbitol would not flow after storage. On the basis of such observations it would appear that glycerin promoted the formation of an o/w emulsion whilst propylene glycol favoured a w/o emulsion ; their use in the wrong types leading to instability. Sorbitol was apparently midway, in such properties, between these other two humectants. Cessna, Ohlmann and Roehm (*ibid.*, 5 Dec. 1946, p. 20) also reported that the three polyols, glycerin, propylene glycol and sorbitol undoubtedly effected the fundamental emulsion properties of the preparations tested in different manners, since glycerin and propylene glycol appeared to have opposite effects in emulsions of the same type.

Griffin, Behrens and Cross (*loc. cit.*) report in this connection that some recent work in their laboratories had indicated that for some formulae the amount and type of polyol had little or no influence on the choice of emulsifier and that it would appear that the variable emulsification effects noted with different polyols, occurred with formulae having only mediocre or poorly balanced emulsifiers. They add, however, that in some instances a change in kind or amount of humectant prevented the formation of the cream. Their observation has been that a notable difference between formulae that are, or are not, sensitive to humectants is that the former always " takes " well during emulsification whereas the latter does not.

TOXICITY OF HUMECTANTS

The three humectants widely employed in the cosmetic and toilet industry at the present time—and which have been discussed in this chapter—namely, glycerin, sorbitol and propylene glycol, are non-toxic and dermatologically innocuous.

Ethylene glycol is not considered safe, since it is oxidised in the body to oxalic acid and any absorption through the skin might lead to renal calculus ; for the same reason diethylene glycol is considered toxic. The mono-ethyl ether of diethylene glycol (" Carbitol ") has been widely used in cosmetic and toilet preparations and because of its " ether " grouping does not constitute, so far as is known, a hazard when used externally in cosmetic and toilet preparations.

Footnotes to Humectants, Table I and Text

[1] *Amines*, Carbon & Carbide Co., New York, 1944.
[2] *Average Temperature and Humidity*, American Maize-Products Co., Twelve Maps (months of year), New York, 1939.
[3] *Atlas Sorbitol*, Atlas Powder Company, 1947.
[4] Cl. Bauschinger, *Fette u. Seifen.*, 1939, **46**, 723.
[5] *Carbowaxes*, New York : Carbon & Carbide Co., 1946.
[6] O. C. Cessna, E. O. Ohlmann and L. S. Roehm, *Proc. Sci. Sect., T.G.A.*, 1946, No. 6, p. 20.
[7] *Dow Glycols*, Dow Chemical Co., 1947.
[8] A. F. Gallagher and H. Hibbert, *J. Amer. chem. Soc.*, 1936, **58**, 813.
[9] *Glycols*, Carbon & Carbide Co., New York, 1941.
[10] T. C. Gregory, ed. *Condensed Chemical Dictionary*, New York : Reinhold, 1942.
[11] W. C. Griffin, *Ind. Engng. Chem.*, 1945, **37**, 1126.
[12] Hangen and Watson, *Chemical Process Principles*, Part I, p. 158, New York : John Wiley and Sons, 1943.
[13] I. M. Heilbron, ed., *Dictionary of Organic Compounds*, New York : Oxford University Press, 1934.
[14] C. Hodgman, ed., *Handbook of Chemistry and Physics*, pp. 351-847, Cleveland : Chemical Rubber Publishing Co., 1939.
[15] *J. Ass. off. agric. Chem.*, 1925, **8**, 255.
[16] J. Kamlet, U.S. Patent, 2,483,418.
[17] G. M. Kline, *J. Res. nat. Bur. Stand.*, 1935, **14**, 67.
[18] N. A. Lange, ed., *Handbook of Chemistry*, pp. 314-654, Ohio : Handbook Publishers, Sandusky, 1944.
[19] J. W. Lawrie, *Glycerol and the Glycols*, pp. 155-207, 369-374, ACS Monograph, No. 44, New York : Chem. Cat. Co., 1928.
[20] M. A. Lesser, *Proc. Sci. Sect., T.G.A.*, 1945, No. 3, pp. 7-12.
[21] S. M. Livengood, *Chem. Ind.*, 1948, **63**, 948.
[22] deNavarre, *Proc. Sci. Sect., T.G.A.*, 1945, No. 4, p. 22.
[23] J. H. Perry, ed., *Chem. Engng. Handbook*, pp. 271-574, New York : McGraw-Hill, 1941.
[24] W. H. Rinkenbach, *Ind. Engng. Chem.*, 1927, **19**, 474.
[25] M. L. Sheeley, *ibid.*, 1932, **24**, 1060.
[26] M. E. Spaght, S. B. Thomas and G. S. Parks, *J. phys. Chem.*, 1932, **36**, 882.
[27] *Synthetic Organic Chemicals*, Carbon & Carbide Co., New York, 1945.
[28] E. W. Washburn, ed., *International Critical Tables*, vols. III and V.

CHAPTER 45

MODUS OPERANDI

This chapter is intended merely as a very brief guide or outline of the mechanical processes involved in the manufacture of cosmetic and allied preparations. It does not purport to be complete, but gives an outline of the operations which may be involved in the making of cosmetics and a brief reference to the types of equipment commonly used.

Production and Packaging of a Simple Lotion

This involves solution or dispersion of the constituents of the lotion in the solvent to be employed, agitation to ensure adequate dispersion and clarification.

Alcoholic-aqueous lotions may be prepared by (*a*) agitating the constituents in the alcohol-water mixture of the same concentration as the final product until solution occurs, or (*b*) dissolving any of the constituents which are readily soluble in alcohol (but not in dilute alcohol) in the concentrated alcohol and then gradually diluting this solution by the addition of the requisite amount of water, ensuring by agitation that no local concentration of water, high enough to throw the substance out of solution, occurs.

Whichever method is employed agitation has to be provided either by means of an electrically operated propeller which can be clamped on the sides of the mixing tank, or in the case of very large-scale production, permanently built into the side of the mixing tank near the floor. It has been shown that by the use of two propellers, the pitch of the lower one being reversed, powerful upward streaming from the bottom of the vessel comes into collision with an equally powerful downward flow occasioned by the upper propeller, and by adjusting these propellers on their shaft, the best conditions for adequate dispersion (or emulsification) can be obtained. This type of mixer is often called a push-pull mixer. To obtain maximum efficiency the mixing tank should be cylindrical and may be either glass-lined, or of pure nickel, aluminium, Monal metal or stainless steel according to the materials to be mixed.

In non-alcoholic lotions, gum mucilages, etc., the mixing vessel may be steam-jacketed, or, alternatively, hot distilled water may be run directly into the mixer, the substances to be dissolved added and agitation continued until complete solution is effected.

The product thus obtained requires clarification which usually involves filtration, though in some cases adequate chilling followed by syphoning off the clear liquid under slight vacuum is employed, the layer drawn off depending upon whether the impurities which it is desired to remove are on the surface or deposited.

Small-scale filtration may be carried out by ordinary laboratory methods, using filter papers of the required size, paper and asbestos pulp or filter cloth. This method is not suitable, however, for products containing a relatively high proportion of alcohol or another volatile solvent, because of the loss of solvent occurring by slow filtration in air. Gravity filtration may be of value in the filtration of certain aqueous soapless detergents which froth under the application of vacuum.

The usual method employed by the manufacturer, however, for lotions in general is filtration under negative pressure in which the substance is filtered through a suitable medium (sintered glass disc, paper pulp, asbestos or fine cloth) under reduced pressure. On the small scale a pressure flask and water-operated filter pump may be used. This method, when used with a suitable negative pressure, can be used for the sterilisation of solutions decomposed by heat, and in which the incorporation of germicides has to be avoided.

After filtration or other clarification, the solution so obtained may be filled directly into the package in which it is to be marketed or transferred to containers, preferably glass-lined, either to mature or simply to store until required. Glass-lined tanks are eminently suitable for the majority of cosmetic and toilet products except those containing alkali in relatively large concentrations, i.e. cuticle remover, etc. (Nickel when pure has high resistance to alkaline solutions.)

All bottles and other containers require cleansing unless they are purchased already cleaned and capped. In most cases after several months' storage an alkali bloom is deposited on ordinary glass, and many manufacturers allow new bottles to age for a while before cleaning them. An air blower can be utilised. However, the best method is that employing hot water, followed by rinsing and drying.

The smaller manufacturer may fill his preparations into bottles of every type, including sprinkler bottles by simple gravity, the head of filling liquid exerting sufficient pressure for comparatively rapid filling. This method is not only cheap but is advisable in cases of shampoos and other soapless or soapy detergents which are inclined to foam badly under pressure, and also for alcoholic preparations which tend to lose solvent if the pressure is reduced. A more rapid and elegant method of filling for toilet preparations in general, however, is by vacuum by which gangs of bottles, sprinkler neck included, can be readily and rapidly filled to a definite height, thus allowing for expansion, and at the same time avoiding the undesirable attention which may be drawn to bottles containing varying amounts of the same preparation.

Capping of the finished bottled product may be carried out by the use of a mechanically (or hand-) operated chuck equipped with a friction clutch which grips and rotates the cap until the requisite degree of tightness has been attained, upon which the clutch disengages. In cases of volatile products the cap may be covered with a viscose or other enclosure, applied in the moistened state and allowed to constrict by drying.

EMULSIONS

The production of liquid o/w emulsions is very similar to the above except in so far as it is necessary to dissolve any fat-soluble constituents in the oil phase, and water-soluble constituents in the aqueous phase before emulsification which may be produced by the push-pull type of agitator already discussed. It is then usual to homogenise the product. (*See also* Ultrasonic Emulsifiers, Chapter 41.)

The fat-soluble constituents should be melted with any oils and fats in a stainless steel steam-jacketed kettle, and when dissolved, run into the mixing vessel. The water, containing any water-soluble constituents, is heated separately and when both solutions are between 70°-80° C., depending on the particular preparation being made and the melting point of the fats involved, the aqueous solution is run into the melted fats with constant agitation. The product is finally homogenised and filled in a manner similar to that already described for lotions.

Solid o/w emulsions, which include vanishing creams and a great many of the modern cold creams, are prepared in a similar way. The mixing equipment, however, is different, the mixing paddle being of design such that it produces the minimum of aeration. The slowest speed of stirring which will produce effective mixing is employed. Mixing is continued with the heat shut off, until the temperature of the mix falls to 50° C. Perfume may then be added, and the product stirred from time to time by hand, or, if on a large scale, with an occasional mechanical stir of short duration, to prevent formation of a crust. Many manufacturers run their products, after emulsification and while still hot, through a homogeniser and then allow the product to cool with an occasional stir. Vanishing cream should not be stirred when cold, except for a short period, as the cream becomes very thin owing to the breaking down of the crystallised particles of stearic acid which impart the characteristic sheen and the desired consistency. The final adjustment of these characteristics are very largely dependent upon the mixing methods employed, particularly in regard to the handling of the cold product. Cold cream may be similarly prepared. Here, however, in the majority of cases, the final product is not so sensitive to thinning by mixing when cold, as is a vanishing cream.

If a colloid mill is used for such products, care should be taken to avoid excessive aeration.

By suitable technique, w/o creams may also be prepared in a similar manner, save that the aqueous solution is incorporated into the fatty phase a little at a time. Such creams are often rather sensitive, and while most are rendered very much more satisfactory by being mixed and then homogenised, some may be better made in an ointment mill.

The filling of solid creams may be carried out either while they are still hot enough to flow, or in the cold. Vanishing creams are almost invariably filled by the latter method. In many cosmetic and toilet creams the choice is optional. In general, hot filling, particularly in the case of a cold cream, produces a product with a high gloss, while cold filling produces a cream of a pleasant short crisp texture. In the latter case, the excess cream has to be removed from the jar by means of a wiper, operated either mechanically or by hand. Cold filling may be accomplished by the use of the ram type of filler, in which a plunger is mechanically moved along a cylindrical tube containing the cream whose only outlet is through a nozzle of the requisite size which is introduced into the container to be filled. This should be cylindrical in shape in order to avoid air pockets in filling. Cold filling is cheap, and the product does not have to undergo any long period of cooling with risk of subsequent contamination, either microbiological or otherwise.

Warm filling from a jacketed container may be carried out either by simple gravity or by vacuum. In gravity and vacuum filling the temperature should be as low as will allow free flow of the product, and precautions must be taken to ensure that the nozzle of the filler is jacketed. In some models which the author has inspected, though the container has been well jacketed, the issuing nozzle has been ignored with consequent stoppage owing to solidification of the cream. If jacketing is impracticable, solidification may be prevented by focusing the rays from a special infra-red heater on the nozzle outlet. A mixing device should be included in the jacketed container to keep the product homogeneous, and means provided such as a closing plunger or stop cock for stopping delivery of cream while changing from one container to the next.

Pastes

The liquid or solid medium into which the powder or other insoluble substance is to be incorporated is prepared according to one of the methods discussed above, and appropriate to the substance used, whether simple solution, or a liquid or solid emulsion, or fat. Incorporation of the powder may then be carried out in a poney mixer, or a dough mixer.

Powders

Powder mixing is usually carried out in a semi-circular trough equipped with a spiral agitator on which two flights of ribbons cause the mix to travel in opposite directions, thus producing considerable tumbling. They are extremely good for bath salts and other crystalline materials and are very widely employed for face powders. It is my experience, however, that better dispersion with less risk of bleeding occurs when the product, in the case of face powders, is finally pulverised and ground in a ball mill or treated in some other way in which a " rubbing " effect accompanies simple mixing. In *small* batches even an ointment mill can be used to achieve this. On a larger scale pin disc mills of the " Periflo " type are quite suitable.

APPENDICES

ANNUAL MEAN MAXIMA AND MINIMA TEMPERATURES AND ANNUAL MEAN HUMIDITIES IN VARIOUS PARTS OF THE GLOBE

DURING investigations into the stability of toilet creams, etc., it is often necessary to determine the mean maxima and minima temperatures to which these products might be subjected in different parts of the world.

The usual temperature tables give only the average monthly temperatures, which differ considerably from the data required.

The following temperature tables have therefore been compiled and alphabetically arranged from Geophysical Memoirs No. 44, M.O. 307*d*, "The Distribution of Mean Annual Maxima and Minima Temperatures over the Globe," by Brooks and Thorman, H.M. Stationery Office, 1928, whilst the average humidities are those given by Barker and Hirst, *J. Soc. Dyers and Colourists* (1927), Vol. XLIII, 9, 301. Average humidities are given only as a matter of interest, as the majority of cosmetic and toilet products are contained in air-tight containers, and the humidity inside the container is then purely a function of the temperature to which the container is subjected.

	Maximum (annual) temperature °C.	(°F.)	*Minimum (annual) temperature* °C.	(°F.)	*Mean humidity per cent.*
AFRICA					
Aden	43	(109)	18	(65)	—
Alexandria	44	(111)	3	(38)	—
Algiers	43	(109)	− 2	(28)	67
Berbera	41	(106)	15	(59)	—
Cairo	46	(115)	2	(36)	50
Capetown	39	(103)	0	(33)	72
Durban	36	(97)	0	(32)	70
Johannesburg	32	(90)	− 4	(25)	65
Khartoum	47	(117)	7	(45)	28
Kimberley	39	(103)	− 6	(21)	—
Lagos	40	(104)	15	(60)	—
Nairobi	31	(88)	1	(34)	—
Port Sudan	47	(117)	12	(54)	—
Pretoria	39	(103)	− 5	(23)	—
Tunis	40	(104)	2	(37)	68
AMERICA—NORTH					
Nome (Alaska)	26	(79)	−44	(−47)	—
Sitka (Alaska)	26	(80)	−20	(−4)	—
St. Johns	50	(87)	−29	(−20)	—
Toronto	39	(103)	−30	(−22)	—
Winnipeg	37	(99)	−41	(−42)	—

	Maximum (annual) temperature °C.	(°F.)	Minimum (annual) temperature °C.	(°F.)	Mean humidity per cent.
AMERICA—UNITED STATES					
Chicago	39	(103)	−22	(−16)	—
New York	39	(103)	−25	(−13)	—
San Diego	43	(110)	− 4	(25)	—
San Francisco	38	(101)	0	(33)	79
Washington	41	(106)	−25	(−13)	—
AMERICA—CENTRAL					
Bermuda	32	(90)	6	(43)	—
Colon (Panama)	33	(93)	20	(68)	—
Havana (Cuba)	34	(94)	10	(50)	—
Mexico City	33	(91)	− 4	(24)	—
Montserrat	37	(99)	15	(59)	—
AMERICA—SOUTH					
Buenos Aires	39	(103)	− 6	(22)	79
Montevideo	43	(109)	− 4	(25)	—
Rio de Janeiro	37	(99)	−12	(55)	78
Santiago	37	(99)	− 4	(25)	—
AUSTRALIA					
Adelaide	45	(113)	0	(33)	53
Brisbane	41	(106)	2	(36)	68
Hobart (Tasmania)	39	(102)	− 4	(25)	—
Melbourne	42	(107)	− 1	(29)	68
Perth	43	(109)	1	(34)	62
Port Darwin	38	(101)	15	(59)	—
Sydney	41	(106)	3	(37)	70
AUSTRIA					
Vienna	33	(92)	−11	(3)	—
BALKANS					
Athens	43	(109)	− 5	(23)	62
Bucharest	40	(104)	−24	(− 9)	—
Budapest	39	(103)	−19	(− 2)	—
BELGIUM					
Brussels	37	(99)	−16	(+ 2)	82
CHINA					
Hankow	40	(104)	− 7	(19)	—
Hong-Kong	34	(94)	4	(39)	77
Shanghai	39	(103)	−11	(+12)	—
Tientsin	40	(104)	−19	(− 2)	—

	Maximum (annual) temperature °C.	(°F.)	Minimum (annual) temperature °C.	(°F.)	(Mean) humidity per cent.
DENMARK					
Copenhagen	29	(84)	−16	(3)	—
FINLAND					
Helsingfors	31	(88)	−30	(−23)	—
FRANCE					
Marseilles	36	(97)	− 9	(16)	—
Nantes	36	(97)	−11	(12)	—
Paris	38	(101)	−16	(4)	79
GERMANY					
Hamburg	33	(92)	−16	(+ 2)	—
Potsdam	35	(96)	−22	(−10)	—
GIBRALTAR	35	(97)	2	(36)	—
IRAN					
Baghdad	50	(123)	− 4	(24)	—
Teheran..	—	—	−12	(+10)	—
INDIA AND BURMA					
Allahabad	46	(116)	3	(37)	66
Bangalore	37	(99)	10	(50)	78
Bombay	36	(96)	15	(59)	78
Calcutta	41	(107)	7	(45)	83
Hyderabad	49	(121)	− 3	(26)	—
Karachi	45	(113)	6	(43)	—
Mandalay	44	(112)	8	(48)	—
Quetta	40	(104)	−15	(3)	—
ITALY					
Rome	35	(96)	− 4	(25)	—
JAPAN					
Tokyo	34	(94)	− 8	(17)	74
NEW ZEALAND					
Christchurch	34	(94)	− 5	(23)	—
Wellington	29	(85)	− 1	(29)	—
NORWAY					
Bergen	30	(86)	−14	(+ 7)	—
Trondheim	33	(91)	−23	(− 9)	—
POLAND					
Warsaw	37	(99)	−23	(− 9)	—

	Maximum (annual) temperature °C.	(°F.)	Minimum (annual) temperature °C.	(°F.)	Mean humidity per cent.
PORTUGAL					
Lisbon	40	(103)	0	(32)	—
RUSSIA					
Archangel	33	(92)	−39	(−38)	—
Astrakan	38	(100)	−29	(−20)	—
Leningrad	33	(91)	−32	(−26)	—
Moscow	36	(98)	−36	(−33)	—
Omsk	36	(98)	—	—	—
Vladivostock	33	(92)	−30	(−22)	—
SCOTLAND					
Aberdeen	29	(83)	−22	(7)	—
Lerwick..	20	(69)	− 9	(16)	—
SPAIN					
Madeira (Canary Islands) ..	38	(101)	5	(41)	—
Madrid	43	(109)	−10	(14)	—
Palma (Balearic Islands) ..	37	(99)	− 2	(27)	—
SWEDEN					
Spitzbergen	14	(58)	−50	(−57)	—
Upsala	34	(92)	−26	(−15)	—
SWITZERLAND					
Zurich	36	(98)	−16	(3)	—

The above figures represent extremes of temperature variation.[1] In the British Isles stability in a temperature range of 32°-95° F. should be adequate.

[1] In assessing possible maximum temperatures it should be remembered that the above readings are not indicative of the maximum temperature to which a preparation may be subjected by misuse—as, for example, being placed in direct sunlight in a shop window or under tropical conditions in a ship's hold.

SPECIFIC GRAVITY, BAUME AND TWADDELL, OF CAUSTIC SODA AND CAUSTIC POTASH SOLUTIONS, AT 15° C. AND PERCENTAGES OF Na_2O, NaOH, K_2O AND KOH

Specific Gravity	*Baumé*	*Twaddell*	*Per cent. Na_2O*	*Per cent. NaOH*	*Per cent. K_2O*	*Per cent. KOH*	*Specific Gravity*	*Baumé*	*Twaddell*	*Per cent. Na_2O*	*Per cent. NaOH*	*Per cent. K_2O*	*Per cent. KOH*
1·007	1	1·4	0·47	0·61	0·7	0·9	1·220	26	44·0	15·18	19·58	20·2	24·2
1·014	2	2·8	0·93	1·20	1·4	1·7	1·231	27	46·2	15·96	20·59	21·1	25·1
1·022	3	4·4	1·55	2·00	2·2	2·6	1·241	28	48·2	16·76	21·42	21·9	26·1
1·029	4	5·8	2·10	2·71	2·9	3·5	1·252	29	50·4	17·55	22·64	22·7	27·0
1·036	5	7·2	2·60	3·35	3·8	4·5	1·263	30	52·6	18·35	23·67	23·5	28·0
1·045	6	9·0	3·10	4·00	4·7	5·6	1·274	31	54·8	19·23	24·81	24·2	28·9
1·052	7	10·4	3·60	4·64	5·4	6·4	1·285	32	57·0	20·00	25·80	25·0	29·8
1·060	8	12·0	4·10	5·29	6·2	7·4	1·297	33	59·4	20·80	26·83	25·8	30·7
1·067	9	13·4	4·55	5·87	6·9	8·2	1·308	34	61·6	21·55	27·80	26·7	31·8
1·075	10	15·0	5·08	6·55	7·7	9·2	1·320	35	64·0	22·35	28·83	27·5	32·7
1·083	11	16·6	5·67	7·31	8·5	10·1	1·332	36	66·4	23·30	29·93	28·3	33·7
1·091	12	18·2	6·20	8·00	9·2	10·9	1·345	37	69·0	24·20	31·22	29·3	34·9
1·100	13	20·0	6·73	8·68	10·1	12·0	1·357	38	71·4	25·17	32·47	30·2	35·9
1·108	14	21·6	7·30	9·42	10·8	12·9	1·370	39	74·0	26·12	33·69	31·0	36·9
1·116	15	23·2	7·80	10·06	11·6	13·8	1·383	40	76·6	27·10	34·96	31·8	37·8
1·125	16	25·0	8·50	10·97	12·4	14·8	1·397	41	79·4	28·10	36·25	32·7	38·9
1·134	17	26·8	9·18	11·84	13·2	15·7	1·410	42	82·0	29·05	37·47	33·5	39·9
1·142	18	28·4	9·80	12·64	13·9	16·5	1·424	43	84·8	30·08	38·80	34·4	40·9
1·152	19	30·4	10·50	13·55	14·8	17·6	1·438	44	87·6	31·00	39·99	35·4	42·1
1·162	20	32·4	11·14	14·37	15·6	18·6	1·453	45	90·6	32·10	41·41	36·5	43·4
1·171	21	34·2	11·73	15·13	16·4	19·5	1·468	46	93·6	33·20	42·83	37·5	44·6
1·180	22	36·0	12·33	15·91	17·2	20·5	1·483	47	96·6	34·40	44·38	38·5	45·8
1·190	23	38·0	13·00	16·77	18·0	21·4	1·498	48	99·6	35·70	46·15	39·6	47·1
1·200	24	40·0	13·70	17·67	18·8	22·4	1·514	49	102·8	36·90	47·60	40·6	48·3
1·210	25	42·0	14·40	18·58	19·6	23·3	1·530	50	106·0	38·00	49·02	41·5	49·4

By courtesy of " S.P.C. Buyers' Guide and Cyclopædia ", p. 33 (1939).

SPECIFIC GRAVITIES OF PURE GLYCERIN (TEMPERATURE 15° C.)

Sp. gr.	*Per cent. water.*	*Sp. gr.*	*Per cent. water.*	*Sp. gr.*	*Per cent. water.*	*Sp. gr.*	*Per cent. water.*
1·262	0	1·2142	19	1·160	38	1·109	57
1·261	1	1·211	20	1·157	39	1·106	58
1·258	2	1·207	21	1·155	40	1·103	59
1·255	3	1·203	22	1·152	41	1·1006	60
1·2515	4	1·2004	23	1·149	42	1·088	65
1·250	5	1·198	24	1·1464	43	1·075	70
1·2467	6	1·195	25	1·1437	44	1·0623	75
1·245	7	1·1923	26	1·141	45	1·049	80
1·243	8	1·189	27	1·1377	46	1·0365	85
1·241	9	1·183	28	1·1353	47	1·0243	90
1·237	10	1·1846	29	1·1326	48	1·0218	91
1·235	11	1·182	30	1·1304	49	1·0192	92
1·2324	12	1·179	31	1·127	50	1·0168	93
1·229	13	1·176	32	1·125	51	1·0147	94
1·2265	14	1·1734	33	1·1224	52	1·0125	95
1·2245	15	1·171	34	1·1204	53	1·01	96
1·2225	16	1·168	35	1·117	54	1·0074	97
1·2185	17	1·165	36	1·114	55	1·0053	98
1·2174	18	1·163	37	1·112	56	1·0026	99

RULES FOR CONVERTING THERMOMETER SCALES

Degrees F into C. First subtract 32, then multiply by 5 and divide by 9.
„ F „ R. First subtract 32, then multiply by 4 and divide by 9.
„ C „ F. Multiply by 9, divide by 5 and add 32.
„ C „ R. Multiply by 4 and divide by 5.
„ R „ F. Multiply by 9, divide by 4 and add 32.
„ R „ C. Multiply by 5 and divide by 4.

THERMOMETER TABLES

Cent.	*Réaum.*	*Fahr.*	*Cent.*	*Réaum.*	*Fahr.*	*Cent.*	*Réaum.*	*Fahr.*
0	0·0	32·0	34	27·2	93·2	68	54·4	154·4
1	0·8	33·8	35	28·0	95·0	69	55·2	156·2
2	1·6	35·6	36	28·8	96·8	70	56·0	158·0
3	2·4	37·4	37	29·6	98·6	71	56·8	159·8
4	3·2	39·2	38	30·4	100·4	72	57·6	161·6
5	4·0	41·0	39	31·2	102·2	73	58·4	163·4
6	4·8	42·8	40	32·0	104·0	74	59·2	165·2
7	5·6	44·6	41	32·8	105·8	75	60·0	167·0
8	6·4	46·4	42	33·6	107·6	76	60·8	168·8
9	7·2	48·2	43	34·4	109·4	77	61·6	170·6
10	8·0	50·0	44	35·2	111·2	78	62·4	172·4
11	8·8	51·8	45	36·0	113·0	79	63·2	174·2
12	9·6	53·6	46	36·8	114·8	80	64·0	176·0
13	10·4	55·4	47	37·6	116·6	81	64·8	177·8
14	11·2	57·2	48	38·4	118·4	82	65·6	179·6
15	12·0	59·0	49	39·2	120·2	83	66·4	181·4
16	12·8	60·8	50	40·0	122·0	84	67·2	183·2
17	13·6	62·6	51	40·8	123·8	85	68·0	185·0
18	14·4	64·4	52	41·6	125·6	86	68·8	186·8
19	15·2	66·2	53	42·4	127·4	87	69·6	188·6
20	16·0	68·0	54	43·2	129·2	88	70·4	190·4
21	16·8	69·8	55	44·0	131·0	89	71·2	192·2
22	17·6	71·6	56	44·8	132·8	90	72·0	194·0
23	18·4	73·4	57	45·6	134·6	91	72·8	195·8
24	19·2	75·2	58	46·4	136·4	92	73·6	197·6
25	20·0	77·0	59	47·2	138·2	93	74·4	199·4
26	20·8	78·8	60	48·0	140·0	94	75·2	201·2
27	21·6	80·6	61	48·8	141·8	95	76·0	203·0
28	22·4	82·4	62	49·6	143·6	96	76·8	204·8
29	23·2	84·2	63	50·4	145·4	97	77·6	206·6
30	24·0	86·0	64	51·2	147·2	98	78·4	208·4
31	24·8	87·8	65	52·0	149·0	99	79·2	210·2
32	25·6	89·6	66	52·8	150·8	100	80·0	212·0
33	26·4	91·4	67	53·6	152·6			

PERCENTAGE INTO LB. PER CWT., AND INTO CWT. AND LB. PER TON

Per cent.	Per cwt.	Per ton	Per cent.	Per cwt.	Per ton	Per cent.	Per cwt.	Per ton
	Lb.	*Cwt. lb.*		*Lb.*	*Cwt. lb.*		*Lb.*	*Cwt. lb.*
1	1·12	22·4	**41**	45·92	8 22·4	**81**	90·72	16 22·4
2	2·24	44·8	**42**	47·04	8 44·8	**82**	91·84	16 44·8
3	3·36	67·2	**43**	48·16	8 67·2	**83**	92·96	16 67·2
4	4·48	89·6	**44**	49·28	8 89·6	**84**	94·08	16 89·6
5	5·60	1 0	**45**	50·40	9 0	**85**	95·20	17 0
6	6·72	1 22·4	**46**	51·52	9 22·4	**86**	96·32	17 22·4
7	7·84	1 44·8	**47**	52·64	9 44·8	**87**	97·44	17 44·8
8	8·96	1 67·2	**48**	53·76	9 67·2	**88**	98·56	17 67·2
9	10·08	1 89·6	**49**	54·88	9 89·6	**89**	99·68	17 89·6
10	11·20	2 0	**50**	56·00	10 0	**90**	100·80	18 0
11	12·32	2 22·4	**51**	57·12	10 22·4	**91**	101·92	18 22·4
12	13·44	2 44·8	**52**	58·24	10 44·8	**92**	103·04	18 44·8
13	14·56	2 67·2	**53**	59·36	10 67·2	**93**	104·16	18 67·2
14	15·68	2 89·6	**54**	60·48	10 89·6	**94**	105·28	18 89·6
15	16·8	3 0	**55**	61·60	11 0	**95**	106·40	19 0
16	17·92	3 22·4	**56**	62·72	11 22·4	**96**	107·52	19 22·4
17	19·04	3 44·8	**57**	63·84	11 44·8	**97**	108·64	19 44·8
18	20·16	3 67·2	**58**	64·96	11 67·2	**98**	109·76	19 67·2
19	21·28	3 89·6	**59**	66·08	11 89·6	**99**	110·88	19 89·6
20	22·40	4 0	**60**	67·20	12 0	**100**	112·00	20 0
21	23·52	4 22·4	**61**	68·32	12 22·4			
22	24·64	4 44·8	**62**	69·44	12 44·8			
23	25·76	4 67·2	**63**	70·56	12 67·2			
24	26·88	4 89·6	**64**	71·68	12 89·6			
25	28·00	5 0	**65**	72·80	13 0			
26	29·12	5 22·4	**66**	73·92	13 22·4			
27	30·24	5 44·8	**67**	75·04	13 44·8			
28	31·36	5 67·2	**68**	76·16	13 67·2			
29	32·48	5 89·6	**69**	77·28	13 89·6			
30	33·60	6 0	**70**	78·40	14 0			
31	34·72	6 22·4	**71**	79·52	14 22·4	**0·1**	0·112	2·24
32	35·84	6 44·8	**72**	80·64	14 44·8	**0·2**	0·224	4·48
33	36·96	6 67·2	**73**	81·76	14 67·2	**0·3**	0·336	6·72
34	38·08	6 89·6	**74**	82·88	14 89·6	**0·4**	0·448	8·96
35	39·20	7 0	**75**	84·00	15 0			
36	40·32	7 22·4	**76**	85·12	15 22·4	**0·5**	0·560	11·20
37	41·44	7 44·8	**77**	86·24	15 44·8	**0·6**	0·672	13·44
38	42·56	7 67·2	**78**	87·36	15 67·2	**0·7**	0·784	15·68
39	43·68	7 89·6	**79**	88·48	15 89·6	**0·8**	0·896	17·92
40	44·80	8 0	**80**	89·60	16 0	**0·9**	1·008	20·16

From *Bayley's Chemists' Pocket Book.* *By courtesy of E. & F. N. Spon Ltd., 1929*

INTER-CONVERSION TABLES

Kilograms and Pounds (Avoir.)
Short tons and Long tons
Short tons and Metric tons

Kilo-grams		*Av. pounds*	*Short tons*		*Long tons*	*Metric tons*		*Long tons*	*Metric tons*		*Short tons*
0·454	**1**	2·205	1·12	**1**	0·892	1·016	**1**	0·984	0·907	**1**	1·102
0·907	**2**	4·409	2·24	**2**	1·785	2·032	**2**	1·968	1·814	**2**	2·205
1·361	**3**	6·614	3·36	**3**	2·677	3·048	**3**	2·953	2·722	**3**	3·307
1·814	**4**	8·818	4·48	**4**	3·570	4·064	**4**	3·937	3·629	**4**	4·409
2·268	**5**	11·023	5·60	**5**	4·462	5·080	**5**	4·921	4·536	**5**	5·512
2·722	**6**	13·228	6·72	**6**	5·354	6·096	**6**	5·905	5·443	**6**	6·614
3·175	**7**	15·432	7·84	**7**	6·247	7·112	**7**	6·889	6·350	**7**	7·716
3·629	**8**	17·637	8·96	**8**	7·139	8·128	**8**	7·874	7·257	**8**	8·818
4·082	**9**	19·842	10·08	**9**	8·032	9·144	**9**	8·858	8·165	**9**	9·921
4·536	**10**	22·046	11·20	**10**	8·924	10·161	**10**	9·842	9·072	**10**	11·023
9·072	**20**	44·092	22·40	**20**	17·848	20·321	**20**	19·684	18·144	**20**	22·046
13·608	**30**	66·139	33·60	**30**	26·772	30·482	**30**	29·526	27·215	**30**	33·069
18·144	**40**	88·185	44·80	**40**	35·696	40·642	**40**	39·368	36·287	**40**	44·092
22·680	**50**	110·231	56·00	**50**	44·620	50·803	**50**	49·211	45·359	**50**	55·116
27·215	**60**	132·277	67·20	**60**	53·545	60·963	**60**	59·053	54·431	**60**	66·139
31·751	**70**	154·323	78·40	**70**	62·469	71·124	**70**	68·894	63·503	**70**	77·162
36·287	**80**	176·370	89·60	**80**	71·393	81·284	**80**	78·737	72·574	**80**	88·185
40·823	**90**	198·416	100·80	**90**	80·317	91·444	**90**	88·579	81·646	**90**	99·208
45·359	**100**	220·462	112·00	**100**	89·241	101·605	**100**	98·421	90·718	**100**	110·231

From *Whitaker's Almanack*, 1944. *By courtesy of J. Whitaker & Sons Ltd.*

[*Note.*—The central figure in heavy type represents either of the two adjacent columns as the case may be, viz. 1 kilogram = 2·205 pounds (avoirdupois) or 1 pound (avoir.) = 0·454 kilogram.]

INTER-CONVERSION TABLES

Litres and Pints
Litres and Gallons
English gallons and U.S. gallons

Litres		*Pints*	*Litres*		*Gallons*	*U.S. gallons (liquid)*		*English gallons (liquid)*
0·568	**1**	1·760	4·546	**1**	0·220	1·200	**1**	0·833
1·136	**2**	3·520	9·092	**2**	0·440	2·401	**2**	1·666
1·705	**3**	5·279	13·638	**3**	0·660	3·601	**3**	2·499
2·273	**4**	7·039	18·184	**4**	0·880	4·802	**4**	3·332
2·841	**5**	8·799	22·730	**5**	1·100	6·002	**5**	4·165
3·409	**6**	10·559	27·276	**6**	1·320	7·203	**6**	4·998
3·978	**7**	12·319	31·822	**7**	1·540	8·403	**7**	5·831
4·546	**8**	14·078	36·368	**8**	1·760	9·603	**8**	6·664
5·114	**9**	15·838	40·914	**9**	1·980	10·804	**9**	7·497
5·682	**10**	17·598	45·460	**10**	2·200	12·004	**10**	8·330
11·365	**20**	35·196	90·919	**20**	4·399	24·009	**20**	16·661
17·047	**30**	52·794	136·379	**30**	6·599	36·013	**30**	24·991
22·730	**40**	70·392	181·838	**40**	8·799	48·017	**40**	33·321
28·412	**50**	87·990	227·298	**50**	10·999	60·022	**50**	41·652
34·094	**60**	105·588	272·758	**60**	13·198	72·026	**60**	49·982
39·777	**70**	123·186	318·217	**70**	15·398	84·030	**70**	58·312
45·459	**80**	140·784	363·677	**80**	17·598	96·034	**80**	66·642
51·142	**90**	158·382	409·136	**90**	19·797	108·039	**90**	74·973
56·824	**100**	175·980	454·596	**100**	21·997	120·043	**100**	83·303

From *Whitaker's Almanack*, 1944. *By courtesy of J. Whitaker & Sons Ltd.*

[*Note.*—The central figure in heavy type represents either of the two adjacent columns as the case may be. Example: 1 litre = 1·760 pints or 1 pint = 0·568 litre; 1 litre = 0·220 English gallon or 1 gallon = 4·546 litres.]

*p*H RANGE AND COLOUR CHANGES OF INDICATORS

(As determined by Clark and Lub, Cray and Westrip)

Indicator	*p*H range	*Colour change*	
		Acid	*Alkaline*
Alizarin	11·0–13·0	lilac	blue
„	5·5– 6·8	yellow	red
„ blue S.	5·5– 7·0	yellow	green yellow
„ red S.	4·0– 6·0	yellow green	red
„ yellow G.	10·1–12·1	yellow green	red
Amino-azo-benzene	1·9– 3·3	orange	—
Benzyl-aniline-azo-benzene sulphonic acid	1·9– 3·3	orange	yellow
Benzene-azo-naphthylamine	3·7– 5·0	pink	yellow
Benzoylauramine	3·7– 5·9	blue green	yellow
„	1·0– 3·7	yellow	blue green
Brilliant yellow	6·4– 9·4	yellow	orange
Brom cresol green	4·0– 5·6	yellow	blue
„ „ purple (*p*H 5·5 yellow, 6·0 brown-green, 6·5 violet, 7·0 purple)	5·2– 6·8	yellow	purple
Brom phenol blue (*p*H 3·5 dull green, 4·0 brown-green, 4·5 violet)	2·8– 4·6	yellow	blue
Brom thymol blue (*p*H 6·0 yellow, 6·5 green-yellow, 7·0 green, 7·5 blue)	6·0– 7·6	yellow	blue
o-carboxy-benzene-azo α-naphthylamine	5·6– 7·0	pink	yellow
o-carboxy-benzene-azo-benzyl α-naphthylamine	2·0– 3·7	mauve	heliotrope
Chlor-amino-azo-benzene	1·0– 3·0	red	colourless
Clayton yellow	12·0–13·0	red	colourless
Cochineal	5·0– 6·0	brown pink	lilac
Congo red	3·0– 5·0	blue	scarlet
o-cresol-phthalein	8·2– 9·8	yellow	violet
Cresol red	7·2– 8·8	yellow	red
m-cresol purple	0·5– 2·5	red	yellow
„ „	7·1– 9·2	yellow	purple
Diethyl red	4·4– 6·2	yellow	pink
Dimethyl-amino-azo-benzene	2·9– 4·0	red	yellow
Ethyl orange	3·5– 4·5	pink	yellow
Hæmatoxylin	0 - 1·0	pink	yellow
„	6·0–11·0	pink	blue violet
Hydroxy-amino-azo-benzene	1·0– 3·0	red	yellow

pH RANGE AND COLOUR CHANGES OF INDICATORS—*continued*

Indicator	*pH range*	*Colour change*	
		Acid	*Alkaline*
Iodo-eosin	0·3–14·0	green yellow	pink
Iso picramic acid	4·4– 5·6	yellow	pink
Lacmoid	0 – 7·0	pink violet	violet blue
Litmus	5·0– 8·0	red	blue
Magdala red	0 – 3·6	orange	pink
Methyl orange	3·1– 5·0	red	yellow
Methyl red (*p*H 4·5 violet, 5·0 red, 5·5 orange, 6·0 yellow)	4·4– 6·2	red	yellow
Methyl thymol blue	4·0–10·0	red	yellow
a-naphthol benzene	8·5– 9·8	yellow	green
„ phthalein	7·3– 8·7	red	blue
„ sulphone phthalein	7·5– 9·0	red	blue
Neutral red	6·8– 8·0	red	yellow
p-nitrophenol	5·0– 8·0	colourless	yellow
Phenacetolin	5·0– 6·0	brown red	pink
Phenolphthalein (*p*H 8·5 pale pink, 9·0 deep pink, 9·5 violet-red)	8·3–10·0	colourless	pink
Phenol red (*p*H 6·5 yellow, 7·0 orange-yellow, 7·5 orange, 8·0 red, 8·5 violet-red)	6·8– 8·4	yellow	red
Phenol thymol phthalein ..	8·3–11·0	colourless	violet
Phenol violet	8·0–10·0	colourless	violet
Picramic acid	3·0– 5·0	yellow	orange
Propyl red	4·6– 6·6	red	yellow
Resazurine	5·0– 7·0	red	yellow
Rosolic acid	6·9– 8·0	brown yellow	red
Sodium sulphalizaride	5·0– 6·8	yellow	pink
Tetra brom phenolphthalein ..	0·3– 8·0	colourless	violet
Thymol blue	1·2– 2·8	red	yellow
„ „	8·0– 9·6	yellow	blue
„ phthalein	9·3–10·5	colourless	blue
„ violet	9·0–13·0	colourless	blue
Tropœolin o	11·1–12·7	yellow	red orange
„ oo	1·4– 2·6	pink	yellow
„ ooo	7·0– 8·9	yellow	pink
Turmeric	—	yellow	red brown

INTERNATIONAL ATOMIC WEIGHTS

Name	*Symbol*	*Atomic number*	*Atomic weight*
Actinium	Ac	89	(227)
Aluminium	Al	13	26·97
Americium	Am	95	(241)
Antimony	Sb	51	121·76
Argon	A	18	39·944
Arsenic	As	33	74·91
Astatine	At	85	(210)
Barium	Ba	56	137·36
Berkelium	Bk	97	(243)
Beryllium	Be	4	9·02
Bismuth	Bi	83	209·00
Boron	B	5	10·82
Bromine	Br	35	79·916
Cadmium	Cd	48	112·41
Calcium	Ca	20	40·08
Californium	Cf	98	(244)
Carbon	C	6	12·010
Celtium (Hafnium)	Hf	72	178·6
Cerium	Ce	58	140·13
Cesium	Cs	55	132·91
Chlorine	Cl	17	35·457
Chromium	Cr	24	52·01
Cobalt	Co	27	58·94
Columbium (Niobium) ..	Cb	41	92·91
Copper	Cu	29	63·54
Curium	Cm	96	(242)
Dysprosium	Dy	66	162·46
Erbium	Er	68	167·2
Europium	Eu	63	152·0
Fluorine	F	9	19·000
Francium	Fr	87	(223)
Gadolinium	Gd	64	156·9
Gallium	Ga	31	69·72
Germanium	Ge	32	72·60
Gold	Au	79	197·2
Hafnium (Celtium)	Hf	72	176·6
Helium	He	2	4·003
Holmium	Ho	67	164·94
Hydrogen	H	1	1·008
Indium	In	49	114·76
Iodine	I	53	126·92
Iridium	Ir	77	193·1
Iron	Fe	26	55·85

An atomic weight value given in parentheses is the mass number of the most stable isotope of the element which possesses only unstable isotopes.

INTERNATIONAL ATOMIC WEIGHTS—*continued*

Name	*Symbol*	*Atomic number*	*Atomic weight*
Krypton	Kr	36	83·7
Lanthanum	La	57	138·92
Lead	Pb	82	207·21
Lithium	Li	3	6·940
Lutetium	Lu	71	174·99
Magnesium	Mg	12	24·32
Manganese	Mn	25	54·93
Mercury	Hg	80	200·61
Molybdenum	Mo	42	95·95
Neodymium	Nd	60	144·27
Neon	Ne	10	20·183
Neptunium	Np	93	(237)
Nickel	Ni	28	58·69
Niobium (Columbium) ..	Nb	41	92·91
Nitrogen	N	7	14·008
Osmium	Os	76	190·2
Oxygen	O	8	16·000
Palladium	Pd	46	106·7
Phosphorus	P	15	30·98
Platinum	Pt	78	195·23
Plutonium	Pu	94	(239)
Polonium	Po	84	(210)
Potassium	K	19	39·096
Praseodymium	Pr	59	140·92
Prometheum	Pm	61	(147)
Protactinum	Pa	91	231·0
Radium	Ra	88	226·05
Radon	Rn	86	222·0
Rhenium	Re	75	186·31
Rhodium	Rh	45	102·91
Rubidium	Rb	37	85·48
Ruthenium	Ru	44	101·7
Samarium	Sm	62	150·43
Scandium	Sc	21	45·10
Selenium	Se	34	78·96
Silicon	Si	14	28·06
Silver	Ag	47	107·880
Sodium	Na	11	22·997
Strontium	Sr	38	87·63
Sulphur	S	16	32·066
Tantalum	Ta	73	180·88
Technetium	Tc	43	(99)
Tellurium	Te	52	127·61
Terbium	Tb	65	159·2

An atomic weight value given in parentheses is the mass number of the most stable isotope of the element which possesses only unstable isotopes.

INTERNATIONAL ATOMIC WEIGHTS—*continued*

Name	*Symbol*	*Atomic number*	*Atomic weight*
Thallium	Tl	81	204·39
Thorium	Th	90	232·12
Thulium	Tm	69	169·4
Tin	Sn	50	118·70
Titanium	Ti	22	47·90
Tungsten (Wolfram)	W	74	183·92
Uranium	U	92	238·07
Vanadium	V	23	50·95
Wolfram (Tungsten) ..	W	74	183·92
Xenon	Xe	54	131·3
Ytterbium	Yb	70	173·04
Yttrium	Y	39	88·92
Zinc	Zn	30	65·38
Zirconium	Zr	40	91·22

An atomic weight value given in parentheses is the mass number of the most stable isotope of the element which possesses only unstable isotopes.

INDEX

D

G

H

M

Q

R

S

U